Bruce-Chwatt's essential malariology

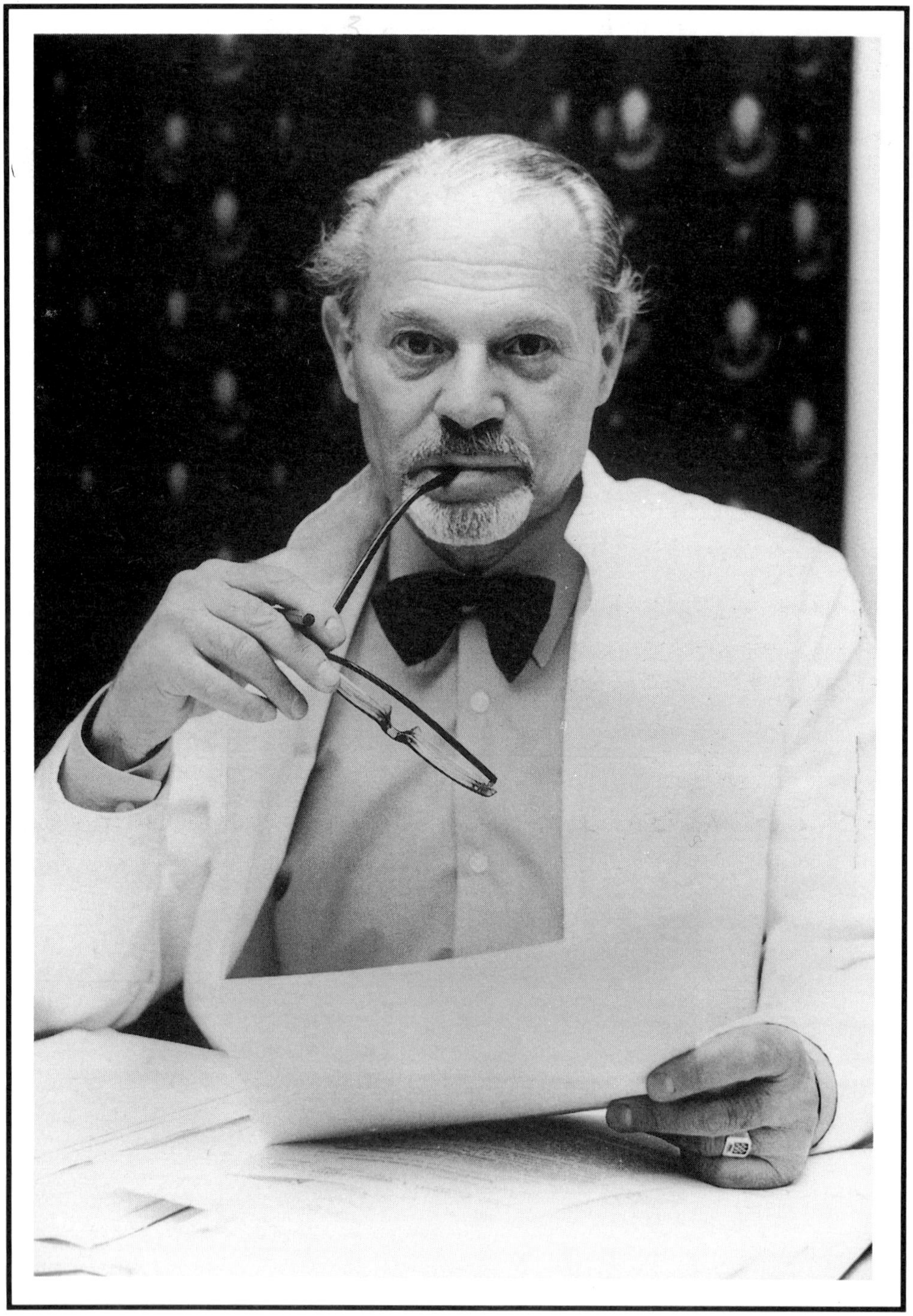

In memory of Leonard Jan Bruce-Chwatt, 9.6.1907–18.5.1989

Bruce-Chwatt's essential malariology

Third edition

Herbert M. Gilles
Emeritus Professor of Tropical Medicine, University of Liverpool
Formerly Professor of Tropical Medicine and Dean, Liverpool School of Tropical Medicine
Honorary Senior Research Fellow, Department of Clinical Pharmacology and Therapeutics, University of Liverpool
Visiting Professor of Public Health, University of Malta

David A. Warrell
Professor of Tropical Medicine and Infectious Diseases and Director of the Centre for Tropical Medicine, University of Oxford

Edward Arnold
A division of Hodder & Stoughton
LONDON BOSTON MELBOURNE AUCKLAND

First published in Great Britain 1980
Second edition 1985
Third edition 1993

Distributed in the Americas by Little, Brown and Company
34 Beacon Street, Boston, MA 02108

British Library Cataloguing in Publication Data
Bruce-Chwatt, Leonard Jan
Bruce-Chwatt's Essential Malariology. –
3Rev.ed
I. Title II. Gilles, Herbert M.
III. Warrell, D. A.
616.9362

ISBN 0-340-57190-X

Whilst the advice and information in this book is believed to be true and accurate at the date of going to press, neither the author nor the publisher can accept any legal responsibility or liability for any errors or omissions that may be made. In particular (but without limiting the generality of the preceding disclaimer) every effort has been made to check drug dosages; however, it is still possible that errors have been missed. Furthermore, dosage schedules are constantly being revised and new side effects recognised. For these reasons the reader is strongly urged to consult the drug companies' printed instructions before administering any of the drugs recommended in this book.

Typeset in 10/11½pt Linotron Baskerville by Rowland Phototypesetting Limited, Bury St Edmunds, Suffolk.
Printed and bound in Great Britain for Edward Arnold, a division of Hodder and Stoughton Limited, Mill Road, Dunton Green, Sevenoaks, Kent TN13 2YA by Butler and Tanner Limited, Frome, Somerset.

Contents

Foreword to the first edition (abridged)

In 1955 the World Health Organization began a malaria eradication campaign that was strongly supported by the Pan-American Health Organization, the United Nations Children's Fund, the US Public Health Service, the US Agency for International Development and its predecessors, and by many national health departments. Directly and indirectly this programme resulted in the eradication of malaria from the USA, most of Europe, much of the Middle East, important areas in the Caribbean and South America.

But today malaria is tragically resurgent in Asia and elsewhere. The reasons for the present situation are technical, administrative, financial and others. Most importantly, adequate training of malariologists has been rare, and there has been a crippling decline in the attention devoted to malaria control by international, national and philanthropic agencies. Other health problems have seemed more urgent or more interesting.

Very likely, the demonstration of malaria's power of damaging human health and slowing down socio-economic advance will stimulate a revival of interest in malaria control.

In my opinion, few men are so well prepared to write *Essential Malariology* as Professor Bruce-Chwatt, whom I first met in 1950. He was for many years in the service of the Federal Government of Nigeria and of the World Health Organization. He then became Director of the Ross Institute and Professor of Tropical Hygiene at the London School of Hygiene and Tropical Medicine.

I welcome this concise and authoritative book, especially at a time when malaria is increasingly prevalent and neglected.

North Edgecomb, Maine, USA
July 1978

Paul F. Russell, MD, MPH
Formerly, Member Field Staff,
Rockefeller Foundation;
Chief Malariologist,
Allied Military Government, Italy;
Malaria Consultant to
Surgeon General, US Army and
to the World Health Organization.

Dr Paul F. Russell died on 2 November 1983.

Introduction to the first edition

No one who has followed over the past five years the annual reports of the World Health Organization on the situation of malaria, can doubt that the former rapid progress of the eradication of this disease has now come to a halt and that the resurgence of the infection causes much concern. Malaria continues to be a major problem of tropical developing countries and the recent years have seen the return of it to areas freed from the disease in the 1960s.

The causes of this setback to a unique international health endeavour have often been analysed and commented upon. Certainly, technical factors such as resistance of insect vectors to insecticides played a major role in these reverses of fortune. Not less and probably more important were other, often imponderable factors. Inadequacy of planning, administrative shortcomings, financial stringency, shortage of personnel, poor training were equally responsible for the recent shift of strategy from malaria eradication to malaria control in countries not equipped for the undertaking of a complex and difficult programme of eradication.

With the general recognition of the magnitude of our unfinished task came the understanding of pressing needs for further research into methods of malaria control and the return to the provision of adequate information on many essential aspects of parasitology, entomology, epidemiology, prevention, treatment and control of malaria. It is a fact that the older generation of malariologists has largely disappeared and the number of professional workers in tropical community health competent in the field of malaria control is woefully inadequate, while the need for them is steadily growing. In the context of factors related to the inadequacies of personnel and training, good leadership is an essential ingredient of success. Leadership is often an innate quality of an individual but it may be enhanced by judicious selection and proper training. The renewed concentration of both the national governments and international organizations on the provision of and assistance to training centres in malaria control is a good augury for the future.

The provision of concise and up-to-date description of clinical and public health aspects of human malaria is the purpose of this book. It attempts to present in a factual and readable form the principles and practice of prevention, diagnosis, treatment and control of malaria in individuals and in communities of both advanced and developing countries.

Its approach has been inspired by Dr Paul F. Russell's most successful primer, published a quarter of a century ago. Like Russell's *Malaria: Basic Principles Briefly Stated*, the present book does not intend to elaborate on all, often highly specialized and increasingly complex branches of applied science, which contribute to the sum total of the discipline of malariology. For this, some of the books quoted in the references are still unsurpassed, while much of the newer knowledge will be found in publications and other documents of the WHO, that form an admirable source and constant stream of authoritative information.

It is apposite and perhaps significant that the need for the present book arose at the time when we are about to commemorate in November 1980 the centenary of the discovery of the malaria parasite by Alphonse Laveran. The readers of *Essential Malariology* will be able to judge how much has been achieved since that date, but they may also realize what remains to be done to free the world from malaria.

Leonard Jan Bruce-Chwatt
Wellcome Museum of Medical Science
London NW1

Introduction to the second edition

During the few years that have elapsed between the first and the present edition of this book the world's malaria situation has deteriorated. This is particularly evident in many developing countries situated in the tropics, where the revised strategy of malaria control (seen as an alternative to malaria eradication) has not been implemented because of adverse social and economic conditions, due either to the general recession or to various internal difficulties. Technical problems of resistance of mosquito vectors to insecticides or the continuing spread of resistance of some malaria parasites to the available drugs, have contributed to the universal concern about mankind's ability to maintain the achievements of the past 25 years, when malaria receded from large parts of the temperate areas of the world. A tremendous amount of scientific advance on all aspects of malaria and its control has been achieved during the past few years when the UNDP/World Bank/WHO Special Programme for Research and Training in Tropical Diseases increased its activity. This offers reasonable hope that better weapons for attacking both the wily *Plasmodium* and the elusive *Anopheles* will be discovered. The main difficulty in preparing the present text lay in selecting the practical information of value in the field from an avalanche of recent publications. However, since many prospective methods of malaria control are based on fundamental studies of the parasite, its vector and the immune response of the human host, some of these topics have been outlined in order to stress the close relationship between basic research and its application.

The change of World Health Organization's strategy from malaria eradication to more realistic aims of malaria control has now been given the emphasis for the association of these activities with the overall responsibilities of primary health care. Various patterns of such close or loose integration have been developed in different countries, depending on their epidemiological, administrative, and socio-economic conditions or systems of government. While some of such programmes are undoubtedly successful, many others have not fulfilled their role, mainly because of the absence of a core of technical expertise in guiding the specific antimalaria operations.

The fact is that some 1600 million people throughout the world are still exposed to considerable risk of malaria infection. In areas of endemic malaria this disease causes high mortality of infants and children, and is an adverse factor of the social and economic advance of the Third World. Any country that undertakes a malaria control campaign must see it as a component part of its whole health system, but with a nucleus of professional expertise. To meet the challenge of the disease, research and intensive training of medical and health personnel are the best guarantee of success. It is for the new generation of malariologists and sanitarians that this second edition of *Essential Malariology* has been prepared.

Leonard Jan Bruce-Chwatt

Introduction to the third edition

About a year or so before Leonard Bruce-Chwatt died, he kindly invited me to collaborate with him in the production of the third edition. Unfortunately his terminal illness was a good deal more severe than he had anticipated and little had been done by the time he died. We had, however, several discussions about the book and came to some clear decisions.

The first was that we would leave *intact* as much of the script as possible providing it was still valid. We would merely update and/or correct portions which in the light of new knowledge were erroneous or incomplete. The second was that it would continue to be aimed at the same readership as in the past.

His death left me with the daunting task of tackling the whole revision on my own, an endeavour for which I realized I was totally unprepared. I therefore decided to solicit and was fortunate to acquire the help of several colleagues – all friends of Leonard – who accepted as far as possible the decisions that he and I had originally made. Many readers will therefore recognize Leonard's inimitable style in large portions of the book.

David Warrell agreed to be co-editor and to revise the chapters on clinical features, pathology and treatment; Kevin Marsh accepted to revise the immunology chapter which, in the light of the rapid advances in this field, required a great deal of rewriting; Michael Service updated the section on the vectors, while Erminio Onori and Peter Beales helped me with the revision of Chapters 10 and 11.

It is my earnest hope that the third edition will prove to be a worthy tribute to Leonard – one of the great malariologists of the 20th century – whose life was so wrapped up in malaria that he even composed a ballad to the *Plasmodium* which is reproduced over.

Herbert M. Gilles

Acknowledgement

We are grateful to SmithKline Beecham for their generous contribution towards the cost of the coloured plates.

The Ballad of the Plasmodium

Plasmodium has a lot in store
And works in stages by the score.
Anopheles that probes your skin
Pumps many sporozoites in,
    They lose no time, move into liver
    And settle down before you shiver,
    Some hypnozoites go to sleep
    A late relapse intending keep.
But others grow, divide like mad
And move from liver into blood.
In red cells do their very worst
Expanding to make each cell burst
    As merozoites they are vexed
    By being greatly undersexed.
    Their life is tedious, rather stale
    Without a female and a male
This truth they soon will realize
And change assuming larger size
So now, when a mosquito bites
It must suck up gametocytes
    And microgametes being sucked
    Can now perform the amorous act
    When in the stomach of the gnat
    They find a macrogamete fat.
Their love's great feat is now complete
As female forms öokinete
Then losing all her self-control
She goes through insect's stomach wall.
    And there encysted feels more able
    To raise a new plasmodial stable
    When thousand sporozoites fit
    Will prove that she has done her bit
To salivary glands they wend
And start again; there is no end.
The moral of this age-old story
Is that we can't aspire to glory
    Until our principal objective
    Will make control much more effective
    And faced with chloroquine resistance
    We must depend on more assistance
And find a new medicament
To solve our great predicament
A compound that in all event
Is active, cheap, polyvalent.

Perhaps we need a proper vaccine
With antigens that science mucks in
And adjuvants that will not itch
And antibody God knows which.
    Or to develop other means
    To fight those vicious little fiends
    That no one who is from Mankind
    Could e'er defend, if sound of mind.

Leonard Bruce-Chwatt

Contributors

P. F. Beales, World Health Organization, Division for the Control of Tropical Diseases, Geneva

N. Francis, Senior Lecturer in Histopathology and Cytopathology, Charing Cross and Westminster Medical School, Westminster Campus, London

K. Marsh, Wellcome Trust Senior Research Fellow in Clinical Medicine, Wellcome Trust Research Laboratories, Kilifi, Kenya

E. Onori, formerly World Health Organization Staff Member Malaria Action Programme, Geneva

M. W. Service, Professor of Medical Entomology, Liverpool School of Tropical Medicine, University of Liverpool

Chapter 1

Historical outline

H. M. Gilles

It is assumed that the evolutionary history of mammalian plasmodia started with the adaptation of Coccidia of the intestinal epithelium to some tissues of the internal organs and then to the invasion of free cells in the blood. The next step was the possibility of transmission of the parasites from one animal to another by bloodsucking arthropod vectors. The great antiquity of malarial infection is confirmed by the fact that well over 100 parasite species similar to those of humans are found in a wide range of vertebrates from reptiles or birds to higher apes. None of the parasites, except for those found in some monkeys, can be transmitted to humans. This high host specificity indicates a long association between the human species and the four particular species of plasmodia that infect humans.

Prehistoric man in the Old World was subject to malaria. It is probable that the disease originated in Africa, which is believed to be the cradle of the human race. Fossil mosquitos were found in geological strata 30 million years old and there is no doubt that they have spread the infection through the warmer regions of the globe, long before the dawn of history. Malaria followed in the wake of human migrations to the Mediterranean shores, to Mesopotamia, the Indian peninsula and South-east Asia. How malaria established itself in the New World is subject to speculation, as no reliable historical or other data exist on this point. It is possible that *Plasmodium vivax* and *P. malariae* were brought from South-east Asia by early trans-Pacific voyages, while *P. falciparum* is of post-Columbian origin, through the African slaves brought by the Spanish colonizers of Central America.

References to seasonal and intermittent fevers exist in the ancient Assyrian, Chinese and Indian religious and medical texts but their true identity with malaria is uncertain. These afflictions, usually ascribed to the punishment of gods or vengeance by evil spirits, were met by incantations or sacrificial offerings. Hippocrates, who lived in Greece in the fifth century BC, was the earliest physician to discard superstition for logical observation of the relationship between the appearance of the disease and the seasons of the year or the places where his patients lived. He was also the first to describe in detail the clinical picture of malaria and some complications of the disease. Galen and other Greek and Roman physicians also left various references to malaria in the second century AD. Non-medical writers alluded to fevers that affected those who lived in marshy areas. Malaria or 'Roman fever' was common in the vicinity of Rome and cyclical epidemics of malaria continued in Greece, Italy, many parts of Europe and other continents throughout many centuries.

For nearly 1500 years no additional knowledge of the extent, cause or treatment of malaria was forthcoming. However, the awareness of the association of fevers with stagnant waters and swamps led to various methods of drainage practised by the Greeks and Romans already in the sixth century BC and continued, for the improvement of agricultural land and better health conditions, throughout the Middle Ages in Italy, France, Holland, England and elsewhere.

However, the main breakthrough in the long history of malaria was connected with the first real therapeutic advance. At the beginning of the seventeenth century came the discovery of the value of 'Peruvian bark' for treatment of fevers. The use of this remedy spread rapidly all over Europe and it soon became obvious that only certain fevers were easily cured by this drug. In the seventeenth century, Morton and Sydenham in England and later Torti in Italy differentiated between the true intermittent fevers and others that failed to respond to the drug, which was then known under the name 'Jesuit's powder'.

These specific fevers known in England as 'agues' received in the eighteenth century the Italian name 'mal'aria', since it was then widely believed that their cause was related to the foul air common near marshy areas. The French term 'paludisme' indicating a close connection with swamps was introduced much later. In 1735 the tree producing the Peruvian bark was given, by Linnaeus, its scientific name of Cinchona. But quinine, the active principle of it, was not isolated until 1820 by Pelletier and Caventou in France.

The most important events in the history of malaria took place towards the end of the nineteenth century, when the sciences of bacteriology and pathology were discovering the causes of infectious diseases, observing the morbid changes in the organs and tissues and also perceiving the role of insects in the transmission of some infections. It was in 1880 that Laveran, a French army surgeon in Algeria, first saw and described malaria parasites in the red blood cells of human beings. Soon after that Romanowsky in Russia developed a new method of staining the malaria parasites in blood films and this, together with the improvement of the microscope, made further studies of plasmodia very much easier.

However, the way in which the disease was transmitted from person to person was still a mystery although a few early and inspired guesses pointed to the possible association between swamps, mosquitos and fevers.

Patrick Manson, a Scotsman who was practising medicine in China, discovered in 1878 that mosquitos are arthropod hosts of human filarial parasites found in the blood. Soon after that, David Bruce demonstrated in Africa that tsetse flies can transmit the trypanosome, a blood parasite of horses and cattle, from one animal to another. This provided a new clue for considering mosquitos as possible vectors of malaria. But the final elucidation of the actual mode of transmission was not forthcoming until 1897 when Ronald Ross working in Secunderabad (India) found a developing form of the malaria parasite in the body of a mosquito that had previously fed on a patient with the plasmodia in his blood. The whole complex picture of the cycle of development of malaria parasites in humans and in the female Anopheles mosquito became clear as a result of further studies by the Italians Amico Bignami, Giuseppe Bastianelli and especially Battista Grassi in 1898–99. A striking confirmation of the fact that malaria is transmitted by Anopheles mosquitos was based on the combined field experiment carried out by Patrick Manson and his colleagues near Rome and in London in 1900. This proved that protection from the bites of Anopheles prevents the occurrence of the infection; conversely, Anopheles obviously infected in Italy and brought to England were capable of transmitting the disease by their bite.

During the twentieth century much research was devoted to malaria control. Larvicides in the form of oil or Paris green were introduced to prevent the breeding of mosquitos in various types of waters. Wider use of these and other methods of mosquito reduction demonstrated the practicability of controlling malaria and yellow fever in Cuba and the Panama Canal Zone, where two American campaigns organized by General William Crawford Gorgas proved to be outstanding successes. These were followed in Malaya by Malcolm Watson who introduced the concept of 'naturalistic control' based on the knowledge of the breeding habits of species of *Anopheles* involved in the local transmission of the disease.

The ravages of malaria experienced during the First World War and the difficulties of securing cheap supplies of quinine stimulated a line of research in Germany aimed at the discovery of synthetic antimalarial drugs. This was brilliantly accomplished in 1924 by Schulemann's discovery of pamaquine. However, a much more valuable drug – Atabrin (mepacrine) – was prepared in 1930 by Kikuth, Mietzsch and Mauss. There can be no doubt that the availability of this compound played an immense role during the Second World War. Other valuable synthetic drugs developed by the Germans, the French, the Americans and the British followed in 1934 (chloroquine), 1944 (proguanil), 1946 (amodiaquine), 1950 (primaquine) and 1952 (pyrimethamine).

In the meantime, another major discovery was to revolutionize the technique of malaria control by spraying insecticides against adult mosquitos. The possibility of the new method was foreshadowed in South Africa, where De Meillon's use of pyrethrum sprays greatly reduced the amount of malaria in rural areas.

At the beginning of the Second World War, Paul Muller discovered in Switzerland the high insecticidal action of a synthetic compound, dichlorodiphenyl-trichloroethane, which was given the abbreviated name of DDT when samples of it were sent in 1942 to the UK. The value of this compound for control of flies and mosquitos was soon confirmed, and in 1944 the first field tests were carried out in Italy. Other projects followed and in 1945 Venezuela and Guyana became the first countries where malaria control on a large scale was instituted (Fig. 1.1).

Among other residual insecticides which were introduced soon after DDT, hexachlorocyclohexane (BHC or HCH) and dieldrin should be mentioned. Their general use in malaria control was less effective than first anticipated because of some unexpected difficulties related to the developing resistance of mosquitos.

The possibility of global extension of malaria control activities to bring about the final eradication of the disease was contemplated in the 1950s when the results of the application of DDT in Venezuela, Italy, Greece, Guyana, Ceylon and the USA showed great promise.

In the meantime, parasitological studies on the cycle of development of the malaria parasites continued although little progress had been made since 1901 when Grassi formulated the idea that there is a third, cryptic tissue phase following the inoculation of sporozoites by the bite of *Anopheles*. Raffaele in Italy was the first to demonstrate in 1934 the existence of this phase in bird malaria. This was soon followed by similar findings in other species of avian and monkey parasites. Then in 1948 the exo-erythrocytic stages, first of monkey malaria (*P. cynomolgi*), then of human (*P. vivax*) malaria, were discovered in the UK by Shortt and Garnham. This explained what happens to the parasite during the incubation period, how the relapses of malaria infection occur and gave new impetus to the chemotherapeutic research which was soon to develop new and powerful drugs.

The characteristics of DDT and other residual insecticides, namely, their high potency against the

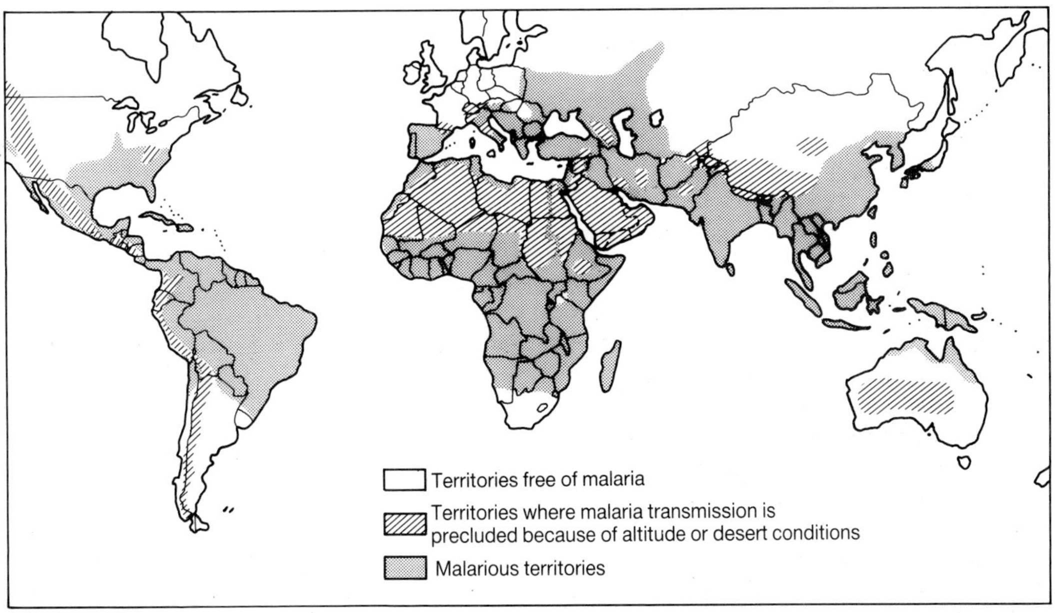

Fig. 1.1 Geographical distribution of malaria before 1946 (before residual insecticides were used). (WHO, 1991.)

mosquitos, low toxicity to humans, ease of application in rural areas and relatively low cost, encouraged many health workers to press for malaria eradication. The examples of Greece and Italy where in 1951 a temporary interruption of house spraying with DDT had not interfered with the elimination of the disease, confirmed the apparent practicability of malaria eradication, without necessarily eliminating the main *Anopheles* vector.

The concept of malaria eradication was adopted by the World Health Assembly in 1955, and two years later the World Health Organization (WHO) launched a global campaign. Its results over the next 15 years were excellent in Europe, North America, some parts of Asia, the former USSR and Australia and less good in tropical countries. The causes of this lack of progress are many and will be fully dealt with in the appropriate section of this book. In 1969 the World Health Organization revised the strategy of malaria eradication by stressing the need for greater involvement of general health services and for extension of research on new insecticides, improved surveillance, development of new antimalarial drugs and alternative methods of malaria control.

However, during the past decade there has been a considerable increase of malaria in several tropical areas, where in the past the eradication programmes appeared to advance satisfactorily. This resurgence of the disease was greatest in southern and south-eastern Asia, but there was also a higher incidence in Central America and parts of South America; a serious epidemic of malaria occurred in the Asian part of Turkey. In tropical Africa, the malaria situation has deteriorated. Severe outbreaks have occurred in several countries, with a high mortality and a shift of morbidity to older age groups. Uncontrolled and rapid urbanization has created pockets of transmission in the cities, thus increasing the size of vulnerable groups. Chloroquine resistance of *P. falciparum* has spread throughout the continent. In South-east Asia multidrug resistance is now commonly encountered. Political concern and will to reduce morbidity and mortality from malaria has been mobilized at a Ministerial Conference held in Amsterdam in 1992.

Remarkable progress of scientific activity related to malaria has been seen during the past ten years when the United Nations Development Programme (UNDP)/World Bank/WHO Tropical Diseases Research and Training Programme increased its activity and widened its aims. Research on malaria was extended over the whole range of the host–parasite relationship, not excluding the mosquito vector or the socio-economic impact of the disease. Considerable advance has been made in the drug development and field-testing of some new chemical compounds. Some progress has also been made in the development of a prospective vaccine.

The large number of cases of malaria imported from tropical areas into Europe, the USA and other countries presents the medical and health authorities with a potentially serious problem, wherever the local anopheline population remains high. The speed and constantly rising volume of international travel have created new conditions for massive influx of various communicable diseases into countries where these infections were unknown or from which they had disappeared.

The present concern with the problem of malaria is justified from the viewpoint of general practitioners and other clinicians in developed and developing parts of the world. The specialist in community health is equally concerned since he recognizes that there can be no complete safety from this disease and no satisfactory socio-economic advance of underprivileged countries as long as vast areas of the tropical world remain in the grip of an enormous accumulation of plasmodial infections.

Milestones in the history of malaria and its control

The main chronological landmarks in the advance of our knowledge of malaria and the control or eradication of this disease followed three different and yet related roads. This list of major events related to the history of malaria is necessarily arbitrary and incomplete. Its purpose is to indicate the continuous research activity and an increasing effort to overcome the present obstacles to the treatment of malaria in individual cases, and to its control in large areas of the tropical world. A fuller summary of events will be found in periodic reports issued by the UNDP/World Bank/WHO Special Programme for Research and Training in Tropical Diseases and the WHO Division for the Control of Tropical Diseases.

Malaria parasites and their transmission

1847 Dempster in India introduced spleen palpation of children as an index of epidemicity of malaria.

1848 Virchow and Frerichs in Germany recognized that the presence of pigment in internal organs may be related to deaths from intermittent fevers.

1878 Manson in China showed that a mosquito (*Culex fatigans*) can act as a vector of human filaria.

1880 Laveran in Algeria discovered and described malaria parasites in human blood.

1886 Golgi in Italy described in detail two species of human malaria parasites (*P. vivax* and *P. malariae*)

1889 Danilewski in Russia described the morphology of avian parasites and indicated their wide distribution.

1889–90 Celli and Marchiafava in Italy described *P. falciparum*.

1889–93 Smith and Kilborne in the USA demonstrated the role of the arthropod vector (tick) in the transmission of Texas fever (piroplasmosis) of cattle.

1891 Romanowsky developed his polychrome staining method for demonstrating plasmodia in blood smears.

1894–96 Bruce, in Zululand, working on nagana, a disease of horses and cattle, showed that an infection caused by a protozoan parasite can be transmitted by a true insect (tsetse fly).

1894 Manson put forward the theory that malaria is transmitted from person to person by mosquitos.

1897 Ross discovered pigmented cysts (oöcysts) on the stomach wall of an Anopheles mosquito (probably *A. stephensi*) in Secunderabad, India.

1897 MacCallum in the USA described the sexual phase of *Haemoproteus* in the blood of a crow, and observed exflagellation of a male gametocyte in *P. falciparum* and the penetration of a female gametocyte by a 'flagellum'.

1898 Ross worked out the complete cycle of bird malaria in naturally infected sparrows in Calcutta.

1898 Grassi, Bignami and Bastianelli in Italy described the cycle of human malaria parasites in Anopheles mosquitos.

1900 Manson, by experiments with human volunteers in the Roman Campagna and in London, confirmed the mosquito–malaria transmission theory.

1901 Grassi forecast the existence of a third phase in the life cycle of the malaria parasite.

1902 Schaudinn announced, incorrectly, the penetration of a red blood cell by a sporozoite, thus apparently refuting Grassi's theory and retarding this line of research for many years.

1922 Stephens identified and described *P. ovale*.

1931 James revived Grassi's theory, and suggested that the sporozoite, soon after entering the body, invades reticuloendothelial cells or cells lining the capillary blood vessels.

1934 Raffaele, in Italy, described tissue forms in *P. elongatum* and concluded that in avian malaria there is a schizogonic cycle of development in the reticuloendothelial system as well as in the red blood cells.

1937 James and Tate described schizogonic development of *P. gallinaceum* in fixed tissue cells of the fowl, and showed that the brain is an important place for the localization of the endothelial stages.

1947 Garnham described exo-erythrocytic forms of *P. kochi* (now classed as *Hepatocystis*) in parenchyma cells of the liver of lower monkeys in East Africa.

1948 Shortt, Garnham and Malamos, in England, described pre-erythrocytic forms of *P. cynomolgi* in parenchyma cells of the liver of *Macaca mulatta* (rhesus) monkeys. Shortt and Garnham also described persistent exo-erythrocytic forms of *P. cynomolgi* in a monkey's liver.

1948 Vincke and Lips in the former Belgian Congo (Zaire) discovered *P. berghei*, the first plasmodium of rodents.

1948	Shortt, Garnham, Covell and Shute described pre-erythrocytic forms of *P. vivax* in the human liver.
1948	Rodhain showed that the chimpanzee is a host of *P. malariae* in Central Africa.
1949	Nikolaev described *P. vivax hibernans* with a long incubation period.
1949	Shortt, Fairley, Covell, Shute and Garnham described pre-erythrocytic forms of *P. falciparum* in the human liver.
1950	Garnham described pre-erythrocytic forms of *P. inui*, a quartan-like parasite, in a simian liver.
1953	Garnham described pre-erythrocytic forms of *P. ovale* in the human liver.
1965	Elucidation by Cohen and McGregor of the humoral transfer of protective antibodies of *P. falciparum*.
1966	Discovery by Young of the experimental transmissibility of human plasmodia to the Colombian owl monkey (*Aotus trivirgatus*).
1973	First attempt by Clyde at immunizing humans with irradiated sporozoites of *P. falciparum* and *P. vivax*.
1976	Continuous *in vitro* culture of *P. falciparum* developed by Trager and Jensen in the USA.
1977	Characterization by Carter and Walliker of the genetic diversity of strains of *P. falciparum* using enzyme electrophoresis.
1978	Demonstration by Aikawa of the mechanism of penetration of merozoites into erythrocytes.
1980	Discovery of hypnozoites of *P. cynomolgi* and suggestion of the role of hypnozoites of *P. vivax* in delayed relapses of human malaria. *In vitro* production of mature gametocytes of *P. falciparum*, infective to mosquitos. Production and use of monoclonal antibodies against *P. falciparum* antigens.
1982	Characterization of polypeptides specific to surface antigens in sporozoites and erythrocytic stages of several animal and human plasmodia.
1983	Isolation of mRNA from *P. falciparum* and cloning of its DNA into a bacterium (*Escherichia coli*).
1987	Recombinant DNA *P. falciparum* sporozoite vaccine and synthetic peptide sporozoite vaccine both tested in volunteers.
1988	Synthetic asexual stage *P. falciparum* peptide vaccine tested in volunteers.
1992	Field trials of asexual stage vaccine and of sporozoite vaccine.

Treatment of malaria

1600	Juan Lopez, a Jesuit missionary, recorded the use of the 'fever tree bark' by Peruvian Indians.
1643	Cardinal Juan de Lugo carried out trials of the Peruvian bark at the Santo Spirito Hospital in Rome.
1649	Cardinal de Lugo supported a wide use of the bark which became known as 'Jesuit's powder'.
1637–98	Morton and Sydenham in England noted the specific action of the bark in curing certain fevers (agues).
1712	Torti in Italy clearly described the specific action of the bark on intermittent (but no other) fevers.
1735	Condamine leading the French expedition to Peru identified the 'Quina-quina' tree.
1742	Linnaeus in Sweden described the tree and gave it the name of Cinchona.
1820	Pelletier and Caventou in France isolated the alkaloids quinine and cinchonine from the bark of Cinchona.
1854	Hasskarl, a Dutch botanist, brought the seeds of Cinchona to Java and began large-scale cultivation in Indonesia.
1872	Markham, an English geographer, started Cinchona plantations in the Nilgiri Hills in India.
1914–18	Events during the First World War indicated the shortage of quinine, especially in countries without direct access to Cinchona plantations.

1924 Development of pamaquine (Plasmoquine) in Germany by Schulemann and his colleagues.
1930 Development of mepacrine (Atabrin) in Germany by Mietzsch and Kikuth.
1934 Development of chloroquine (Resochin) in Germany.
1944 Development of proguanil (Paludrine) by Curd, Davey and Rose in England.
1952 Development of pyrimethamine (Daraprim) by Hitchings in the USA and his coworkers in England.
1952 Development of primaquine by Elderfield in the USA.
1956 Development of quinocide by Braude and Stavrovskaya in the former USSR.
1961–65 Reports from Colombia and Brazil on strains of *P. falciparum* resistant to chloroquine. Similar reports from South-east Asia.
1960–66 Rediscovery of the value of sulfones and sulfonamides as antimalarial compounds.
1967–74 Development by the US Army Medical Research and Development Command of a number of new synthetic antimalarials.
1971–75 Development and introduction of mefloquine into treatment of malaria.
1978 Introduction by Rieckmann of a microtest for detection of chloroquine resistance in *P. falciparum*. Development by Schmidt of the Aotus monkey model for advanced studies of antimalaria compounds.
1974–82 Series of amino-alcohol compounds, as possible antimalaria drugs developed by US Walter Reed Army Institute for Research.
1979–82 Development of new antimalarials by the Qinghaosu Antimalaria Coordinating Group in China.
1979–82 Confirmation of the appearance of chloroquine resistance in *P. falciparum* in several countries in East Africa.
1976–83 Development of a series of derivatives of 8-amino-quinolines with high activity for radical cure of relapsing malaria; still not commercially available.
1986 Confirmation of the appearance of chloroquine resistance in *P. falciparum* in several countries in West Africa.
1987 Reversal of *in vitro* chloroquine resistance in *P. falciparum* by Verapamil and other compounds.
1988 Development of trioxane derivatives as potential antimalarials. Development of novel bicyclic peroxide antimalarials related to Yingzhaosu.
1989 Introduction of halofantrine.
1990 Clinical trials of artesunate and artemether in countries outside China and Burma.

Epidemiology and control of malaria

1899 Ross initiated antilarval measures in Sierra Leone.
1899 Large-scale demonstration of successful mosquito control by Gorgas and Le Prince in Cuba.
1901–03 Malaria control by antilarval measures in Malaya initiated by Malcolm Watson. Antimosquito campaign organized by Ross in Ismailia, Egypt.
1904–14 Malaria control campaign carried out by Gorgas and Le Prince in the Panama Canal zone.
1908 Ross carried out a survey of malaria in Mauritius and originated the mathematical approach to the transmission of the infection.
1924–26 Roubaud in France, Swellengrebel and Van Thiel in the Netherlands, and Falleroni in Italy differentiated the cryptic species of *A. maculipennis* complex and elucidated the importance of mosquito behaviour in the transmission of malaria.
1927 First instance of eradication of an invading vector species (*A. albimanus*) in Barbados.
1935–39 First large-scale control of rural malaria by imagicidal measures (using pyrethrum spraying) in South Africa, the Netherlands and India.
1936–39 Discovery of insecticidal action of DDT (synthesized by Zeidler in Germany in 1874) by Muller and Wiesman in Switzerland.

1939–40 Eradication of an invading African mosquito (*A. gambiae*) from Brazil.
1942–45 Eradication from northern Egypt of *A. gambiae*.
1942–46 Development of new synthetic insecticides (HCH, dieldrin, chlordane etc.) with residual action.
1946–51 Antimalaria campaign in Cyprus, Sardinia, Guyana, Venezuela and Greece, followed by interruption of transmission.
1947 Beklemishev introduced the concept and practice of landscape epidemiology in the former USSR.
1950–57 Macdonald in the UK and Moshkowski in the former USSR expanded Ronald Ross's mathematical approach to the understanding of epidemiology of malaria.
1955 Adoption of the principle of malaria eradication by the Fourteenth World Health Assembly.
1957 Definition of the concept and practice of malaria eradication by the WHO.
1979 WHO Expert Committee developed the strategy of malaria control and its tactical variants.
1985 The Thirty-eighth World Health Assembly adopted resolution WHA 38.24 which recommended that malaria control should be developed as an integral part of the national primary health care system.
1986 Stratification of malaria situations in tropical Africa for the development of malaria control within primary health care.
1991 Strategy for malaria control based on major prototypes.
1992 Ministerial Conference on Malaria, Amsterdam.

World Declaration on the Control of Malaria

The Ministerial Conference on Malaria, meeting in Amsterdam this twenty-seventh day of October in the year Nineteen hundred and ninety-two,

expressing the urgent need for commitment to malaria control by all governments, all health and development workers, and the world community,

hereby makes the following declaration:

I

The conference recognizes that malaria constitutes a major threat to health and blocks the path to economic development for individuals, communities and nations. Almost half the world's population are at risk from this disease, which causes one hundred million clinical cases and over one million deaths each year.

II

While over 80% of malaria cases and deaths occur in Africa, malaria is a problem in every region of the world. It affects young and old. Children are particularly at risk, malaria being one of the major childhood killers in tropical Africa, taking the life of 1 out of 20 children before the age of 5 years. The disease causes anaemia in children and pregnant women and increases the vulnerability to other diseases. It afflicts the poor and underprivileged most severely, sapping productivity and causing chronic ill health. The social and economic impact is staggering.

III

Social, political and economic changes all contribute to the worsening malaria problem, particularly through large scale uncontrolled population movements and ecological disturbances. Non-immune populations entering malaria endemic zones within the frontiers of economic development are paying an exorbitant price in disease and disability.

IV

Construction and environmental change brought about by development are creating environments favourable for malaria transmission, exacerbating existing problems and opening the way for devastating epidemics in areas which were previously malaria free, leading to many deaths and profound impoverishment of communities.

V

The spread of drug resistance is making malaria treatment more complicated, often requiring newer drugs that may be more expensive or more toxic than chloroquine. These characteristics place higher priority on personal and community action to protect against mosquito bites and actually render malaria drug prophylaxis a less useful tool.

VI

Despite these problems, the situation can and must be controlled with the tools now available. We have learnt that the key to success is to apply the right strategies in the right place at the right time, and to apply the appropriate strategies on a sustained basis. In most endemic countries, the goal will be to prevent malaria mortality and to reduce morbidity and the social and economic losses provoked by this disease through the progressive improvement and strengthening of local and national capabilities. The challenge will be especially great in the least developed countries.

VII

We, recognizing the above:

- endorse the Global Malaria Control Strategy, acknowledging the need to focus upon strengthening local and national capabilities and to adapt it to specific country circumstances;
- support the four technical elements of this strategy:
  - to provide early diagnosis and prompt treatment;
  - to plan and implement selective and sustainable preventive measures;
  - to detect early, contain or prevent epidemics; and
  - to strengthen local capacities in basic and applied research to permit and promote the regular assessment of a country's malaria situation, in particular the ecological, social and economic determinants of the disease;
- support and decentralize structures of programme management in which those closest to the problem are delegated the responsibilities to employ available resources most appropriately;
- accept the crucial role of a core group of national specialists in defining and evolving national strategies and in implementing effective systems of training and supervision and of health education which incorporate them. These systems are needed to assure that new knowledge especially from operational research and from routine monitoring and evaluation, is continuously made available to those in the best position to utilize it;
- know that the problem of malaria will continue to evolve, and know that malaria control strategies must too evolve. We support the need for continuous research and development, including basic research to develop better tools for malaria control and applied research to permit the optimal use of existing resources under the widely varying conditions in

which malaria flourishes. We recognize that there is need for science in the service of the social sectors to be supported far more extensively, putting it to work for all mankind.

VIII

We commit ourselves and our countries to control malaria, and

- will review our current efforts, acknowledging the better use of existing resources is possible and that existing resources along with the clear identification of unmet needs are prerequisites to obtaining any additional resources required to expand current activities;
- will plan for malaria control as an essential component of health development and will incorporate health development as an essential component of national development. We know that the potential for development projects to spread malaria and other tropical diseases can far exceed the ability of the health and social sectors to take remedial action. Health concerns must be incorporated in such projects if they are to contribute positively to social and economic development for the communities concerned;
- will involve the communities concerned as partners in our efforts, as well as the sectors concerned with education, water resources, sanitation, agriculture and development; and
- will implement malaria control in the context of primary health care, seeing it as an opportunity to strengthen health and social interstructures and to promote the fundamental right of all populations affected by malaria to have access to early diagnosis and appropriate treatment.

IX

While recognizing the primary responsibility of affected countries to take the actions essential for malaria control, we draw attention to the fact that the problem is often greatest in the very countries or areas which can least afford to take action. Recognizing also that external support will inevitably be limited in time and directed at building up self-reliance within a reasonable period, we call upon international development partners, including the United Nations system, bilateral agencies, and nongovernmental organizations to increase their support to malaria control efforts, contributing their resources so as to strengthen sustainable national malaria control plans in accordance with the global strategy and to increase support to research that will lead to new malaria control tools, including vaccines. We base this call on grounds of social justice and equity as well as on the conviction that such support will contribute specifically to social and economic development and to alleviating world poverty.

X

We call on the World Health Organization in fulfilment of its constitutional function to act as the coordinating authority on international health work, to exercise leadership in providing support for national implementation of this global strategy.

Therapeutic malaria

Hippocrates and Galen mentioned that malaria seemed occasionally to have beneficial effects on other diseases. In England, John Macculoch (1828) described an attempt to 'acquire an ague for removing a previous chronic disorder'. Deliberate infection with malaria for treatment of general paralysis was proposed by Wagner von Jauregg in Vienna in 1887, although the first trials only started in 1918. The initial method consisted of infecting patients by injection of blood obtained from other persons suffering from malaria.

In 1922 Warrington Yorke in Liverpool began inducing malaria by the bites of infected mosquitos since this method had many advantages over blood inoculation. Therapeutic malaria has been widely used in many countries and with generally satisfactory results. The explanation of the beneficial effects of malaria on late neurosyphilis is not clear. In addition to the possible effect of febrile paroxysms it is likely that the plasmodial infection stimulates some specific defence mechanism against *Treponema pallidum*. The benefit depends on the degree of fever and on the number of paroxysms.

Many aspects of transfusion malaria were studied in the course of therapeutic malaria. The main difference between the two is that in the former the infection is accidental and presents an added hazard to the recipient of the blood. In therapeutic malaria the induced infection is deliberate; the species of the parasite is known in advance, the dosage of plasmodia as well as the number of injections are related to the state of health of the patient, and the course of the infection can be easily moderated by the use of appropriate drugs.

It is obvious that the 'incubation period' of therapeutic malaria induced by blood injection depends on the species of the parasite and on the numbers of plasmodia used; it varies between 3 days (0.5–1 million plasmodia) and 10 days (1000–2000 million plasmodia). On the other hand, the true incubation period related to the mosquito transmission of the infection depends primarily on the species of the malaria parasite involved.

Therapeutic malaria was widely practised in many countries between 1920 and 1950. In the past, many thousands of patients have benefited from this treatment. The advent of penicillin for treatment of syphilis has greatly reduced the demand for therapeutic malaria and the procedure is now employed only in exceptional cases or for scientific purposes.

Plasmodium vivax has been used in preference to any other species, largely because of the relatively benign infection that it causes. (It should be remembered that in malaria induced by injection of infected blood there are no relapses due to the absence of exo-erythrocytic forms in the liver, since the infection takes place without the involvement of sporozoites. Thus the treatment of induced malaria is relatively simple.) However, in some cases *P. malariae*, *P. falciparum* or *P. ovale* have been employed. A simian malaria parasite, *P. knowlesi*, has been used occasionally; it causes moderate fever and is easily controlled by drugs.

Various species of *Anopheles* have been preferred by different specialists for transmission of induced malaria by mosquitos. In Europe *A. atroparvus* has been most commonly used, although more recently the Indian *A. stephensi* proved to be an efficient vector. In the USA *A. quadrimaculatus* was generally employed.

Therapeutic malaria provided great opportunities for research in various fields of parasitology, immunology, and chemotherapy.

In the USA much of the advance of chemotherapy of malaria during the past 30 years was due to the existence of 'human malaria research centres' where the infection could be induced in volunteers. In Brazil, induced malaria was tentatively given for treatment of non-syphilitic psychiatric disorders.

In the UK over the past 50 years the scientific contribution of the malaria therapy unit, later known as Malaria Reference Laboratory, Horton Hospital, has been immense. The characteristics of various strains of the three species of plasmodia were determined, the development of the parasite in different *Anopheles* species was elucidated, the pattern of relapses in malaria became clearer, much knowledge of the immune response to the infection in humans was gained in the course of long-term observations; the action of various drugs on the course of the disease and its prevention contributed substantially to the development of synthetic antimalarials. In 1948 the discovery of pre-erythrocytic stages of *P. vivax* was made after the infection of a volunteer with the Madagascar strain of *P. vivax* and subsequent biopsy of his liver.

A few years later an international collaborative project studied the parasitological and epidemiological characteristics of *P. vivax* North Korean strain on patients infected with malaria for therapeutic purposes.

With the discovery in the 1960s that human malaria can be transmitted to the owl monkey (*Aotus trivirgatus*) and other South American monkeys the importance of deliberately induced malaria to human volunteers declined still further. Nevertheless, for the final testing of some new antimalarial drugs, vaccines or immunological methods, the value of the study of the course of infection in humans is essential.

Chapter 2

The malaria parasites

H. M. Gilles*

The microorganisms causing malaria are commonly referred to as malaria parasites; this term is restricted to the family Plasmodiidae within the order Coccidiida, sub-order Haemosporidiidea, which comprises various parasites found in the blood of reptiles, birds and mammals. The classification of Haemosporidiidea as a sub-order of the Coccidiida is complex and controversial, since an alternative system has been proposed by Levine (1978). However, Garnham's (1969) classification of Haemosporidiidea into Plasmodiidae, Haemoproteidae and Leucocytozoidae has been maintained here. The zoological family of Plasmodiidae includs the parasites which undergo two types of multiplication by asexual division (*schizogony*) in the vertebrate host and a single sexual multiplication (*sporogony*) in the mosquito host. The genus *Plasmodium* has been defined on the basis of one type of the asexual multiplication by division occurring in cells other than the erythrocytes of the vertebrate host (*exo-erythrocytic schizogony*); the other characteristic of this genus is that the mosquito hosts are various species of *Diptera*.

There are nearly 120 species of *Plasmodia*, including at least 22 species found in primate hosts and 19 in rodents, bats or other mammals. About 70 other plasmodial species have been described in birds and reptiles. *Plasmodia* of the primate hosts are divided into three sub-genera and within the sub-genus of *Plasmodium* there are four groups classified according to the periodicity of their erythrocytic schizogony and some other characteristics (Table 2.1).

The zoological classification of *Plasmodia* is complex, and even today there is some difference of opinion with regard to the taxonomic position of the parasite causing falciparum malaria. In this malaria parasite the crescentic shape and lengthy

Table 2.1 *Plasmodia* of primates and other mammals

Genus: *Plasmodium*		
Sub-genus: *Plasmodium*		
Group: Vivax,	Species:	*P. vivax,* P. cynomolgi, P. eylesi, P. gonderi, P. hylobati, P. jefferyi, P. pitheci, P. schwetzi, P. simium, P. sylvaticum, P. youngi*
Group: Ovale,	Species:	*P. ovale,* P. fieldi, P. simiovale*
Group: Malariae,	Species:	*P. malariae,* P. brazilianum, P. inui*
Group: Uncertain,	Species:	*P. coatneyi, P. fragile* (both with tertian periodicity) *P. knowlesi* (quotidian periodicity)
Sub-genus: *Laverania*,	Species:	*P. falciparum,* P. reichenowi*
Sub-genus: *Vinckeia*,	Species:	Large number of species (some of them of uncertain taxonomic status) infecting lemurs, rodents, bats and other animals

*Signifies *Plasmodia* of humans.

***The help of Dr David Payne in the revision of this chapter is gratefully acknowledged.**

development of sexual erythrocytic forms has been accepted by some authors as a valid argument for recognition of the parasite as belonging to a separate genus, *Laverania falcipara*. While this view may be correct in a context of zoological systematics, the rejection of the familiar name *Plasmodium falciparum* might be confusing and since the use of this well-known name is still taxonomically permissible it is proposed to retain it in the present text.

There are four generally recognized species of malaria parasites of humans:

P. malariae (Laveran, 1881)*
P. vivax (Grassi and Feletti, 1890)
P. falciparum Welch, 1897
P. ovale Stephens, 1922

of which only *P. malariae* may naturally infect non-human primates. Infections caused by the various human species of *Plasmodia* have been given a number of colloquial names:

P. vivax	Benign tertian, simple tertian, tertian
P. malariae	Quartan
P. falciparum	Malignant tertian (MT), subtertian, aestivo-autumnal, tropical, pernicious
P. ovale	Ovale tertian

These colloquial names have now become obsolete. Their replacement by the unitalicized specific names of the relevant plasmodia is recommended. Thus, one refers to vivax malaria, ovale malaria, falciparum infection etc. An exception may be made with regard to 'malariae' as this could be confusing; a term such as 'quartan malaria' is acceptable.

Some authors refer to the mosquito as the definitive host, while humans and animals are regarded as intermediate hosts of the malaria parasite. This nomenclature may be zoologically correct, since the sexual development of plasmodia is the more important function in the perpetuation of the species. However, this terminology gives rise to some confusion and it may be preferable to speak of invertebrate and vertebrate hosts.

It is not uncommon to observe that some morphological or other characteristics of one well-defined species of malaria parasite may vary somewhat from one geographical area to another. The best known differences are biological variations which may be so distinctive that they provide an acceptable basis for referring to these parasite populations as 'strains'. A parasite strain has been defined as 'a population of common stock descending from a single ancestor or derived from a single source and maintained without intermixture from other sources through a number of generations'. This definition is not easily applicable to the designation of a group of parasites in field conditions. At the present time, the term 'isolate' is favoured when we refer to a sample of parasites, not necessarily genetically homogeneous, collected on a single occasion from an infected host and preserved in the laboratory either by passaging to other hosts or maintained in a culture or in deep frozen state.

The differentiation of strains of malaria parasites, based in the past on morphological characteristics, relapse pattern, drug response, infectivity to various vectors and immunological differences has been given recently more attention thanks to a new biochemical and genetic approach.

The composition of a 'strain' depends on knowledge of the basic genetic organization of the parasite and on the way in which the genetic factors are inherited and distributed within the parasite population.

Life cycle and morphology of human malaria parasites

The life cycle of all species of human malaria parasites is essentially the same. It comprises an exogenous sexual phase (*sporogony*) with multiplication in certain Anopheles mosquitos, of which worldwide, about 60 are important malaria vectors in nature, and an endogenous asexual phase (*schizogony*) with multiplication in the vertebrate host. The latter phase includes the development cycle in the red corpuscles in the blood (*erythrocytic schizogony*) and the phase taking place in the parenchyma cells in the liver (*exo-erythrocytic schizogony*).

***In formal zoological nomenclature the binary designation of species is completed by adding the name of the author of the original description and the relevant date. If the generic placing is not that of the original author then the name of the author and the date of description are given in parentheses.**

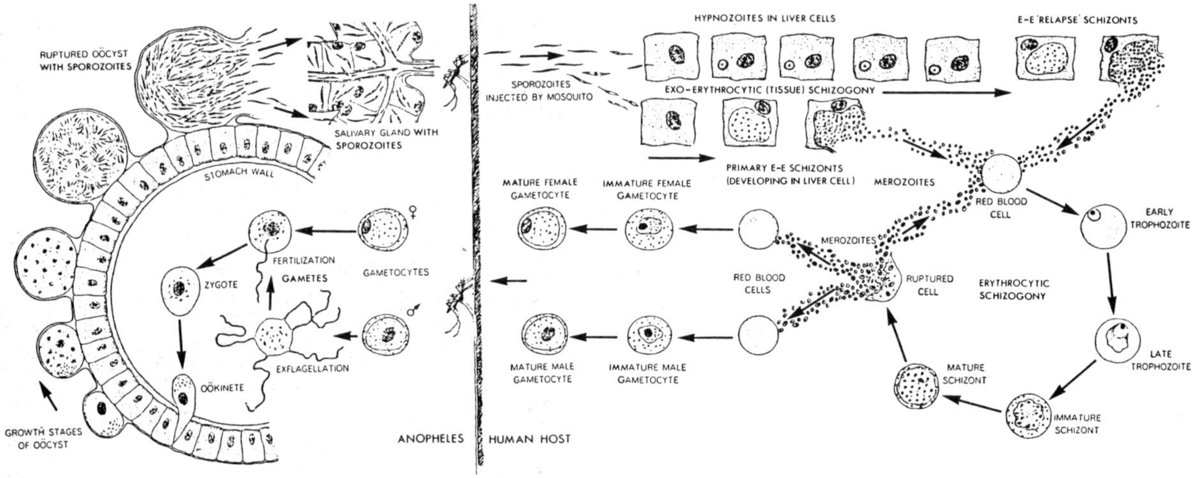

Fig. 2.1 The life cycle of malaria parasites in the mosquito and in the human host, according to present views on the exo-erythrocytic schizogony.

In the latter, often referred to as the *tissue stage*, one should distinguish between the primary or *pre-erythrocytic schizogony* which follows the development of the sporozoite without delay and the delayed *exo-erythrocytic schizogony* which is related to relapses (Fig. 2.1).

The parasite in the mosquito host

When a female Anopheles mosquito ingests the blood of a human host with malaria parasites in the circulation the asexual parasites are digested together with the red blood cells while the mature sexual cells (*gametocytes*) undergo further development. In the male gametocytes the nucleus divides into four to eight nuclei, each of which then forms a long thread-like structure 20 to 25 μm in length (*flagellum*); they shoot out from the original cell, lash about for a while and then break free. This process (*exflagellation*) takes only a few minutes at the appropriate temperature and can be seen in a fresh blood drop under the microscope.

The female gametocyte undergoes a maturation process and forms a *female gamete* or *macrogamete*; the flagellum or *male gamete* is called a *microgamete*.*

In the stomach of the mosquito a microgamete is attracted by a macrogamete; the latter forms a small projection through which the microgamete enters and thus completes the fertilization. The product of fusion of male and female gamete is called a *zygote*. This is at first a motionless globular body, but within 18 to 24 hours of its formation it elongates and becomes mobile; this worm-like stage measuring 18 to 24 μm in length is known as *oökinete* (Fig. 2.2).

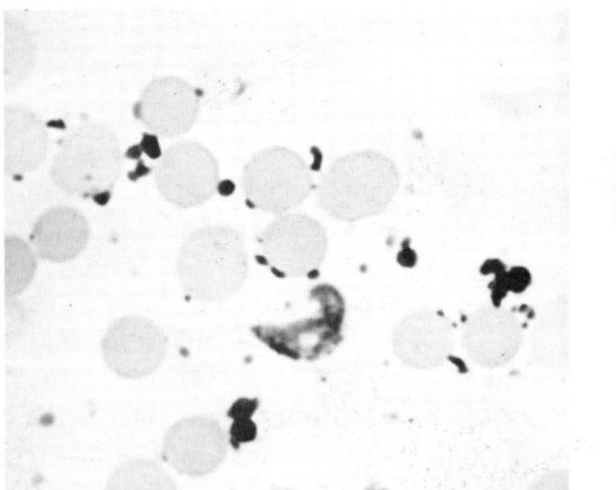

Fig. 2.2 An oökinete in the stomach of an *Anopheles* mosquito; this stage of the malaria parasite proceeds to the outer epithelium of the mid-gut of the mosquito to form an oöcyst. (Wellcome Museum of Medical Science.)

***French, German and Russian authors often use the term 'gamont' for gametocyte.**

The oökinete soon forces its way to the stomach wall, passes between epithelial cells to the outer surface of the stomach and settles down. It becomes rounded up into a small sphere with an elastic membrane and is now called an *oöcyst*. The number of oöcysts on the stomach of an *Anopheles* may vary between a few and several hundreds (Fig. 2.3).

The oöcyst gradually increases in size and appears on the stomach as a semi-transparent globular body, some 40 to 80 μm in size containing grains of pigment. The distribution and size of pigment grains, and their colour are characteristic for the given species of *Plasmodium*. As the oöcyst enlarges and the nucleus divided repeatedly the pigment is obscured. Recent studies using electron microscopy have revealed many details of the process of maturation of the oöcyst. The cytoplasm sub-divides into a number of interconnected lobes, in which budding centres of radiating spindle-shaped bodies appear. The divided nuclei of the sporoblast then form elongated sporozoites each 10–15 μm in length with a central nucleus. Being motile, they burst through the weakened or ruptured wall of the oöcyst and invade the body cavity of the mosquito (Fig. 2.4). In old infections of the insect host the oöcyst wall may remain attached to the midgut and becomes chitinized, forming the so-called 'Ross's black spores'. Sporozoites released into the body cavity reach the salivary glands of the female *Anopheles* which now becomes infective. When the mosquito feeds on blood after piercing the human skin the sporozoites are injected into the wound and pass into the bloodstream of the vertebrate host (Fig. 2.5). It has been estimated that on average one single oöcyst of *P. falciparum* may produce and release about 1000 sporozoites.

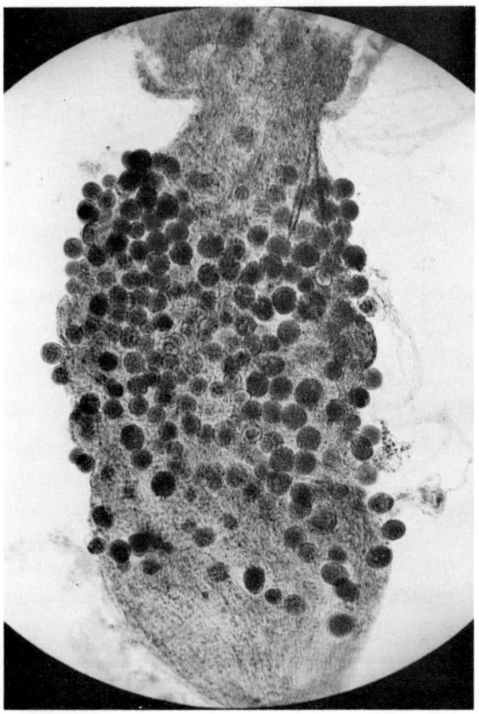

Fig. 2.3 Midgut of an *Anopheles* mosquito heavily infected with oöcysts of *P. vivax*. × *c*. 40. (Wellcome Museum of Medical Science.)

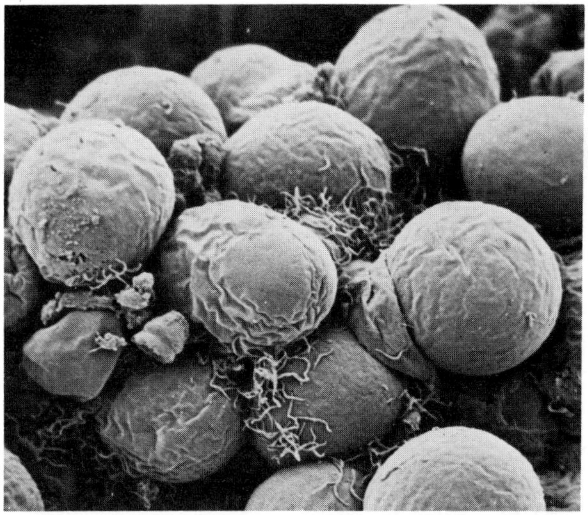

Fig. 2.4 Scanning electron photomicrography of mature oöcysts of *P. yoelii* on the midgut of *A. stephensi* with numerous emerging sporozoites. × 2730. (Professor R. E. Sinden, Department of Pure and Applied Biology, Imperial College, London.)

The parasite in the vertebrate host

Tissue phase

Following the inoculation of sporozoites by the mosquito there is a brief period of about half an hour when the blood is infected. Later the sporozoites disappear from the blood. Many are destroyed by phagocytes, but some enter the parenchymal cells of the liver (hepatocytes) directly or via the Kupffer cells and undergo a process of development and multiplication known as *pre-erythrocytic schizogony*.

The detailed follow-up of this process has been

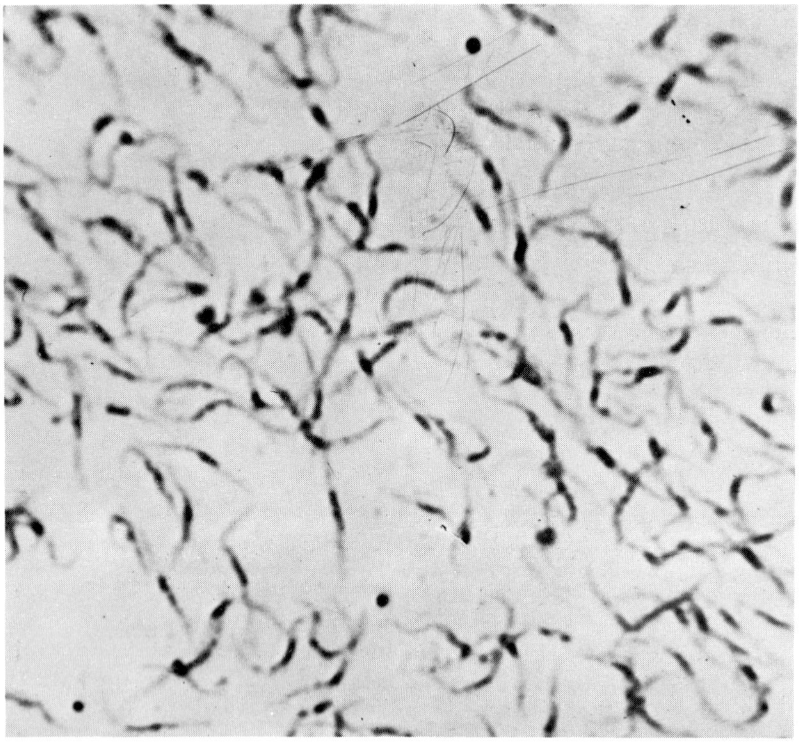

Fig. 2.5 Sporozoites of *P. falciparum* released from a ruptured mature oöcyst. × 1420. (Wellcome Museum of Medical Science.)

described only recently. Within 40–48 hours after the infective bite, tiny parasites, about 3 µm in diameter and consisting of a single nucleus with a narrow cytoplasmic rim can be seen (in *P. cynomolgi* experimental infection of monkeys). These *hypnozoites*, discovered in 1980, seem to exist only in relapsing types of malaria infection, namely in *P. vivax* and probably *P. ovale*. In *P. falciparum* or *P. malariae* the sporozoites do not form hypnozoites, but develop directly into pre-erythrocytic schizonts. The growth of the latter unpigmented tissue forms takes between 6–16 days, and this period varies according to the parasite species. Mature tissue schizonts range in size from 30 to 70 µm in diameter and greatly enlarge the host cell, pushing its nucleus to one side. No inflammatory reaction of the surrounding cells is evident until the mature schizont bursts, to release into the blood thousands of merozoites, each measuring about 1 µm in diameer (Fig. 2.6). The duration of this phase, the size of the fully grown schizont and the number of merozoites it contains, depend on the species of the malaria parasite.

Some comparative characters of the stages of sporogony in the *Anopheles* and of the pre-erythrocytic schizogony in human liver are given in Table 2.2.

At the end of the pre-erythrocytic stage, after about 6 to 16 days from the time of infection, the envelope of the cell containing the schizont ruptures; the merozoites are set free into the surrounding tissue and thence into the blood circulation. Most of them invade the red blood cells present in the sinusoids of the liver, but some are phagocytosed.

It was thought at one time that the completion of the pre-erythrocytic or *primary exo-erythrocytic schizogony* may be followed by the *secondary exo-erythrocytic schizogony* during which merozoites of *P. vivax*, *P. ovale* and perhaps *P. malariae* re-enter fresh liver cells and repeat the process of schizogony, thus causing relapses of these infections at a later date.

It was discovered in 1980 that the sporozoites of the relapsing species of malaria parasites, namely *P. vivax*, *P. ovale* of humans and probably some simian *Plasmodia*, of tertian periodicity, differentiate either into *hypnozoites* or into developing tissue schi-

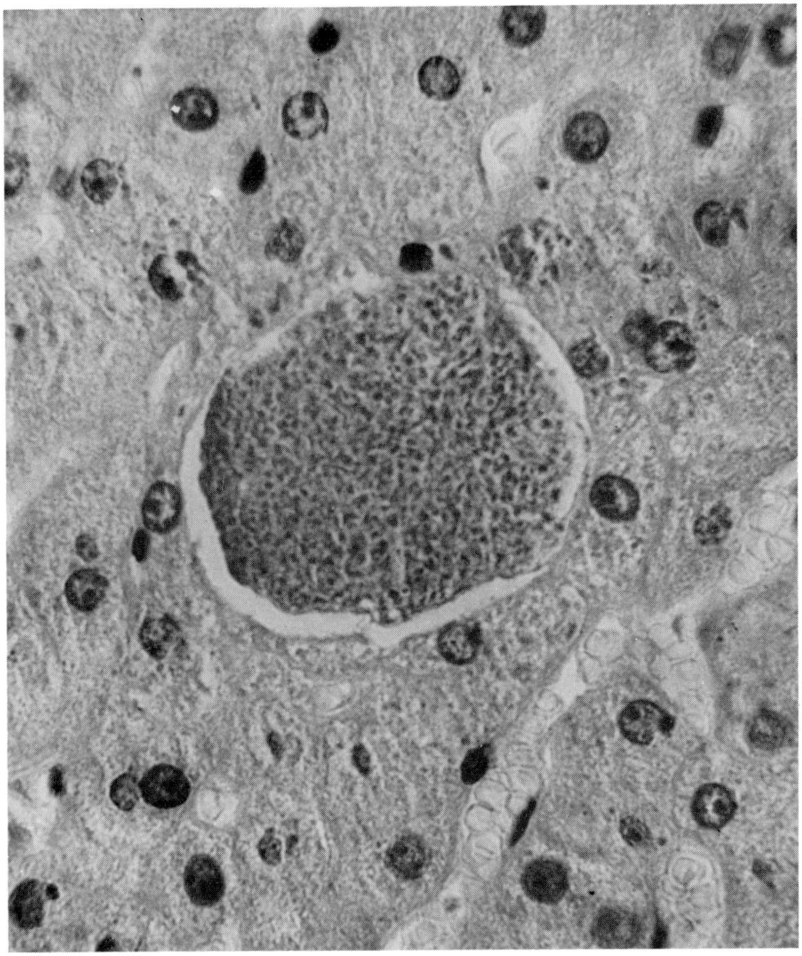

Fig. 2.6 Pre-erythrocytic schizont of *P. falciparum* in the liver. × 760. (Wellcome Museum of Medical Science.)

Table 2.2 Some comparative characters of sporogonic and schizogonic stages of four species of human *Plasmodia*

Species	Duration of sporogony in *Anopheles* (at 28°C)	Diameter of mature oöcyst	Appearance of pigment in oöcyst	Duration of pre-erythrocytic stage (in humans)	Mean diameter of mature pre-erythrocytic schizont	Number of merozoites in pre-erythrocytic schizont
P. vivax	8–10 days	50 μm	Feathery	6–8 days	45 μm	*c.* 10000
P. malariae	14–16 days	40 μm	Clusters at periphery	14–16 days	55 μm	*c.* 15000
P. ovale	12–14 days	45 μm	Crossed lines	9 days	60 μm	*c.* 15000
P. falciparum	9–10 days	55 μm	Rows and chains	$5\frac{1}{2}$–7 days	60 μm	*c.* 30000

Note: Previous data on *P. malariae* based on experimental studies on *P. inui* suggested that the number of pre-erythrocytic merozoites was of the order of 2000. The above information derives from the study of *P. malariae* (Bray and Garnham, 1982).

zonts in varying proportions, depending on the strain. The hypnozoites remain dormant in hepatocytes as uni-nucleated forms, 4–5 μm in diameter, for considerable periods. At a predetermined time the hypnozoites begin to grow and undergo exo-erythrocytic schizogony forming a wave of merozoites that invade the blood, and produce a clinical relapse. Additional populations of hypnozoites may cause further relapses in the same way, according to the relapse pattern of the species and strain of *Plasmodium*.

There is no evidence of true relapses in *P. falciparum* and *P. malariae* (or similar parasites of apes and monkeys) since their sporozoites do not differentiate into hypnozoites but undergo normal rapid pre-erythrocytic schizogony in the liver.

Erythrocytic phase

The interval between the date of the infection and the time when the malaria parasites are detectable in the peripheral blood is known as the *pre-patent period*. This should be distinguished from the *incubation period* which is related to the first appearance of clinical symptoms of the disease.

The merozoites released from the tissue schizont invade the erythrocytes. This process has now been observed and analysed with the help of the electron microscope. Merozoites contain at their apex certain organelles (rhoptries and micronemes) which, after having come into contact with the erythrocyte, cause an invagination of its surface; the resulting dimple deepens gradually, so that the merozoite slips into the erythrocyte. During this process the merozoite loses two of its three membranes and, on entering the erythrocyte, assumes a rounded form. Antibodies present in the blood of partially immune patients may cause mature merozoites to cluster and this prevents invasion of fresh erythrocytes. The merozoite enters the cell by five stages: initial recognition and attachment, formation of a junction, creation of a vacuole membrane continuous with the red cell membrane, entry into the vacuole through the moving junction, and sealing of the erythrocyte after entry (see Fig. 2.8, p. 21).

The youngest stages in the red blood cell are small, more or less rounded bodies, some of which contain a vacuole which displaces the cytoplasm to the periphery, while the nucleus is situated at the pole. In optical section the cytoplasm has an annular appearance and the young parasites are known as *ring forms*. As these grow in size they become more irregular in shape. All these early stages of the parasite are termed *trophozoites*. In the course of their development they absorb the haemoglobin of the red blood cell, leaving as the product of digestion a pigment called *haemozoin*, a combination of haematin with protein. The enzyme involved is probably cysteine proteinase. This iron-containing pigment is seen in the body of the parasite in the form of dark granules, which are more obvious in the later stages of development.

The early studies confirmed that the erythrocytic parasites are intracellular, within vacuoles formed by the erythrocytic internal membrane; they feed by pinching off small amounts of the cytoplasm of the host, through a mouth-like structure (*cytostome*). The ring appearance of young trophozoites is due to the distribution of the cytoplasm and the nucleus in the form of a concave disk. As it grows the trophozoite becomes globular and is filled with ribosomes, while the pigment from the ingested haemoglobin accumulates in the form of granules. The trophozoites grow through the proliferation of endoplasmic reticulum; the vacuole's membrane increases in area and small particles of it accumulate on the inner membrane of the infected erythrocyte, producing the characteristic stippling seen in stained films. In *P. falciparum* the vacuole membrane forms longer loops touching the cytoplasm of the host cell and this may explain the aspect of 'Maurer's dots' seen in stained blood films. The effect of chloroquine is to disrupt the action of the food vacuole and, to a lesser extent, the mitochondria and other organelles. Much research has recently been carried out in the use of calcium channel blockers (such as verapamil and its analogue desipramine) which appear to inhibit the resistant strains of *P. falciparum* from preventing this disruption and thus, potentially, revert chloroquine to its potency.

After a period of growth the trophozoite undergoes an asexual dividing process of erythrocytic *schizogony*. The nucleus of the parasite divides 3–5 times into a variable number of small nuclei. This is soon followed by the division of cytoplasm forming a *schizont*. *Mature schizonts* are fully developed forms in which, as a result of the segmentation of the nucleus and the cytoplasm, a number of small rounded forms (*merozoites*) are produced.

When the process of schizogony is completed the red blood cell bursts and the merozoites are released into the blood stream. The merozoites then invade fresh erythrocytes in which another generation of parasites is produced by the same process. This *erythrocytic cycle of schizogony* is repeated over and over again in the course of infection, leading to a progressive increase of parasitaemia until the process is slowed down by the immune response of the host.

The development of parasites in the red blood cell brings about certain changes of it; among these abnormal appearances the most important are *enlargement*, *decolorization* and certain forms of *stippling*, now thought to be associated with the transport of malaria proteins through the membranes to the surface of the erythrocyte. These changes are characteristic for the particular species of *Plasmodium* involved.

The length of the erythrocytic phase is known as *schizogonic periodicity*. It differs according to the species of the parasite, being 48 hours in vivax, ovale and falciparum malaria and 72 in quartan. In the early stage of infection there may be groups ('broods') of parasites developing at different times so that the febrile symptoms show no characteristic periodicity. Later, the schizogonic periodicity is better synchronized and the febrile paroxysms assume a more definite 3- or 4-day pattern.

While merozoites originating from pre-erythrocytic schizogony may also give rise to sexually differentiated forms (gametocytes), it is usually only after several rounds of blood schizogony that these forms are produced in greater numbers. After invading fresh erythrocytes these sexual forms grow, but the nucleus remains undivided. The mature gametocytes have different forms in different species of *Plasmodia*; in *P. falciparum* they are usually crescent-shaped when mature, while in other species they are round. In all species of *Plasmodia* the female (*macrogametocyte*) has a deeply stained cytoplasm and a small compact nucleus while the male (*microgametocyte*) stains pale blue or pink and has a larger, diffuse nucleus. Both contain numerous pigment granules.

In synchronous infections of some species of *Plasmodia* gametocytes mature at night and it has been suggested that this represents an adaptation of the parasite to the nocturnal feeding habits of Anopheles mosquitos.

Ultrastructure

The study of the inner structure of all stages of development of malaria parasites has been revolutionized by the techniques of electron microscopy. The ultrastructure of different human *Plasmodia* is generally similar, with a few exceptions of the blood stages, in which the parasites depend essentially upon the uptake and digestion of nutrients from the host cells. Only the main aspects of the recent findings can be given here.

The *oökinete* is surrounded by a double pellicle; its anterior end is conical with a nucleus in the centre. The process of penetration of the oökinete through the epithelial layer of the midgut of the mosquito is effected by secreting a proteolytic substance.

The *oöcyst* is enclosed in a globular envelope, about 1 μm thick; it contains a nucleus, abundant ribosomes (granules of protein and RNA), mitochondria and pigment. Nuclear division takes place during maturation; vacuoles are formed which coalesce dividing the oöcyst's cytoplasm into several sporoblasts where sporozoites develop and emerge by a budding process.

All plasmodial *sporozoites* have the same internal structure. They measure about 11 μm in length and 1 μm in diameter. The pellicle has two membranes with 15–16 underlying microtubules; there are also paired organelles, long rhoptries, convoluted rods (*toxonemes*) and a cytostome; the sporozoites contain a nucleus, mitochondria and endoplasm with ribosomes (Fig. 2.7). The external pellicle of sporozoites, when incubated with immune serum, forms a dense coat along the surface; this is the evidence of its antigenic nature. *Exo-erythrocytic stages* of human *Plasmodia* have not been well studied for obvious reasons. In infections of monkeys with *P. cynomolgi* the tissue stages have a number of vacuoles which form clefts separating the cytoplasm into lobes. Merozoites bud off from these lobes, but there is no evidence that cytostomes are involved in the absorption of nutrients. When the maturing trophozoite approaches the schizont stage a mitotic spindle and a centriole are formed in the nucleus and, as the nuclear division proceeds, cytoplasmic organelles develop in the growing merozoites. This process is repeated 3–5 times until the erythrocytic schizont reaches its maturity, when all the merozoites are formed and the pigment concentrates into a single residual mass, from which merozoites eventually separate.

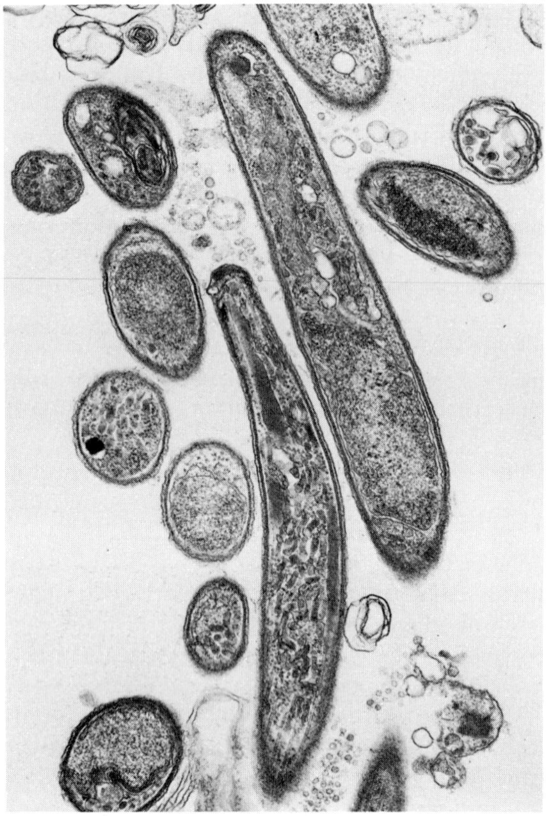

Fig. 2.7 Sporozoites of *P. cynomolgi*. Electron photomicrograph of longitudinal and cross-sections. × 20 000. (Dr M. Aikawa, Institute of Pathology, Case Western Reserve University, Cleveland, Ohio; Published by Cochrane *et al.*, 1976.)

Merozoites of mammalian *Plasmodia* are pear-shaped bodies, 1.5 μm in length, with an apical end that has a polar ring and two vesicle-like bodies (*rhoptries*). The coat of the merozoite is composed of three layers. The spectacular entry of the merozoite into the erythrocyte starts with the former orientating itself, so that the apex is close to the cell membrane. After the contact, some substance (probably a 60 kD merozoite protein) is released by the rhoptries of the merozoite and forms a deep pit in the red blood cell; the merozoite then enters the cell maintaining a contact-ring with the body of the erythrocyte (*endocytosis*); when the entry is completed the red cell membrane seals itself, the whole process taking about 30 seconds. Once within the cell, the merozoite rounds up and loses its various internal organelles (Fig. 2.8).

The development of *gametocytes* seems to be stimulated by a stress due either to rising immunity or nutrient depletion (Fig. 2.9). The small, rounded parasite forms a pellicle and produces an accumulation of microtubules; within the nucleus a mitotic spindle is formed and DNA replication takes place. As the maturation proceeds, differences between the male and female gametocytes become apparent. The numbers of ribosomes and mitochondria are reduced in the male gametocytes while the females retain them at high density. When ingested by the mosquito or seen on a fresh blood film under the microscope, the exflagellation of the male gametocyte is dramatic (Fig. 2.10). The red cell membrane surrounding the parasite is disrupted, a single mitotic spindle forms in the nucleus, it then divides rapidly producing a total of eight peripheral haploid genomes and further complex changes take place forming flagella-like male gametes which are suddenly ejected from the parent body, though initially attached to it at one end; they remain motile for up to 1 hour *in vitro*. When the male gamete contacts the female, the tail-like axoneme of the former enters the female cytoplasm, the two nuclei fuse and produce a zygote.

Human *Plasmodia*

Plasmodium vivax

This species of malaria parasite of humans occurs throughout most of the temperate zones and also in large areas of the tropics. It is much less common in tropical Africa, especially so in West Africa. It causes so-called 'benign tertian' malaria with relapses, the pattern of which varies, in relation to various strains of *P. vivax*.

The existence of the *pre-erythrocytic cycle* of development of this parasite was proved experimentally in 1948 by Shortt, Garnham, Covell and Shute, thus confirming the early hypothesis of Grassi and refuting the notoriously erroneous description by Schaudinn (1902) of the penetration of an erythrocyte by a sporozoite.

Sporozoites of *P. vivax* differentiate, after invading the liver, either into early, primary tissue schizonts or into hypnozoites, the latter being responsible for late relapses of the infection (see Fig. 2.1, page 14).

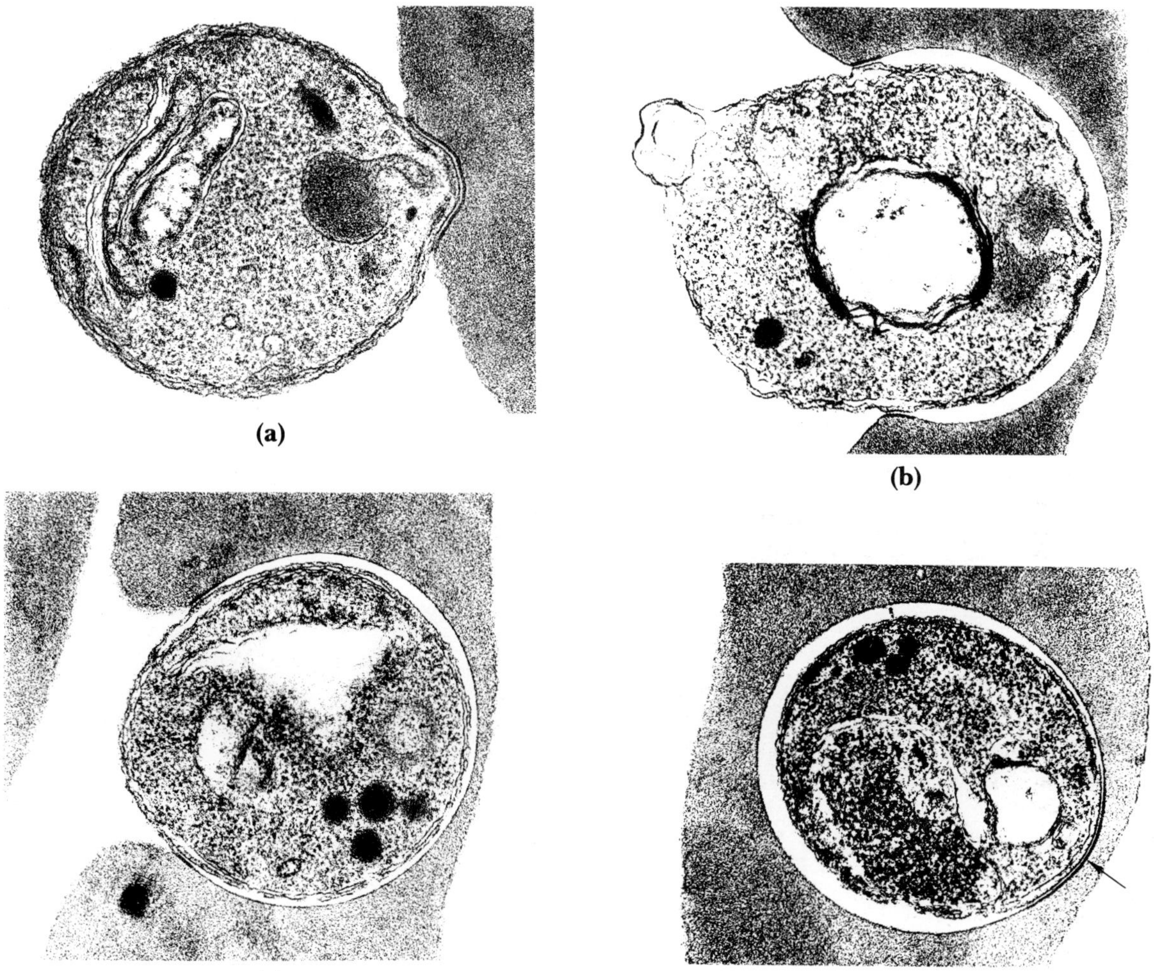

(a) (b) (c) (d)

Fig. 2.8 (a) Electron photomicrograph of a longitudinal section of a merozoite of *P. knowlesi* soon after its contact with the erythrocyte. The erythrocyte membrane is thickened and forms a junction with the plasma membrane of the merozoite. The darker, bottle-shaped part of the merozoite near the junction is the rhoptry which releases its contents on the erythrocyte membrane at the point of attachment. × 48 000. (Dr M. Aikawa, Institute of Pathology, Case Western Reserve University, Cleveland, Ohio; published by Aikawa *et al.*, *Malaria and the Red Cell*, CIBA Foundation Symposium, 1983.) (b) Electron photomicrograph of a merozoite of *P. knowlesi* entering an erythrocyte at an advanced stage of the interiorization process. The moving junction formed between the thickened membrane of the erythrocyte and the merozoite brings the latter within the invagination of the erythrocyte. A small projection still connects the apical end of the merozoite and the erythrocyte membrane. × 54 000. (Dr M. Aikawa, Institute of Pathology, Case Western Reserve University, Cleveland, Ohio; published by Aikawa *et al.*, 1978.) (c) Electron photomicrograph of a section of a merozoite of *P. knowlesi* entering an erythrocyte. The merozoite is located within an invagination of the erythrocyte; at the junction points there is a distinct thickening of the erythrocyte membrane (which is about to seal itself). × 54 000. (Dr M. Aikawa, Institute of Pathology, Case Western Reserve University, Cleveland, Ohio; published by Aikawa *et al.*, 1981.) (d) Completion of the entry of the merozoite into the erythrocyte. The membranes of the erythrocyte are sealed leaving the merozoite within a vacuole lined by the erythrocyte membrane. × 50 000. (Dr M. Aikawa, Institute of Pathology, Case Western Reserve University, Cleveland, Ohio; published by Aikawa *et al.*, 1978.)

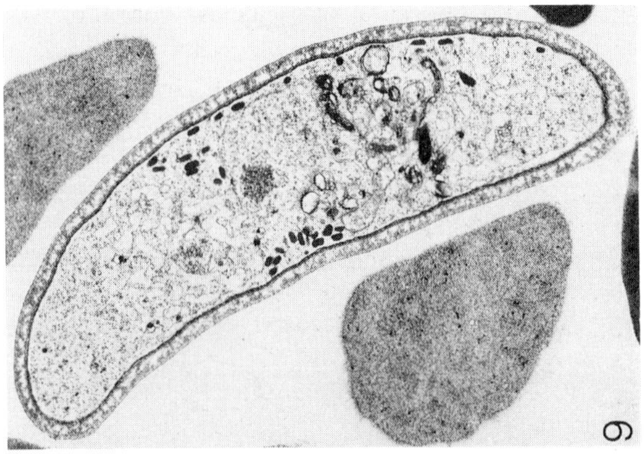

Fig. 2.9 Electron micrograph of a longitudinal section through a macrogametocyte of *P. falciparum*. (Professor R. E. Sinden, Department of Pure and Applied Biology, Imperial College, London.)

The mean duration of the pre-erythrocytic stage of the early tissue schizonts is 8 days; the existence of secondary exo-erythrocytic forms, developing from tissue schizonts and causing relapses of the infection, has now been disproved. The number of merozoites in a mature tissue schizont on the eighth day is between 8000 and 20 000.

Some strains of *P. vivax* in the northern hemisphere (such as the Russian one, given the subspecific name of *P. vivax hibernans* by Nikolaev in 1949) do not produce primary attacks soon after infection, and the first clinical symptoms occur 8–9 months after the infective bite. On the other hand, tropical strains of *P. vivax* tend to cause a number of randomly distributed short-term relapses following an early primary attack. A delay of primary attack due to *P. vivax* or *P. ovale* infections may also be

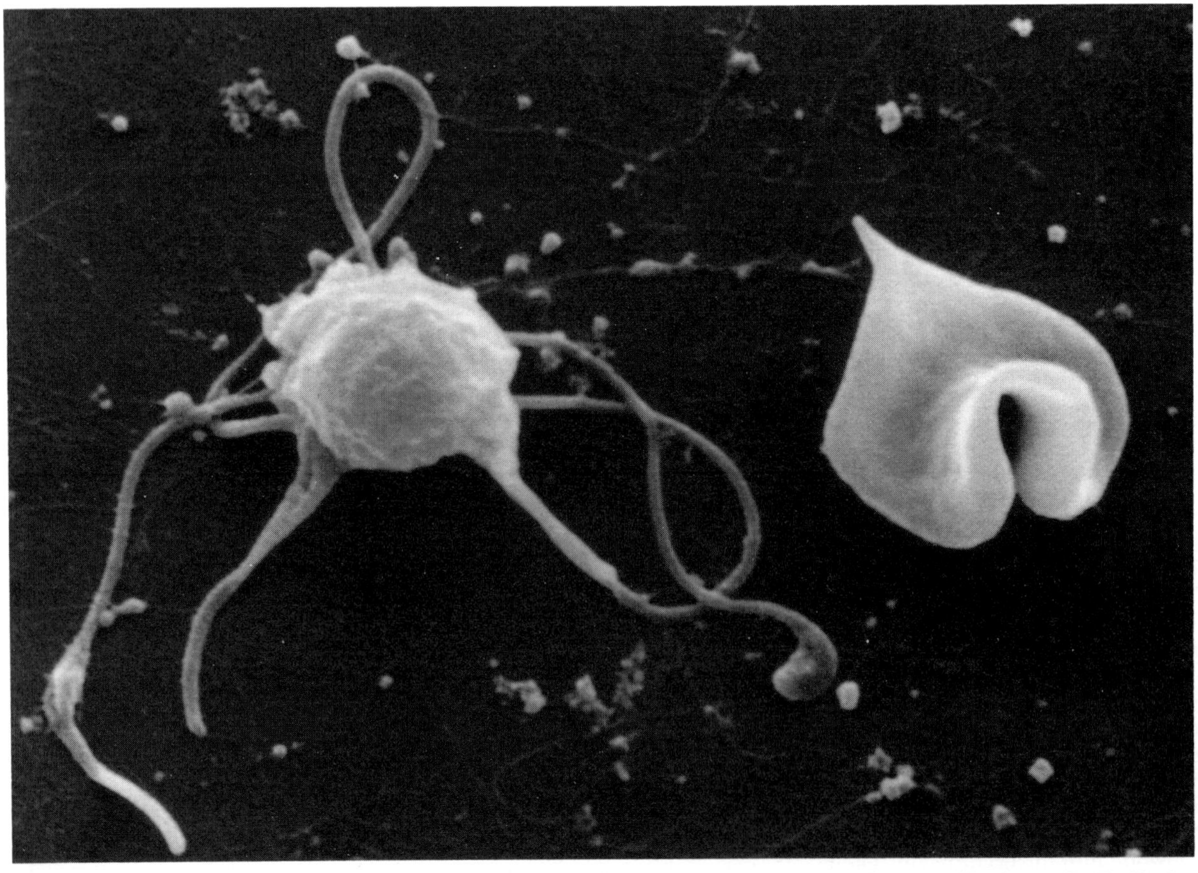

Fig. 2.10 Scanning electron micrograph of exflagellation of a male gametocyte of *P. yoelii*. (Professor R. E. Sinden, Department of Pure and Applied Biology, Imperial College, London.)

caused by inadequate chemotherapeutic suppression. There are also so-called intermediate subtropical strains with a delayed primary attack or a relapse after 9 months, following an infection. It seems that the chronological pattern of the primary attack and subsequent relapses depends on the relative proportion of the early and late sporozoites in a given strain of *P. vivax*. It has been suggested that the two types of sporozoites should be designated as 'tachy-sporozoites' (fast) and 'brady-sporozoites' (slow), although we cannot distinguish them morphologically. The latter type presumably develop into hypnozoites that remain latent for 8–9 months before developing into tissue schizonts.

Although the involvement of hypnozoites in the origin of relapses has been supported by much experimental evidence, there are still some unanswered questions. Thus, the stimulus which may activate the latent hypnozoite and provoke the relapse is unknown. The experimental possibility of observing the change of hypnozoite into a growing exo-erythrocytic schizont has yet to be achieved.

During the erythrocytic development of *P. vivax* all blood forms can be found in the circulation and most stages are larger than in the other species of human *Plasmodia*. The young trophozoite or ring grows rapidly and soon exhibits the characteristic malaria pigment. The parasite when alive has a pronounced amoeboid activity and the presence of cytoplasmic 'pseudopodia' seen in a stained blood film is typical for this species. A large vacuole forms a 'hole' in the ring until the division of the nucleus begins. After the nuclei have ceased to divide the mature schizont, which has on average 12 to 18 merozoites, fills the entire host cell. Segmentation is followed by the rupture of the infected erythrocyte and release into the blood of merozoites and pigment. The merozoites, each measuring about 1.5 μm, invade fresh erythrocytes and the entire asexual erythrocytic cycle is repeated approximately every 48 hours; certain strains show a somewhat shorter periodicity. The degree of infection in vivax malaria rarely exceeds 50 000 per μl of blood as the merozoites can only invade reticulocytes. Infections of one erythrocyte by two or more parasites may be seen but are not very common.

Plasmodium vivax has a striking effect on the invaded red blood cell, which gradually enlarges and becomes decolorized. A characteristic *stippling* in the form of small reddish points appears in the infected erythrocyte and is known as *Schüffner's dots* (Fig. 2.11).

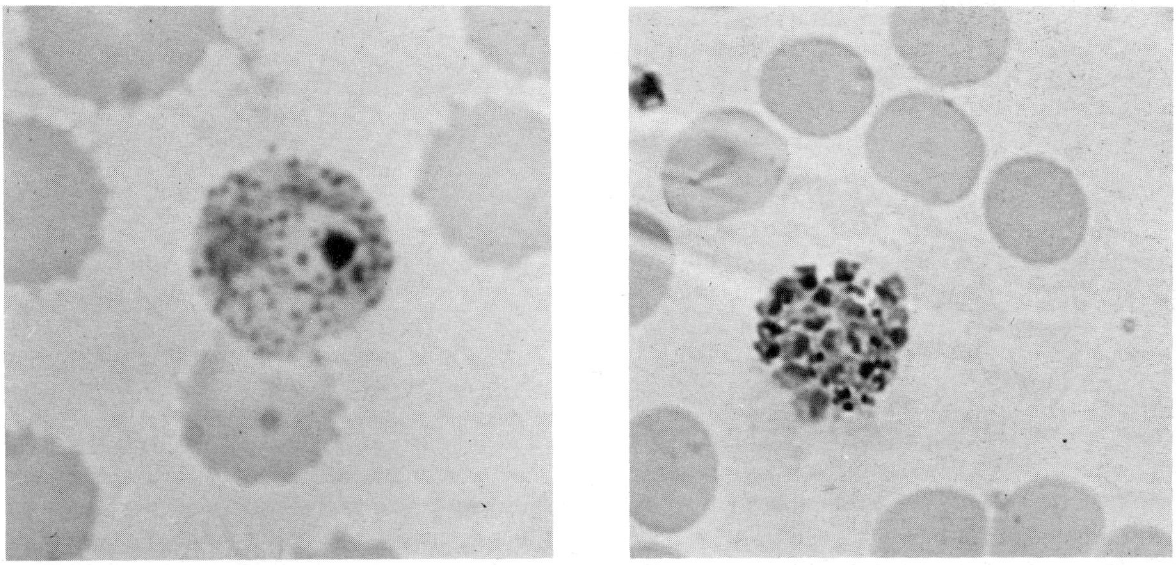

(a) (b)

Fig. 2.11 *Plasmodium vivax*. (a) Trophozoite with pronounced Schüffner's stippling in an enlarged erythrocyte. (b) Fully developed schizont with about 20 merozoites ready to burst and to invade new red blood cells. (a) × 1144, (b) × 800. (Wellcome Museum of Medical Science.)

Gametocytes may appear in the blood within 3 days after the first appearance of asexual parasites. Both male and female gametocytes are large, round or oval, filling nearly the whole enlarged and 'stippled' host cell. The *macrogametocyte* has a dense cytoplasm, staining dark blue and a small compact nucleus; the *microgametocyte* has a greyish-blue cytoplasm and a large diffuse nucleus. Both contain numerous pigment granules.

The periodicity of the asexual cycle of *P. vivax* is typically tertian with gametocytes developing in the peripheral blood. The course of development of the parasite is well synchronized.

The gametocytes develop into gametes in the midgut of the *Anopheles*. After the exflaggellation of the male and fertilization of the female gamete the sexual cycle takes 16 days at 20°C, and 8–10 days at 28°C. Below 15°C the completion of the sporogonic cycle is unlikely.

The young oöcyst has a light brown pigment distributed in the form of fine granules without any distinctive pattern. In older oöcysts the granules are often arranged in a single or triple line (Table 2.2).

Plasmodium ovale

Plasmodium ovale infection produces a tertian type of fever similar to that of vivax malaria, but often with prolonged latency, a lesser trend to relapse and generally milder clinical symptoms. It was described only in 1922 by Stephens who saw it in the blood of a soldier who had returned from East Africa. *Plasmodium ovale* has been recorded chiefly from tropical Africa, in the west of which it is quite common. It has been reported sporadically from the west Pacific region and from southern China, Burma and South-east Asia. Some of these identifications are not absolutely certain and may relate to simian *Plasmodia*.

The asexual erythrocytic cycle of development of *P. ovale* is similar to that of *P. vivax* and extends over 48 hours. The pre-erythrocytic stage has a general period of 9 days and the mature liver schizonts, some 60 μm in diameter, contain about 15 000 merozoites; the nucleus of the schizont-containing hepatocyte is often enlarged. The changes produced by the parasite on the infected erythrocytes are similar to those seen in *P. vivax*. The young trophozoites measure about one-third the diameter of the red blood cell. Schüffner's stippling appears quite early and is more pronounced than in the case of *P. vivax*. As the trophozoites grow they show some resemblance to *P. malariae*; most of them are round and compact with granules of pigment coarser than in *P. vivax* but not as coarse as in *P. malariae*. At this stage many erythrocytes are slightly enlarged and in thin films many of them assume an oval shape with ragged or fimbriated margins and heavy stippling.

The schizonts may resemble those of *P. malariae*. They are rounded, compact and when mature contain 8–10 nuclei which are arranged peripherally around the central clump of pigment granules. Occasionally the number of merozoites may be as high as 16.

The gametocytes of *P. ovale* resemble those of *P. malariae*, but the erythrocyte that contains them rarely assumes the oval shape. The female gametocyte has a small, compact, bluish nucleus, the male's diffuse nucleus stains pale blue with a reddish tinge.

The pigment in the oöcyst is dark brown and the granules have a tendency to form chains which cross each other in the centre of the cyst. The completion of the sporogonic cycle in the mosquito takes 12–14 days at 28°C (Table 2.2).

Plasmodium malariae

Plasmodium malariae is the causal organism of quartan malaria, so named because the paroxysms recur on the fourth day, after an interval of 2 days. The parasite differs from the other species affecting humans by its morphological characters and also by its slow development in both the human and the insect host. The course of the disease is not unduly severe but its long persistence is notorious. The geographical range of quartan malaria extends over both tropical and subtropical areas, especially West and East Africa, Guyana and parts of India, but its presence in various zones tends to be patchy.

No direct evidence is available of pre-erythrocytic stages of *P. malariae* after the inoculation of sporozoites into the human host but the evidence of such a stage has been obtained indirectly by infecting Anopheles mosquitos on human *P. malariae* and inoculating sporozoites into a chimpanzee in whose liver exo-erythrocytic schizonts were demonstrated. *Plasmodium malariae* occurs naturally in chimpanzees and these animals may be potential reservoirs of quartan malaria. The old name of *P. rodhaini*, a parasite naturally found in chimpanzees, is synonymous with *P. malariae*. The pre-erythrocytic schizonts in the liver do not reach maturity until the fourteenth day after inoculation of sporozoites. When the mature schizont discharges the merozoites into the blood circulation, the asexual erythrocytic cycle begins and shows a 72 hour periodicity.

The infection with *P. malariae* has a tendency to persist in the human host for many years, perhaps even for a lifetime; this led to the hypothesis of a succession of several secondary exo-erythrocytic cycles in the liver. However, no late relapse forms of this parasite have been found in livers of chimpanzees infected with quartan *Plasmodia* and the infection is as persistent after inoculation of infected blood as it is after an injection of sporozoites. This seems to confirm that hypnozoites responsible for late relapses do not exist in *P. malariae* infections and that re-appearance of parasitaemia with clinical symptoms after periods of latency is presumably due to the recrudescence of the primary attack from erythrocytic forms persisting in very small numbers in internal organs.

The young trophozoites in the blood are not very different from those of *P. vivax* although their cytoplasm is thicker and they stain more deeply. Older trophozoites, when rounded, are about half the size of the host cell. In thin films, the trophozoites may stretch across the entire width of the cell; such *band forms* are a characteristic feature of *P. malariae*. The pigment granules are numerous, large and dark.

The entire development of the trophozoite takes about 54 hours and during the succeeding 18 hours the parasite undergoes the schizogonic development. Young schizonts divide repeatedly and finally the mature schizont has an average of eight merozoites. The merozoites occupy almost the entire erythrocyte and form either an irregular cluster or are arranged symmetrically around the centre, in the form of a daisy. The term *rosette* is often applied to such schizonts.

Plasmodium malariae produces no evident changes in the host cells although they may often appear somewhat smaller than uninfected erythrocytes. A special staining may show the presence of discrete stippling, often called Ziemann's stippling.

The degree of parasitaemia in quartan malaria is lower than in any other plasmodial infections and in naturally acquired infections the parasite count rarely exceeds 10 000 per µl of blood.

The gametocytes probably develop in the internal organs and appear in the peripheral blood when fully grown. The female gametocyte has a deep blue cytoplasm and a small, dense nucleus; the male stains pale blue and has a diffuse larger nucleus.

The 72 hour periodicity of the asexual cycle of development is usually well synchronized with the forms of parasite seen in the blood.

The sporogonic cycle in the *Anopheles* takes 30–35 days at 20°C; at 28°C it may be as short as 14 days although the average period is usually longer.

The pigment in the oöcysts is in the form of large dark-brown ganules and has a characteristic peripheral distribution. The clumping of the pigment in a small area of the oöcyst is of value in identifying the infection in the mosquito (Table 2.2).

Plasmodium (Laverania) falciparum

Of all the species of *Plasmodia*, *P. falciparum* is the most highly pathogenic, as indicated by the name *malignant* often applied to the type of malaria associated with it. This, in a non-immune subject, usually runs an acute course, and unless promptly treated with specific drugs, frequently terminates fatally. It is the chief infection in areas of endemic malaria in Africa, and is also responsible for the great regional epidemics which were a feature of malaria in north-west India and Sri Lanka. It is generally confined to tropical or subtropical regions because the development in the mosquito is greatly retarded when the temperature falls below 20°C. Even at this temperature, about 3 weeks are required for maturation of sporozoites.

The asexual development of *P. falciparum* in the liver involves only a pre-erythrocytic phase and the hypnozoites do not occur. The earliest forms hitherto seen in the liver are schizonts measuring about 30 µm in diameter on the fourth day after infection. The number of merozoites in a mature schizont, which reaches some 60 µm in size, is about 30 000.

The young ring forms of *P. falciparum*, as usually seen in the peripheral blood, are very small, measuring about one-sixth of the diameter of a red blood cell. In many of the ring forms there may be two chromatin granules, and marginal (*accolé*) forms are fairly common. There are frequently several ring forms to be seen in a single host cell.

Although marginal forms, rings with double chromatin dots and multiple infections of red cells may occur in other human *Plasmodia*, they are much more common in *P. falciparum* and their presence is an important aid to diagnosis.

Later in the attack the ring forms of *P. falciparum* may be considerably larger, measuring one-quarter and sometimes nearly one-half the diameter of a red cell, and may be mistaken for parasites of *P. malariae*. They may have one or two grains of pigment in their cytoplasm.

In acute infections with numerous parasites, atypical forms are sometimes seen and these have erroneously been described under different specific names. These amoeboid forms have been designated under the name *P. tenue*, but this is not regarded as a valid species.

The succeeding developmental stages of the asexual erythrocytic cycle do not generally occur in the blood, except in severe 'pernicious' cases. The presence of maturing or mature schizonts of *P. falciparum* in a blood film is therefore often an indication for prompt and vigorous treatment. Segmenting forms of *P. falciparum* are easily recognized by having one or at most two solid grains of pigment. In other species of human malaria parasites beyond the half grown stage there may be 20 or more pigment granules; the form of these pigment granules is affected by antimalarial drugs: chlorquine causes clumping and mefloquine causes them to disappear entirely.

The ring forms and older trophozoites usually disappear from the peripheral circulation after 24 hours and are held up (*sequestered*) in the capillaries of the internal organs, such as the brain, heart, placenta, spleen, intestine or bone marrow, where their further development takes place. This sequestration may be caused by an adherence between endothelial lining cells and the distorted shape of the infected erythrocytes, showing knob-like projections 40 × 80 nm in size. It is likely that these 'knobs' have special antigenic properties and are more common in some strains. In the course of 24 hours the parasites in the capillaries multiply by schizogony. When the schizont is fully grown it occupies about two-thirds of the red cell. Finally, it undergoes segmentation giving rise to from 8 to 24 merozoites, the average number being 16. The mature schizont of *P. falciparum* is smaller than that of any of the other malaria parasites. The degree of infection of this type of malaria is considerably higher than in the other forms, the density of parasites sometimes exceeding 300 000 per μl of blood.

The distribution of the parasites in organs and tissues of the human body varies in different cases, thus accounting for the diversity of clinical manifestations observed in falciparum malaria. Most of the severe and fatal cases show blocking (occlusion) of the capillaries by clumps of red blood cells harbouring developing parasites, enormous numbers of which can be seen in smears and sections of *post-mortem* material (see pp. 51–2). The presence of high levels of *P. falciparum* antigen and IgG deposits in the adjacent capillary basement membrane may suggest that the damage to cerebral capillaries could be due to immunopathological mechanisms.

In falciparum malaria the infected red cells retain their normal size throughout all stages of development of the parasites. Cells harbouring the older trophozoites and schizonts are frequently stippled with a few coarse reddish dots (Maurer's dots), scattered over about two-thirds of the erythrocyte. The clustering around infected erythrocytes of non-infected erythrocytes *in vitro* is a variable genetic trait.

The development of the gametocytes takes place in the inner organs, but sometimes young forms are seen in the blood. The young gametocytes tend to be elongated, becoming spindle-shaped or elliptic as they grow. Finally, they assume the characteristic curved shape of the mature gametocytes. These first appear in the peripheral blood after several broods have undergone schizogony, usually about 10 days after the initial invasion of the blood. The body of the mature gametocytes may be sausage-shaped, banana-shaped or crescentic; they are usually referred to as *crescents*. The female form or macrogametocyte is usually more slender and somewhat longer than the male, and the cytoplasm takes up a deeper blue colour with Romanowsky stains. The nucleus is small and compact, staining dark red, while the pigment granules are closely aggregated round it. The male form or microgametocyte is broader than the female and is more inclined to be sausage-shaped.

The cytoplasm is either pale blue or tinted with pink, and the nucleus, which stains dark pink, is large and less compact than in the female, while the pigment granules are scattered in the cytoplasm around it. The number of gametocytes present in falciparum infections is variable, occasionally amounting to 50 000 to 150 000 per µl of blood.

Although erythrocytic schizogony in *P. falciparum* is completed in 48 hours and the periodicity of development is therefore of typically tertian type, there frequently occurs in this species two or more broods of parasites, the segmentation of which is not synchronized, so that the periodicity of symptoms in the patient tends to be irregular.

The sexual cycle of *P. falciparum* in the mosquito conforms with that described for mammalian *Plasmodia* in general. Its duration at 20°C is 22 days; at 23°C, 15 to 17 days; and at 28°C, 9 to 10 days (Table 2.2). The pigment in the oöcyst is almost black and the granules are relatively large. It usually forms a double circle around the periphery, but it may be arranged as a small circle in the centre, or even as a double straight chain. By the eighth day much of the pigment becomes obscured, but a few grains can still be seen.

Mixed infections

Infections due to two or more species of malaria parasites are not uncommon, but they are often overlooked. In endemic malarious areas mixed infections are particularly frequent; there is a tendency for one species of the parasite to predominate over the other. The most common types of mixed infections are *P. falciparum* and *P. vivax* in subtropical areas while in tropical Africa *P. falciparum* and *P. malariae* are prevalent, although *P. falciparum* and *P. ovale* are also frequent. On rare occasions all three species can be found in one blood film.

The best way of diagnosing a mixed infection with more than one species of *Plasmodia* is by a careful and longer than usual microscopical examination of the blood film. Some characteristics of infection with the four species of human *Plasmodia* are given in Table 2.3.

Table 2.3 Some characteristics of infection with four species of human *Plasmodia*

	Species			
	Plasmodium vivax	*Plasmodium ovale*	*Plasmodium malariae*	*Plasmodium falciparum*
Pre-erythrocytic stage (days)	6–8	9	14–16	5½–7
Pre-patent period (days)	11–13	10–14	15–16	9–10
Incubation period (days)	15 (12–17) or up to 6–12 months	17 (16–18) or longer	28 (18–40) or longer	12 (9–14)
Erythrocytic cycle (hours)	48 (about)	50	72	48
Parasitaemia per µl (mm^3)				
Average	20 000	9000	6000	20 000–500 000
Maximum	50 000	30 000	20 000	2 000 000
Primary attack*	Mild to severe	Mild	Mild	Severe in non-immunes
Febrile paroxysm (hours)	8–12	8–12	8–10	16–36 or longer
Relapses	++	++	–	–
Period of recurrence†	Variable	Variable	Very long	Short
Duration of untreated infection (years)	1½–5	Probably the same as *P. vivax*	3–50	1–2

*The severity of infection and the degree of parasitaemia are greatly influenced by the immune responses. Chemoprophylaxis may suppress an initial attack for weeks or months.

†Patterns of infection and of relapses vary greatly in different strains.

Animal *Plasmodia*

Simian *Plasmodia*

The presence of malaria parasites in the blood of monkeys was observed already in 1893 and one of these parasites found in an East African monkey received the name of *P. kochi* (later renamed *Hepatocystis kochi* by Garnham). In 1907 the discovery of *P. cynomolgi* in *Macaca irus* from Java was of particular interest because of its resemblance to the *P. vivax* of humans, and during the first quarter of the present century a series of other simian *Plasmodia* were found in monkeys in the field or in the zoos in various parts of the world. Much of the early work on simian malaria was done in India where *P. knowlesi* was isolated in 1932 from *Macaca irus* and subsequently transmitted to humans. The study of *Plasmodia* of higher apes (chimpanzees and gorillas) was given great impetus by Rodhain who showed in 1940 the identity of *P. malariae* of humans with that of *P. rodhaini* of chimpanzees.

In 1947 Garnham demonstrated the true nature of *Hepatocystis kochi* in the East African monkey *Cercopithecus aethiops*. He showed that the blood forms of this parasite are composed of gametocytes only and discovered the presence, in the liver of infected monkeys, of the exo-erythrocytic stages of the parasite. The final stage of development in the tissue is a merocyst with a large vacuole; the numerous merozoites present in a simple merocyst invade the blood stream.

This finding was the first step to the subsequent discovery of exo-erythrocytic stages of the true malaria parasites. The vector of *H. kochi* is a *Culicoides* as found by Garnham in 1951.

The importance of studies on simian malaria was brilliantly demonstrated by Shortt and Garnham in 1948. The discovery of exo-erythrocytic stages in the liver of monkeys infected with *P. cynomolgi* pointed the way to finding the tissue stages of *P. vivax* in humans.

Although the relationship between the *Plasmodia* of monkeys and those of humans had already become obvious in the 1930s, when *P. knowlesi* was used in Romania for malaria therapy by blood infection, the question of simian malaria as a zoonosis became important in the 1960s. In those years American workers described the case of an accidental laboratory infection by *P. cynomolgi bastianellii* transmitted from *Macaca irus* through mosquitos. The tertian periodicity of the febrile illness and the presence of vivax-like parasites in the blood of the accidentally infected individual drew attention to the possibility of natural transmission of the disease from monkeys to humans.

Plasmodium cynomolgi infections in the rhesus monkey have occupied an important place in the search for new antimalarials between 1950 and 1960. This model offered a precise biological and chemotherapeutic counterpart of *P. vivax* infection of humans. It was due to this model that identification of primaquine as an answer to radical cure of relapsing malaria became possible.

Further work especially in Malaysia and Brazil was responsible for a surge of new knowledge of simian malaria. Within 5 years the number of species of *Plasmodia* of lower monkeys increased to about a dozen.

It was soon found that in addition to the confirmed possibility of transmission to humans of *P. cynomolgi* through mosquitos, other *Plasmodia* of lower monkeys such as *P. brazilianum* and *P. inui* could also be transmitted in the same way.

It is of interest that persons of African descent are refractory to infections with *P. cynomolgi*, *P. inui*, *P. knowlesi* and *P. schwetzi* in analogy to *P. vivax*; this is due to the absence of some specific receptors on the erythrocytes of these people.

Although the possibility of the two-way transmission (monkey – vector – humans) of simian malaria in natural conditions was experimentally established, the proof that it can happen in nature was provided in three cases of human infection with *P. knowlesi* in Malaya and in another case of a similar infection with *P. simium* in Brazil. These exceptional occurrences, while stressing the close relationship between human and some simian *Plasmodia*, do not invalidate the fact that in nature the only true reservoir of human malaria parasites is the infected human being.

During the past 20 years, an increasing amount of research has shown not only that some *Plasmodia* of monkeys or apes can be transmitted to humans, but also that human malaria parasites can be successfully transmitted to some lower primates and especially to several species of neotropical monkeys.

The latter finding by Young and his colleagues in Panama in 1960 was of special significance since it opened an entirely new field for experimental chemotherapy of malaria.

Thus, *P. vivax*, *P. falciparum* and *P. malariae* can now be transmitted to the Colombian night monkey *Aotus trivirgatus*. Inoculation with blood forms is the usual procedure. Receptivity is greatly enhanced by splenectomy. Transmission by sporozoites is rarely successful even in splenectomized *Aotus* monkeys. Other South American monkeys (*Ateles*, *Cebus*, *Saimiri*, *Saguinus*) are also susceptible to infection with human *Plasmodia*, but the *Aotus* is by far the most useful experimental animal in this respect. A retransmission of *P. falciparum* from *Aotus* to humans has been achieved.

The value of this species is so great that its wide use in various research centres has now led to a great shortage of *Aotus* and to an embargo imposed by some South American governments on trapping and exportation of these animals.

Some characteristics of the main species of simian malaria parasites are shown in Table 2.4.

Plasmodia of other mammalian hosts

These parasites of the genus *Plasmodium* are now classified under the sub-genus *Vinckeia* which comprises some 20 species, occurring in various murine and non-murine rodents, lower primates (lemurs), bats and other mammals. The first of the above groups is of special interest and importance.

The discovery of *P. berghei*, a new species of malaria parasite in a rodent, was made in 1948 by Vincke and Lips in the former Belgian Congo (now Zaire). It was not a chance discovery but a purposeful search for an animal host which might have infected an Anopheles mosquito (*A. dureni*) commonly found in a gallery forest in the Katanga province. This animal host was eventually discovered and proved to be a tree rat *Thamnomys surdaster*. It was soon found that the new parasite could be easily transmitted by injection of blood to laboratory mice and rats.

However, experimental, cyclical transmission of *P. berghei* through its original vector or through other *Anopheles* was not successful until 1964 when Yoeli demonstrated that three conditions must be fulfilled: (1) a newly isolated strain of the parasite is needed, (2) the mosquitos must be fed on the animal during the early stage of parasitaemia, and (3) the mosquitos must be maintained at a comparatively low temperature of 19–20°C. The latter factor corresponds to the environment of the gallery forest in Katanga.

Exo-erythrocytic stages of *P. berghei* become mature about 50 hours after sporozoite inoculation. They are present (as in primate malaria) in parenchymatous cells of the liver.

The asexual cycle in the blood, from trophozoites to schizonts, averages 24 hours; multiple infections of the red blood cells are common and occur particularly in young erythrocytes. The number of merozoites in fully developed schizonts varies between six and twenty. Gametocytes have a typical appearance but their numbers decline markedly after a series of blood passages.

Further studies of rodents in various areas of tropical Africa led in 1952 to the discovery of *P. vinckei* by Rodhain; this was followed by the isolation of *P. chabaudi* in 1965 and *P. yoelii* in 1966. All four species are infective to mice by blood inoculation and by mosquito transmission, but there are some differences in the susceptibility of laboratory animals such as hamsters and white rats, which are more resistant to *P. chabaudi* and *P. vinckei*. Six sub-species of these murine *Plasmodia* have been described and there have been some successes in adapting other laboratory animals to the infection. Cyclical transmission by mosquitos commonly uses *Anopheles stephensi*, which is easily maintained in the laboratory.

All *Plasmodia* of murine rodents, and *P. berghei* in particular, have rapidly become most valuable experimental models for research on parasitology, immunology and chemotherapy of malaria. More than 2500 papers have been published on these studies and most of the primary screening in some 300 000 compounds developed during the past 20 years in the USA was done using *P. berghei* which is lethal to mice and young rats.

For chemotherapeutic studies rodent *Plasmodia* have some limitations since their biochemical characteristics are somewhat different from those of human parasites.

Avian *Plasmodia*

Malaria parasites of birds are found in nearly every country in the world. This is largely due to the migratory flights of birds and the ample facilities for transmission of the infection by many genera

Table 2.4 Important species of simian *Plasmodia* [partly after Garnham (1966) and Wernsdorfer (1980)]

Species	Natural host	Geographical distribution	Natural vector	Periodicity	Remarks
P. brazilianum	*Alouatta* P. *Ateles* sp. *Cebus* sp. *Lagotrix* sp. and others	Brazil Colombia Panama Peru Venezuela	*A. (Kerteszia) cruzii*	Quartan	Several Central and South American monkeys found naturally infected. Transmissible to humans
P. coatneyi	*Macaca fascicularis*	Malaysia	*A. hackeri*	Tertian	
P. cynomolgi	*Macaca* sp. *Presbytis* sp.	South-eastern Asia	*A. hackeri* *A. balabacensis* and others	Tertian	Sub-species known as *bastianellii*. Laboratory infections of humans
P. fieldi	*Macaca nemestrina* *Macaca follicularis*	Malaysia	*A. balabacensis* *A. hackeri*	Tertian	
P. fragile	*Macaca radiata*	Sri Lanka, Southern India	*A. elegans*	Tertian	
P. inui	*Macaca* sp. *Presbytis* sp.	South-east Asia	*A. balabacensis*	Quartan	Sub-species known as *shortti*
P. knowlesi	*Macaca* sp. *Presbytis* sp.	India South-east Asia	*A. hackeri*	Quotidian	Transmissible to humans. Natural infection reported from Malaysia
P. pitheci	*Pongo pygmeu* (orangutan)	Borneo	Unknown	Possibly tertian	
P. (Laverania) reichenovi	*Pan satyrus* (chimpanzee) *Gorilla* sp.	Equatorial Africa Sierra Leone Liberia	Unknown	Tertian	Not transmissible to humans
P. rodhaini Synonymous with *P. malariae*	*Pan satyrus* *Homo sapiens*	West and Central Africa	Presumably the same that transmit human malaria	Quartan	
P. schwetzi	*Pan satyrus* *Gorilla* sp.	West Africa Cameroon Lower Congo	Unknown	Tertian	Transmissible to humans
P. simium	*Alouatta* sp. *Brachyteles* sp.	Brazil	Unknown	Tertian	Natural infection of humans reported

Note: Other species of simian *Plasmodia* not mentioned in this table are: *P. eylesi*, *P. jefferyi*, *P. youngi* from Malaysia; *P. gonderi* from West Africa and Cameroon; *P. simiovale* from Sri Lanka and *P. sylvaticum* from Borneo.

and species of mosquitos. It was Danilewsky in Russia who first observed, in 1884, malaria parasites in the blood of birds. His major work published in 1894 indicated the wide distribution of these parasites. Ross in 1897 demonstrated the development of *P. relictum* in Culicine mosquitos fed on infected sparrows. Grassi and other Italian workers described in 1899–1900 a number of avian malaria parasites and their transmission by mosquitos.

The main characteristics that distinguish avian malaria parasites from those of primates are as follows. (1) Avian parasites are found in nucleated erythrocytes. (2) They are transmitted mainly by mosquitos of the genera *Aedes* and *Culex* and very rarely by *Anopheles*. (3) The exo-erythrocytic stages of avian parasites are found in mesodermal tissue, the primary cycle occupies two generations and can arise from blood stages.

Over 450 species of birds have been found infected with malaria parasites. Avian malaria parasites are classified into the sub-genera: *Haemamoeba*, *Giovannolaia*, *Novyella* and *Huffia*; they comprise over 40 species, the identification of which is not easy and must be based on observation of various stages of the life cycle and certain biological features.

After the discoveries of Ross and Grassi it seemed that the knowledge of the life cycle of the malaria parasites was complete, but it soon became obvious that there must be an unknown phase between the introduction of the sporozoite and the appearance of parasites in the blood. Grassi formulated this idea in 1906, but there was no definite proof of the presence of these forms in the body of the host. It was not until 1934–36 that Raffaele described the exo-erythrocytic forms of *P. elongatum* and *P. relictum* in the bone marrow and brain of birds. These findings were soon confirmed in *P. gallinaceum* by James and Tate and were a precursor to the discovery of exo-erythrocytic schizogony in malaria parasites of primates.

In 1926 Roehl in Germany introduced quantitative methods of assessment of antimalarial action of new compounds. Roehl's test was based on infecting canaries with *P. relictum*; untreated birds showed parasites in the blood after 4–5 days, while birds given quinine by a stomach tube showed no parasitaemia. This method was used as a primary screening test of a number of antimalarial drugs developed by the Germans during the 1930s.

Experimental chemotherapy of malaria benefited greatly from the discovery of avian *Plasmodia*. *Plasmodium cathemerium*, *P. circumflexum*, *P. gallinaceum*, *P. lophurae* and *P. relictum* were most widely used for this purpose, especially in 1940–45, and are still of some value, even though rodent and simian malaria parasites are increasingly employed at the present time.

Plasmodia of other animals

Among other species of animal *Plasmodia* two were found in Madagascar lemurs, one was discovered in an Indian buffalo, three in African and Malaysian deer; one each in an African squirrel and a fruit bat have been described.

At least 41 species of malaria parasites have been described in reptiles such as lizards, iguanas, skinks and snakes from various, but mainly tropical, parts of the world. The classification of these parasites is difficult because their schizogony takes place in blood cells other than erythrocytes, and their morphology varies according to the host. It is probable that some Culicine mosquitos and Phlebotomid flies are the usual vectors. None of these *Plasmodia* infects the common laboratory animals.

Biochemistry of *Plasmodia* and their genetics

The metabolic requirements of *Plasmodia* are obtained from the haemoglobin of the host erythrocytes and from the nutrients available to the plasma. The presence of the parasite in the red cell increases its permeability through the membrane for the passage of nutrients, but the biochemical exchanges are very complex. Energy required for intracellular growth is obtained from glucose, which is converted into lactate by phosphorylation. The oxidative processes are maintained by oxyhaemoglobin of the infected erythrocyte. The process is different in bird malaria. Protein synthesis is achieved from the essential amino acids, including cystine and methionine, present in the plasma. The degradation of haemoglobin is incomplete, leaving the malaria pigment as residue. Lipids are synthesized from the components of the host's plasma. Nucleic acids are partly synthesized by the *Plasmodia* and partly obtained by other pathways. A cofactor, tetrahydrofolate (THF), is important for the conversion of certain amino acids and for the synthesis of purine nucleotides; this enzyme is produced by malaria parasites through a reaction in which another enzyme, dihydrofolate reductase (DHFR), is involved. It is this particular pathway which is the point of action of some antimalarial drugs such as pyrimethamine and sulfonamides.

Malaria parasites contain DNA and RNA; the first is double-stranded and its base components are characteristic for each group of *Plasmodia*. RNA is ribosomal and messenger RNA has a composition similar to other protozoa.

Recently, much interest has been concentrated on the membranes of the parasite and of the infected red blood cell. Morphological criteria are inadequate for characterization of these membranes, and biochemical studies, involving specific markers, are being carried out. These studies indicate that the major reactions, taking place between these membranes, are related to the transfer of glycoproteins. Alterations in erythrocyte membrane proteins, carbohydrates and lipids might be responsible for the increased osmotic fragility and greater permeability which are characteristic of infected red blood cells. Recent research shows that a very large malaria protein (erythrocytic membrane protein, EMP, which has a molecular weight of approximately 30 000) is exported from the parasite and deposited on the surface of the erythrocytic membrane.

Research on the biochemistry of malaria parasites is aimed at finding possibilities for development of antimalaria drugs. The introduction of *in vitro* culture methods for some species of *Plasmodia* should greatly assist these investigations, which are of notorious complexity and difficulty.

Obviously, the state of nutrition of the host has an important bearing on the multiplication of *Plasmodia*. It has been found that para-amino-benzoic acid (PABA) must be present in the diet of the host or in the culture medium, since this is one of the essential building stones of the molecule of the folic acid needed for the growth of mammalian *Plasmodia*. The importance of this and other biochemical studies is considerable for the understanding of the action of antimalarial compounds.

Biochemical changes produced by the ageing of the red blood cells have an important bearing on their susceptibility to invasion by *Plasmodia*. Thus, *P. vivax* and *P. ovale* are predominantly found in young erythrocytes. *Plasmodium malariae* seems to prefer mature red blood cells while *P. falciparum* appears to be indifferent to the age of its host cell. Some new evidence derived from the study of *in vitro* cultures indicates, however, that the rate of invasion of *P. falciparum* is higher in young than in old red cells. Explanations for the failure of older red cells to be invaded is three-fold: (a) loss of specific receptors on the membranes of older cells, (b) loss of metabolic activity, and (c) greater rigidity of the older cells' membranes, which cannot be penetrated by merozoites during the invasion process.

Recent studies indicate that the receptor for merozoites of *P. falciparum* is glycophorin, a glycoprotein component of the erythrocyte membrane.

Our present knowledge of the genetics of *Plasmodia* comes mainly from the studies of malaria parasites of rodents. The sexual stages of *Plasmodia* give rise to gametes in the stomach of the mosquito, where fertilization takes place and where a diploid zygote is formed. However, it is not known where the meiotic (reduction) division takes place, because chromosomes have never been detected as distinct structures, although some observations suggest that there are 8–10 haploid chromosomes. Genetic studies require cloning techniques, namely, producing from a single organism a progeny that has a genetic marker. Such markers are enzyme polymorphisms and differences of the antigenic structure, but resistance to some drugs or degrees of virulence can also be used as characteristics. Much use of these studies has been made of enzyme variation and of the pattern of inheritance of various markers following interbreeding of different isolates. Previously all genetic work on malaria parasites was based on strain hybridization and progeny analysis. Important advances have been made by the application of techniques of molecular genetics. Thus, biochemical characteristics of DNA may reveal differences in the genetic composition of the parasite. Much progress has been made by using enzyme electrophoresis which reveals subtle differences between strains related to these products of separate gene loci.

Recently, extensive use has been made of various enzymes which are inherited in *Plasmodia* according to Mendelian principles and remain stable over many generations. The most useful plasmodial enzymes have been: glucose-phosphate isomerase (GPI), 6-phosphogluconate dehydrogenase (PGD), lactate dehydrogenase (LDH), adenosine deaminase (ADA) and peptidase E (PEPE). These studies are of importance as they may reveal different characteristics of parasite strains of varying sensitivity to antimalarial drugs.

Most of this research has been done on various species of rodent *Plasmodia*, but some of it was carried out on *P. falciparum*, thanks to the present possibility of maintaining it *in vitro*. In the latter species it was found that many enzymes were common in all geographical 'strains', but some were present at fairly characteristic and identifiable frequencies.

Recent studies on *P. falciparum* have revealed

great diversity among genetically derived characters of various isolates from different parts of the world. This diversity extends to six enzyme variants, to DNA sequence arrangements, to variant protein forms, to antigenic determinants, and to levels of sensitivity of parasites to antimalarial drugs. The application of monoclonal antibody techniques may yield more information in this respect. The present conclusion is that while *P. falciparum* is a single worldwide species, many isolates contain mixtures of genetically diverse organisms with geographical differences in the frequencies with which variant genetic markers occur. Extensive rearrangements occur in the parasite genome after cross-fertilization between these genetically diverse parasites and this determines characters such as antigens, enzymes and drug resistance. It may be assumed that the degrees of antigen diversity are related to the intensity of transmission in a particular area.

Present advances of our knowledge of genetics of malaria parasites explain their adaptability to adverse conditions encountered in the external environment or in the body of their hosts. Drug resistance is the result of gene mutation selection pressure. The spread of resistant genes in a parasite population depends on many internal factors such as the immune response of the host, but external factors, namely, the mobility of the mosquito vector and the human host, also play a role in spreading the resistance far from the initial area of its development. Currently, with the exception of reports from Australia of *P. vivax* infections contracted in Papua New Guinea and Indonesia showing poor response to the standard treatment regimen of 25 mg/kg body weight of chloroquine, chloroquine continues to provide adequate treatment for *P. vivax*, *P. malariae* and *P. ovale*.

A surface coat which is present in both sporozoites and merozoites of *Plasmodia* consists of glycoproteins, and it has been suggested that the changes of this coat in merozoites may be responsible for antigenic variations of strains such as seen in trypanosomes. A circumsporozoite-like protein has also been detected in mature merozoites although at a much lower level than in sporozoites.

Cryopreservation of parasite isolates at −70°C in carbon dioxide snow (dry ice) or at −196°C in liquid nitrogen has been of great value for genetic and other studies. This technique has been used for storing blood forms of *Plasmodia* and sporozoites for up to 10 years, with little or no loss of viability. Storage at −20°C in a domestic freezer is adequate for short periods. However, different types of cells require different rates of cooling and thawing; moreover, both procedures depend on the type of medium used for preservation. Blood stages of *Plasmodia* survive freezing better with the use of preservatives such as glycerol or dimethylsulfoxide; other stages (sporozoites) are generally less tolerant of cryopreservation.

Preservation of strains of malaria parasites in viable condition for a limited period of 1–3 days, such as may be necessary for transporting a blood sample by air, is not difficult. All it requires is to place the 5–10 ml of infected blood, prevented from clotting by heparin or other anticoagulant, in a small, well-stoppered vial. The vial should be placed in a plastic, well-sealed bag. Another larger plastic bag should be inserted in a good quality Thermos flask, and then filled with chipped ice; if the loss of ice by melting is made up by new chips of ice the blood should remain infective for the whole time of air transport. To preserve viable infected blood for longer periods by freezing at −70°C or lower, carbon dioxide snow or liquid nitrogen in special containers are available, but this requires slightly different techniques of preparation of frozen samples.

Cultivation of malaria parasites

In vitro cultures of malaria parasites were attempted in 1912 by Bass and Johns; they and their followers obtained a limited multiplication of human *Plasmodia*. In 1945 a medium for maintenance of cultures of the avian *P. gallinaceum* was devised by Hawking and subsequently Trager improved the methods for culture of *P. lophurae*. In the 1950s Ball and Geiman were able to keep for limited periods cultures of the simian *P. knowlesi*, in a complex nutrient medium, but long-term sub-cultures were not possible.

Thus, the discovery in 1976 by Trager and Jensen of an extremely simple method of *in vitro* culture of *P. falciparum* came as a great surprise; the subsequent rapid adoption of this method and its various improvements can be considered as a milestone in the history of malaria research. These methods have since been used for cultivation of the erythrocytic stages of four species of *Plasmodia* of monkeys: *P. knowlesi*, *P. cynomolgi*, *P. inui* and *P. fragile*. There have also been reports of partial success with *P. malariae* and *P. vivax*. However, most work continues to be done with *P. falciparum* in human erythrocytes, using the original method of Petri dishes in candle jars. The Petri dish method has been used to study the metabolism of malaria parasites, their growth in red blood cells with genetic variants such as sickle cell haemoglobin, the effects of antimalarial drugs and the degree of resistance of *Plasmodia*. Many other applications of this technique are being developed. A continuous flow method devised by Trager and improved by others permits the maintenance of stock cultures for a long time. Moreover, recent developments of computer-controlled culture systems provide a steady supply of antigenic material for extensive studies.

The principle of the original 'candle-jar' method is to maintain the infected erythrocytes in a relatively simple culture medium, with the addition of human (or rabbit or calf) serum in an atmosphere of 3–4% carbon dioxide and 16% oxygen, such as can be provided in a closed jar in which a candle has been extinguished. Fresh red blood cells can be added for the continuation of the growth, division and multiplication of *Plasmodia* (Fig. 2.12).

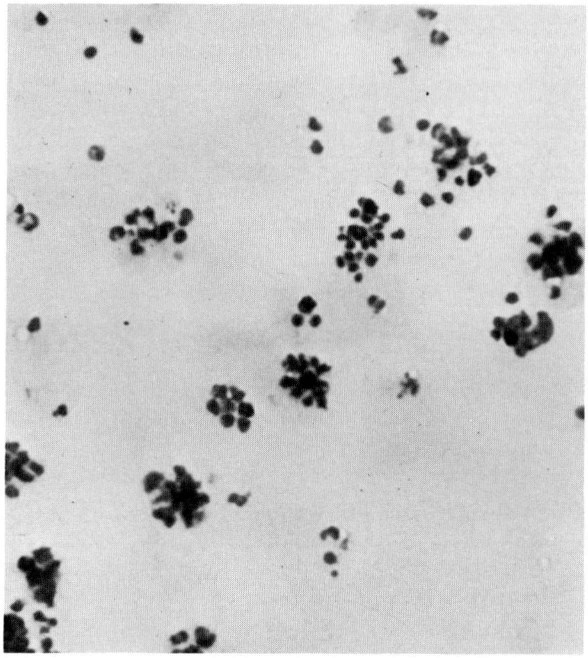

Fig. 2.12 *In vitro* culture of *P. falciparum* using the technique of Trager and Jensen (1976). Note a number of fully grown schizonts, some ruptured schizonts and scattered free merozoites in this 48-hour culture. × 880. (Dr A. J. Sulzer, Centers for Disease Control, Atlanta.)

A large number of culture lines have been established in various laboratories, either from blood of infected Aotus monkeys or more often directly from human infections. Claims that parasites from some regions are difficult to culture have been discounted, and it seems that this is more often the result of an inadequate technique. There is evidence that chloroquine-resistant parasites are much easier to cultivate under the more marginal culture conditions of the *in vitro* test system as evidenced by the much higher schizont counts in the control wells of tests of resistant strains.

There seems to be no loss of infectivity after a prolonged culture *in vitro*, but some culture lines may show certain morphological changes of parasites. Culture methods, combined with cloning from a single *Plasmodium*, give much information on the nature and presence of strains resistant to various drugs, especially chloroquine. Production of gametocytes in culture varies with the isolate and the time of culture; when tested for their infectivity to *Anopheles* most gametocytes fail to develop into sporogonic forms. However, some recent improvements of the composition of culture media and techniques produced infective gametocytes and this should provide a convenient source for further studies aimed at obtaining sporozoites and, eventually, at an *in vitro* cultivation of sporogonic stages. Although exo-erythrocytic stages of avian malaria parasites were obtained in tissue cultures of chick or turkey brain cells some 25 years ago, this is much more difficult in mammalian malaria. Nevertheless, success in producing pre-erythrocytic forms of the rodent parasite *P. berghei* by inoculation of sporozoites into various tissue cultures (hepatoma cells, human embryonic lung fibroblasts) has paved the way for the recently achieved *in vitro* cultivation of pre-erythrocytic stages of primate malaria parasites.

Chapter 3

Clinical features of malaria

D. A. Warrell

Malaria causes an acute febrile illness which may be characterized by periodic febrile paroxysms occurring every 48 or 72 hours with afebrile asymptomatic intervals and a tendency to recrudesce or relapse over periods of months to many years. The severity and course of an attack of malaria depends on the species and strain of infecting parasite and hence on the geographical origin of the infection; on the age, genetic constitution, state of immunity, general health and nutritional status of the patient and on any chemoprophylaxis or chemotherapy which has been used. There are no absolutely diagnostic clinical features of malaria except for the regular paroxysms of fever with virtually asymptomatic intervals (Fig. 3.1).

The *incubation period* is the interval between infection and the first clinical sign, usually fever, of the primary attack. The *pre-patent period* extends from the time of infection to the first discovery of malaria parasites in the blood (Table 3.1). It is important to remember the minimum incubation period, about 7 days in the case of falciparum malaria, because this is the earliest time after arrival in a malarious country that symptoms can be attributed to malarial infection. Theoretically, there should be no pre-patent period and the incubation period should be a few days shorter when infection is with asexual parasites (when transplacental, from blood transfusions, organ/tissue transplants and needlestick injuries) since no preliminary hepatic cycle need occur before infection of erythrocytes. Shorter incubation periods have been observed in a large series of cases injected with infected blood but, usually, the non-mosquito routes of infection are associated with longer pre-patent and incubation periods because of the relatively small inoculum of parasites. Since asexual erythrocytic cycle parasites cannot invade the liver no true relapses will follow *Plasmodium vivax* and *Plasmodium ovale* infections by these unusual routes. Incubation may be prolonged by immunity, chemoprophylaxis or chemotherapy.

The best known symptom of malaria is the febrile paroxysm, ague attack or ague fit which resembles, clinically and pathophysiologically, 'endotoxin reactions' in other infections (for example, lobar pneumonia and pyelonephritis), response to typhoid vaccine and the Jarisch–Herxheimer reaction of syphilis, relapsing fevers and other infections.

For 2 or 3 days before the first malarial paroxysm, the patient may have experienced prodromal symptoms such as malaise, fatigue and lassitude, with, according to Manson, a desire to stretch the limbs and yawn, headache, dizziness especially on trying to stand up, pain or aching in the chest, back, abdomen, joints and bones, anorexia, nausea, vomiting, a sensation of cold water trickling down the back and slight fever. Fever may be detectable for 2 or 3 hours before the paroxysm. The patient looks ill, and may be clinically anaemic and mildly jaundiced with tender enlargement of the liver and spleen. The conjunctivae are suffused. There are no focal signs, lymphadenopathy or rash (except for cold sores). The *cold stage* starts with a sudden inappropriate feeling of cold and apprehension. Mild shivering quickly turns into violent teeth chattering and shaking of the whole body. The patients try to cover themselves with all available

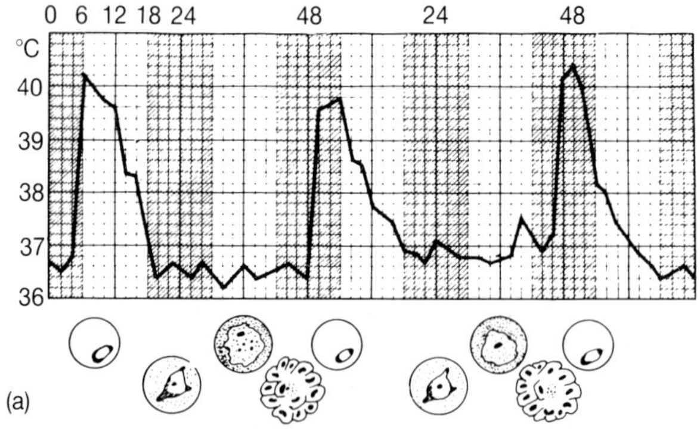

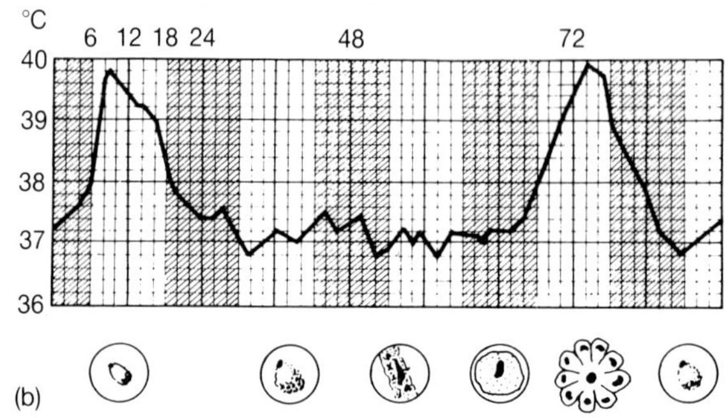

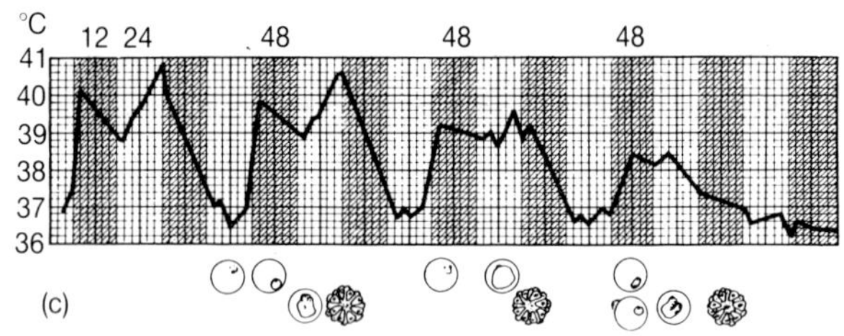

Fig. 3.1 (a) Typical temperature chart of *Plasmodium vivax* infection showing tertian periodicity related to the maturation and rupture of erythrocytic schizonts. (b) Typical temperature chart of *Plasmodium malariae* infection showing quartan periodicity. (c) Typical temperature chart of *Plasmodium falciparum* infection showing irregular tertian periodicity and the influence of successful treatment.

Table 3.1 Main features of the human malarias

	P. falciparum	*P. malariae*	*P. vivax*	*P. ovale*
Pre-patent period (days)	9–10	15–16	11–13	10–14
Incubation period (days)	9–14 (12)	18–40 (28) or longer	12–17 (15) or up to 6–12 months	16–18 (17) or longer
Fever periodicity (hours)	24, 36, 48 (quotidian, tertian, sub-/bi-tertian)	72 (quartan)	48 (tertian)	48 (tertian)
Relapses	–	–	++	++
Recrudescences	+	+	–	–
Invasion requirements	?	?	Duffy -ve blood group	?
Drug resistance	+ (multiple, widespread)	–	+ (chloroquine, New Guinea)	–

bedclothes. Although the core temperature is high and rising quickly, there is intense peripheral vasoconstriction; the skin is cold, dry, pale, cyanosed and goose-pimpled. The pulse is rapid and of low volume. The patient may vomit and febrile convulsions may develop at this stage in young children. These rigors last for 15–60 minutes after which the shivering ceases, the patient feels some waves of warmth and the *hot stage* (flush phase) ensues. Patients quickly become unbearably hot and throw off all their bed clothes. A severe throbbing headache, palpitations, tachypnoea, prostration, postural syncope, epigastric discomfort, nausea and vomiting, and thirst develop as the temperature reaches its peak of 40–41°C (104–106°F) or more. During this phase the patient may become confused or delirious. The skin is flushed, dry and burning. The pulse is rapid, full and bounding. Splenic enlargement may be detected for the first time at this stage. The hot stage lasts from 2 to 6 hours. In the *sweating stage*, defervescence or diaphoresis, the patient breaks out into a profuse drenching sweat. The fever declines over the next 2 to 4 hours, symptoms diminish and the exhausted patient sleeps.

The total duration of the typical attack is 8 to 12 hours. Most paroxysms start between midnight and midday or, at the latest, in the early afternoon.

The classical periodicity of febrile paroxysms develops only if the patient is untreated until the infection becomes synchronized so that sufficient numbers of erythrocytes containing mature schizonts rupture at the same time. The interval is determined by the length of the asexual erythrocytic cycle: 48 hours in *P. falciparum*, *P. vivax* and *P. ovale*, producing febrile paroxysms on alternate days (or days 1 and 3, hence tertian); 72 hours for *P. malariae*, causing febrile paroxysms on days 1 and 4 (hence quartan). However, intermittent fever is usually absent at the beginning of the disease, when headache, malaise, fatigue, nausea, muscular pains, slight diarrhoea and slight increase of body temperature, are the predominant and vague symptoms which are easily mistaken for influenza or a gastrointestinal infection. Tertian periodicity is rarely seen in falciparum malaria: persistent spiking fever or a daily (quotidian) febrile paroxysm is more usual.

The start of a *primary attack* marks the end of the incubation period. The attack is composed of a number of febrile paroxysms. Unless the parasites are eliminated by adequate treatment the attack is followed by a more or less prolonged period during which the trend of the infection depends on a balance between multiplication of parasites and the counteraction of the immune response of the host (Fig. 3.2).

Relapses of *P. vivax* and *P. ovale* result from reactivation of hypnozoite forms of the parasite in the liver. Precipitants may include cold, fatigue, trauma, pregnancy, infections including intercurrent falciparum malaria and other illnesses. *Recrudescences* of *P. falciparum* and *P. malariae* result from exacerbations of persistent undetectable parasitaemias in the absence of an exo-erythrocytic cycle.

Falciparum malaria ('malignant', tertian or sub-tertian malaria)

Falciparum malaria is responsible for almost all of the 2 million or more deaths attributed to malaria each year worldwide. People who live in endemic areas and have been frequently infected acquire some immunity so that they can tolerate *P. falciparum* parasitaemia with trivial or no symptoms. However, in non-immune people, such as expatriate travellers in malarious regions, falciparum infection nearly always causes debilitating symptoms and must be regarded as a potentially fatal disease. Experience with malaria induced for the treatment of neurosyphilis indicated that the shortest pre-patent period following a mosquito

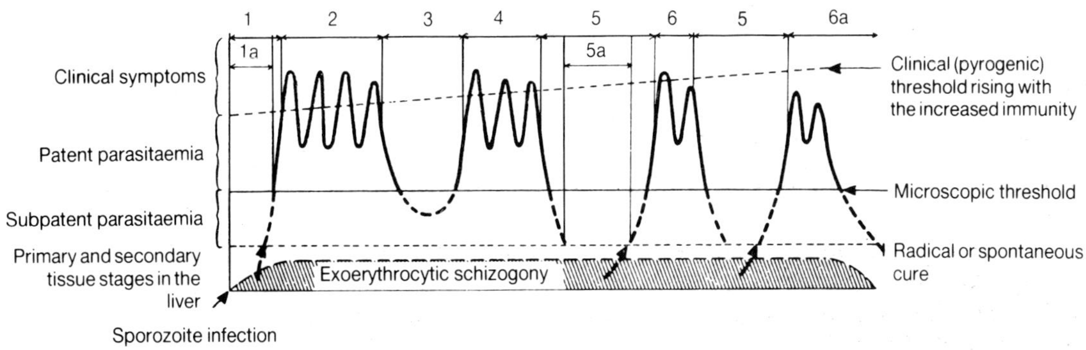

1. Incubation period
1a. Pre-patent period
2. Primary attack composed of paroxysms
3. Latent period (clinical latency)
4. Recrudescence (short-term relapse)
5. Latent period
5a. Parasitic latency
6. Clinical recurrence (long-term relapse) followed by parasitic recurrence
6a. Parasitic relapse

Fig. 3.2 Diagram of the course of a malaria infection showing the primary attack and relapses or recrudescences. (WHO, 1963.)

bite was 5 days, and the shortest incubation period was 7 days. These periods were inversely proportional to the dose of sporozoites. The incubation period is prolonged by immunity, chemoprophylaxis and partial chemotherapy. In western countries, 65–95% of patients with imported falciparum malaria develop symptoms within 1 month of arriving back from the tropics. A few present up to 1 year later, but none after more than 4 years.

The classical febrile malarial paroxysm followed by an afebrile asymptomatic interval is not a feature of falciparum infection. The illness starts with headache, dizziness, pains in the back and limbs, malaise, anorexia, nausea, vague abdominal pain, vomiting or mild diarrhoea and a feeling of chill. There are intermittent chills rather than a clearly circumscribed cold phase and the fever is continuous or remittent as in enteric fevers. When periodic febrile paroxysms do occur they are daily (quotidian), every third day (tertian) or twice every 3 days (sub- or bi-tertian). The physical findings like the symptoms are non-specific and include fever, prostration, postural hypotension, a tinge of jaundice and tender hepatosplenomegaly. The finding of a rash, other than febrile *Herpes simplex* of the lips, lymphadenopathy and focal signs suggests a diagnosis other than malaria. In non-immune people the disease can progress very rapidly to severe life-threatening malaria unless appropriate treatment is started, and in some cases despite treatment. Some patients have died within 24 hours of their first symptom, but this is most unusual and may have been explained by their having a very high symptom threshold.

During the past decade new attempts have been made to describe and define more precisely the life-threatening manifestations and complications of falciparum malaria so that patients found to have these problems could be given special treatment (Table 3.2).

Table 3.2 Severe falciparum malaria: manifestations and complications

Cerebral malaria
Repeated generalized convulsions
Malarial anaemia
Hyperpyrexia
Hyperparasitaemia
Hypoglycaemia
Renal failure
Hepatic dysfunction
Fluid, electrolyte and acid base disturbances
Pulmonary oedema (adult respiratory distress syndrome)
Circulatory collapse (algid malaria)
Haemostatic abnormalities
Massive intravascular haemolysis ('Blackwater fever')
Splenic rupture

Cerebral malaria

This is the most notorious form of severe malaria. In most parts of the world about 90% of patients will become comatose sometime before dying of malaria. In adults, there is commonly a preceding history of several days of fever and non-specific symptoms (see above) before gradual impairment of consciousness or a generalized convulsion followed by persisting coma. Drowsiness is always a worrying symptom but since high fever alone can cause confusion, irritability, obtundation, delirium, psychosis and, in children, febrile convulsions, the term cerebral malaria, which implies an encephalopathy specifically related to *P. falciparum* infection, should be restricted to patients with unrousable coma (Tables 3.3 and 3.4). Patients with cerebral malaria may be open-eyed but unseeing (Fig. 3.3), may lie immobile or toss about restlessly, flailing their head from side to side (Fig. 3.3) and grinding their teeth ('bruxism'). Spontaneous movement implies lighter coma and so its absence is a sign of poor prognosis. Various involuntary movements and muscular spasms are seen. The term extensor posturing covers a number of bizarre neurological signs including decerebrate (Fig. 3.4) and decorticate (Fig. 3.5) rigidity with extension of the neck and back, so that the patient

Table 3.3 Cerebral malaria: definitions

Practical definition
Any impairment of consciousness or convulsions in a patient exposed to malaria

Research definition
1. Unrousable coma (see Table 3.4) persisting for at least 30 minutes after a generalized convulsion
2. Asexual forms of *P. falciparum* in the blood smear
3. Exclude other causes of encephalopathy (see Table 3.5)
(4. Fatal cases only. Confirmation of typical brain histopathology [see pp. 51–2, Plates 9–12])

Table 3.4 Definition of unrousable coma: modified Glasgow coma scale

		Score
Adults		
Best verbal response:	Oriented	5
	Confused	4
	Inappropriate words	3
	Incomprehensible sounds	2
	None	1
Best motor response:	Obeys commands	6
	Localizes pain	5
	Flexion to pain:	
	withdrawal	4
	abnormal	3
	Extension to pain	2
	None	1
	Total	2–1
	'unrousable coma'	≤7
Children ('Blantyre scale', Molyneux *et al.*, 1989)		
Eye movements:	Directed (e.g. follows mother's face)	1
	Not directed	0
Verbal response:	Appropriate cry	2
	Moan or inappropriate cry	1
	None	0
Best motor response:	Localizes painful stimulus	2
	Withdraws limb from pain	1
	Non-specific or absent response	0
	Total	0–5
	'unrousable coma'	≤2

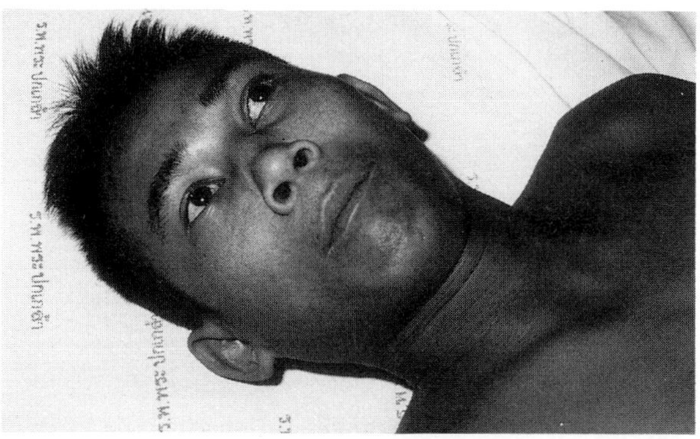

Fig. 3.3 Thai man with cerebral malaria: unrousable coma, open-eyed but non-seeing. (© D. A. Warrell.)

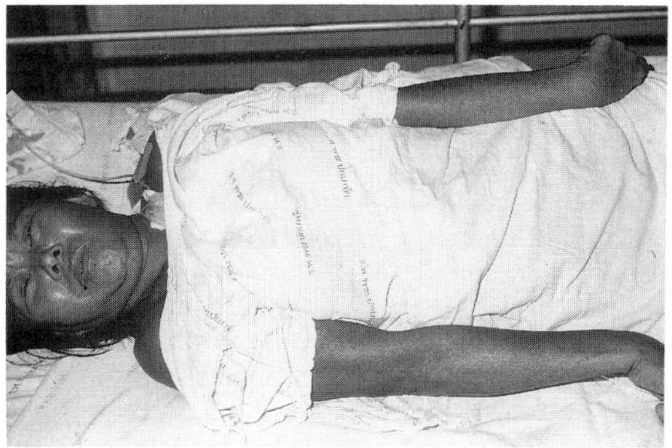

Fig. 3.4 Thai woman with cerebral malaria and profound hypoglycaemia showing extensor posturing (decerebrate rigidity). Note extension of upper limbs and neck, flexion of wrists and sustained upward gaze with facial grimacing. (© D. A. Warrell.)

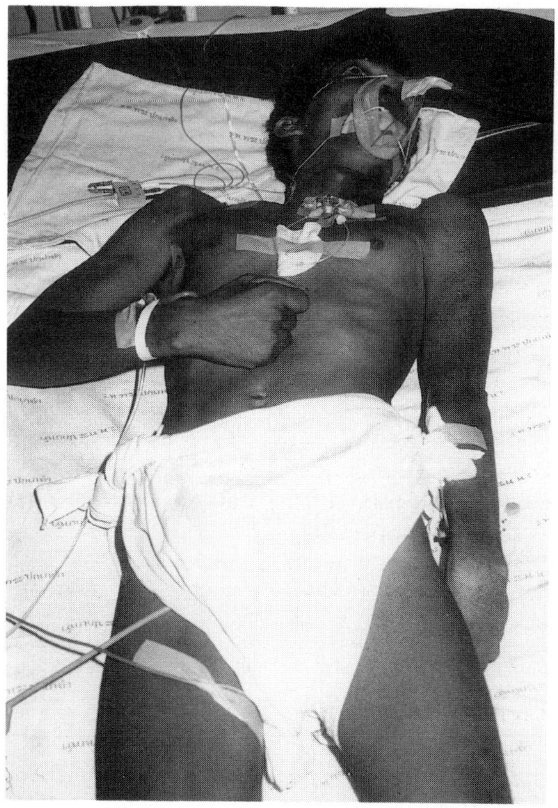

Fig. 3.5 Thai man with cerebral malaria uncomplicated by hypoglycaemia showing extensor posturing (decorticate rigidity). Note extension of neck and sustained upward gaze, extension of lower limbs and flexion of elbows and wrists. (© D. A. Warrell.)

assumes a position of opisthotonos, sustained upward deviation of the eyes and pouting with laboured, grunting respirations. Unless prophylactic anticonvulsants are given early, about half the adult patients and even more of the child will convulse. Convulsions are usually generalized, but Jacksonian-type or persistent focal seizures also occur. There may be mild meningism but no neck rigidity or photophobia. Papilloedema is very rarely seen in cerebral malaria, but retinal haemorrhages (Plate 1) are found in about 15% of adults and are sometimes associated with exudates. In most parts of the world, this retinopathy is associated with established or imminent coma and carries a bad prognosis.

Dysconjugate gaze (internuclear ophthalmoplegia) is common (Fig. 3.6) and convergent spasm (Fig. 3.7), transient ocular bobbing, horizontal and vertical nystagmus and VIth nerve palsies (Fig. 3.8) are described. In adults corneal, eyelash, pupillary, oculocephalic ('doll's eye') and oculovestibular (caloric) reflexes are usually normal in contrast to the findings in African children (see below). The mouth is often kept forcibly closed. The jaw jerk may be brisk. A pout reflex can usually be elicited indicating frontal release, but a grasp reflex is rare. The gag reflex is normal. The usual neurological picture in adults is of a symmetrical upper motor neuron lesion with increased muscle tone, brisk tendon reflexes, ankle clonus and extensor plantar responses. However, muscle tone and reflexes are sometimes decreased especially in children (Fig. 3.9). The brisk abdominal reflexes usually found in younger people with fevers of other causes and with hysteria distinguish these conditions from cerebral malaria in which these reflexes are absent.

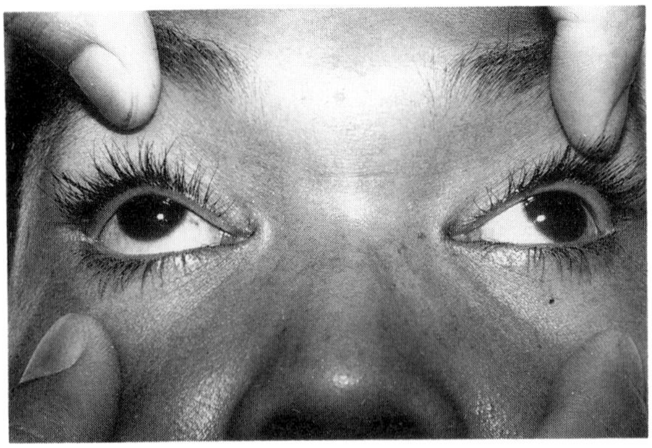

Fig. 3.6 Dysconjugate gaze in a Thai patient comatose with cerebral malaria. The optic axes are divergent. (© D. A. Warrell.)

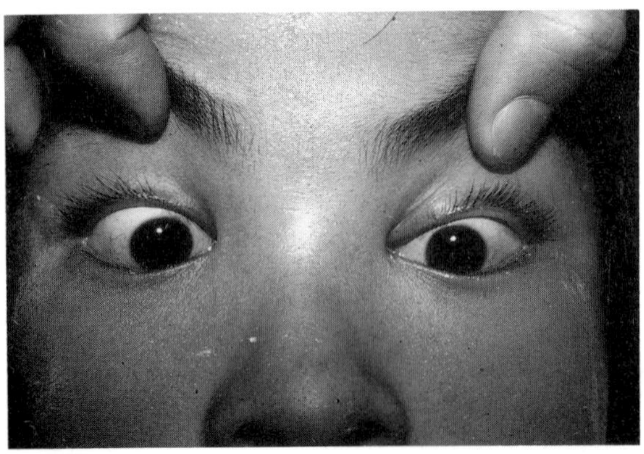

Fig. 3.7 Convergence spasm in a Thai girl comatose with cerebral malaria. (© D. A. Warrell.)

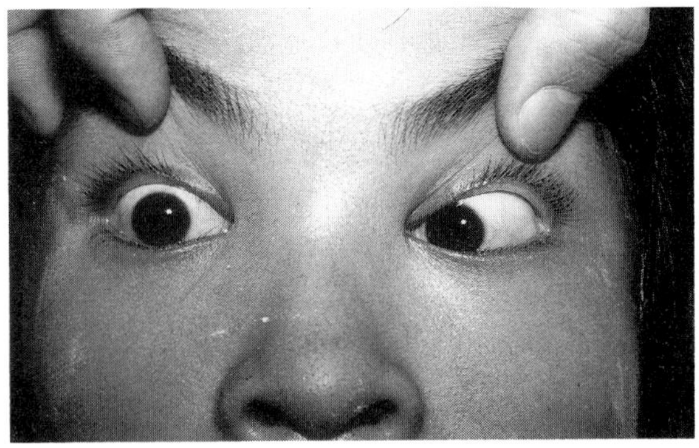

Fig. 3.8 Right VIth cranial nerve palsy in a Thai girl convalescent from cerebral malaria. (© D. A. Warrell.)

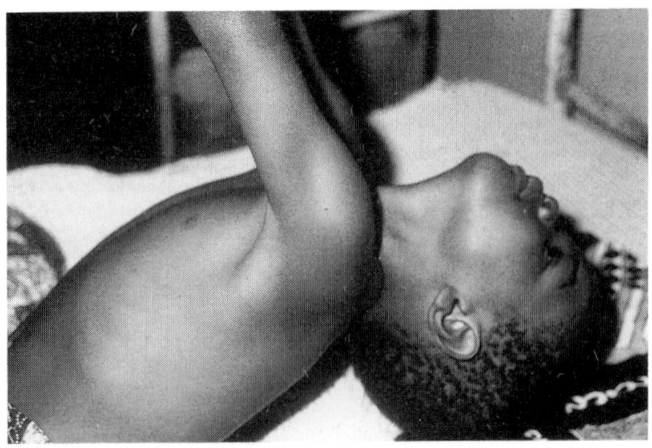

Fig. 3.9 Generalized reduction in muscle tone ('broken neck sign') in a Kenyan child recovering from cerebral malaria. (© D. A. Warrell.)

Those who recover from cerebral malaria usually become rousable after about 40 hours of coma and are fully conscious within the ensuing 18 hours. Recovery after prolonged unconsciousness, for 1 week or even longer, has been observed but is very uncommon. The mortality of cerebral malaria, as defined above, is about 15–20% where good standards of hospital care can be provided. In a series of 200 patients with severe malaria studied in eastern Thailand, 95% of the deaths were evenly spaced over the first 4 days of hospital admission.

Neurological sequelae are common in African children (see below) but are detected in less than 10% of adults. They include psychosis, extrapyramidal tremor, cranial nerve lesions, polyneuropathy, mononeuritis multiplex, Guillain–Barré syndrome and focal epilepsy.

Other manifestations of central nervous dysfunction

Delirium and brief reactive psychosis

Malarial psychoses have been observed following recovery of consciousness in patients with cerebral malaria and in patients convalescent from milder attacks of malaria. Most of these disturbances were transient, lasting only a few days. Auditory hallucinations, paranoid delusions, mental confusion, amnesia, depressive elements, attempted suicide (as in the case of Orde Wingate of the Chindits) and aggressive behaviour have been described. It may be difficult to separate the effects of drugs, including antimalarial drugs, and other psychological factors in attributing these symptoms to malaria.

Cerebellar syndrome

Cerebellar ataxia has been described as a complication of a variety of infections, notably typhoid. The cerebellar syndrome of falciparum and vivax malaria may present as part of the acute illness, in convalescence or after an asymptomatic interval of a few weeks ('delayed cerebellar ataxia'). The clinical features include dysarthria, nystagmus, opsoclonus, ataxia, intention tremor and hypotonia. The syndrome seems to be particularly common in Sri Lanka and the Indian subcontinent. In all reported cases, full neurological recovery took place over a period of a few weeks to several months.

Cerebral malaria in children

In holoendemic areas of Africa cerebral malaria can occur in children less than 6 months old but is most common in 2 to 3 year olds. Early symptoms include fever, irritability or apathy, failure to feed, convulsions, cough, vomiting and, rarely, diarrhoea. Children become unrousable a few hours or more, usually 1–2 days, after their first symptom. Convulsions are very common and are of generalized tonic clonic, focal clonic or bilateral clonic type. *Petit mal* 'absences' and tonic eye deviation have also been observed. Subtle partial seizures detected by electroencephalogram monitoring may be clinically inapparent. Unlike adults with cerebral malaria, children may show abnormalities of corneal, oculovestibular (Fig. 3.10) and oculocephalic reflexes, but the pupillary light reflexes are usually normal. Muscular hypotonia is more common in children than in adults (Fig. 3.9). Intracranial hypertension has recently been documented in Kenyan children with cerebral malaria. Tensely bulging fontanelles may be found in young children (<18 months old) and cerebrospinal fluid opening pressures measured at lumbar puncture are usually raised. Neurological evidence of cerebral herniation was seen, especially in fatal cases. Most deaths occur within the first 24 hours after admission to hospital. In survivors, the duration of coma is shorter than in adults and averages about 30 hours to regain full consciousness. Neurological sequelae are persistent in more than 10% of cases. These

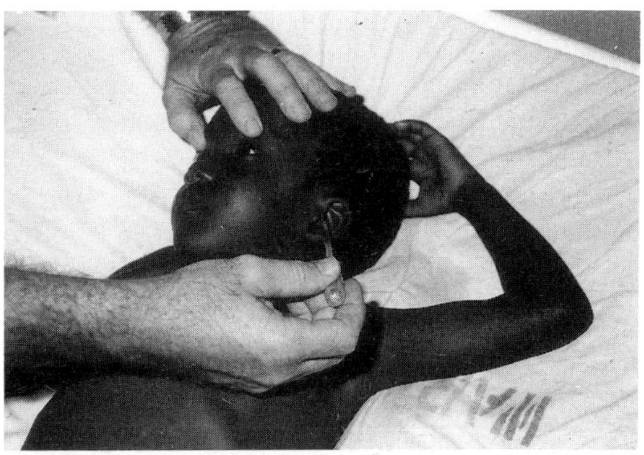

Fig. 3.10 Eliciting the ocular vestibular reflex in a Kenyan child recovering from cerebral malaria. Cold saline is introduced into the external auditory meatus and the eyes observed for nystagmus. (© D. A. Warrell.)

include hemiplegia, cortical blindness, epilepsy, inability to speak, cerebellar ataxia, extensor posturing, generalized spasticity or hypotonia, psychosis, tremors, mental retardation and behavioural disturbances. In the Gambia, three-quarters of the children with sequelae had improved or recovered after 6 months.

More adults than children show neurological improvement after intravenous glucose. The mortality and incidence of neurological sequelae is greatly increased in African children found to be hypoglycaemic on admission to hospital. Hypoglycaemia also complicates other severe infections such as bacillary dysentery.

Other features of severe falciparum malaria

Anaemia

In parts of Africa malarial anaemia (Plate 2) kills as many children as cerebral malaria, its peak incidence being at the younger age of less than 2 years. It is also common in pregnant women. The severity of anaemia correlates with parasitaemia and schizontaemia. Clinical associations are with retinal haemorrhages, hepatic and renal dysfunction and secondary bacterial infections.

Jaundice and hepatic dysfunction

Jaundice (Plate 3) is far more common in adults than children. The liver and spleen are commonly enlarged and tender, especially in young children and non-immune adults. Liver failure, with features of hepatic encephalopathy such as asterixis and clinical and biochemical evidence of severe liver cell damage does not occur unless there is concomitant viral hepatitis.

Hypoglycaemia

Anxiety, breathlessness, feelings of coldness, light-headedness, tachycardia, impairment of consciousness, extensor posturing and seizures, the classical symptoms of hypoglycaemia, are likely to be attributed to the malaria infection. This may have been why hypoglycaemia was overlooked for so many years. Hypoglycaemia is detected in more than 5% of children with severe malaria on admission to hospital. It is common and may be asymptomatic in pregnant women with severe or uncomplicated falciparum malaria, and in patients with severe malaria and hyperparasitaemia, and is an important complication of treatment with the cinchona alkaloids, quinine and quinidine.

Renal dysfunction

This is another of the complications of falciparum malaria which is much commoner in adults than children. About one-third of non-immune adults with severe malaria develop biochemical evidence of renal dysfunction which is associated with hypoglycaemia, jaundice, prolonged coma, pulmonary oedema, hypovolaemia, hyperparasitaemia and increased mortality. In only a minority of cases is there progression to acute renal failure.

Haemostatic abnormalities

Petechiae of the skin and mucosae (Plate 4) and spontaneous bleeding from the gingival sulci (Plate 5), nose and gastrointestinal tract, are seen in less than 10% of adults and rarely in children.

Shock, 'algid malaria' and other cardiovascular abnormalities

'The algide forms of pernicious attack, as indicated by the name, are characterized by collapse and extreme coldness of the surface of the body, and a tendency to fatal syncope. These symptoms usually coexist with elevated axillary and rectal temperature' (Manson, 1898). Manson's description of algid malaria is strongly reminiscent of bacteraemic shock, and in some patients with this clinical picture, Gram-negative rod bacteraemia can be detected by blood culture. However, in most patients with malaria the blood pressure is at the lower end of the normal range. Mild supine hypotension with a postural drop in blood pressure is usually attributable to vasodilation and hypovolaemia. Hypotension and shock are also seen in patients who develop pulmonary oedema, metabolic acidosis and haemorrhage into the gastrointestinal tract or from a ruptured spleen. Cardiac arrhythmias and evidence of myocardial failure are hardly ever seen in malaria.

Pulmonary oedema (See Fig. 3.11.)

This most dreaded complication of malaria may develop at any stage of the disease. When precipitated by excessive parenteral fluid therapy it may present late when the patient appears to be recovering. It is a common terminal event and was found in all the patients in Spitz's autopsy series. The earliest warning is an increased respiratory rate, dyspnoea and detection of crepitations. Central venous pressure will be high when the mechanism is fluid overload, but in the majority of patients the clinical picture is that of adult respiratory distress syndrome (ARDS) with normal right heart pressures. A chest radiograph will help to distinguish bronchopneumonia and the hyperpnoea of metabolic acidosis.

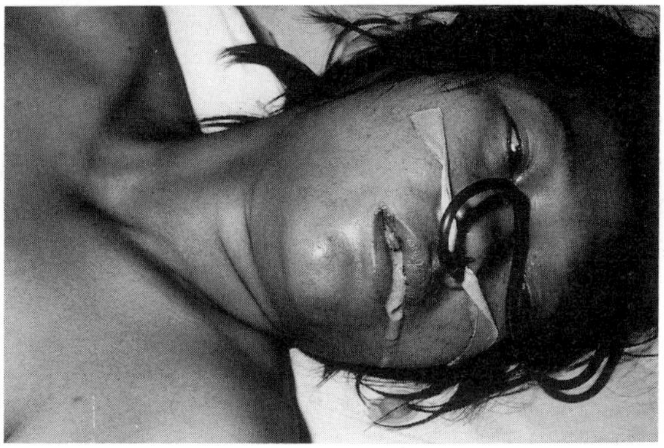

Fig. 3.11 Acute pulmonary oedema in a Vietnamese woman with cerebral malaria complicated by hypoglycaemia. Despite the very poor prognosis of this complication, this patient made a complete recovery. (© D. A. Warrell.)

Malarial haemoglobinuria and Blackwater fever

Blackwater fever was a common manifestation of severe falciparum malaria in long-term European expatriates, particularly in Africa in the earlier part of the century. Typically, the patient had lived in a malarious area for months or longer, had had previous attacks of malaria and was taking quinine sporadically for prophylaxis and treatment. The next attack of malaria began with the familiar symptoms but after a few days the patient developed pain in the abdomen or loin, bilious vomiting, diarrhoea, polyuria followed by oliguria or anuria. The urine became mahogany-coloured or even black. The signs included fever, tachycardia, tender hepatosplenomegaly, profound anaemia, jaundice and prostration. Renal failure was a common feature as was hypertension and coma, but the parasitaemia and fever were mild or absent. Severe intravascular haemolysis in the absence of hyperparasitaemia was usually attributed to immune haemolysis of quinine-sensitized erythrocytes but this was never proved. More commonly these days, patients with inherited abnormalities of the erythrocyte enzymes such as glucose-6-phosphate dehydrogenase deficiency haemolyse and develop haemoglobinuria in response to oxidant antimalarial drugs such as primaquine or chloroquine (Plate 6). Such patients may not even be infected with malaria.

Laboratory investigations in severe falciparum malaria

Microscopical diagnosis and measurement of parasite density are described in Chapter 6. Anaemia is usual and serum haptoglobins may be undetectable indicating haemolysis. Neutrophil leucocytosis is associated with a bad prognosis and occurs whether or not there is a complicating bacterial infection. Thrombocytopenia is usual and does not correlate with severity. Prolonged prothrombin and partial thromboplastin times and other evidence of disseminated intravascular coagulation are found in less than 10% of patients. Plasma total and indirect (unconjugated) bilirubin concentrations are increased consistent with haemolysis, but in some patients with very high total bilirubin concentrations, conjugated bilirubin predominated indicating hepatocyte dysfunction. In some patients there is evidence of cholestasis. Serum albumin concentration is reduced. Serum aminotransferases 5′ nucleotidase and especially lactic dehydrogenase are moderately elevated but not into the range seen in viral hepatitis. Metabolic acidosis is usually explained by a lactic acidosis. Mild hyponatraemia is associated with increased plasma osmolality. Mild hypocalcaemia and hypophosphataemia have been described especially when the patient had been given blood or glucose infusions. Biochemical evidence of generalized rhabdomyolysis (elevated serum creatine phosphokinase concentration, myoglobinaemia and myoglobinuria) has frequently been found in Gambian children.

In cerebral malaria, the cerebrospinal fluid (CSF) shows a mild lymphocyte pleocytosis (rarely more than 15 cells/μl) and increased protein concentration. The CSF glucose concentration is appropriate to the blood glucose but may be very low or undetectable in patients with profound hypoglycaemia. The urine may contain protein, erythrocytes, haemoglobin and red cell casts.

Gram-negative rod bacteria including *Escherichia coli* and *Pseudomonas aeruginosa* have been cultured from the blood of adult patients with severe falciparum malaria, some of whom had clinical features of bacteraemic shock ('algid malaria'). In children, blood cultures are very rarely positive, but in the Gambia there is an association between malaria and non-typhoid Salmonella septicaemia.

Vivax malaria

The incubation period for vivax malaria in non-immune people is usually between 12 and 17 days but may be prolonged to 8 to 9 months or even longer. Some strains of *P. vivax*, especially from temperate regions, show consistently long incubation periods of 250–637 days (for example, *P. v. hibernans* from Russia north of latitude 52°N, and *P. v. multinucleatum* in central and north China). Only about one-third of imported cases of vivax malaria present within a month of returning from the malarious area and in 5–10% symptoms are delayed for more than a year after their return. The primary attack begins with headache, pain in the neck, nausea and general malaise; these prodromal symptoms are mild or absent in relapses. The fever is irregular for 2 to 4 days, but soon becomes 'intermittent', i.e. with marked swings between the morning and the evening. At first there is no regularity in the pattern of fever because several broods of the parasite are not synchronized, but soon the 48-hour periodicity becomes established. Febrile paroxysms occur chiefly in the afternoon or evening and the classical cold, hot and sweating stages become evident. The temperature may rise to 40.6°C (105°F) or higher. Nausea and vomiting may be distressing and herpes of the lips is common. Dizziness and mild impairment of consciousness may occur but is transient. Cerebral vivax malaria has occasionally been reported, especially with the long incubation period of *P. v. multinucleatum* in China, but in none of the reported cases has mixed falciparum infection or another encephalopathy been adequately excluded. Severe vivax malaria has been described in the past (for example, in Europe) possibly related to malnutrition and other intercurrent diseases. However, although the symptoms may be severe and temporarily incapacitating, especially in non-immune people, the acute mortality of vivax malaria is very low. For example, there were no deaths during the 1969 Sri Lanka epidemic of half a million cases of vivax malaria. It is important to remember that most people of West African origin are resistant to *P. vivax* infection because of the rarity of Duffy blood group antigen alleles Fy^a and Fy^b required for erythrocyte invasion. Mild anaemia is a common result of vivax malaria but it may become severe and even life-threatening in children and debilitated patients after relapsing infections. Thrombocytopenia is common. Patients may become mildly jaundiced with tender hepatosplenomegaly. Splenic rupture, which carries a high mortality rate, is more common with vivax than falciparum malaria. It results from acute rapid enlargement of the spleen with or without trauma. Chronically enlarged spleens are less vulnerable. Splenic rupture presents with abdominal pain and guarding, haemorrhagic shock, fever and a rapidly falling haematocrit, features which may be misattributed to malaria itself.

During the early phase of the primary attack, parasites are scanty in the peripheral blood, but they are common when the tertian rhythm of fever is established. Gametocytes appear in the blood about 1 week after the onset of the primary attack.

Relapses of vivax malaria

A single untreated attack consists of a week or more of repeated febrile paroxysms. In about 60% of untreated or inadequately treated cases, clinical symptoms recur after a period of quiescence which depends on the strain of parasite: 'short-term' relapses are seen during the first 8–10 weeks after the primary attack; 'long-term' relapses between the 30th and 40th weeks after the primary attack. Vivax infections acquired in different parts of the

Plate 1 Retinal haemorrhages in a Thai patient with cerebral malaria showing typical 'Roth's spot' pattern with pale centres clustered around the macula (© D. A. Warrell.)

Plate 2 Profound anaemia (haemoglobin 1.2 g/dl) in a young Kenyan boy with heavy *Plasmodium falciparum* parasitaemia (© D. A. Warrell.)

Plate 3 Deep jaundice in a Vietnamese man with severe falciparum malaria (© D. A. Warrell.)

Plate 4 Palatal petechiae in a British patient with imported falciparum malaria complicated by severe thrombocytopenia (© D. A. Warrell.)

Plate 5 Bleeding from the gingival sulci in a Thai patient with cerebral malaria complicated by disseminated intravascular coagulation (© D. A. Warrell.)

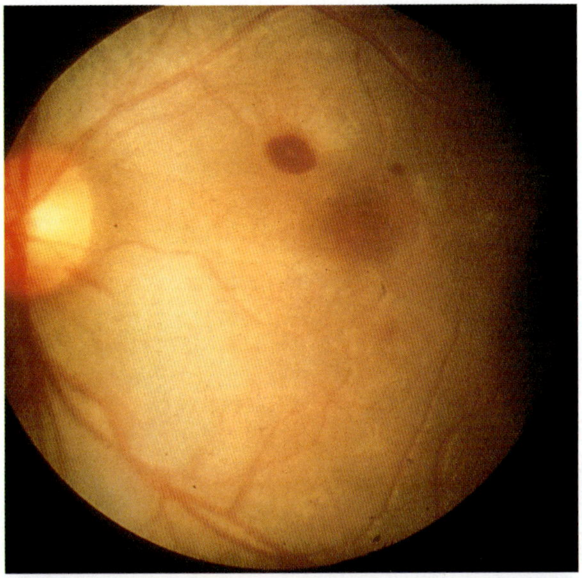

1

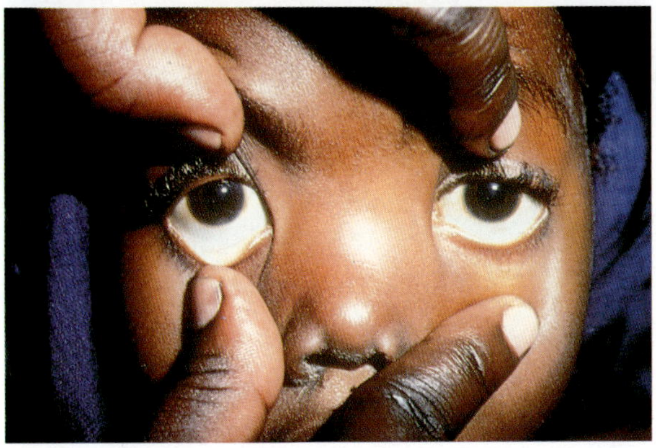

2

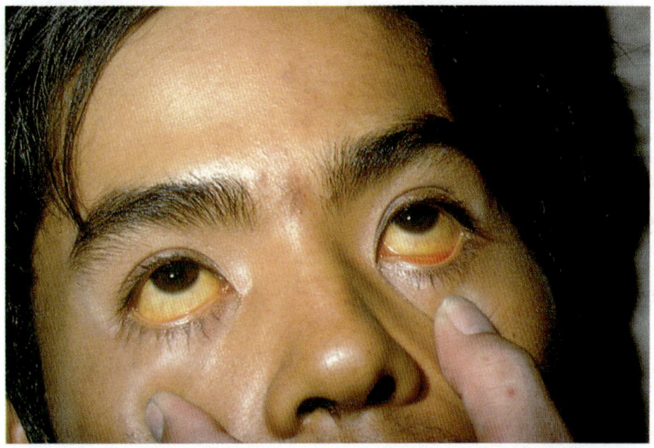

3

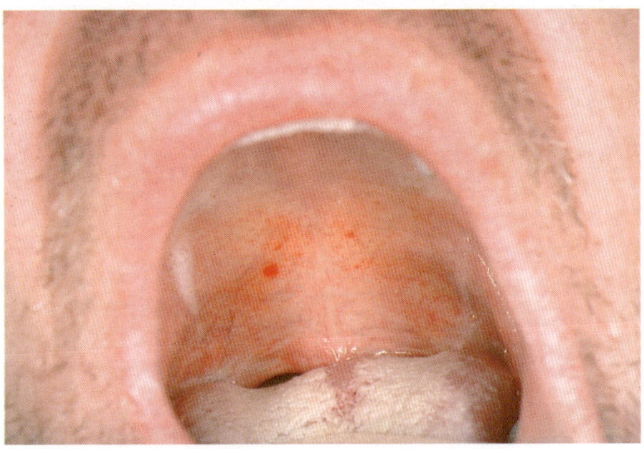

4

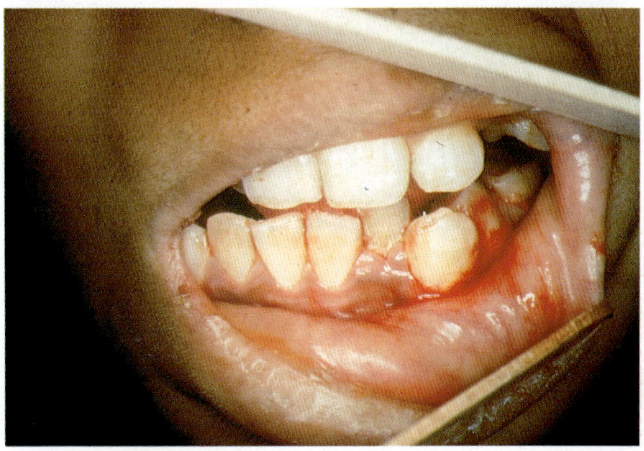

5

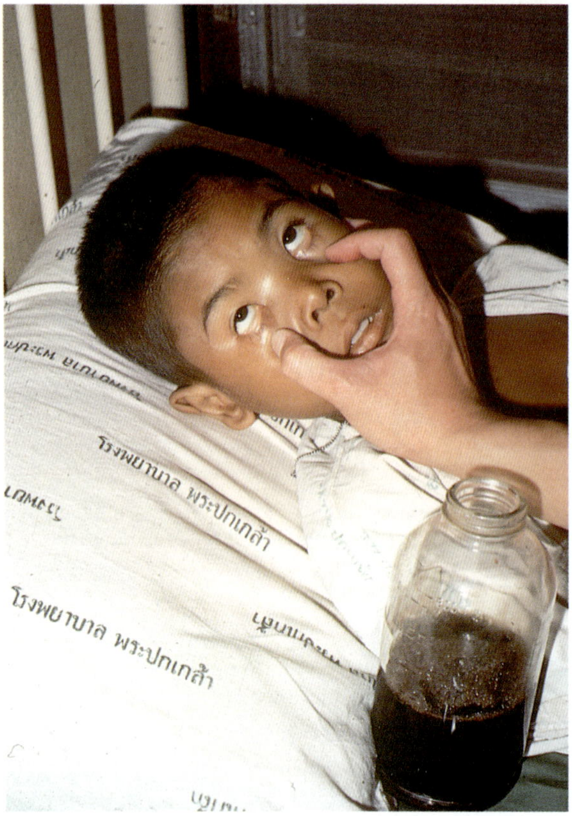

6

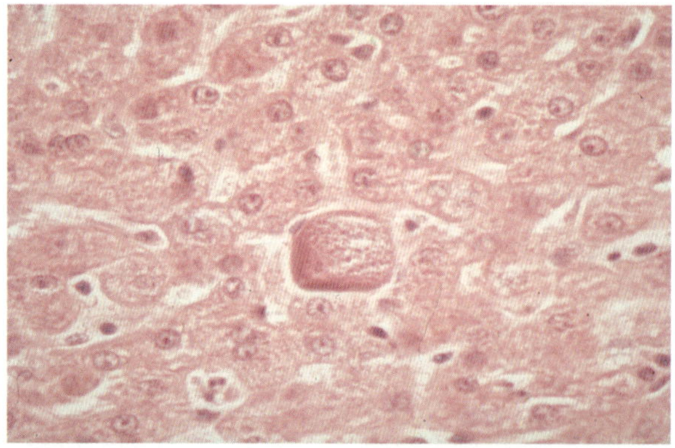

7

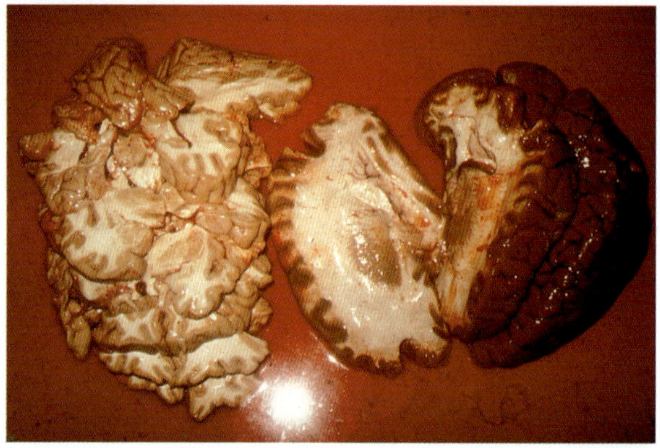

8

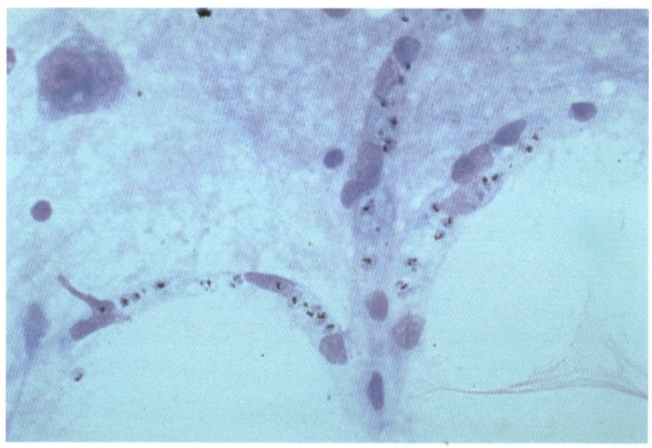

9

Plate 6 Haemoglobinuria in a Thai patient with glucose-6-phosphate dehydrogenase deficiency who took an oxidant antimalarial drug (primaquine) (© D. A. Warrell.)

Plate 7 Central liver cell swollen with merozoite development in extra-erythrocytic phase. H & E (© N. Francis.)

Plate 8 Characteristic macroscopic appearance of the brain in cerebral malaria (right) showing leaden/slatey or plum-coloured cortex and petechial haemorrhages in the white matter compared with a normal brain (left) (Reproduced by courtesy of Dr U Hla Mon.)

Plate 9 Smear from *post-mortem* needle necropsy of brain in a victim of cerebral malaria showing choking of small capillaries and venules with erythrocytes containing mature forms of the parasite with pigment (Reproduced by courtesy of Dr M. J. Warrell.)

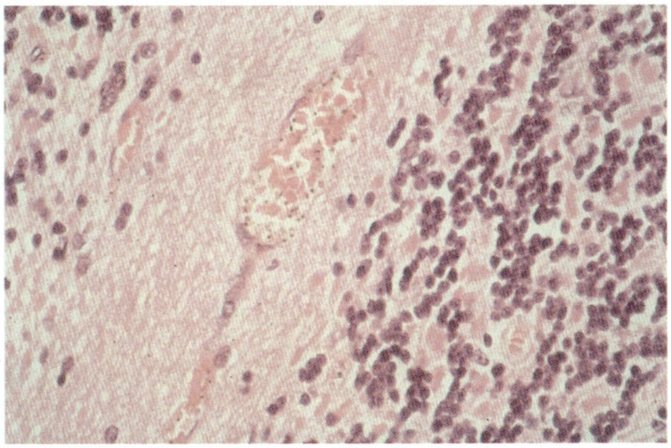

10

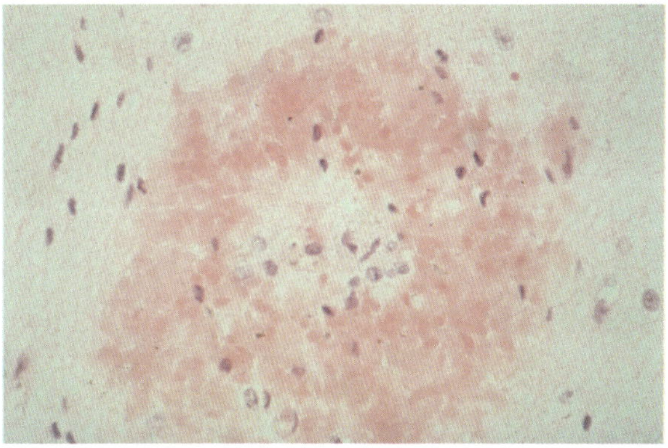

11

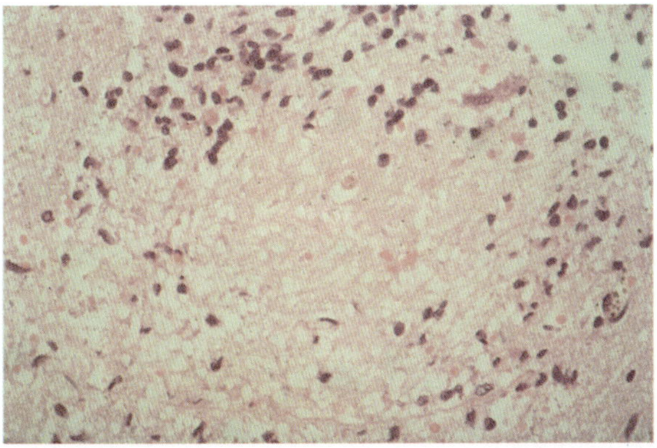

12

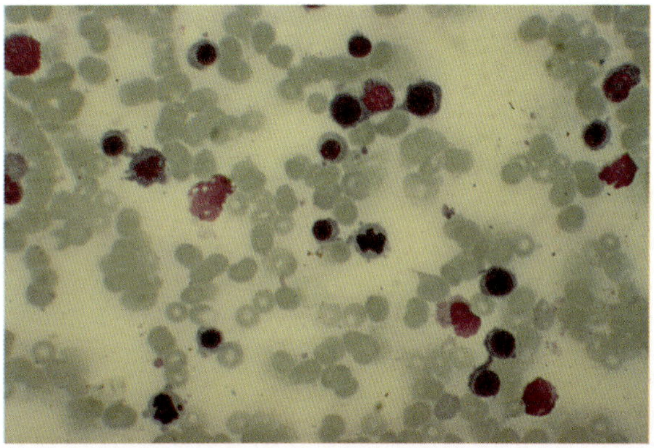

13

Plate 10 Section from cerebellum with parasitized red cells marginating in vessel. Note lack of oedema and lack of any inflammatory response. H & E (© N. Francis.)

Plate 11 Brain showing ring haemorrhage: small central vessel contains parasitized erythrocytes with pigment. Extravasated erythrocytes are largely non-parasitized, a few contain pigment. H & E (© N. Francis.)

Plate 12 Dürck's granuloma: demyelinized central part with ring of microglial cell proliferation. The small central vessel lumen is visible and parasitized erythrocytes in marginal small vessels are also visible. H & E (© N. Francis.)

Plate 13 Dyserythropoietic changes in the bone marrow of a patient with severe falciparum malaria. Normoblasts show intercytoplasmic bridging and multinuclearity (Reproduced by courtesy of Dr Szu Hee Lee.)

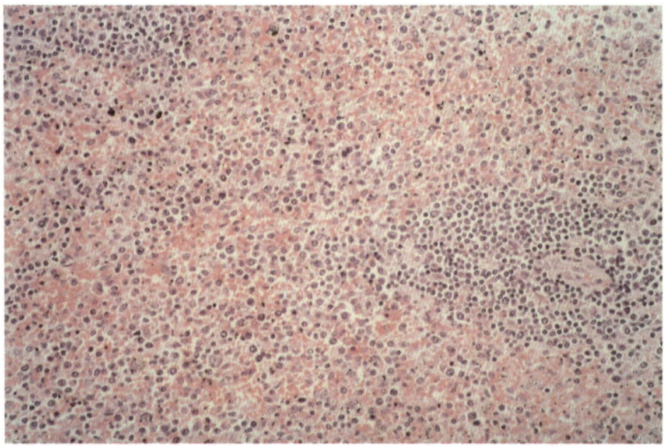

14

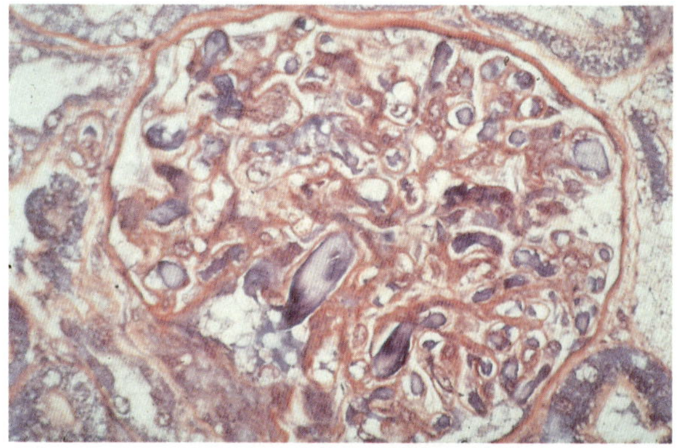

15

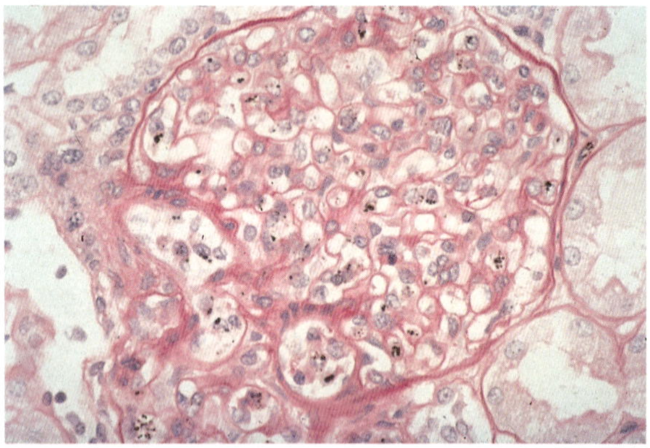

16

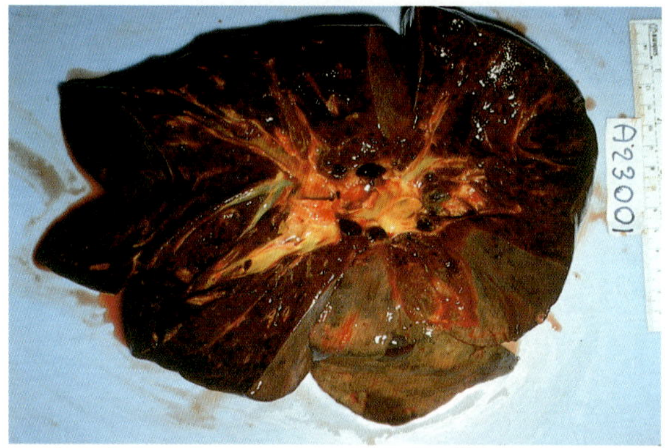

17

Plate 14 Spleen showing expanded red and white pulp. Red pulp shows increased white cells and macrophages plus diffuse pigment deposition. H & E (© N. Francis.)

Plate 15 Kidney showing case with extensive capillary fibrin thrombi PTAH stain. (© N. Francis.)

Plate 16 Kidney: hypercellular glomerulus with pigment-laden macrophages in capillary lumina. Periodic acid–Schiff (© N. Francis.)

Plate 17 Haemorrhagic lung in a patient dying of severe falciparum malaria (© D. A. Warrell.)

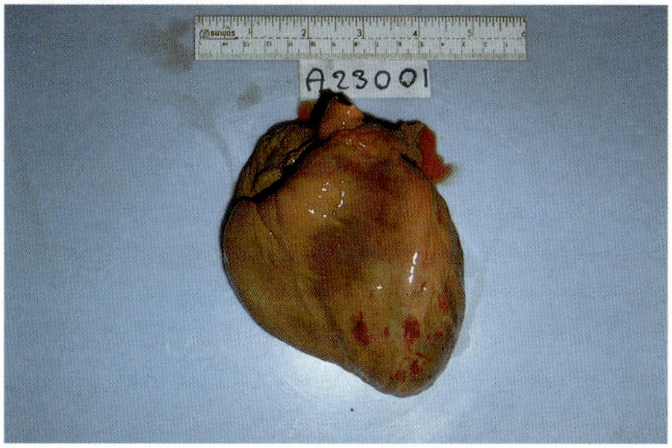

18

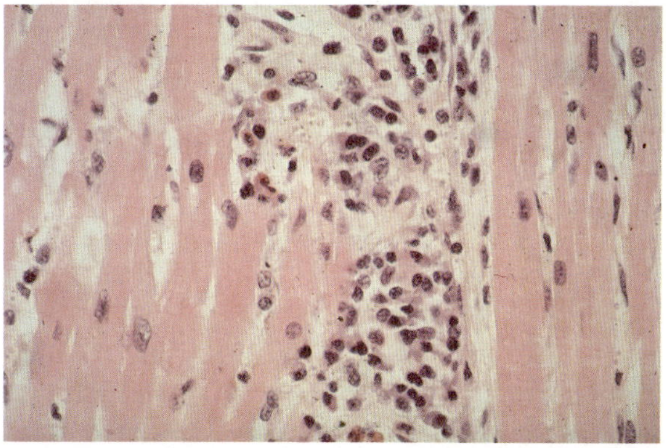

19

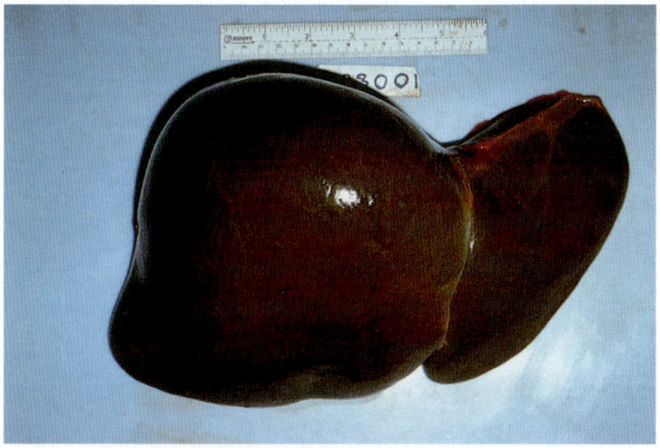

20

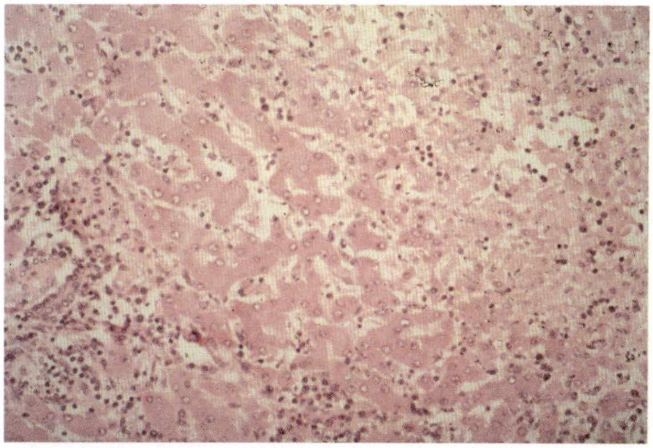

21

Plate 18 Epicardial petechial haemorrhages in a fatal case of algid malaria. (© D. A. Warrell.)

Plate 19 Heart: interstitial chronic inflammation between myocardial fibres and small vessels (upper centre) showing parasitized erythrocytes. H & E (© N. Francis.)

Plate 20 Characteristic enlarged black liver in severe falciparum malaria (© D. A. Warrell.)

Plate 21 Liver with portal and sinusoidal inflammation and marked pericentral necrosis (mid right) (© N. Francis.)

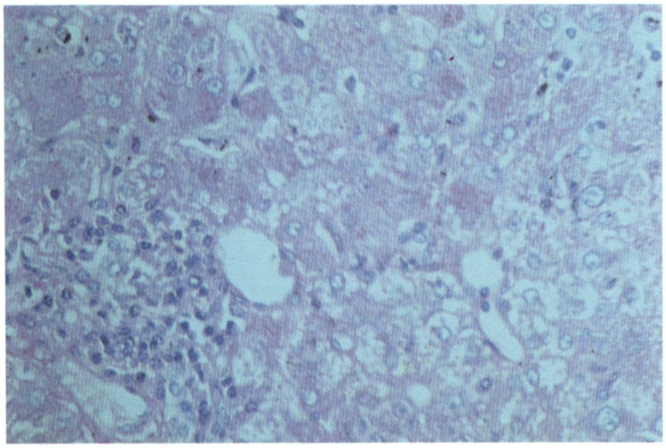

22(a)

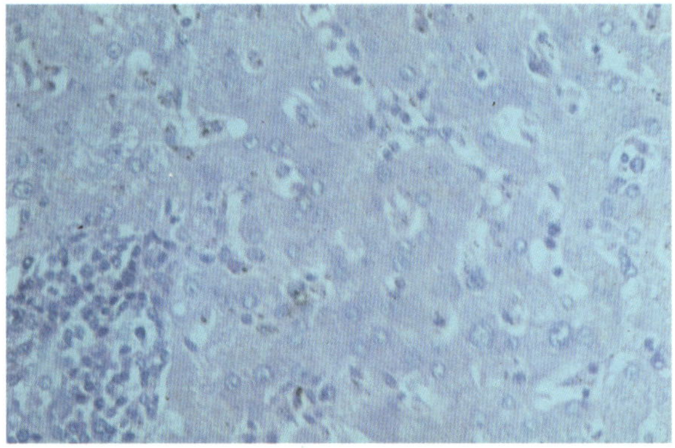

22(b)

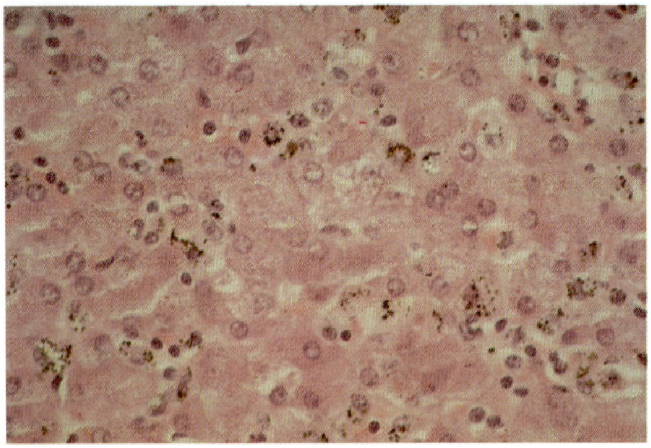

23

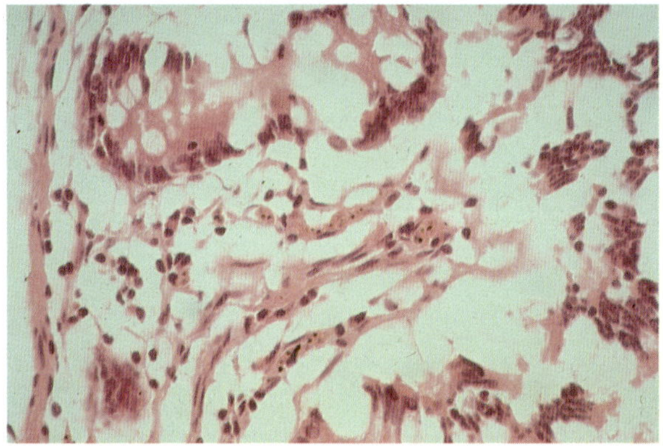

24

Plate 22 Liver from a fatal case of falciparum malaria showing periodic acid–Schiff stain for glycogen (a) before and (b) after digestion of glycogen with diastase (Reproduced by courtesy of Dr M. S. Dunnill.)

Plate 23 Liver showing extensive pigment granule deposition in hepatic sinusoids with parasitized erythrocytes discernible and minimal liver cell damage. H & E (© N. Francis.)

Plate 24 Small intestine showing *postmortem* autolysis but numerous parasitized erythrocytes in lamina propria capillary vessels. H & E (© N. Francis.)

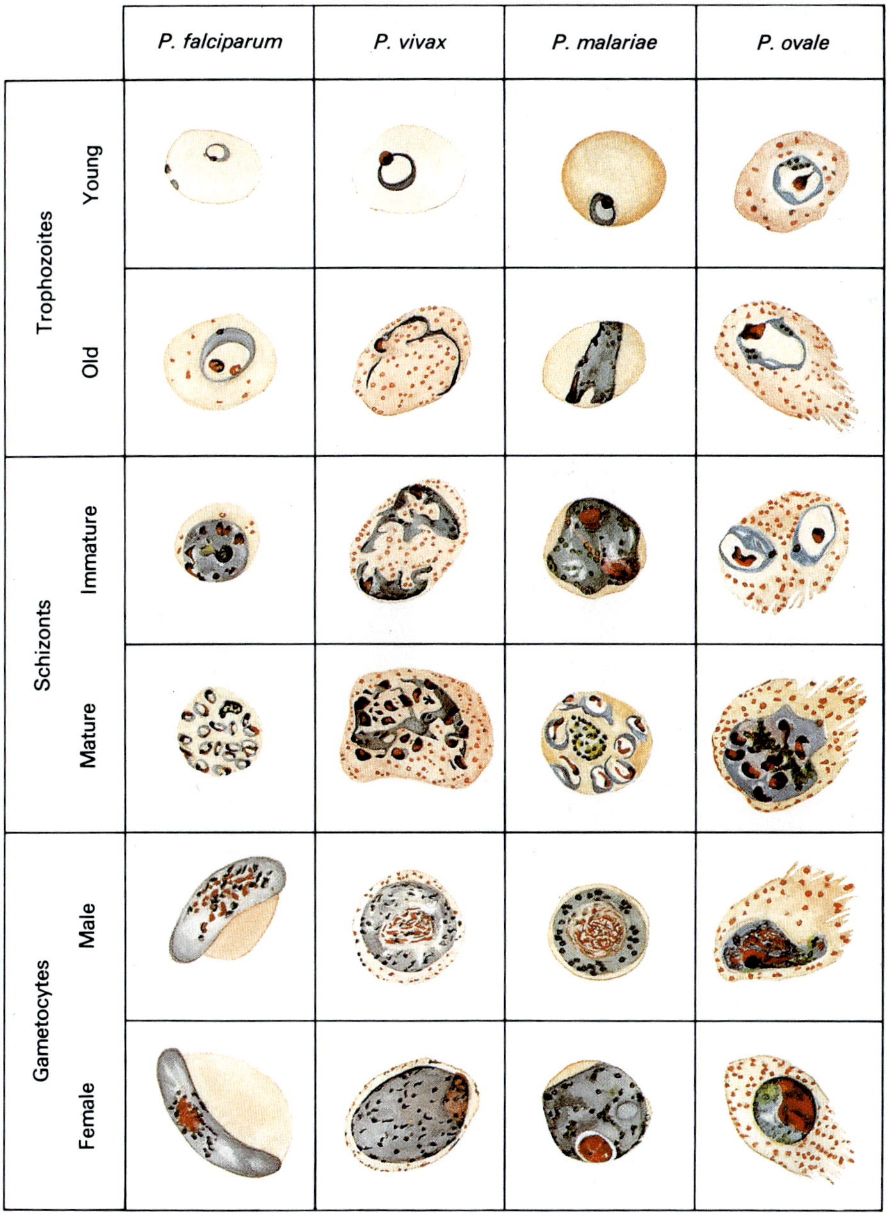

25

Plate 25 Appearance of parasite stages in Giemsa-stained film

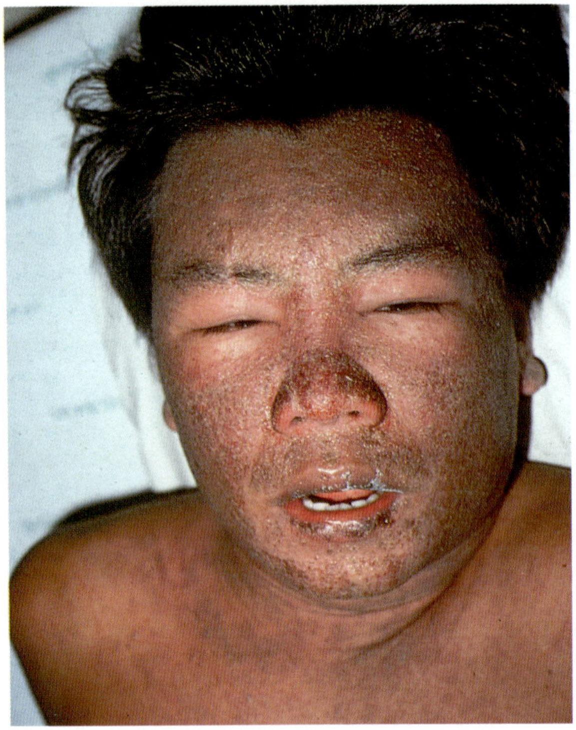

26

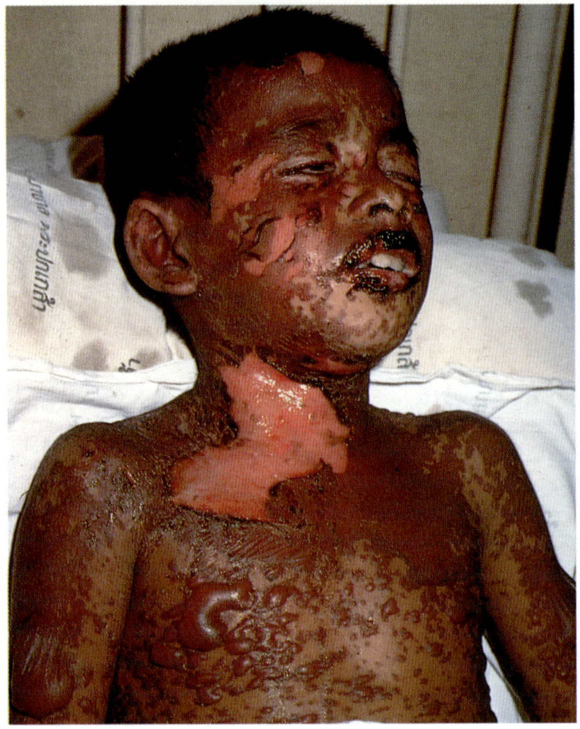

27

Plate 26 Stevens–Johnson syndrome in a patient who took sulfonamide–pyrimethamine (© D. A. Warrell.)

Plate 27 Toxic epidermal necrolysis in a child who took sulfonamide–pyrimethamine. (© D. A. Warrell.)

Plate 28 Global distribution of multidrug-resistant malaria 1992 (Reproduced by courtesy of Dr Shapira.)

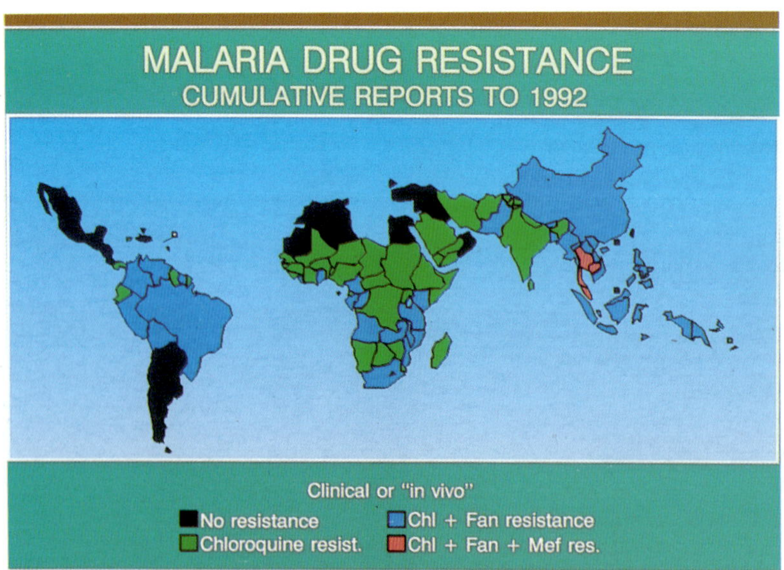

28

world show striking differences in the duration of the incubation period and the occurrence of periods of latency. These differences have been broadly correlated with climatic zones. Prolonged latency has been observed chiefly in temperate regions.

In most of the temperate or subtropical areas the incidence of vivax malaria shows a bimodal curve, with a peak in the spring and another in the summer. The first peak is composed of long-term relapses or of delayed primary attacks of those infections contracted in the previous summer; the second peak consists of primary attacks of recent infections. Prolonged primary latency must not be confused with the delayed appearance of the infection produced by the use of suppressive antimalarial drugs. Tropical strains of vivax malaria show a different pattern of relapses with short latencies.

Ovale malaria

The clinical picture of ovale malaria closely resembles that of vivax malaria. The febrile paroxysms may be as severe but spontaneous recovery is more common and there are fewer relapses. The parasite often remains latent and is easily suppressed by other more virulent species of *Plasmodia*. It may appear in the blood when the others have declined. Mixed infections in which *P. ovale* is found are common in those exposed to malaria in tropical Africa. Anaemia and splenic enlargement are less severe than in vivax malaria and the risk of splenic rupture is lower.

Quartan (malariae) malaria

The incubation period of quartan malaria is never less than 18 days and may be as long as 30–40 days. The clinical picture of the primary attack resembles that of vivax malaria but prodromal symptoms and rigors may be more severe. The febrile paroxysms are more regularly spaced and often occur in the late afternoon. Anaemia is less pronounced and although splenomegaly may be particularly gross, the risk of splenic rupture seems to be lower than with vivax malaria.

Plasmodium malariae has no hypnozoite form or persisting hepatic cycle. However, undetectable parasitaemia may continue with symptomatic recrudescences, frequent during the first year and then at longer intervals up to 52 years after the last exposure to infection. Asymptomatic parasitaemia may be detected in blood donors or as a result of transplacental spread to a neonate. All stages of asexual parasites are usually present in the peripheral blood at the same time, but parasitaemia rarely exceeds 1% of the erythrocytes.

Quartan malarial nephrosis

In parts of East and West Africa, Guyana in South America, India, South-east Asia and Papua New Guinea, there is strong epidemiological evidence that *P. malariae* is an important cause of nephrotic syndrome. Only a small minority of those exposed to repeated *P. malariae* infections develop the condition, suggesting that additional factors are involved. The histological appearances, which are not entirely specific, are of glomerulosclerosis with glomerular deposits of *P. malariae* antigen in about 25% of the cases examined. Half the cases develop nephrotic syndrome before the age of 15 years. The prognosis is poor. Few patients respond to corticosteroids, but there is some response to azathioprine and cyclophosphamide in patients whose renal biopsies show coarse or mixed granular patterns of immunofluorescence. Antimalarial treatment does not reverse the lesion, but the condition could be prevented by antimalarial prophylaxis and has disappeared in countries such as Guyana following eradication of *P. malariae.*

Monkey malarias

Human erythrocytes can be infected with strains of at least six species of simian malaria parasites (*Plasmodium brazilianum*, *Plasmodium cynomolgi*, *Plasmodium inui*, *Plasmodium knowlesi*, *Plasmodium schwetzi* and *Plasmodium simium*). Zoonotic infections of humans and accidental laboratory infections are rare. High fever and other generalized symptoms have been described but no cerebral or other severe complications. No human mortality has been reported. Parasitaemia may remain undetectable for 2 to 6 days after the start of symptoms. The periodicity of fever is quotidian for *P. knowlesi* and tertian for *P. simium* and *P. cynomolgi*. Infectivity and virulence may be enhanced by repeated passage in humans.

Malaria in pregnancy and the puerperium

In those parts of the tropics where malarial transmission is unstable and young women have a poor degree of acquired immunity, malaria remains a major cause of maternal death, abortion, stillbirth, premature delivery and low birthweight. In some holoendemic areas the clinical symptoms and parasitaemia are more severe in primiparous than multiparous women, but in many parts of Africa the only definite consequence of malaria in pregnancy seems to be reduced birthweight of the infant. In non-immune people, cerebral and other forms of falciparum malaria are more common in pregnancy and the mortality is higher than in other patients. Malaria contributes to the severe anaemia which complicates pregnancy in many tropical countries. Progressive anaemia resulting from chronic hookworm infection, malnutrition and repeated attacks of malaria may result in cardiac failure with generalized oedema in late pregnancy. Pregnant women are particularly vulnerable to quinine-induced hyperinsulinaemic hypoglycaemia even when their malaria is otherwise uncomplicated. Hypoglycaemia, which may be misleadingly asymptomatic, may also develop in the absence of treatment with cinchona alkaloids.

Congenital and neonatal malaria

Vertical transmission of malaria across the placenta from mother to foetus is diagnosed when parasitaemia is found in the neonate within 7 days of birth, or later if there is no possibility of post-partum infection by mosquito bite or blood transfusion. In malaria endemic regions, the incidence of congenital malaria is usually extremely low despite the high prevalence of placental infection. The incidence is much higher in infants born to non-immune mothers and increases during malaria epidemics. All four species can produce congenital infection; *P. falciparum* and *P. vivax* are most commonly reported, but outside the endemic area *P. malariae* causes a disproportionate number of cases because of its very long persistence. Clinical features include fever, irritability, feeding problems, anaemia, hepatosplenomegaly and jaundice.

Malaria in children

The child at first appears restless or drowsy, refuses food and may complain of headache and nausea. There may be pallor of the skin or, in dark-skinned races, of the nails and mucous membranes with slight cyanosis. As the temperature rises thirst may be marked; breast-fed infants make frequent attempts to suck the breast but this is soon abandoned, possibly because of nausea. A clear-cut cold stage and a definite rigor are uncommon in infants and children. Vomiting of bile-stained material is common and may make oral therapy impossible, but it is seldom sufficient to result in severe dehydration or electrolyte depletion. The stools are often loose and dark green with mucus but there is no blood or pus cells. Infants may appear to have an acute abdomen and older children may refer pain to the liver or spleen and may be constipated.

The temperature is very variable; in some it is only moderate but in the majority it is high (40°C), often continuous or irregular and the child is flushed and sweaty. Febrile convulsions may occur even when the temperature is only moderately elevated. They usually last only a few minutes followed by a quick recovery of consciousness, but if the postictal coma lasts more than about 30 minutes cerebral malaria must be suspected. There is no easy distinction between prolonged impairment of consciousness associated with frequent febrile convulsions and true cerebral malaria, implying an underlying encephalopathy. The liver often enlarges and may be slightly tender. Many days may pass before splenic enlargement can be detected clinically, especially in the primary attack in non-immune children. Splenomegaly develops earlier in vivax malaria, less rapidly in falciparum malaria and very slowly in quartan malaria. In most cases the urine shows no specific abnormalities; mild albuminuria, scanty casts and a few red and white cells might also be found in fevers of other causes.

The manifestations of malaria in infants and children inhabiting highly endemic areas are even more variable. In tropical Africa, a small proportion of infants may be found with a low-grade parasitaemia and few if any symptoms apart from slight restlessness, lack of appetite, sweating, anaemia and occasional rises of temperature. After a variable interval, immunity acquired passively from the mother declines and the clinical attacks become more severe. Children living in a highly endemic malarious area without chemoprophylaxis or any protection from mosquito bites and continuously exposed to the infection are, until the age of about 5 years, at a particularly critical stage of their host–parasite relationship. Many of them die of cerebral malaria, severe malarial anaemia or with repeated generalized convulsions and prostration. Some, after several successive attacks, achieve a relative tolerance to the infection and in these the clinical picture of malaria may be mild consisting of fever, fretfulness, tiredness, cough and diarrhoea. Many indigenous children, particularly in tropical Africa, have enlarged spleens and livers and malaria parasites in their blood without any other signs of the disease other than a degree of anaemia to which other factors such as malnutrition, schistosomiasis and intestinal parasites may contribute. Cerebral and other severe forms of falciparum malaria (described above) occur most commonly between the ages of 6 months and 3 years in children growing up in endemic regions. They are responsible for the very high mortality of malaria, which amounts to more than a million deaths a year in Africa alone.

Tropical splenomegaly syndrome

(Also known as hyperreactive malarial splenomegaly or 'big spleen disease'.)

In the malaria endemic regions of Africa, Asia, South America and the western Pacific, some young adults show a progressive, sometime massive, enlargement of the spleen instead of the usual reduction in splenic size after childhood. The prevalence of this condition reaches 80% in some parts of Papua New Guinea. There is a past history of repeated attacks of fever or malaria but parasitaemia is often not detectable when the patient presents with abdominal distention, a vague dragging sensation and occasional episodes of severe sharp pain with peritonism, suggesting perisplenitis or splenic infarction. Anaemia, which may be exacerbated by haemolytic episodes especially in pregnancy, may become severe enough to cause the features of high output cardiac failure. The spleen may be enormous, filling the left iliac fossa, extending across the midline and anteriorly producing a visible mass with an obvious notch (Fig. 3.12). In 80% of patients there is non-tender hepatomegaly, especially on the left lobe. Patients may become cachectic and show chronic ulceration of the legs. The untreated mortality rate is high and is usually attributable to overwhelming infection arising in the skin or respiratory system.

A definition of this syndrome, which varies in different parts of the world, includes gross splenomegaly (more than 10 cm below the costal margin), elevation of serum IgM and clinical and immunological response within 3 months of starting continuous antimalarial prophylaxis. Evidence of immunity to malaria and hepatic sinusoidal lymphocytosis are additional criteria.

The syndrome seems to be an abnormal immune response to recurrent malaria infections with excessive IgM production, formation of macromolecular IgM aggregates and hypertrophy of the splenic reticuloendothelial system which phagocytoses these immune complexes. In Africa, peripheral lymphocytosis results from increased circulating B lymphocytes, whereas T cell numbers are normal. In Flores Island, Indonesia, T8 cells were reduced and there was no increase in B cell numbers.

The blood picture is that of hypersplenism (normochromic, normocytic anaemia, reticulocytosis, thrombocytopenia and leucopenia) and, especially in West Africa, peripheral lymphocytosis which may

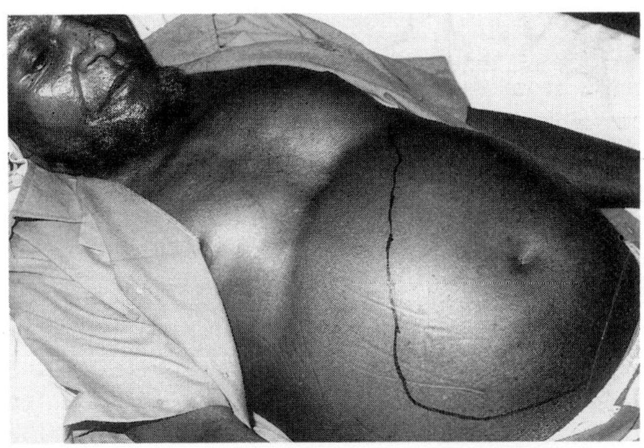

Fig. 3.12 Papua New Guinean man with tropical splenomegaly syndrome. (© D. A. Warrell.)

Table 3.5 Differential diagnosis of malarial syndromes

Symptom	Diagnosis
1. Acute fever	Heat stroke, hyperpyrexia of other causes, other infections, other causes of fever
[Pregnant woman]	Infection of urinary tract, uterus, adnexa, breast
2. + Paroxysms (rigors)	Other infections, especially lobar pneumonia, ascending cholangitis, pyelonephritis and viral hepatitis, acute intravascular haemolysis
3. + Confusion, obtundation, coma ('Cerebral malaria')	Viral, bacterial, fungal, protozoal (e.g. African trypanosomiasis) or helminthic meningoencephalitis, cerebral abscess Head injury, intracranial bleed/thrombosis/embolism, intoxications (e.g. insecticides), poisonings (e.g. antimalarial drugs), metabolic (diabetes, hypoglycaemia, uraemia, hepatic failure, hyponatraemia) Septicaemias, 'cerebral' typhoid
4. + Convulsions	Encephalitides, metabolic encephalopathies, hyperpyrexia, cerebrovascular accidents, epilepsy, drug and alcohol intoxications, poisoning
[Pregnant woman]	Eclampsia, literiosis
[Children]	Febrile convulsions, Reye's syndrome
5. + Bleeding/clotting abn	Septicaemias (e.g. meningococcaemia), viral haemorrhagic fever, rickettsial infection
[Pregnant woman]	Postpartum defibrination syndrome
6. + Abnormal behaviour ('Malarial psychosis')	Psychosis, alcohol intoxication/withdrawal, other drugs and poisons, viral encephalitis (e.g. *Herpes simplex*, rabies etc.)
7. + Jaundice	Viral hepatitis, yellow fever, leptospirosis, relapsing fevers, septicaemias, haemolysis, biliary obstruction, hepatic necrosis (drugs, poisons)
[Pregnant woman]	Acute fatty liver, cholestasis
[Neonate]	Rhesus incompatibility, other intrauterine infections (e.g. cytomegalovirus, *Herpes simplex*, rubella, toxoplasmosis, syphilis)
8. + Nausea, vomiting, diarrhoea ('Bilious remittent fever')	Travellers' diarrhoea, dysentery, enteric fever, other bacterial infections, inflammatory bowel disease
9. + Abdominal pain	Ruptured spleen, enteric fevers, amoebic liver abscess, acute pancreatitis, perforation, peritonitis
[Pregnant woman]	Ruptured ectopic pregnancy
10. + Haemoglobinuria ('Blackwater fever')	Drug-induced haemolysis (e.g. oxidant antimalarials in glucose-6-phosphate dehydrogenase-deficient patient), favism, transfusion reaction, dark urine of other causes (e.g. myoglobinuria, urobilinogen, porphobilinogen)
11. + Acute renal failure	Septicaemias, yellow fever, leptospirosis, drug intoxications, poisonings, prolonged hypotension
12. + Shock ('Algid malaria')	Septicaemic shock, haemorrhagic shock (e.g. massive gastrointestinal bleed, ruptured spleen), perforated bowel, dehydration, hypovolaemia, myocarditis

cause confusion with chronic lymphatic leukaemia. There is a lymphocytic infiltration of the bone marrow. The raised serum IgM is polyclonal. Immune complexes, cryoglobulins, rheumatoid factor-like antiglobulins and other autoantibodies have been detected. Levels of both IgM and IgG antimalarial antibodies are raised.

Differential diagnosis of malaria

The parasitological diagnosis of malaria is discussed in Chapter 6. Malaria must be considered in the differential diagnosis of any acute febrile illness in a patient who could have been exposed to malaria by mosquito bite or from the rare routes of transmission such as transplacental (in a neonate), blood transfusion, contact with blood-contaminated needles and organ/tissue transplants. Malaria presents many different clinical features, none of which is specific. Patients with fever and prostration have often been misdiagnosed as having influenza. Those with cerebral malaria presenting with altered behaviour, impaired consciousness or convulsions have been misdiagnosed as having viral encephalitis or psychosis. Those with jaundice have been misdiagnosed as viral hepatitis and those with bleeding and clotting abnormalities as having viral haemorrhagic fever.

The discovery of parasitaemia provides an explanation for symptoms in non-immune patients, but in those who are immune, parasitaemia may be an incidental finding with no diagnostic relevance to the patient's current illness. Failure to discover parasites even after repeated examinations, does not exclude the diagnosis of malaria and should not delay the start of a therapeutic trial in patients with severe disease who could have been exposed to the infection.

Some of the commoner and more important differential diagnoses of the various clinical syndromes caused by malaria are given in Table 3.5.

Chapter 4

Pathology and pathophysiology of human malaria

N. Francis and D. A. Warrell

Introduction

Following mosquito transmitted infection by all four species of human malaria the sporozoites injected by the mosquito invade the liver where they undergo an initial pre- or exo-erythrocytic cycle. In the case of *Plasmodium vivax* and *Plasmodium ovale* infections, arrested development of some sporozoites results in latent or dormant forms (hypnozoites) from which the infection may later relapse. The pre-erythrocytic stage of infection produces minimal histopathological changes (Plate 7) and absolutely no detectable symptoms or functional disturbances in the host. Pathological processes in malaria are the result of the erythrocytic cycle. Merozoites invade erythrocytes where they develop through ring forms to trophozoites and eventually schizonts. In the case of *Plasmodium falciparum* this process results in the following changes to the infected erythrocyte: altered membrane transport mechanisms, decreased deformability and other mechanical and rheological changes, development (in some strains) of protuberances or knobs beneath the surface membrane, expression of variant surface (strain specific) neoantigens, development of cytoadherent and rosetting properties and digestion of haemoglobin to pigment.*

***Malarial pigment is a blackish brown acid haematin with characteristic birefringency with polarized light but without any positive staining characteristics with special staining techniques. Ultrastructurally it can be identified by its rectangular crystalline structure and solubility in alkaline lead citrate, leaving electron-lucent clear spaces.**

The secondary effects of these changes are related to the host's immunological response to parasite antigens and altered red cell surface membranes such as the stimulation of the reticulo-endothelial system, changes in regional blood flow and vascular endothelium and systemic complications of altered biochemistry, anaemia, tissue and organ hypoxia and cytokine production.

The fever, febrile paroxysms, headache, a variety of aches and pains and prostration, the most familiar and consistent symptoms of an acute malaria attack, are probably the result of cytokines released from macrophages at the time of schizont rupture. Recent studies suggest that the malarial 'toxin' released at schizont rupture is the lipid, glycosyl phosphatidyl inositol (GPI), anchor of a parasite membrane protein (possibly MSP-1). Of the various cytokines, including interleukins and interferons, released by activated macrophages, tumour necrosis factor (TNF or cachexin) has been implicated as the cause of malarial fever. Earlier work in the pre-cytokine era had detected the release of 'endogenous pyrogen' at the time of the febrile paroxysm. Recently, an antiTNF monoclonal antibody was found to produce dose-related suppression of fever in Gambian children with cerebral malaria.

Pathological and pathophysiological changes in organs and tissues in malaria

Brain

Cerebral involvement appears to be confined to *P. falciparum* infection. More than 95% of adults and more than 85% of children who recover from cerebral malaria show no persistent neurological sequelae which suggests that much of the pathology must be transient and reversible. Interpretation of pathology should be carefully considered in relation to the clinical picture which falls into three broad groups: (a) cerebral malaria, as defined by strict clinical criteria (see Chapter 3) and from which the patient makes a full or partial recovery, (b) fatal cerebral malaria, and (c) malaria without clinical evidence of cerebral involvement. Obviously, studies of *postmortem* brain tissue confines our knowledge of the pathology to severe cases of cerebral malaria or those dying of other complications of severe malaria. The brains of some but not all cases of fatal cerebral malaria have been described as oedematous. Cerebral oedema is detected less commonly during life, using such techniques as computed tomographic (CT) and nuclear magnetic resonance (NMR) scans. In two of ten unusually severe cases of cerebral malaria in Thailand, cerebral oedema developed as an agonal phenomenon. Engorgement of arachnoid blood vessels with erythrocytes containing mature pigmented parasites results in the classical leaden or plum-coloured brain (Plate 8). Pigment deposition causes a grey cortex and there are numerous petechial haemorrhages in the white matter. Infarction, necrosis and large haemorrhages are, however, rare. In fatal malaria without neurological symptoms the brain usually shows no detectable macroscopic abnormalities.

Common to all pathological descriptions is the presence of large numbers of parasitized red cells, undergoing schizogony, in the small capillaries and venules (Plate 9; Fig. 4.1) and to a lesser extent margination of infected red cells in the medium-sized vessels (Plate 10). Although fibrin thrombi have been described in these vessels, they are not common and some detailed studies have failed to detect them. It may be that the presence of significant fibrin thrombi in the brain or elsewhere is a manifestation of disseminated intravascular coagulation rather than a direct consequence of malarial infection. The reduced deformability of the infected red cells together with their cytoadherence to endothelium and to uninfected cells (rosetting) leads to impairment of blood flow. Histological evidence of oedema and local inflammatory response to these plugged vessels is minimal. A consequence of sequestration is the local production of lactate and the systemic induction of interleukin-1 and tumour necrosis factor by macrophages. Ultrastructurally, cerebral endothelial cells show formation of microvillous cytoplasmic projections, some of which link to red cell membrane knobs via thin electron-dense strands (Fig. 4.2). The cause of these changes is not known but they have been seen in experimental

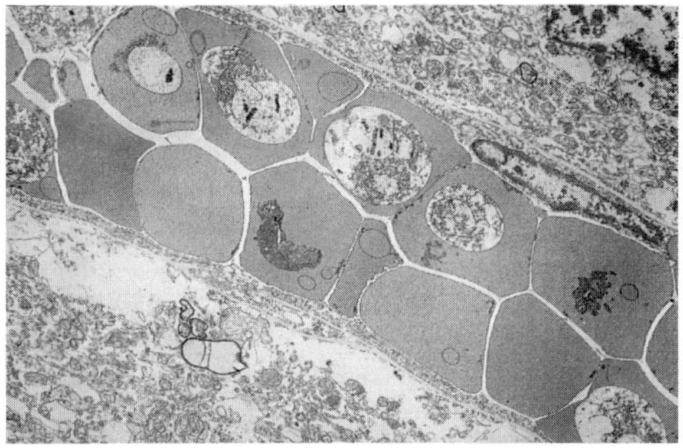

Fig. 4.1 Cerebral malaria electron micrograph showing numerous parasitized erythrocytes packing cerebral vessels. (© N. Francis.)

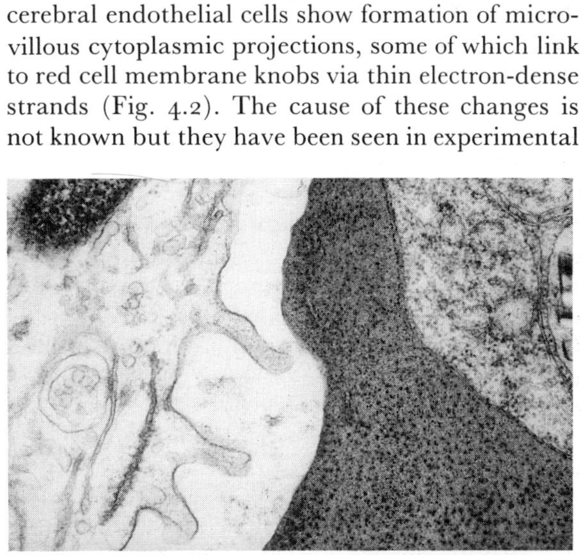

Fig. 4.2 Cerebral malaria electron micrograph showing formation of endothelial cell microvilli extending towards parasitized erythrocyte with parasites seen upper right. (© N. Francis.)

systems in association with free oxygen radical production.

In many patients focal ring haemorrhages are seen centred on small subcortical vessels (Plate 11). The reparative process following the ring haemorrhage leads to a small nodule or Dürck's granuloma, composed of microglial cell aggregates around the area of demyelination associated with the vessel (Plate 12). The pathogenesis of the haemorrhages is not known but may relate to increased capillary permeability resulting from the mechanisms indicated above. In foci of haemorrhage with extravasated parasitized red cells an inflammatory response is quite common in contrast to the findings around apparently intact vessels.

Clinical evidence of cerebral herniation in African children with cerebral malaria (see Chapter 3) has prompted a search for grooving of the midbrain by the free edge of the notch of the tentorium cerebelli and damage to the cerebellar tonsils caused by their herniation through the foramen magnum. So far, very little evidence has emerged that herniation of the brain is an important terminal event in patients dying with cerebral malaria.

Pathophysiology of cerebral malaria

Several hypotheses have been proposed to explain the development of coma. The permeability hypothesis arose from studies of *Plasmodium knowlesi*-infected rhesus monkeys which suggested that a circulating malarial toxin, possibly a kinin, caused increased cerebral vascular permeability, leakage of plasma across the blood–brain barrier, cerebral oedema and resulting coma. However, there is now considerable evidence against the permeability hypothesis, at least in South-east Asian adults. The passage of ^{125}I-labelled human serum albumin across the blood–cerebrospinal fluid (CSF) barrier in comatose humans was 300 times less than in the rhesus monkey model and did not decrease during convalescence. Cerebral oedema is demonstrable in only a small minority of comatose human patients and the CSF opening pressure measured at lumbar puncture was normal in 80% of patients; in a few of whom it was measured repeatedly during coma. Finally, dexamethasone, the most potent anti-inflammatory drug in experimental bacterial meningitis, did not prove beneficial to patients with cerebral malaria. However, the recent finding of elevated CSF opening pressures in African children with cerebral malaria indicates that, in this age group at least, intracranial pressure is usually elevated. This could be the result of raised intracranial blood volume, perhaps caused by massive sequestration of parasitized erythrocytes and vasodilation caused by their products, or of cerebral oedema.

There is increasing evidence in support of the mechanical hypothesis which postulates cytoadherence of parasitized erythrocytes to the endothelium of cerebral venules resulting in the sequestration and tight packing of infected cells in these vessels. This might lead to reduction in the supply of oxygen and other nutrients to the brain causing coma, or to local release of cytokines and activation of endothelial cells to release nitric oxide which can disturb neurotransmission. The appearance of cerebral capillaries choked with parasitized erythrocytes in patients dying of cerebral malaria illustrated above (Figs 4.1 and 4.2; Plates 11 and 12) has been familiar since the end of the nineteenth century. Ultrastructural studies have shown that up to 70% of erythrocytes in cerebral vessels were parasitized and that these cells were more tightly packed than in other organs and tissues. The degree of sequestration of parasitized erythrocytes in the cerebral microvascular has been found to correlate with depth of coma. No animal model yet described reproduces adequately the clinical and histopathological features of human cerebral malaria. However, some predictions of the mechanical hypothesis are testable in human patients. In Thai adults, comatose with cerebral malaria, cerebral blood flow was reduced relative to arterial oxygen content, one of its principal physiological determinants. Cerebral oxygen consumption and cerebral arteriovenous oxygen content differences were decreased and cerebral venous pO_2 increased. Arterial lactate concentration and cerebral lactate production were significantly higher while the patients were comatose than when they had just recovered consciousness and the CSF lactate concentration was elevated in patients with cerebral malaria and was significantly higher in fatal cases than survivors. These results confirm a switch to anaerobic cerebral glycolysis in patients comatose with cerebral malaria. The molecular basis for cytoadherence is currently of great interest and importance because of the possibility of preventing or reversing this key pathogenic process with competitively binding antibodies to the adhesin on the surface of the infected erythrocyte or against the ligand on the endothelial cell, or with a synthetic peptide fragment of these receptors. One possible adhesin is the large malarial protein PfEMP1 which shows appropriate properties and strain-specific diversity. Parasite-induced changes to the band 3 protein of the erythrocyte surface membrane may also allow binding to endothelial receptors. Candidate endothelial ligands are three glycoproteins – CD36, intercellular adhesion molecule-1 (ICAM-1) and the multifunctional adhesive protein thrombospondin. Clones of *P. falciparum* show a high rate of antigenic variation (perhaps 2% per generation) allowing them to express in successive generations adhesins to bind with a repertoire of endothelial receptors including the ones so far identified. Rosetting, the adhesion of non-parasitized to parasitized erythrocytes, is a property exhibited *in vitro* and *ex vivo* in the rat's mesoappendix model by some strains of *P. falciparum* and some sequestering animal malarias (*Plasmodium chabaudi*, *Plasmodium fragile* and *Plasmodium coatneyi*). Rosetting is affected by heparin (including non-anticoagulant analogues), divalent cations, pH and antibodies directed against the malarial protein HRP-1. In Gambian children with cerebral malaria all parasite isolates were able to form rosettes *in vitro* and the sera of these children lacked antirosetting antibodies.

The cytokine hypothesis is based on the observation that in African children with cerebral malaria, plasma concentrations of TNF, interleukin-1α and other cytokines correlate with disease severity, as judged by parasitaemia, hypoglycaemia, case fatality and the incidence of neurological sequelae. Cytokines released by macrophages under the influence of a malarial toxin (possibly GPI anchor) released at schizont rupture could be involved in enhancing cytoadherence by increasing the expression of endothelial receptors such as ICAM-1 and CD36, and can induce fever, hypoglycaemia, coagulopathy, dyserythropoiesis and leucocytosis.

Haematological changes

Anaemia is an inevitable consequence of erythrocyte parasitization as all infected cells are destroyed at schizogony. The survival of non-parasitized erythrocytes was found to be reduced for several weeks after clearance of parasitaemia in patients with falciparum and vivax malarias. In Gambian children, initial studies showed a correlation between severe anaemia and a positive direct antiglobulin (Coomb's) test, implying immune haemolysis. Later studies failed to confirm this finding. In Thai adults with falciparum malaria, there was no increase in IgG coating of erythrocytes and no correlation between the number of IgG molecules/cell and the severity of anaemia. However, IgG-coated cells appeared to be cleared more rapidly by the spleen for a period of several weeks after the acute infection. Iron sequestration, erythrophagocytosis and dyserythropoiesis (Plate 13) were found in the acute phase of falciparum malaria. Maturation defects were present in the marrow for at least 3 weeks after clearance of parasitaemia. Survival of radioisotope-labelled compatible donor erythrocytes was significantly shorter than that of the patient's own (autologous) erythrocytes which were presumably survivors or the enhanced splenic clearance of ageing or subtly altered cells. Patients with splenomegaly showed markedly accelerated clearance of labelled heat-damaged erythrocytes and a lower mean haematocrit than those without splenomegaly. In many parts of the tropics, repeated attacks of malaria eventually lead to profound anaemia, especially if there is a background of chronic blood loss from hookworm infection, malnutrition, pregnancy and persisting relapsing or recrudescent parasitaemia.

Thrombocytopenia is common with falciparum and vivax malarias. Its degree, if not its presence, has some prognostic significance. Platelet survival is reduced to 2–4 days in severe falciparum malaria. Platelet-associated IgG and IgG-coating of platelets has not been a consistent finding. Increased numbers of large abnormal-looking megakaryocytes have been found in the marrow and the circulating platelets may also be enlarged suggesting dyspoietic thrombopoiesis. Enhanced splenic uptake or sequestration may contribute to thrombocytopenia and in patients with disseminated intravascular coagulation (DIC), platelets may be removed from the circulation at sites of fibrin deposition. Surprisingly, platelets are rarely found in cerebral blood vessels in patients dying with cerebral malaria.

Mild leucopenia has been described in uncomplicated malarias, but a neutrophil leucocytosis is an important abnormality in patients with severe falciparum malaria and is associated with a bad prognosis. Tumour necrosis factor may be responsible for this leucocytosis which may be associated with a complicating Gram-negative rod or other bacteraemia.

Spleen

In acute falciparum infections, the spleen is enlarged and soft, varying from dark red to dark or slate grey, depending on the duration of the infection and the amount of pigment present. There is congestion with hyperplasia of the red and white pulp. Large numbers of parasitized erythrocytes are present showing all stages of development. Splenic cords and sinuses are filled with monocytes and macrophages containing pigment (Plate 14), infected and non-infected red cells. The red pulp is expanded by lymphocytes, immunoblasts and plasma cells and extramedullary haematopoiesis is common. Focal haemorrhage and infarction may also be seen. Numerous infected red cells are seen by electron microscopy. The part of the erythrocyte containing the parasite may be nipped off during migration through the splenic cords, a process known as 'pitting' (Fig. 4.3). Infected red cells adhere to macrophages via their surface knobs (Figs 4.4 and 4.5) and degenerating forms of parasites may be seen within some macrophages. These features are also seen in bone marrow sinusoids together with morphological abnormalities of erythrocytes, phagocytosis of parasitized red cells and increased numbers of plasma cells and macrophages. In patients with chronic (repeated attacks of) malaria, lymphoid compartments of the white pulp may show considerable depletion. The red pulp still shows reticuloendothelial hyperplasia and the fibrous trabeculae and capsule are thickened. The colour may vary with the amount of pigment and this may persist for a year or more after the last acute attack although it will eventually be removed. The spleen may exceed 20 times its normal weight.

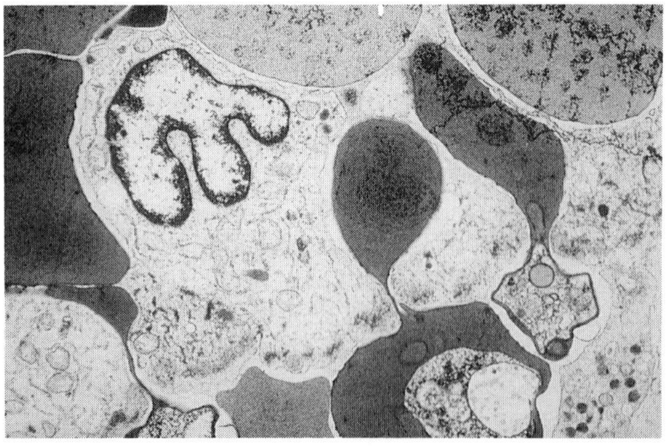

Fig. 4.3 Spleen: electron micrograph showing pitting of parasitized erythrocyte by splenic cord. (© N. Francis.)

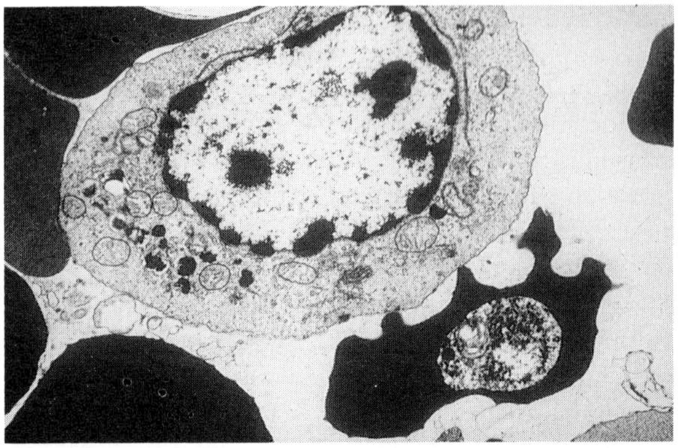

Fig. 4.4 Spleen: electron micrograph showing adherence of infected red cell to splenic macrophage. (© N. Francis.)

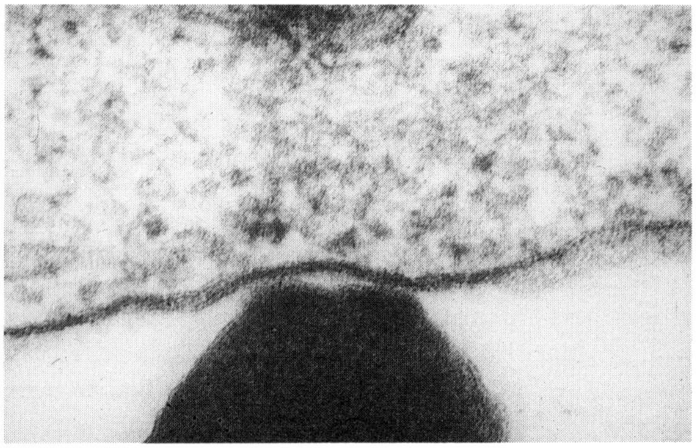

Fig. 4.5 Higher power electron micrograph of Fig. 4.4 showing cytoadherence via knobbed surface to macrophage. (© N. Francis.)

In vivax malaria enlargement of the spleen is more rapid with marked lymphoid hyperplasia and an increased risk of rupture. It also shows active phagocytosis of infected red cells.

Lymph nodes

In acute falciparum infection there is enlargement of nodes (not usually detectable clinically) as a result of paracortical and medullary expansion and the infiltration of subcapsular sinuses by pigmented macrophages and relatively small numbers of parasitized erythrocytes. The cellular proliferation is similar to that in the spleen.

Kidney

There are several distinct patterns of renal involvement in malaria. In acute falciparum malaria an acute and transient self-limiting glomerulonephritis is common whereas in *P. malariae* infection a chronic glomerulonephritis (malarial nephropathy) presents as nephrotic syndrome.

In Blackwater fever and in patients with inherited erythrocyte enzyme defects such as glucose-6-phosphate dehydrogenase deficiency who have been given oxidant drugs, large amounts of haemoglobin are cleared by the kidney following intravascular haemolysis. This may lead to oliguric or anuric acute renal failure. The pathophysiology of Blackwater fever is discussed in Chapter 3.

About one-third of non-immune adults with severe falciparum malaria will show biochemical evidence of renal dysfunction, but this is less common in children and particularly rare in African children. The histopathological changes are those of acute tubular necrosis (Fig. 4.6). Many cases show malarial pigment in circulating macrophages within glomerular capillary lumena and some also show parasitized red cells in peritubular capillaries as well as in the glomeruli (Figs 4.7 and 4.8) and fibrin thrombi (Plate 15). Necrosis of distal and collecting tubules may predominate with tubular casts and pigment-laden macrophages and parasitized erythrocytes in peritubular vessels.

Plasmodium falciparum glomerulonephritis is usually associated with proteinuria with or without microscopic haematuria. The glomeruli are hypercellular with mesangial expansion and the presence of electron-dense deposits in the mesangium, paramesangium and capillary wall (Plate 16; Fig. 4.9). IgM, IgG and β-1c globulin can be demonstrated in the deposits as well as in *P. falciparum* antigens. The presence of circulating immune complexes with reduced serum C3 and C4 also supports the view that this is an immune complex glomerulonephritis. This glomerulonephritis is rarely if ever of clinical significance.

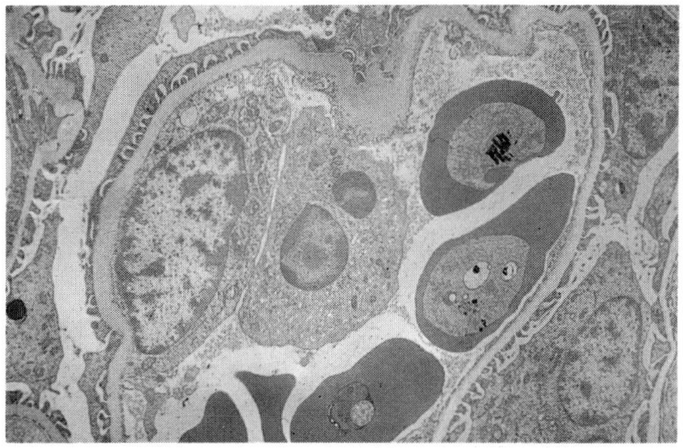

Fig. 4.7 Kidney: electron micrograph showing a capillary loop containing three parasitized erythrocytes (note pigment granules in the parasites) and a circulating mononuclear cell. (© N. Francis.)

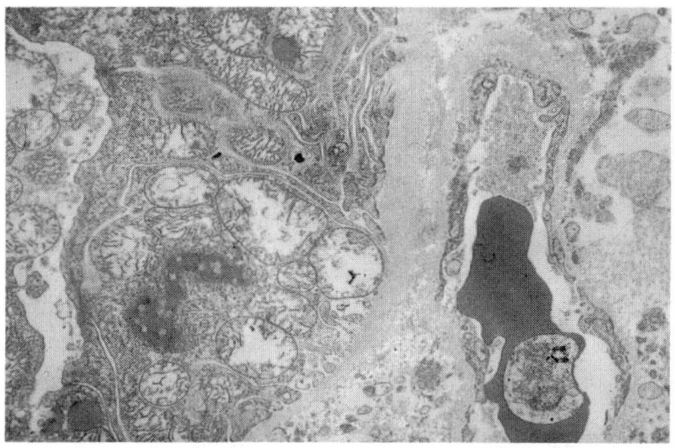

Fig. 4.8 Kidney: electron micrograph showing parasitized erythrocyte in peritubular capillary with apparent adherence to endothelial cell. (© N. Francis.)

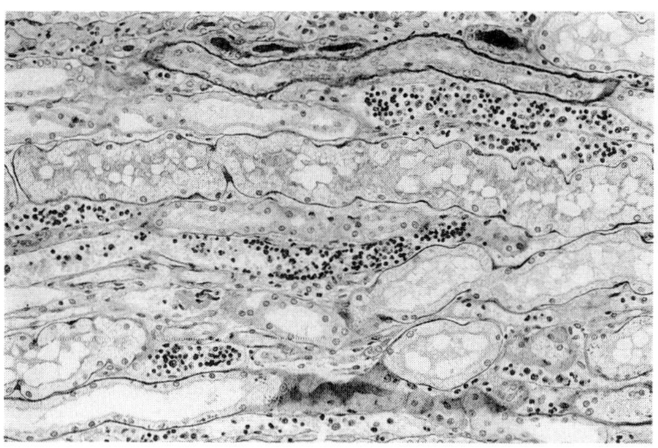

Fig. 4.6 Kidney: electron micrograph of early acute tubular necrosis with congestion of peritubular capillaries by large numbers of mononuclear inflammatory cells. (© N. Francis.)

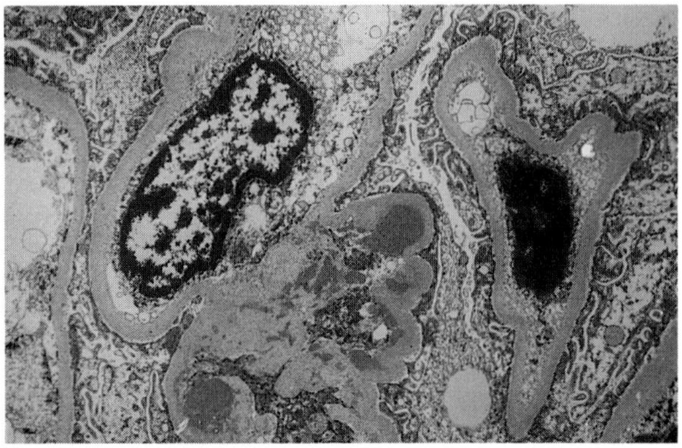

Fig. 4.9 Kidney: electron micrograph illustrating mesangial and paramesangial electron-dense deposits (centre and bottom centre). Capillary loop to right is plugged with fibrin thrombus. (© N. Francis.)

The mechanism of renal dysfunction is uncertain but many of the patients are dehydrated when first admitted to hospital and in some of them renal function is restored to normal by simple rehydration. In patients with hyperparasitaemia, jaundice or haemoglobinuria, renal impairment may persist despite rehydration. Studies of renal cortical blood flow by the ^{133}Xe clearance method and radiological studies (angiography and contrast urography) have demonstrated reduced cortical perfusion during the acute stage of the disease as in other forms of acute tubular necrosis.

Plasmodium malariae infection is associated with a chronic progressive glomerulonephritis presenting as nephrotic syndrome. There is considerable evidence that this is an immune complex disease which may show a variety of microscopic patterns ranging from minimal change to membranous, the latter referred to as quartan malarial nephropathy because of its prominent membrane changes and lack of mesangial proliferation. Immunoglobulins (predominantly IgM), complement components, malarial antigens and electron-dense deposits have been found in the abnormal glomerular tufts. Tubular and medullary changes have not been well described in *P. malariae* infection.

Lung

The older literature contains descriptions of a variety of pneumonic, fibrotic and other syndromes alleged to be related specifically to malaria. Pneumonia is a familiar complication of severe falciparum malaria and is usually attributable to aspiration or bacteraemic spread from another site of infection. Acute pulmonary oedema, whether the result of iatrogenic fluid overload and associated with elevated pulmonary artery wedge pressures, or whether of the adult respiratory distress syndrome (ARDS) type with normal or low hydrostatic pressures in the pulmonary vascular bed, is a grave complication of severe falciparum malaria. Pulmonary oedema was a universal finding among Spitz's autopsy series of American soldiers in the Second World War. Macroscopically the lung is dark with scattered haemorrhages (Plate 17). The alveoli are congested with pigment-laden macrophages, plasma cells, neutrophils and parasitized erythrocytes. The alveoli are lined with a laminated periodic acid–schiff (PAS) positive membrane which eventually destroys and incorporates the alveolar wall within it. This is associated with abundant oedema fluid and may have a marked inflammatory infiltrate. In the case of ARDS the mechanism is thought to be increased pulmonary capillary permeability resulting from leucocyte products released through complement-/cytokine-related mechanisms.

Cardiovascular system

In patients dying of malaria the heart shows little macroscopic abnormality. Petechial haemorrhages of the epi- or endocardial surfaces may be found (Plate 18) but the most striking findings are microscopic. There is congestion of the myocardial capillaries with parasitized erythrocytes, pigment-laden macrophages, lymphocytes and plasma cells (Plate 19). However, the erythrocytes are not tightly packed and there is little evidence of cytoadherence. In a small number of cases fatty changes of the myocardium and capillary fibrin thrombi have been observed and the latter showed well-demarcated myocardial necrosis. Myocardial function appears normal in severe falciparum malaria. Most patients have an elevated cardiac index attributable to cytokine-mediated vasodilation, low systemic vascular resistance and low or normal pulmonary arterial wedge pressures. The mean arterial pressure is usually markedly reduced. Profound hypotension or shock ('algid malaria') is unusual. In some cases it is explained by a complicating Gram-negative rod septicaemia. Cardiac arrhythmias are very uncommon.

Liver and gastrointestinal system

Findings are similar in all forms of malaria but tend to be more severe in *P. falciparum* infection. The major changes are in hepatic sinusoids and lining cells but there is relatively little damage to hepatocytes. The liver is enlarged as a result of oedema and ranges in colour from tan-pink to brown and eventually to black due to deposition of malarial pigment (Plate 20). In acute infection, the liver may be friable, becoming firm with repeated attacks. Lobular accentuation is attributable to pigment in the portal tracts.

The extra- or pre-erythrocytic phase of the life cycle may sometimes be detectable. Intrahepatocyte schizonts and merozoites can be seen with displacement of the liver cell nucleus without inflammatory changes (Plate 8). In vivax malaria, small non-dividing parasites which resemble the hypnozoites of experimental *P. cynomolgi* infection in rhesus monkeys, have been found in human liver biopsies and *in vitro* in cultured hepatocytes. They are 5–6 μm in diameter.

In early infection there is sinusoidal dilation and congestion with Kupffer cell hyperplasia (initially in the periportal zone), parasitized erythrocytes and fine pigment in red cells and Kupffer cells. There is phagocytosis of infected and non-infected erythrocytes by Kupffer cells, endothelial cells and sinusoidal macrophages which are increased in number and are probably recruited from the spleen. Infected erythrocytes fill the sinusoids causing reduced hepatic circulation and associated splanchnic constriction.

Small areas of central liver cell necrosis (Plate 21) are difficult to separate from effects of coexistent shock or disseminated intravascular coagulation and may not be local effects of parasitaemia. There is often reduced hepatocyte glycogen, on PAS staining (Plate 22a and b) and ultrastructurally (Fig. 4.10), which may explain in part the hypoglycaemia in malaria. In general, the histological severity does not correlate well with abnormalities of liver function. Later in the disease pigment becomes clumped, macrophages are increased in the sinusoids (Plate 23) and there is a chronic inflammatory infiltrate and pigment deposition in the portal tracts. Ultrastructurally, most of the infected erythrocytes contain trophozoites, may be knobbed or knobless and contain characteristic crystalline malarial pigment granules (Fig. 4.11). Partially degenerate erythrocytes are also seen. Sites of attachment between knobbed parasitized erythrocytes and phagocytic cells can be demonstrated. The hepatocytes, apart from containing lipofuscin and sometimes haemosiderin, show some fat droplet formation and swollen mitochondria which may become depleted (Fig. 4.12). There is also narrowing of the space of Disse with loss of microvilli of the bile canaliculi, features which have been suggested as the basis for hepatic dysfunction

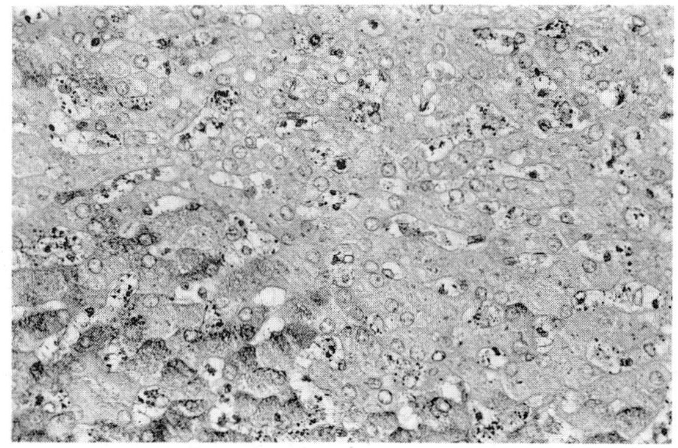

Fig. 4.10 Liver showing extensive pigment in hepatic sinusoids with increased sinusoidal macrophages. Also shown is lack of glycogen in most of field with some residual glycogen in lower left. Periodic acid–schiff. (© N. Francis.)

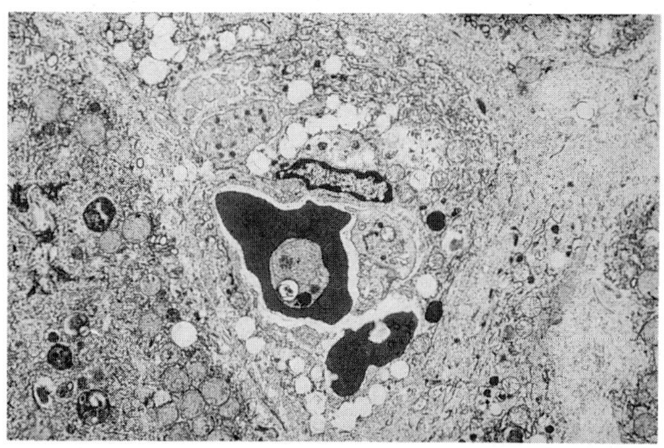

Fig. 4.11 Liver: electron micrograph showing erythrocytes in sinusoid containing trophozoite in one and pigment granule in the other deformed red cell. (© N. Francis.)

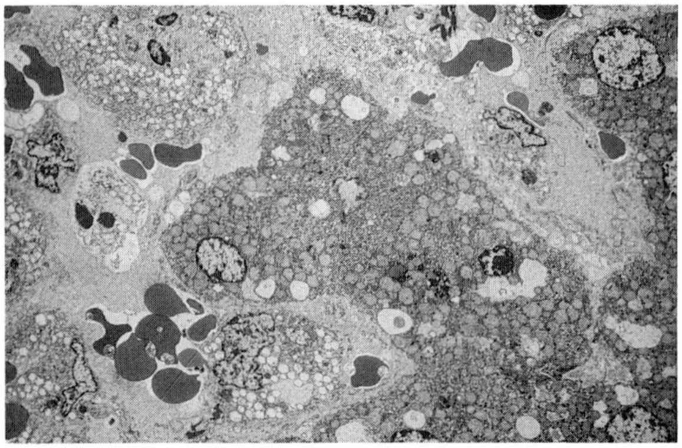

Fig. 4.12 Liver: electron micrograph showing sinusoids containing numerous parasitized erythrocytes, with swollen endothelial cells and fat droplet formation within hepatocytes. (© N. Francis.)

and cholestasis. In patients with DIC, fibrin may be seen in sinusoids and, when there is associated anaemia, extramedullary haematopoiesis is found in the periportal area.

In tropical splenomegaly syndrome there is a characteristically dense lymphocytic infiltrate of the sinusoids which may resemble leukaemia and Kupffer cell hyperplasia with some pigment and variable portral tract chronic inflammation. Infected erythrocytes are not usually seen.

In severe falciparum malaria, hepatic dysfunction is reflected by blood coagulation abnormalities, hypoalbuminaemia and reduced metabolic clearance of many substances including alanine, lactate and antimalarial drugs. Hepatic blood flow measured by an indocyanine green method was reduced during the acute phase of severe noncerebral malaria, returning to normal during convalescence. One possible explanation for this finding would be sequestration or microcirculatory obstruction in the portal circulation. Portal vein constriction was found in rhesus monkeys infected with *P. knowlesi*. The term 'malarial hepatitis' has been applied to jaundiced patients, but histopathological studies rarely provide a basis for the use of this term.

Gastrointestinal disturbances are common in falciparum malaria. Sequestration and cytoadherence have been seen in the small and large bowel, predominantly within the lamina propria capillaries but also in larger submucosal vessels (Plate 24). In a significant proportion of severe cases mucosal ulceration and haemorrhage may ensue and in some of these fibrin thrombi are found in small blood vessels. Malabsorption of amino acids, sugars, fats, chloroquine and quinine have been described although in practice drug absorption from the gut appears to be adequate in all but the most severely ill patients. In the acute phase of falciparum malaria, Thai adult patients showed greatly reduced absorption of sugars which rely on mediated mechanisms and unmediated diffusion. Absorption returned to normal in convalescence. The pattern of reduced absorption was not characteristic of mucosal damage but could have resulted from impaired splanchnic perfusion. Neither sugar absorption nor liver blood flow was reduced in uncomplicated falciparum malaria.

Placenta

In active infection the placenta is black or slatey grey and the sinusoids are packed with infected erythrocytes and increased numbers of pigment-laden macrophages. However, there is no evidence yet that significant cytoadherence occurs to any components of the placenta. Syncytiotrophoblastic necrosis and loss of microvilli, fibrinoid necrosis of the villi and thickening of the trophoblast basement membrane have been observed and may provide a basis for impaired foetal nutrition. In previous or resolved infection, variable amounts of pigment deposition alone are seen in perivillous fibrinoid material and placental bed tissue and, if the infection is recently resolved, may be seen in syncytiotrophoblasts and circulating mononuclear cells or macrophages. Transmission of infection across an intact placenta to the foetus rarely occurs. Parasitized erythrocytes are sometimes seen in foetal vessels in infected placentae.

Mechanism of hypoglycaemia

Hypoglycaemia is an increasingly recognized complication of falciparum malaria. The cinchona alkaloids, quinine and quinidine, release insulin from pancreatic islet cells and this reduces hepatic gluconeogenesis and increases peripheral glucose uptake by tissues, resulting in hypoglycaemia. Inappropriately high plasma insulin concentrations will be found with increased lactate and alanine and low ketone concentrations.

Glucose consumption may be increased in patients with malaria as a result of fever, infection and anaerobic glycolysis in the host tissues and by the parasite burden.

Glycogen reserves may be depleted especially in children and pregnant women as a result of fasting and 'accelerated starvation'. Inhibition of hepatic gluconeogenesis by TNF and other cytokines could be the cause of a common hypoglycaemic syndrome in African children with severe malaria, adult patients with severe disease and pregnant women who have elevated plasma lactate and alanine concentrations and, in some, moderately increased ketone bodies. Counter-regulatory hormone levels are usually very high. Similar disturbances have been found in other severe infections such as bacillary dysentery in children.

Chapter 5

Immunology of human malaria

K. Marsh

Malaria is an important cause of morbidity but not everyone infected with the malaria parasite becomes seriously ill or dies. In areas of stable endemicity repeated exposure to the parasite leads to the acquisition of *specific immunity* which restricts serious problems to young children; malaria in older subjects causing a relatively mild febrile illness. However, even in people exposed to malaria for the first time there is a range of possible outcomes, from death at one extreme to the occasional subject who appears resistant to infection at the other. In this case any resistance is *non-specific*; it does not depend on prior exposure to malaria and may be either *acquired* or *innate*. Of course the situation is not necessarily clear-cut and in any one individual several factors may interact, for instance, when innate genetic factors exert their effect on the acquisition of specific immunity. Most of this chapter is concerned with specific acquired immunity to malaria, how it might work, what goes wrong with it and the possibilities for manipulation by vaccination. However, we begin with a brief outline of important innate and acquired factors which lead to non-specific immunity.

Innate resistance to malaria

The malaria parasite faces a succession of challenges within the host; it has to attach to, enter and thrive in, first, hepatocytes and then erythrocytes, and having overcome these hurdles it has to leave the host to carry on the next part of its cycle in the mosquito. Along its way the parasite is susceptible to a whole range of potential interruptions including simple physical barriers, non-specific protective responses, alterations in the supply of essential nutrients and the operation of specific immune mechanisms. Many host genes will be involved in the control of the internal environment which faces the parasite and the major disadvantages of being parasitized should favour the survival of those host genes that afford any degree of protection against the parasite. Finding out which human genes are important is difficult, although more is probably known about the selective effect of malaria on the human genome than any other infection. This is due not only to malaria having been such a potent selective force but also to the fact that the red cell, the most important host environment for the parasite, is relatively easy to characterize in terms of genetic differences.

The effect of host genetics on other aspects of parasite success such as interactions with the hepatocyte, the generation of immune responses and even the ability to form infective gametocytes are much less well understood.

Red cell polymorphisms and malaria

Hundreds of genetic variations have been described which affect human red blood cells. The variants of most interest are those that have achieved polymorphic status, i.e. alternative versions of the same gene coexist in a population at frequencies well above those that could be explained simply by the repeated occurrence of the mutation which produces the variant. At a time when the only well-recognized red cell polymorphisms were those giving rise to the thalassaemic states, J. B. S. Haldane suggested that their geographical distribution was due to a selective effect of malaria on the heterozygote, i.e. the carriers of the genes enjoyed some advantage which balanced the disadvantage of the homozygotic states. This 'malaria hypothesis' was a key insight into the interaction of human genetics and infectious diseases.

The red cell polymorphisms for which there is now reasonable evidence to support a 'malaria hypothesis' include conditions affecting the structure of the β globin chain of haemoglobin (HbS, HbC and HbE), rates of synthesis of globin chains, (α-thalassaemia and β-thalassaemia), the level of a key red cell enzyme (glucose-6-phosphate dehydrogenase, G6PD) and conditions affecting the red cell membrane and cytoskeleton (Duffy blood group negativity and hereditary ovalocytosis). There are a number of less clear-cut cases affecting both membrane structure and other red cell enzymes where either the degree of polymorphism is less or is not yet clearly established; these will not be discussed.

In most cases the strongest evidence for the malaria hypothesis is epidemiological, although there is clear-cut clinical evidence of protection for sickle cell trait (the carrier state for HbS) and to a lesser extent with β-thalassaemia and G6PD deficiency. Several potential mechanisms of protection have been shown *in vitro*. They include interference with the complex events of red cell invasion and metabolic effects on the parasite, either by not providing the optimum intracellular environment or by increasing the susceptibility of the infected cell to oxidant damage. In many cases it is likely that several mechanisms operate together. There is emerging evidence in a number of cases for increased immunological clearance of infected variant cells, providing a potential 'unified theory' to underpin the malaria hypothesis.

Haemoglobin S

The haemoglobin molecule is a tetramer; the 'normal' haemoglobin of adults (HbA) comprises two α chains and two β chains. Haemoglobin S is formed when there is a particular amino acid substitution (valine for glutamine at position 57) in the β chain. The resulting abnormal β chain can still combine with α chains but the haemoglobin molecule formed has altered physicochemical characteristics. Normally there are two functional β globin genes, one inherited from each parent. Heterozygotes for HbS have one normal and one defective β gene (they are said to have sickle trait and are designated AS). Their red cells, which contain a mixture of HbA and HbS, function fairly normally in most situations. By contrast, red cells of homozygotes (designated SS) contain mainly HbS, as both β globin genes are of the abnormal type. Their cells form an abnormal shape (sickle) under conditions of low oxygen tension which leads to both increased red cell lysis and obstruction of vascular flow as the abnormal cells lodge in small blood vessels. Except under circumstances with a high availability of medical care the homozygous condition (sickle cell disease) is almost uniformly fatal in childhood, indicating that there must be a very high degree of advantage to the heterozygote to maintain the gene at high frequencies.

Haemoglobin S is only found at significant frequencies in malarious areas. It reaches very high levels in parts of Africa where over 20% of the population are heterozygotes. It occurs at lower frequencies in some Mediterranean populations, in the Middle East and in parts of India. The selective advantage is exercised predominantly in childhood and the overwhelming evidence is that this is due to a strong protection against the clinical effects of malaria, rather than an effect on susceptibility to malaria infection *per se*, which is not markedly less common in AS individuals. A number of protective mechanisms have been suggested; infected AS cells sickle more readily than uninfected cells, which may lead to increased reticuloendothelial clearance. Parasite growth is inhibited in AS cells under conditions of low oxygen tension, possibly due to an alteration in red cell potassium levels. However, it is striking that homozygotes, which have even higher levels of HbS, are susceptible to fatal malaria and this would seem to argue against protection in AS individuals being primarily due to an unfavourable intracellular environment and to support the idea that there is an interaction between increased sickling and accelerated removal of infected cells, which may not occur in SS individuals because of their well-known deficits in splenic function.

Haemoglobin C

Haemoglobin C is formed by substitution of a glutamate for lysine at position 6 in the β chain. It is present at high frequencies in a localized part of West Africa, around Burkina Fasso and Ghana. Cells from the homozygote CC are refractory to parasite growth in culture, possibly due to their resistance to bursting and releasing merozoites rather than any deficit in the intracellular environment. AC cells support parasite growth normally. An interesting twist is added by the fact that in West Africa sickle cell gene frequencies are very high and individuals carrying one βS gene and one βC gene (i.e. SC) are not uncommon and parasite growth is particularly poor in SC cells. It seems unlikely that HbC has been maintained by an advantage of AC heterozygotes, nor that homozygote advantage has been the selective force; it is possible that the high frequencies are not even related to malaria. An interesting possibility is that it is SC individuals who have been at a particular advantage, protection against severe malaria more than balancing the reduced fertility of SC females.

Haemoglobin E

Haemoglobin E is probably the commonest haemoglobin variant in the world. It is caused by a single mutation of glutamine to lysine at position 26 in the β chain and is common throughout South-east Asia. The mechanism of protection is not clear, there is evidence of reduced parasite growth in cells from both homozygotes and heterozygotes, possibly exacerbated under conditions of oxidant stress. In addition, both parasitized EE and AE erythrocytes are phagocytosed more readily than parasitized AA erythrocytes, raising the possibility that protection derives in part from an interaction with the host immune system.

The thalassaemias

The thalassaemias are a heterogeneous group of conditions in which there is a reduced rate of production of one or more of the globin chains of haemoglobin. The β-thalassaemias usually result from single base changes or small deletions in the β globin genes. They occur widely in areas that are, or have been, malarious, being common in the Mediterranean basin, the Middle East and South-east Asia. They occur at lower frequencies in sub-Saharan Africa; this has been explained as the result of the β-thalassaemia genes being 'in competition' with the strongly protective sickle cell gene. While this makes sense it is less clear why both β-thalassaemia and HbE genes coexist at such high frequencies in parts of South-east Asia.

Humans have four α globin genes, a duplicated pair being inherited from each parent. The α-thalassaemias result from defects in one or more of these genes. The effects cover a wide spectrum: from asymptomatic individuals with one α gene affected to the absence of all four functional genes, a condition which is incompatible with life and results in stillbirths with Hb Barts hydrops syndrome. Because the more minor forms are without obvious clinical consequences the epidemiology of the α-thalassaemias has had to await the availability of molecular genetic typing techniques. These have shown that α-thalassaemia genes are widely distributed throughout every part of the world that has been endemic for malaria. Particularly high frequencies are reached in parts of South-east Asia and in Melanesia, where detailed microepidemiological studies have provided strong evidence to support the malaria hypothesis.

As with the other red cell polymorphisms the mechanisms by which the thalassaemias protect against malaria are not known with any certainty. There is reduced parasite growth in β-thalassaemia cells, particularly when exposed to oxidant stress. On the other hand, cells from individuals with single or double α gene deletion support parasite growth normally under all conditions. However, infected cells from both α- and β-thalassaemia subjects show enhanced antigen expression at the surface of the infected red cell, possibly leading to enhanced immune clearance.

Glucose-6-phosphate dehydrogenase deficiency

Glucose-6-phosphate dehydrogenase (G6PD) is the first enzyme of the hexose monophosphate shunt and plays a critical role in the production of NADPH. There are numerous variants of the enzyme described, inheritance of some of which leads to deficiency of the enzyme. The gene for G6PD is on the X chromosome and severe deficiency is fully expressed only in male hemizygotes and rare female homozygotes. Under most circumstances the malaria parasite is thought to use host pathways for NADPH production and it should be susceptible to changes in the level of the enzymes. Although variant genes leading to deficiency states have been found all over the world they only reach polymorphic frequencies (with a few puzzling exceptions) in malaria endemic regions, leading to the hypothesis that they, like genes for structural haemoglobin variants, have been selected for by malaria. This is difficult to establish with certainty because deficient individuals are, perhaps surprisingly, not at much of a disadvantage. Epidemiological studies and *in vitro* studies of parasite growth in deficient cells have been contentious. It does appear that heterozygote females in Africa (who usually have *normal* levels of the enzyme) are protected against higher levels of parasitization but that deficient males are fully susceptible to malaria. This fits nicely with mathematical predictions that for a sex-linked gene at equilibrium the selective advantage will be in the heterozygote females, but has to be reconciled with *in vitro* experiments showing reduced growth in deficient cells. An attractive hypothesis, supported by experimental observations, is that parasites can adapt to grow well in either normal or deficient cells but that in heterozygote females they encounter both types and are repeatedly having to readapt at the cost of efficient growth.

Innate resistance and the red cell membrane

The parasite has to gain entry to the red cell to survive. As there are a number of human genetic polymorphisms affecting the structure and function of the red cell membrane it might be expected that some of these will affect the parasite's ability to invade the red cell. The classical example is the Duffy blood group system and *Plasmodium vivax*. The Duffy system is a group of antigenic determinants on the red cell membrane for which there are two principal alleles: Fy^a and Fy^b. Individuals lacking both of these are homozygous for a third allele FyFy. Red cells from Duffy-negative individuals are completely resistant to infection with *P. vivax* implying that this parasite uses the Duffy determinants during invasion. *P. vivax* is not endemic in West Africa, where the majority of people are Duffy negative, and is rare in other parts of Africa. This is usually interpreted as having come about by malaria selecting for humans who are negative, however, *P. vivax* causes little mortality and it would have to be argued either that there was considerable indirect mortality or that *P. vivax* has in the past been more virulent. An alternative possibility is that Duffy negativity was already established in certain populations by other mechanisms and that the selection has been against the parasite invading these areas, rather than the other way round.

Red cell cytoskeletal abnormalities

The only red cell cytoskeletal abnormality known to reach polymorphic frequencies is hereditary ovalocytosis. This is an autosomal dominant condition in which the red cells have an oval shape and a marked increase in membrane rigidity. The molecular basis of the condition appears to be modification of Band III, the major anion transporter of red cells. Ovalocytic red cells are highly, though not completely, resistant to invasion by both *P. vivax* and *Plasmodium falciparum* and this is reflected epidemiologically by lower parasite rates and densities in ovalocytic individuals. The gene frequency is high (up to 30%) in many parts of South-east Asia through into Papua New Guinea. As the condition is not known to cause any ill effects it is a matter of speculation as to whether it is a balanced polymorphism or whether it is moving towards fixation, i.e. will become the 'normal' red cell type with the passage of time if a selective pressure from malaria is maintained in those populations.

Other genetic polymorphisms and malaria

The relationship between malaria and the red cell has played a central role in the development of ideas on the selection of single genes by infective agents but it seems certain that many other host genes will be important, though to date information is more limited. Human leucocyte antigens (HLA) are a highly polymorphic family of proteins which play critical roles in the genesis of immune responses (see below). There is some evidence from studies in Sardinia of selection for particular HLA types in populations historically exposed to malaria when compared with populations of the same ancestral stock living at a higher altitude, where malaria has never been endemic. Currently, evidence is emerging for associations between a few HLA antigens common in African populations and protection from severe disease. An HLA class I antigen, HLA-Bw53, and an HLA class II haplotype, DRB1*1302-DQB*0501, have been associated with reduced susceptibility to severe disease. It is likely that the characterization of polymorphisms in other host molecules involved in critical interactions with the parasite will lead to an increased recognition of the role of host genetics in susceptibility to malarial infection and disease.

Acquired non-specific resistance to malaria

Not all mechanisms of non-specific resistance to malaria are genetic. Nutritional status is a determinant of outcome in many infectious diseases and because poor nutritional status and malaria endemicity often coexist it may be thought that the one leads to the other. In fact the evidence, where there is any, is for the opposite effect. It is extremely unusual to see severe malaria in children with marasmus or kwashiorkor and there have been several reports of exacerbation of malaria when nutritional supplements have been introduced in times of famine. A specific dietary component that has been associated with increased susceptibility to malaria is iron. It is not clear whether iron deficiency *per se* is protective or whether it is iron supplementation of deficient children which increases susceptibility, for instance, by increasing the supply of young red cells. Similarly, there are indications that low riboflavin levels may give some protection against the parasite. Finally, the observation that a diet deficient in para-amino benzoic acid (PABA) suppresses otherwise virulent malaria infections in rodents led to the suggestion that a pure breast milk diet (which is low in PABA) contributes to the protection from malaria enjoyed by young infants in endemic areas but it is difficult to disentangle this from other potentially protective factors.

It may seem strange to mention drugs as an acquired resistance factor but it should be recognized that community use of chloroquine in some areas is now so common that the drug, which has a long clearance time, can be detected in a large proportion of the population at any one time. Quite apart from possible effects on the spread of drug resistance this is likely to have an effect on the epidemiology of malaria in these areas.

Acquired immunity to malaria

In stable endemic areas a heavy toll of morbidity and mortality falls on young children but malaria is a relatively mild condition in adults. This is due to the acquisition of specific immunity. Children born to immune mothers appear themselves to be relatively immune to malaria for a period. It is not rare to find low numbers of parasites in cord blood, but these do not give rise to overt infections. This contrasts with the situation in less stable areas where clinically severe congenital malaria does occur. The child remains relatively protected for a period of between 3 and 6 months following birth. If transmission is heavy the child may become parasitaemic during this period, and sometimes have fever, but rarely manifests any severe features of malaria. In short, they behave rather like immune adults.

Following the period of relative protection children become increasingly susceptible to the more severe clinical manifestations of malaria. The two most important life-threatening complications are severe anaemia and cerebral malaria. It is striking that the age of maximum susceptibility for these two clinical syndromes is different, with anaemia typically being the major life-threatening complication in children under 18 months and cerebral malaria having a peak incidence in the third year of life. However, it should be stressed that even during the period of maximum susceptibility to severe disease children spend the majority of their time parasitized but healthy; immunity at this stage is a slippery concept! From around the fourth year of life the severity of clinical attacks begins to decline, although parasite rates and densities remain high. Death from malaria is rare after the fifth year and thereafter clinical attacks become less frequent and less severe until in adulthood significant disease is rare, although self-limiting attacks of fever and headache are common. This progression is mirrored in declines in population parasite rates and densities. Complete immunity to parasitization is probably never achieved and the cumulative parasite prevalence in adults is near 100%. Once achieved, malaria immunity may not be stable and it is often reported that immune subjects who spend time outside an endemic area are prone to malaria on re-exposure. However, it has to be said that this is an area with far more anecdotes than hard facts and although there is an increased susceptibility to minor symptoms, immunity to life-threatening disease persists. Similarly, it is often said that fully immune individuals may be susceptible to malaria on moving to another endemic area. Again this phenomenon is probably limited to fever and minor symptoms and does not involve a loss of protection against severe disease. Finally, a third situation in which there is some loss of immunity is pregnancy. This is manifest as an increased prevalence and increased density of parasitaemia which may lead to severe anaemia. At delivery the placenta is often parasitized to a degree far beyond that expected from the peripheral parasitaemia and one of the most important public health affects is the associated reduction in birthweight. The placenta seems to be a privileged site for parasites, which then overflow into the peripheral circulation and are dealt with reasonably normally. The mechanisms for this 'immune evasion' are obscure but the fact that it is predominantly a phenomenon of first pregnancies has led some to suggest that it represents a failure of local immunity, presumably cell mediated, in the new placental–uterine unit and that such local immunity is acquired in subsequent pregnancies. An alternative (or possibly complementary) hypothesis is that immunosuppression is mediated by increased levels of steroid hormones.

What general conclusions about the nature of immunity to malaria can be drawn from this epidemiological picture? Firstly, it appears that a substantial degree of protection can be transferred from mother to child, implying an important role for humoral immune mechanisms. This will be discussed further below. A second conclusion drawn by some is that because children pass through a period when they commonly have high parasitaemia without serious disease there is a part of antimalarial immunity which is not directly antiparasitic but is 'antitoxic', either by neutralizing toxic parasite products or by tempering the hosts' acute response to infection. This idea tends to go through historical phases of popularity, and there is currently a re-awakening of interest because of the increasing awareness of the potential role of acute phase responses in the pathogenesis of disease. Certainly, on the face of it, a child walking around with high parasitaemia that would be incompatible with good health in a non-immune child must have some component of 'antitoxic' immunity. On the other hand, the same child may be dead a few weeks later from cerebral malaria. Again, even when there is tolerance of parasites there must also be mechanisms acting to limit parasite multiplication, otherwise the child would die (albeit asymptomatically!) as its red cells were destroyed by the inexorable increase of parasites. The third and most striking conclusion is that immunity to malaria seems to need a long period of exposure to the parasite for induction, and probably continuing exposure for maintenance. The most plausible hypothesis is that immunity to malaria is, at least during early years, largely strain specific. This implies that many strains exist within a species and that immunity is developed to each one as it is encountered. With increasing experience the frequency of attacks would drop as fewer new strains were encountered, although the fact that severity of any given infection is also reduced with time argues for the parallel development of mechanisms which override strain differences.

Lessons from neurosyphilis (See also Chapter 1.)

For a period of around 20 years prior to the discovery of penicillin the mainstay in the treatment of advanced neurosyphilis was malariotherapy, in which repeated controlled attacks of malaria were induced. The whole area makes a fascinating study in the history of medicine and many questions on malaria immunity raised by observations in endemic areas were answered in this more controlled setting. It was clearly established that immunity to malaria is both *species* and *stage* specific. These observations also provide the best evidence for *strain specificity* in human immunity to malaria. Most experience was gained with *P. vivax*, in which it was possible to generate immunity to a given isolate after only one or two exposures. However, subsequent challenge with the same species of parasite from a different geographical area led to attacks of malaria that were as severe as the primary attack. Less experience was gained with *P. falciparum* and immunity often took longer to develop, but the overall conclusions were clearly the same. Strain specificity is a feature of many animal models of malarial immunity and fits in well with the epidemiological picture described above. The degree to which it can be superseded is of critical importance to prospects for vaccine development.

Mechanisms of immunity

Much of the above could just as well have been written in the 1940s as the 1990s. The last 20 years have seen an unprecedented expansion of work on immunity to malaria facilitated by revolutions in biotechnology and driven by the search for malaria vaccines. In the last edition of this book it was felt that the pace and complexity of developments threatened detailed exposition with premature obsolescence. This remains true, but an attempt at an overview is now necessary in order to appreciate some of the important and difficult issues facing malariologists and immunologists. This requires at least a passing familiarity with certain immunological concepts and these are outlined below. Many readers can safely skip the next section but it may prove useful for those who are not quite sure of the difference between an epitope and an antigen or who feel weak at the mention of HLA restriction.

The immune system is made up of more or less specialized cells which act collectively to protect the host against foreign organisms. The cells are produced in the bone marrow and subsequently move freely between the blood and specific sites such as the lymph nodes, spleen and liver. At the hub of the system are lymphocytes, which are responsible for the fundamental properties of specificity and memory and which are divided into sub-populations by the presence of surface markers (which fortunately have a reasonably close correspondence with function). The fundamental process of all immune mechanisms is the same: lymphocytes recognize foreign material by way of specialized surface receptors. The recognition event leads to stimulation of the lymphocyte resulting in the production of specialized effector molecules which either act directly on foreign organisms or recruit other effector cells to do so (Fig. 5.1).

It is convenient to consider the immune system as two interacting parts. The central cell of the *humoral* arm is the B lymphocyte and the specialized effector molecules are the *immunoglobulins* or *antibodies*. T lymphocytes are the central cell of the *cell-mediated* arm of immunity and there is a range of effector molecules, including ones which act to cause immediate damage in the area of release, those that enter the circulation and act at a distance, and those that recruit other less specific cells (such as polymorphs and macrophages) to the site of action. *Antigen* and *epitope* are key concepts in both arms of immunity. *Antigen* is a rather broad term for the thing which elicits a specific immune response; in a loose sense one could call a whole organism the antigen, although it is more conventional to refer to specific molecules as antigens. *Epi-*

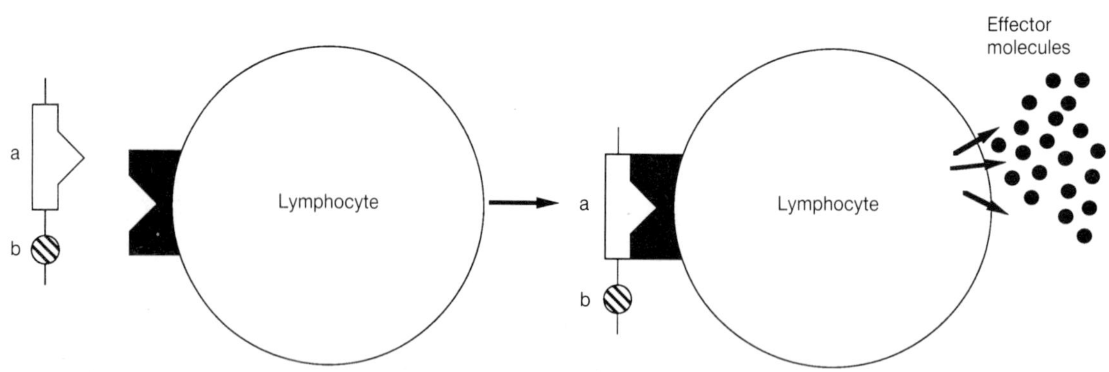

Fig. 5.1 The essential feature of immune responses is the recognition of an epitope 'a' by a specific receptor on the surface of a lymphocyte and the consequent release of effector molecules by that lymphocyte.

tope is a far more precise term for the exact piece of a molecule that is recognized by a given lymphocyte receptor or a given antibody molecule. In the case of a protein molecule an epitope is generally of the order of 5–10 amino acids long and so a single antigenic molecule may contain many different epitopes. Epitopes recognized by T lymphocytes are always linear sequences, i.e. the amino acids are in the order in which they occur in the antigenic molecule. Epitopes recognized by B lymphocytes or antibody may be linear but can also be confirmational where non-contiguous amino acids are brought into close proximity by the three-dimensional structure of the molecule (Fig. 5.2).

Antibody-mediated immunity

Antibodies form a group of specialized proteins that have a shared basic structure of two pairs of polypeptide chains held together by inter- and intrachain disulphide bonds. This basic structure exists in either a monomeric form (of which there are four classes: IgG, IgA, IgD and IgE) or a pentameric form, IgM. Whatever the class the essential feature of antibodies is the possession of a binding site capable of forming strong bonds in a highly specific way with parts (epitopes) of other molecules. There are hundreds of thousands of different epitopes that an organism may potentially encounter in its lifetime, and the extraordinary feature of the humoral immune system is that all human beings possess from birth an equivalently large range of cells of the B lymphocyte lineage capable of recognizing these epitopes. A humoral response comprises the recognition of a foreign antigen by a B cell specific for one of its epitopes, followed by cell division (clonal B cell expansion) and the production of antibody with specificity for that epitope. The receptor by which the epitope is recognized by the B cell has the same structure as the binding site of the antibody which will be produced by that cell (i.e. the B cell receptor is essentially antibody stuck into the cell membrane). Many molecules are capable of being recognized by antibody including carbohydrates and glycolipids but most of the antigens currently of concern in relation to malaria are proteins and the rest of the discussion will be limited to protein antigens.

In the case of challenge with a large complex organism like a malaria parasite there will be hundreds of distinct antigenic molecules and even more potential epitopes. The resulting antibody response will therefore involve numerous distinct B cell clones and antibody specificities. In the absence of continuing antigenic stimulation antibody levels peak and fall off again in a matter of a few weeks; the cells, or their capacity to produce antibody, are short lived. This is the classic primary response, usually the antibody produced is predominantly IgM. Subsequent re-exposure to the antigen results in a secondary antibody response, which is not simply a rerun of the primary response, it is quicker and bigger and the class of antibody is changed, usually to IgG. Furthermore, the antibody response matures, the antibody assuming a progressively better fit with its antigen. This it does by a process of selection: somatic mutation in the expanding B cell clone affecting the fine detail of the binding site is selected for if it leads to a better fit with the epitope.

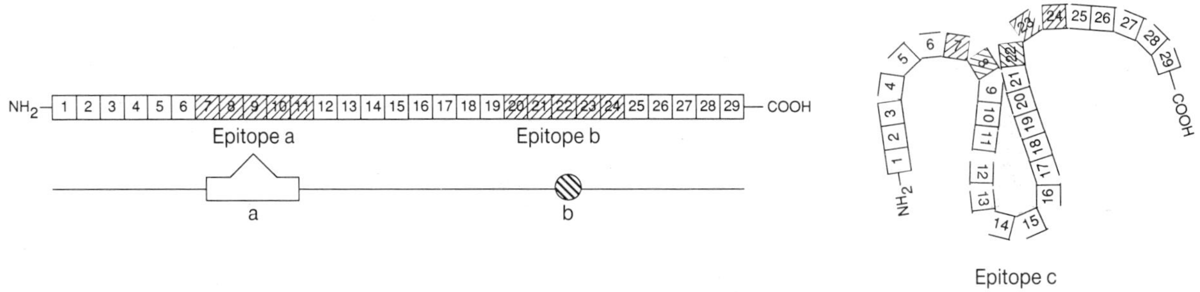

Fig. 5.2 An antigenic molecule comprises one or more epitopes, short sequences that are specifically recognized by antibody or lymphocyte surface receptors. These may be linear epitopes or confirmational epitopes. The schematic diagram shows how individual amino acids may form parts of different epitopes within the same molecule.

We come now to a crucial aspect of antibody production, certainly for understanding some of the most important issues besetting malaria vaccine development. Successful secondary responses to the majority of protein antigens require not only B cells but specific T cells. For many years the nature of the specificity of T cell help was a central problem of immunology. There is now a satisfyingly simple and beautiful explanation illustrated schematically in Fig. 5.3. When the B cell binds a piece of antigen by the epitope for which it has a specific receptor it internalizes the antigen. Here the antigenic molecule is broken down into pieces which are re-exported to the surface of the B cell. It is these fragments which are recognized by specific receptors on T cells (i.e. these fragments are *T cell epitopes*). Thus it can be seen that the specificity of any T cell clone to be able to deliver help to any given B cell clone is determined by sequences in the same molecule that contains the B cell epitope. A further twist to the tale lies in the fact that the T cell epitopes are not exported or recognized in their natural state but rather in association with a class of specialized 'carrier' molecules, the HLA antigens.

Human leucocyte antigen restriction and the immune response

Human leucocyte antigens (HLA) are a polymorphic group of molecules which were first recognized on the surface of white cells but are now known to be produced by most cells in the body and to play a critical role in determining which antigens can elicit an immune response in any one individual. When an antigenic molecule is broken down as described above it first combines with an HLA molecule before being transported to the surface of the cell. The actual determinant recognized by T cell receptors is not the short peptide fragment alone but the three-dimensional combination of *HLA plus peptide*. There are six important HLA genes and each one is present in the human population in numerous polymorphic forms. As one gene is inherited for each locus from both parents everyone has between 6 and 12 different HLA molecules, and for any peptide to be recognized by T cells it has to be able to combine with one of these molecules. Clearly each HLA molecule must be able to combine with a large number of different peptides but many peptides can only combine with

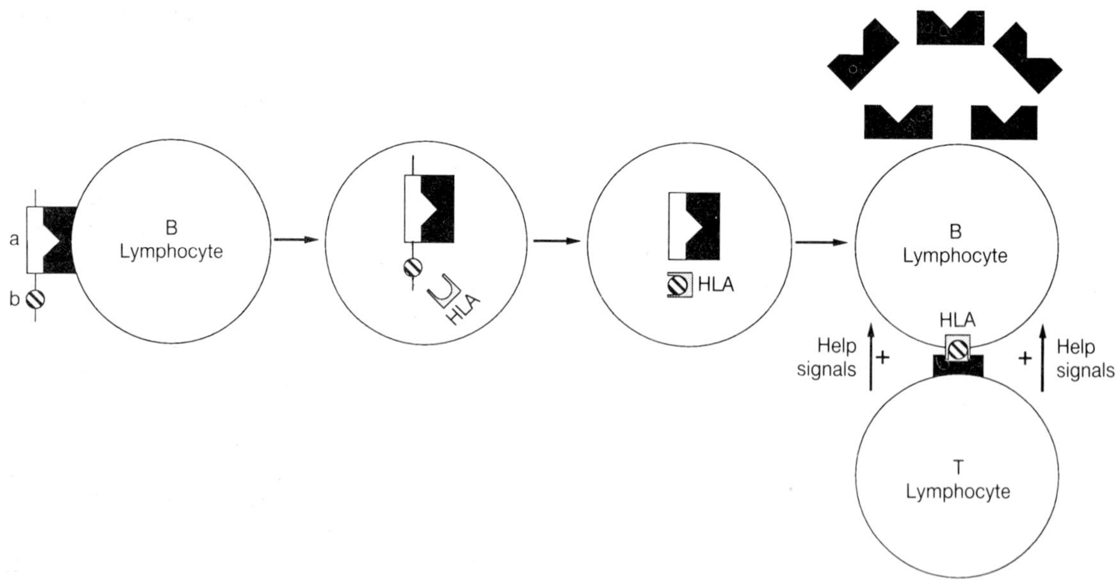

Fig. 5.3 T cell help to B cells. The antigenic molecule is recognized by a B cell through epitope 'a' and internalized. The molecule is broken down and epitope 'b' returned to the B cell surface in specific conjunction with a human leucocyte antigen (HLA) molecule, the combination of which is recognized by a receptor on the surface of a T lymphocyte stimulating it to deliver help signals for the B cell to produce antibody to epitope 'a'.

certain specific HLA molecules; they are said to be *restricted* and the HLA molecule is referred to as the *restriction element* for that peptide. As most antigenic molecules contain several peptide fragments capable of acting as T cell epitopes the chances are that most people can respond to most antigens by using at least one of the potential epitopes. However, when the antigen is reduced in size there will be some individuals who simply cannot make a T cell response (either to help antibody production or as part of a cell-mediated effector mechanism). It may be felt that even a brief outline of HLA restriction such as this is out of place in a book about malaria, but without it it would be impossible to appreciate some of the most important constraints on the immune response, and particularly on the development of malaria vaccines.

It is necessary now to look at how the other part of the immune system works. The best way to understand this is from the mechanism of T cell help discussed above. The ability to process and export small pieces of molecules is not limited to B cells or specialist antigen processing cells, indeed all cells do it and it is probably a way of clearing intracellular debris. Cell-mediated immunity involves the recognition of such fragments by T cells which, instead of delivering a help signal, deliver a damaging response, either the release of *cytolytic* substances (by cytotoxic lymphocytes or CTLs) or the release of *cytokines*, such as g-interferon, which may have a local or more distant effect. Some cytokines act directly on foreign organisms while others attract populations of non-specific effector cells into the area to do the dirty work.

So much for the basic outlines. The questions of concern are: which of the many possible mechanisms in the repertoire of the immune system occur in response to malaria infections? Which ones are protective? What are the molecules responsible for inducing the response and which serve as targets for the response? There are several ways of looking at these problems. One can isolate the constituents of a response for close scrutiny *in vitro*, for example, by placing a particular cellular subset from immune humans in a tissue culture dish with malaria parasites and observing the consequences. Alternatively, one can manipulate the components of the immune response in an animal model of malaria that is selected for its similarities to human infections. Both approaches share the problem that in artificially manipulating the system there is the danger of finding effector responses which are simply not so important in real life. An alternative approach is to take immune effectors, usually antibody from immune individuals, and ask what parasite components do they recognize? Having identified the antigenic molecules one can then build up to a picture of what these molecules do and the mechanisms by which immune responses work. The following sections summarize the potential mechanisms of antimalarial immunity, with an attempt to indicate whether they are likely to be important.

Pre-erythrocytic immunity

Following the bite of the female mosquito sporozoites circulate in the blood stream for a very brief period, some reaching the liver and entering hepatocytes, others being filtered out by a variety of non-specific protective mechanisms. Of the potential immune mechanisms an antibody-mediated attack would seem the most likely. Antibody would necessarily be directed to components on the surface of the sporozoite and having bound could potentially exert its protective effect by any of a variety of mechanisms including opsonization, complement-mediated lysis or neutralization (i.e. blocking the invasion of hepatocytes and thus aborting the infection). Once invasion has taken place the considerations are quite different: now it would be difficult to envisage a role for antibody. On the other hand, the intracellular parasite may be a target for cell-mediated immunity. Hepatocytes have HLA molecules and could therefore present processed antigens derived from the parasite at their surface, leading to recognition and killing by either direct lysis or the range of soluble mediators discussed above.

There is no doubt that pre-erythrocytic immunity can be induced. Experimental immunization with sporozoite preparations has conferred immunity to subsequent sporozoite challenge in a whole range of hosts including mice, monkeys and humans (but such immunization gives no protection against infection initiated by blood stages, confirming the stage specificity of immunity). Much of our knowledge in this area has resulted from the drive to develop a vaccine. Initial interest focussed on the possible roles of antibodies: humans in endemic areas produce antibodies to sporozoites and the pattern at the population level is at least consistent with a role in immunity, levels being low in childhood and rising with age. The development of monoclonal antibodies to the surface of sporozoites and their subsequent use in isolating the genes coding for the major sporozoite surface protein (the *circumsporozoite* or CS protein) was a landmark in parasite immunology. The CS protein of *P. falciparum* was found to have a particularly fascinating structure. Outer parts of the molecule are relatively conventional polypeptides, which are probably important in critical functions such as recognition and attachment to the hepatocyte surface. The central part of the molecule, however, comprises the same sequence of amino acids (NANP) repeated over and over about 40 times. It became apparent that not only were most antisporozoite monoclonal antibodies directed against this central repeating sequence but that the majority of antibodies produced by immune humans seemed to have the same specificity. The demonstration that passive transfer of such antibodies could both protect animals against sporozoite challenge and block the invasion of hepatocytes in *in vitro* models, coupled with the fact that the dominant (NANP) epitope of *P. falciparum* was the same in isolates from all over the world, appeared to offer a perfect vaccine candidate. Furthermore, the candidate vaccine was so simple, comprising repeat blocks of the same four amino acids, that it could even be synthesized chemically. Against the background of such high expectations the results of the first vaccine trials in humans were widely considered disappointing. Particular problems were encountered in raising reasonable levels of antibodies and in boosting responses, however, there was evidence of some protection, albeit in a minority of cases. These results have focussed attention on the question of how to obtain appropriate T cell help for antibody responses with a submit malaria vaccine. It is not surprising that the sequence NANP itself is a rather poor T cell epitope, and many individuals may not have the appropriate HLA restriction molecules to be able to use it as such. It will be necessary to include alternative T cell epitopes in a vaccine, preferably from other parts of the CS protein itself as this would allow boosting by natural exposure to sporozoites.

The problems encountered in the development of the sporozoite vaccine forced a reappraisal of the potential mechanisms of pre-erythrocytic immunity. From the earliest experimental observations there had been a number of clues to suggest that humoral mechanisms may not be the only, or even the most important, aspect. Most notably, successful immunization usually required live sporozoites: an unexpected feature of an antibody-mediated response. It is now clear that cell-mediated responses by T cells recognizing processed antigens on the hepatocyte surface are likely to be important, indeed in some settings they are more important than humoral responses. There is of course no *a priori* reason to expect that the targets for cell-mediated immunity will come from the CS protein, they could just as well be from other parasite proteins, in which case the search for vaccine candidates will have to start again. In fact, so far, it does look as though some important epitopes do come from the CS protein, perhaps because it is produced in large amounts and shed during invasion allowing it to reach the cytoplasm of the hepatocyte.

There remain many unresolved questions over which parts of the CS protein could function as T cell epitopes and to what extent the ability of humans to make a good response will be limited by HLA restriction. Furthermore, whereas the dominant B cell epitope (NANP) is well conserved this is not the case with the putative T cell epitopes which show marked variations in amino acid sequence raising the spectre that the malaria parasite may be able to outwit attempts to vaccinate by its large capacity for generating diversity in key molecules.

Immunity to erythrocytic stages

At first glance it looks as though the malaria parasite ought to be well protected once it leaves the liver and enters the erythrocytic cycle because it spends most of its time inside the host erythrocyte. Only at schizont rupture is the parasite directly exposed, when for a few seconds daughter merozoites have to attach to and enter new red cells. Much attention has therefore been given to the merozoite as a potential target of host immune responses. Antibody-mediated protective responses could be directed against surface proteins of the merozoite, in which case they could act either by blocking key steps in the invasion process or by rendering the merozoite susceptible to secondary effects such as phagocytosis or complement-mediated damage. Alternatively, an antibody-mediated response could be directed at non-surface molecules released transiently as part of the invasion process. In fact there is experimental evidence for all these possibilities and as with the sporozoite the difficulty is in determining which, if any, are important.

Although the intracellular parasite appears well positioned to avoid host responses there are several potential chinks in its defenses. Unlike other intracellular sites there is not really the potential for direct T cell-mediated responses to determinants presented at the host cell surface; the erythrocyte has only low numbers of residual HLA molecules and no mechanism of producing, assembling or transporting new ones. However, the intracellular parasite might clearly be susceptible to soluble products of immune cells. In this case some means of ensuring that parasites were exposed to high concentrations of the cytokine would be needed. A plausible scenario would be: initial parasite clearance by phagocytic cells in fixed parts of the reticuloendothelial system leading to the recruitment of antigen-specific lymphocytes and the production of cytokines. Parasites would then be damaged whenever they passed through this 'cytokine factory'. Such a scenario fits well with the known importance of the spleen in malarial immunity and the massive trafficking of immune cells to the spleen that is seen in experimental models.

Finally, the intracellular parasite is not nearly as unobtrusive as appears at first glance. As the parasite matures it induces a series of morphological, functional and antigenic changes in the host red cell membrane. Some changes are a result of alteration of the host constituents, perhaps by partial disruption of integral membrane proteins, but others result from the parasite inserting its own molecules into the host cell membrane. These 'neoantigens' are potentially important targets for immunity as they advertise the presence of a foreign organism within the cell. The molecular characterization of changes at the host cell surface is considerably less advanced than that for either sporozoites or merozoites but promises to be important in understanding immunity to malaria.

Immunity to sexual stages

In the case of pre-erythrocytic and erythrocytic immunity the observation that immunity occurred naturally provided the impetus for vaccine development. In the case of sexual stages it has been the other way around. The idea is that antibody ingested by the mosquitos when taking a blood meal could act on the parasite stages in the mosquito to interfere with transmission. This would offer no immediate advantage to the immunized person and is sometimes referred to as an 'altruistic' vaccine. The uses of such a vaccine would depend on the level of transmission but in general it is envisaged that they would be just one part of a combined control strategy, for instance, in limiting the transmission of parasites that escape immunity in individuals vaccinated against other stages. The feasibility of this approach has been shown by the experimental blocking of transmission by monoclonal antibodies against surface antigens of gametocytes, zygotes and oökinetes when fed to mosquitos. Antibodies to the surface of gametocytes are found in humans naturally exposed to malaria raising the question of whether antigametocyte immunity has a role in controlling transmission in endemic areas. In the case of *P. vivax* the epidemiological picture in some areas is consistent with such a hypothesis, in the case of *P. falciparum* there is not enough information to be sure, although it may be less likely as antigametocyte responses are a more prominent feature of non-immune persons rather than of individuals living under constant transmission.

Immunity in endemic populations

Does all this information on potential immune responses to the malaria parasite allow us to make any more sense of the epidemiological picture given at the beginning of the chapter? Many studies have been conducted in both immune and non-immune individuals. Malaria infection leads to a brisk and substantial antibody response, with specific antimalarial antibodies of the IgM, IgD and IgG classes being produced. In endemic areas newborns have very high levels of antimalarial IgG as a result of passive transfer across the placenta. The levels decline to almost nil and then rise throughout childhood, the exact kinetics varying with the level of transmission but generally reaching a plateau in late childhood. It is well established that antibodies can protect against malaria in a range of experimental models and the strongest arguments for the importance of humoral immunity in humans are the protection of infants from malaria until they lose passively acquired antibody and the classical observations of Cohen and McGregor on the marked therapeutic effect of gamma globulins from immune adults when given to children with acute malaria. The problems come when one tries to separate out the putative protective responses from the vast majority of the antibody response which is non-protective. Many studies have examined the role of responses to individual parasite components; an example is shown in Fig. 5.4. Some useful conclusions can be drawn from this sort of approach, for example, in the particular case illustrated it is unlikely that antisporozoite antibodies were playing much of a role in protecting children from disease. However, it is easier to draw negative conclusions than positive ones from this kind of study and the goal of identifying critical immune responses remains elusive.

The role of cell-mediated immunity is even less clear. There is no doubting the central importance of T cells in immunity to malaria, and in many animal models this is independent of any role in assisting humoral responses. The question is where on the spectrum do humans lie? All the potential

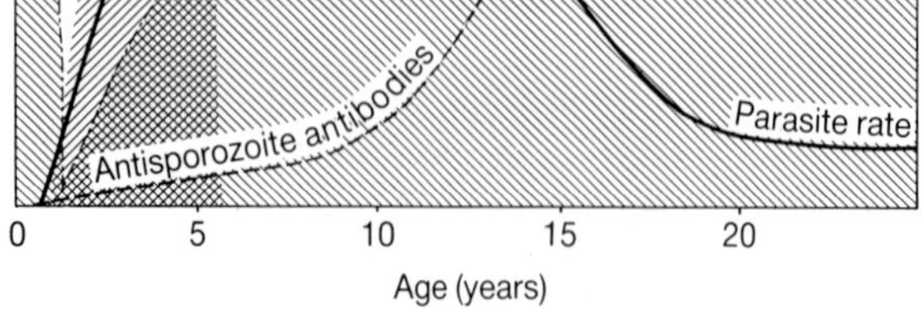

Fig. 5.4 Age-related changes in total antimalarial antibody levels and antisporozoite antibody levels in relation to parasite rates and susceptibility to death in a West African population.

cell-mediated mechanisms discussed have been demonstrated using human material *in vitro* but this is not the same as showing that they are important *in vivo*. Sometimes, earlier observations are worth remembering, for instance, when immune adults have been challenged for various reasons with injections of blood-stage parasites they have been quite capable of exhibiting immunity, indicating that whether or not cell-mediated killing of intrahepatic parasites occurs, immune adults are not relying on it.

The spleen plays a vital role in protection from malaria and its removal renders humans particularly susceptible to infection. The histological picture in humans and experimental animals indicates that it is a site of very active parasite clearance during an acute attack of malaria. Clearance in acute malaria does not necessarily involve the same mechanisms as immunity to future attacks but it is likely that specific antigen recognition and subsequent recruitment of effector cells to the spleen are important. Identifying the critical antigens in this process presents difficulties because, unlike the case with antibody, the possibilities are not narrowed by a requirement to be on the surface of the parasite.

One way in which the molecular characterization of malaria parasites has thrown light on malarial immunity is the revelation of just how much diversity there is within a single species. The majority of malaria antigens examined show considerable polymorphism ranging from single amino acid changes to very extensive deletions and recombinations. Of course not all diversity is related to immune evasion but much of it may be, especially in the light of evidence discussed earlier from experimental infections and the epidemiological picture, which suggest the importance of strain-specific responses. At the simplest level a high level of polymorphism in critical epitopes may allow the parasite population to outflank the human immune response; thus a single amino acid change in a T cell epitope of the CS protein may result in a given host being unable to mount a T cell response, despite already having made good responses to very similar parasites. Other more subtle mechanisms may be important. Many malarial antigens have immunodominant sections made up of short motifs repeated over and over. These often show subtle changes of length and sequence and there are considerable similarities between the repeats of different molecules. It has been suggested that such strongly immunogenic regions may act as decoy or smokescreen antigens and that small changes in otherwise similar sequences prevent the maturation of antibody responses to critical epitopes. A further evasion mechanism of great biological interest is *clonal antigenic variation*, whereby a single clone of parasite has within its genome the capacity to express different versions of a particular antigen sequentially. This is a classical evasion mechanism of African trypanosomes but it is now known to occur in malaria for antigens expressed at the red cell membrane and presumably offers a way for the parasite to keep one step ahead of the host immune system. The importance of this high degree of diversity is two-fold: it makes it even more difficult to study naturally developing immunity and it presents potentially major problems for vaccine development (Fig. 5.5).

It is chastening to realize that our knowledge of the molecular and cellular biological aspects of immunity has not yet taken our understanding of naturally acquired immunity to malaria in humans much beyond that which could be derived from a careful consideration of epidemiological, clinical and experimental evidence available 30 years ago. This is one statement that the present author would

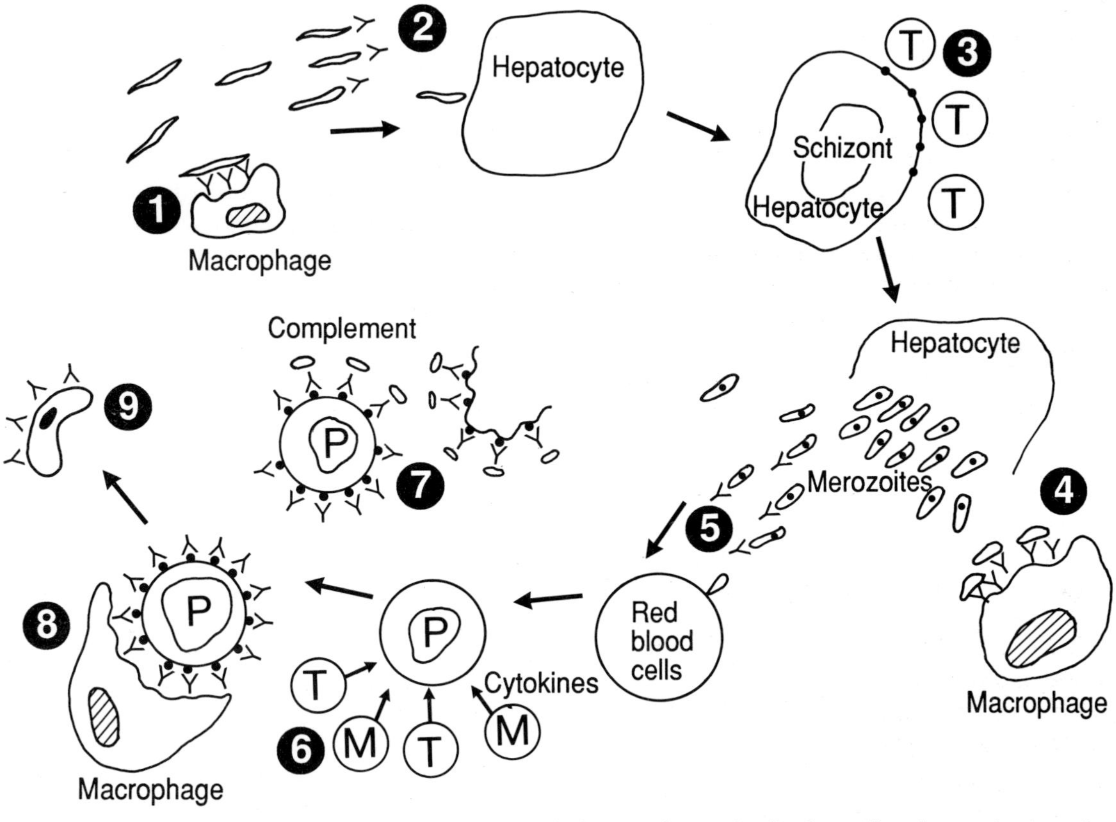

Fig. 5.5 Potential immune mechanisms against the malaria parasite. 1. Antibody-mediated opsonization of sporozoites. 2. Blocking of hepatocyte invasion. 3. Cell-mediated responses to processed antigens at the surface of the infected hepatocyte. 4. Opsonization of merozoites. 5. Blocking of merozoite invasion of red cells. 6. Intracellular killing of parasites by soluble mediators. 7. Complement activation by antibody binding to neoantigens on the surface of infected red cells, leading to lysis. 8. Opsonization of infected red cells. 9. Antibody to the surface of gametocytes (carried into the mosquito where it blocks normal process of fertilization and development). This list is not exhaustive, but indicates the complexity of antimalarial immunity. T, T cell; M, macrophage; P, parasite.

be delighted to see outdated during the lifetime of the current edition of this book!

Prospects for vaccination

Humans in endemic areas do develop immunity to malaria. Increasing difficulties of malaria control and the success of vaccination against other infectious diseases combine to make the development of antimalarial vaccines an attractive goal. The difficulties are enormous. Firstly, no vaccine for human use has been developed against any organism even approaching the complexity of the malaria parasite. For years the major bar to progress was the lack of a practical source of antigen: clearly it is not possible to dissect mosquitos for sporozoites on a large scale and the difficulties of separating parasite components from human red cell components appeared insuperable. The advent of monoclonal antibodies and recombinant DNA technology completely changed these prospects and offered the possibility of defining and artificially producing the specific components of the parasite capable of inducing immunity. The search for such subunit vaccines against all stages of the parasite has dominated immunological research in malaria over the last 10 years. Candidate molecules have been identified for each stage, produced and used in experimental systems with varying degrees of success. As indicated above, the field of sporozoite vaccines moved very rapidly and prototype vaccines have been tried in human volunteers with very limited success to date. Over the next few years the number of candidate vaccine molecules will increase and so will the number and scale of experimental human trials. The technical aspects of malaria vaccine research will change rapidly and probably in unpredictable ways, however, the problems that remain to be overcome are clear. At the most basic level the problems of generating reliable, boostable protective responses given the biological complexities of parasite diversity are formidable but not necessarily intractable. The logistical problems of moving from a potential vaccine through volunteer testing to field trials are often underestimated but again could undoubtedly be solved. Success in producing a practical vaccine would by no means be the end of the road; the toll from easily preventable diseases in childhood continues to be massive in many of the very areas that most need a vaccine. For these reasons optimism over the capacity of human ingenuity to solve the immunological problems must be tempered by a realization that malaria vaccines will not have a major impact on world malaria morbidity and mortality for many years to come.

Immunopathology

As we have seen, infection with malaria induces a broad spectrum of immune responses. Only a small part of the total response is likely to be protective and it might be expected that malaria would be associated with a wide range of immunopathology. It is perhaps surprising that classical immunopathological reactions such as allergic responses or immune complex disease are rare, more important are effects on the regulation of the immune system.

Following an attack of malaria total levels of serum immunoglobulins rise. Only a part of this seems to be specifically antimalarial antibody and in malaria epidemic areas normal individuals are 'hypergammaglobulinaemic'. Although the inhabitants of endemic areas are subjected to many infectious challenges it does seem that hypergammaglobulinaemia is due predominantly to malaria, for when malaria is controlled levels fall remarkably. The mechanisms are unclear: malaria parasites are mitogenetic *in vitro* but other possibilities include immunoregulatory effects of cytokines released during malaria infection and mechanisms such as the reduced ability to control the proliferation of B lymphocytes infected with Epstein–Barr virus that occurs during acute attacks of malaria. Part of the polyclonal antibody response includes the production of a wide range of autoantibodies including antinuclear factor, antibodies against single-stranded DNA and antibodies to intermediate filaments. These are found commonly following an acute attack of malaria and are also common in the population at large in an endemic area. The finding of autoantibodies does not have the significance that it would have in a non-endemic area, indeed autoimmune diseases are generally rare in malaria endemic areas. This appears to be an environmental effect, as the low prevalence is not maintained on migration away from endemic areas. There is intriguing evidence from experimental models that malaria may actually suppress the expression of autoimmune disease.

Immunopathology of acute malaria

It has often been suggested that immune responses play a role in the pathogenesis of disease. Circulating immune complexes (i.e. antigens, in this case from the parasite, bound tightly to antibody) are detectable in the majority of patients, levels rising over the 2 weeks following presentation. It has been reported that levels are higher in patients with cerebral malaria but the significance of this is not clear and there is a divergence of opinions over the possible role of immune complex deposition and local immune responses in the brains of patients with cerebral malaria, some studies having failed to detect any evidence for it. Immune complex deposition in the kidneys is probably common, but in *P. falciparum* it leads only to a subclinical glomerulonephritis; renal failure in acute malaria being predominantly a tubular, rather than a glomerular problem. Immune complex renal disease is important in *P. malariae* infections (see below). Immune complexes may consume complement, and hypocomplementaemia is common during acute attacks of malaria, particularly low levels of C3 and C4. However, this is a transient depression, at least in African children, and normal levels are regained before the appearance of large amounts of immune complexes in the circulation.

Malaria induces a very marked rise in acute phase proteins, for example, levels of C reactive protein and α-1-acid glycoprotein are well above those found in serious bacterial infections. The most compelling evidence for a role of immune mechanisms in pathogenesis is the relationship between the levels of various cytokines, particularly interleukin-1, interleukin-6 and tumour necrosis factor (TNF), and the severity of disease. Thus, for example, there is a gradient in levels of TNF, rising from non-severe disease through cerebral malaria to death. Although it might be suggested that this is an association rather than a causal mechanism the known biological effects of these cytokines argue for a direct role in the genesis of disease.

Malaria is often said to be immunosuppressive and there is much experimental evidence for a whole range of potentially immunosuppressive mechanisms. When malaria is controlled mortality from other causes usually falls too, suggesting that immunosuppression may be important in humans, however, there is surprisingly little *direct* evidence for an important clinical effect in humans. Responses to some, but by no means all, vaccines are reduced in children when given during active infection. There are conflicting views on whether malaria predisposes to other acute infections, for instance, pneumonia, or whether the illnesses observed are in fact part of the clinical spectrum of malaria itself. There is an increased susceptibility to systemic infections with non-typhoid salmonella in children with malaria.

Plasmodium malariae nephropathy

The nephrotic syndrome (a condition in which the normally efficient filtering mechanisms of the kidneys are damaged, resulting in the loss of large amounts of protein in the urine) is common in many malaria endemic areas. That, in a proportion of cases, this is due to *P. malariae* was established by a combination of epidemiological, experimental and clinical observations. The syndrome is associated with a variety of histological pictures. In West African children the findings are sufficiently distinct to allow the description of a specific 'quartan nephropathy'; in contrast, many different histological findings are described in patients in East Africa. It is an immune complex nephropathy, with deposits of both IgG and IgM in the basement membrane. In 50% of cases there is also complement deposition. When antibody is eluted from affected tissues it has specificity for *P. malariae* antigens. The pathogenesis probably requires long-term infection. In a few reported cases where treatment was given as soon as the clinical features of nephropathy were noted a complete cure was obtained. However, the general experience in African children is that once established the syndrome carries a very high mortality (around 80% in 2 years) and progress is not modified by either antimalarial treatment or immunosuppressive drugs. It is striking that, although much more common, *P. falciparum* does not seem to give rise to this syndrome despite commonly causing an asymptomatic glomerulonephritis.

Anaemia

Some degree of anaemia is the rule in malarial infections and it is commonly of greater degree than can be accounted for by destruction of infected red cells. Several mechanisms may operate: during an acute attack of malaria there is usually evidence of increased red cell destruction; at the other extreme a proportion of patients show reduced red cell production, with a markedly dyserythropoetic bone marrow picture. The question of to what extent immunopathological mechanisms play a role in the genesis of malarial anaemia is contentious. Uninfected host red cells commonly have increased levels of antibody bound to their surface after a malaria infection. This could occur by a number of mechanisms including the production of antired cell autoantibodies, the binding of soluble malaria antigen to red cells and subsequent recognition by antimalarial antibodies or the binding of immune complexes (red cells are an efficient clearance mechanism for circulating immune complexes). Increased levels of antibody on uninfected cells could lead to their increased clearance in the spleen and other sites, however, attempts to correlate the degree of antibody binding and anaemia have produced conflicting results and in some communities antibodies on the red cells seem merely to act as a marker of recent malaria infection. It may not be necessary to postulate increased levels of bound antibody as a cause of anaemia, an alternative explanation is that following an attack of malaria the reticuloendothelial system is more efficient, leading to the increased removal of cells carrying the *normal* low levels of antibody. Finally, evidence from experimental models suggests that immune mechanisms could play a role in the abnormal erythropoiesis of malaria through the effects of cytokines such as TNF, however, this remains to be established in human infections.

Hyperreactive malarial splenomegaly

Splenic enlargement is a characteristic feature of malaria infections and in endemic areas palpable splenomegaly is the norm rather than the exception during childhood. However, it is unusual for the spleen to remain palpable into adulthood. In all malaria endemic areas a certain number of subjects, often young adults, are found with marked splenic enlargement. In about half the cases there is no explanation found and these cases are truly idiopathic but others show a constellation of features which form a single identifiable condition originally called tropical splenomegaly syndrome (TSS) and later renamed hyperreactive malarial splenomegaly (HMS). This latter name has not enjoyed complete acceptance and the condition is still often referred to as TSS. The three cardinal features are splenic enlargement, usually to between 6 and 15 cm, elevation of serum IgM to at least two standard deviations above the mean for that population (and often very much higher) and a positive response to antimalarial therapy. This often requires several months of prophylaxis before there is a regression in spleen size. In addition there is commonly marked hepatic enlargement and over 50% of cases show a characteristic feature of hepatic sinusoidal lymphocytosis but this is neither pathognomic or necessary for the diagnosis. The syndrome occurs only in malaria endemic areas and disappears following malaria control. Unlike Burkitt's lymphoma there is not a close correlation with the degree of malaria endemicity nor with any particular malaria species. In parts of South-east Asia and Papua New Guinea the condition is extremely common, with over 50% of the population fulfilling the criteria, i.e. it is almost the 'normal' response to malaria in those communities. In West Africa HMS has a prevalence of around 1 in 1000. Several lines of evidence suggest that there is a strong genetic element to susceptibility. The basic deficit seems to be impaired suppressor T cell function, leading to massive overproduction of IgM. Following splenectomy overproduction of IgM persists and may then be associated with massive hepatomegaly.

Burkitt's lymphoma

Burkitt's lymphoma is the commonest childhood malignancy in Africa. It has a peak prevalence in 4–9-year-old children and presents as a rapidly growing tumour, usually in the jaw or abdomen. Although sporadic cases of lymphoma with the same features occur worldwide, it only reaches high prevalences (endemic Burkitt's lymphoma) in areas of high *P. falciparum* transmission. The evidence that this is due to an interaction between the Epstein–Barr virus (EBV, a herpes virus first discovered in Burkitt's tumour tissue) and malaria is very strong. The basic event appears to be a translocation of an oncogene from its normal position on chromosome 8 to one of several other positions in the genome. In Burkitt's lymphomas the new position is always in the regions that regulate the expression of immunoglobin genes and it is assumed that this allows normal control to be lost over the oncogene and the cell in which the event occurs (a B cell) goes on to divide in an uncontrolled way. The exact role of malaria is contentious but it is clear that during malaria attacks normal immune surveillance of EBV-infected B cells is reduced and it may be that the ensuing proliferation increases the chance of the required translocation taking place.

Chapter 6

Diagnostic methods in malaria

H. M. Gilles*

A definite diagnosis of malaria infection is established on the finding of parasites in the blood. Malaria must be suspected in all cases of fever in endemic areas or in persons who have been exposed to the infection when visiting a tropical country, even after spending a few hours at an exotic airport.

Tentative antimalarial treatment may be advisable when facilities for blood examination are not available or if a laboratory report cannot be obtained immediately. Even in this case, however, a blood slide should be taken for subsequent examination, before the treatment is administered. Failure to control the fever by carefully supervised administration of an adequate drug tends to exclude malaria as the cause of the disease unless resistance to a specific antimalarial drug is suspected.

Malaria may be confused with any other fever and several studies in partially immune African children indicate that almost half of clinically diagnosed malaria patients do not have microscopically detectable parasitaemias. This is particularly so during the low transmission season. A careful history and examination may reveal those in whom symptoms and signs provide a firm basis of differentiation – respiratory and intestinal infections, tonsillitis and meningitis; the latter may occasion difficulties but an examination of the cerebrospinal fluid permits a definite diagnosis. Surgical conditions such as a middle ear infection, an abscess or cellulitis usually direct attention to the affected part. A urinary infection is often misdiagnosed as malaria until the urine is examined. Even more difficult are the initial periods of fever in many virus diseases before the rash and other symptoms appear: measles, smallpox, chickenpox, influenza, poliomyelitis and yellow fever. In fact, some of the virus infections do not cause distinctive physical signs and do not permit a precise diagnosis on clinical grounds. In cases of continued fever, especially if there is no response to antimalarial therapy, there exist many possibilities: tuberculosis in all its manifestations, typhoid, typhus, liver abscess, urinary infections, endocarditis, brucellosis, relapsing fever, trypanosomiasis, kala-azar, severe blood disorders, and rapidly growing tumours.

The diagnosis of malaria is always a matter of clinical judgement; it cannot be merely a matter of uncritically reading a laboratory report, however essential that examination may be. Sound judgement is a supreme virtue in the face of several apparently contradictory facts. Thus, the detection of a few parasites in a blood film of a partially immune indigenous child demonstrates the presence of infection, but it does not necessarily determine the actual disease for which medical aid was sought; this may vary from pneumonia to a fractured femur. On the other hand, many non-immune individuals take antimalarial drugs prophylactically and this (in the case of a breakthrough of malaria) considerably reduces the chance of detecting malaria parasites in the blood. A thorough search of one or several thick blood films should demonstrate parasites in such cases although occasionally the

***The helpful comments and constructive criticism of Dr David Payne are gratefully acknowledged; particularly his section contribution entitled *Molecular Biological Detection Tests*.**

diagnosis of 'clinical malaria' appears justified, especially if fever rapidly subsides after the appropriate treatment. A similar situation is created if antimalarial drugs are given several hours before the examination of the blood. At this stage only the rapid disappearance of all clinical signs lends specious confirmation to the probable diagnosis. Non-immune individuals appear more ill in the presence of a scanty parasitaemia than do partially immune patients who often appear to tolerate with relative equanimity a heavy parasite load. At all times one has to bear in mind the significance of the laboratory report, having regard to the time when the blood film was prepared and the relation to drug administration. One should also remember that many technical mistakes can arise in the long chain of events between the taking of the blood slide and its examination. A microscopical diagnosis is only as reliable as the competence of the workers who prepare the blood slides and examine them.

It is very doubtful whether blood films made from a sternal puncture are superior to blood samples from peripheral circulation. Some authors advocate this controversial and painful procedure, but from personal experience it is not superior to usual skin puncture. Moreover, the presence in the sternal marrow of various immature cells of the erythrocytic series may confuse the picture.

The formerly advocated method of 'provocation' by injection of 0.5 ml of 1:1000 solution of adrenaline, which was supposed to produce a contraction of the spleen and the appearance of parasites in the blood, is of no value for the diagnosis of malaria and may be dangerous when used in patients with high blood pressure. This view has been confirmed by studies on malaria in Vietnam.

Although various modern methods ranging from density gradient high speed centrifugation, through the use of monoclonal antibodies, to the application of magnetic separation techniques, DNA probes and even the newer amplification techniques such as the polymerase chain reaction (PCR) have been tried, in order to detect scanty parasitaemia, it appears that for routine clinical and epidemiological studies the time-honoured thin- and thick-film blood examination by a competent microscopist remains unchallenged when it comes to simplicity and convenience.

Blood examination for malaria parasites

Even with all the serological and immunological techniques currently available and under development, it is probably true to say that the only certain means of diagnosing all four of the human malarias is the detection of the *Plasmodium* spp by microscopical examination of the blood. This examination should be a routine procedure in medical practice not only in all malarious areas, but also in non-malarious countries whatever may be the symptoms of primary diagnosis, if the patient has been travelling abroad within a year.

The main reason for this is that the clinical picture of malaria may be of infinite variety; this infection may also occur as a result of blood transfusion from an infected donor or it may be a complicating factor of other diseases. One should remember that the presence of malaria parasites in the blood is a sign of *infection* but not necessarily a cause of the *disease*; persons who have resided for many years in malarious areas may have scanty malaria parasites in their blood, but the symptoms which made them see the doctor may be due to a different cause.

Biosafety

It is well established that various pathogens such as the hepatitis B virus, the human immunodeficiency virus (HIV) which is the causative agent of AIDS, and malaria itself, can be transmitted by the transfer of infected blood during the taking of blood samples. Accordingly, invasive blood sampling techniques such as venepuncture or finger pricking should only be used when the risk is justified by the potential benefit. Health workers who are required to take blood samples for malaria diagnostic purposes should be aware of the potential risks to their patients and themselves and should always follow the recommended biosafety practices to avoid the possibility of cross- or autoinfection with these blood pathogens. More details of these risks and the recommended precautionary measures are given in the *Bulletin of the World Health Organization* (1991) Vol. 69(2) (see Selected References).

Preparation of blood films

For malaria blood films use perfectly clean 25 mm × 75 mm (1 inch × 3 inch) glass slides that are free of grease and scratches. Blood may be obtained from the ear lobe or (preferably) from the second or third finger of the left hand. In infants the big toe is best. The skin should be cleaned with ether or methylated spirit and be completely dry before being punctured with a special pricker (Microlance) which is sterile and only used once before being safely discarded and destroyed. Squeeze the finger gently until a good blood drop exudes (Fig. 6.1).

For a thick film touch the drop of blood with a glass slide held above the blood drop and then after reversing the slide spread the blood evenly with a corner of another slide to make a square or a circular patch of a moderate thickness that will just allow one to read through it. Keep the slide horizontal while drying and protect it from dust and flies (Figs 6.2 and 6.3).

For a thin film the drop of blood should be smaller than for the thick film. Apply the smooth edge of another clean glass slide to the drop of blood at an angle of 45°, touch the drop of blood till it spreads along the edge. Push the spreader forwards keeping it at the same angle. Dry the thin film by waving it in the air. A properly made thin film should consist of an unbroken layer of single red blood cells with a 'tongue' not touching the edge of the slide (Figs 6.4 and 6.5).

Thin and thick films may be taken on the same slide and details of the patient can be written with ordinary graphite pencil on the thin film before it dries. Blood films may be stained with Leishman's

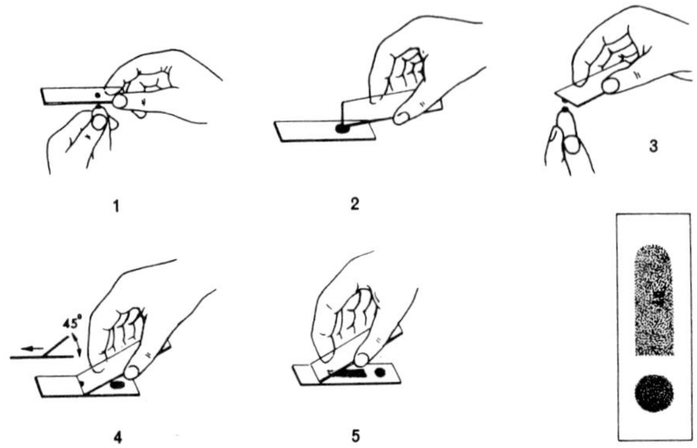

Fig. 6.2 Preparation of a thin and thick blood film on the same slide. 1. The drop of blood is touched with a clean slide. 2. Spread the drop of blood with the corner of another slide to make a circle or a square about 1 cm^2. 3. Touch a new drop of blood with the edge of a clean slide. 4. Bring the edge of the slide carrying a drop of blood to the surface of the first slide, wait until the blood spreads along the whole edge. 5. Holding in at an angle of about 45° push it forward with a rapid but not too brisk movement. Write with a pencil the slide number on the thin film. Wait until the thick film is quite dry. (WHO, 1961.)

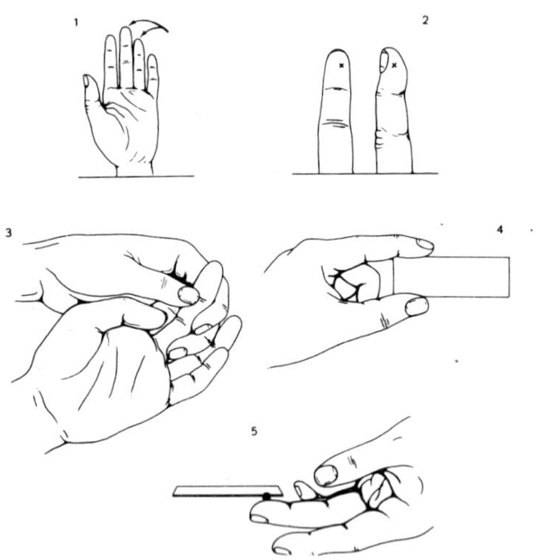

Fig. 6.1 Details of correct technique of blood collection for a thin or thick blood film. 1. The second or third finger of the left hand is generally selected. 2. The site of the puncture is the side of the ball of the finger, not too close to the nail bed. 3. If the blood does not well up from the puncture, a gentle squeeze will bring it up. 4. The slide must always be grasped by its edges. 5. The size of the blood drop is controlled better if the finger touches the slide from below. (WHO, 1961.)

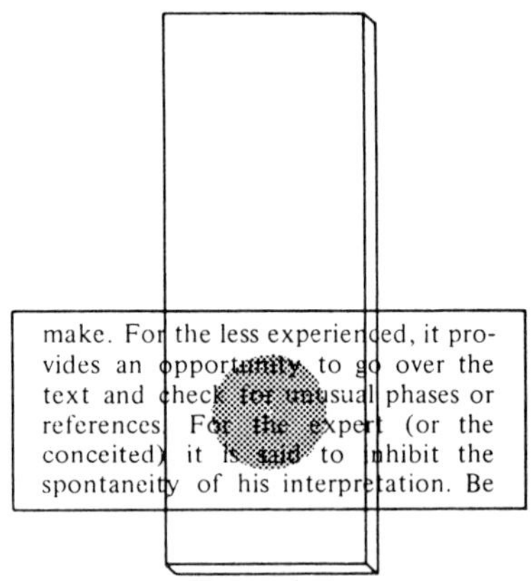

Fig. 6.3 The correct thickness of the thick film can be judged by the legibility of the printed text seen through the slide. It should be just legible.

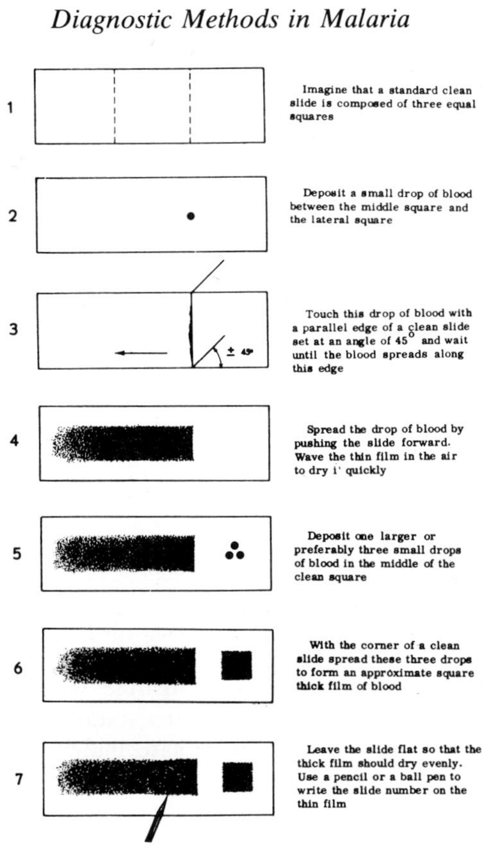

Fig. 6.4 Preparation of thin and thick blood film on the same slide (alternative method). (WHO, 1961.)

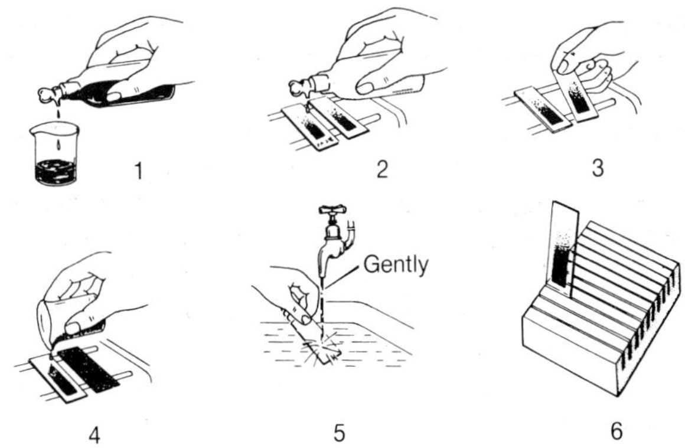

Fig. 6.6 Staining a thin blood film with Giemsa stain. 1. Prepare the staining solution by diluting the Giemsa stock solution with buffered water in a small beaker. The best solution for reasonably fast staining is 2–3 drops of Giemsa to each ml of water. One slide requires about 3–4 ml of the diluted stain. 2. Fix the thin film by pouring a few drops of methyl alcohol for a few seconds. 3. Pour off the alcohol and pour on the diluted stain before the film is dry. 4. Stain for 20–30 minutes. 5. Do not pour off the stain but flush off and rinse by holding the slide in a large container with tap water or under a gentle stream of tap water for 10–15 seconds. 6. Place the slide on end in the slide rack to dry. (WHO, 1961.)

or with Giemsa stain, the second one being preferred in the tropics. A rapid method of staining thick films is that of Field's, using buffered, isotonic Romanowsky stain with a counterstain by eosin (Figs 6.6 and 6.7).

Detailed instructions for preparation of stains will be found in manuals by Wilcox (1960), Shute and Maryon (1960) or Field *et al.* (1963). Only the most important methods are given here.

Giemsa stain

The stock solution of Giemsa stain is easily prepared from Giemsa powder available commercially.

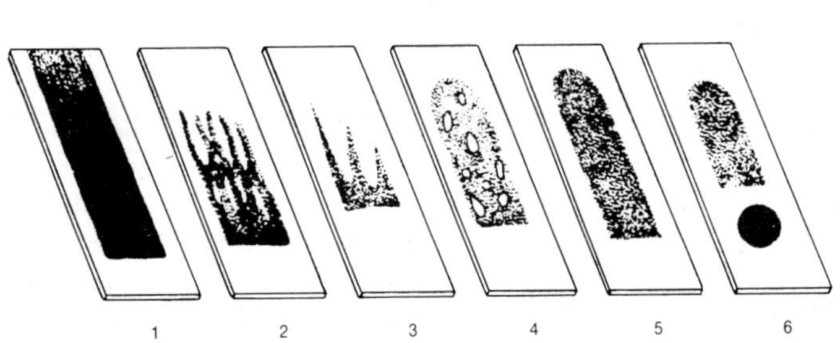

Fig. 6.5 Common faults of a thin blood film. 1. Too much blood – the end of the thin film is lost and the film itself is too thick. 2. Old, devitrified slide or the blood was clotting when the film was made. 3. Uneven contact of the spreader or the edge of the spreader ragged. Film too short. Too little blood. 4. Greasy slide. 5. Good thin film. 6. Thick and thin film on the same slide. (WHO, 1961.)

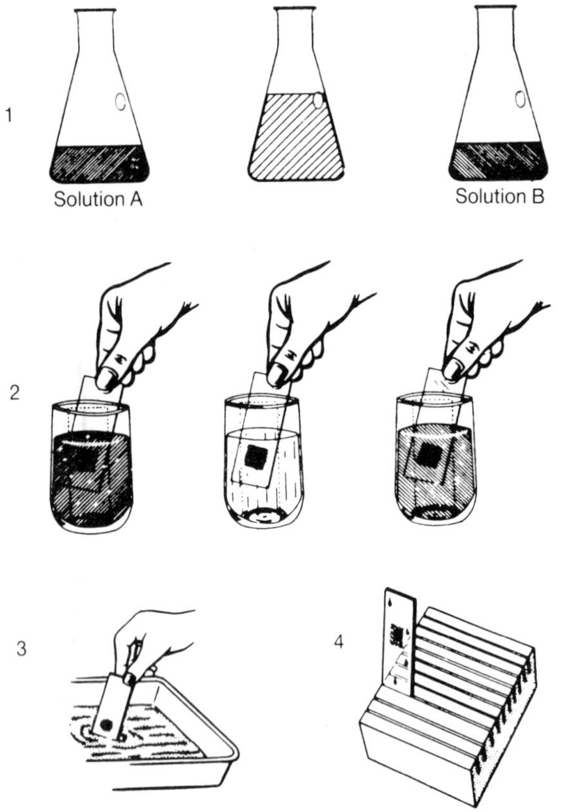

Fig. 6.7 Staining a thick blood film with Field's rapid stain. 1. Prepare three containers with solution A, water and solution B. 2. Dip the blood film into solution A and count slowly up to 'five' (about 2–3 sconds). Remove and wash in a beaker with distilled water or suitable tap water, counting slowly up to 'ten' (4–6 seconds) or until the stain ceases to run from the slide and film. Dip into solution B and count up to 'two' (1 second). 3. Remove and again wash, waving gently in tap water and counting slowly up to 'ten'. 4. Place on slide rack to dry. (WHO, 1961.)

Giemsa powder (Azure B type)	3.8 g
Glycerol, pure	250 ml
Methyl alcohol (certified pure)	250 ml

The stain is prepared best by mixing alcohol and glycerol and then adding gradually small quantities of powder in a porcelain mortar and grinding until most of the powder is dissolved. Some residue may remain and by leaving the mixture for about a week without filtering, the maximum amount of the stain will be absorbed. The prepared stock solution can then be filtered and should be kept in a bottle of hard glass with a close-fitting ground-glass stopper and away from the sunlight.

Stock solutions of Giemsa may be purchased commercially, but some brands seem to be better than others.

Note: When acquiring stain powders or solutions, small trial quantities should be bought for evaluation before bulk orders are made. It should be noted that while cheaper non-branded stains are available on the market they often have to be used at a far higher concentration than the standard well-known products, and any saving in cost is more apparent than real. Also the quality over time of the cheaper stains may be significantly inferior; particularly under tropical conditions.

Dilutions of Giemsa stain

Stock solutions of Giemsa stain must always be diluted by mixing an appropriate amount of it with distilled neutral or slightly alkaline water. The water for dilution can be kept at a standard degree of alkalinity, by using phosphate buffer salts. A buffer solution which gives a pH of 7.2 is prepared as follows:

Potassium dihydrogen phosphate KH_2PO_4	0.7 g
Disodium hydrogen phosphate Na_2HPO_4	1.0 g
Distilled water	1 litre

This solution should be tested after its preparation to make sure that its reaction is correct. It remains stable for a long time provided that it is kept in a well-stoppered bottle of neutral glass.

Tablets of phosphate buffer salts can be obtained commercially for 100 ml or 1000 ml of water.

Technique of staining thin films using Giemsa stain (Fig. 6.6)

1. The thin film should be fixed in absolute methyl alcohol for 30 seconds. This can be done simply by immersing the film in methyl alcohol or by putting a few drops on it by means of a pipette.
2. The staining solution must be freshly prepared by mixing 5 ml of stock solution with 100 ml of buffered water. For one or two slides, less staining solution is adequate providing that it will contain 5% of stock stain.
3. Transfer slide to staining solution or pour it on

the slide lying flat on two glass rods. Stain for 20–30 minutes.

4. Flush slide with tap water and stand upright to dry.

Technique of staining thick films using Giemsa stain

1. The thick film should be dry (but not by heating the slide). If it is to be stained within 1 hour of taking it, then it can be gently heated on top of a microscope lamp for a few minutes.
2. The staining solution must be freshly prepared by diluting 3–5 ml of stock solution of Giemsa to 100 ml of distilled water adjusted to neutral or to pH 7.2 when using phosphate buffer as above.
3. The single slide with the blood film can be stained either horizontally or vertically in a staining trough. In the first case cover the whole slide without any previous fixation with the diluted stain and allow to act for 30 minutes.
4. The slide is then gently flushed with distilled water (tap water may suffice), care being taken not to wash the blood film away.
5. Stand the slide upright to dry.

Note: Some authors advise the use of normal (0.85%) saline solution buffered to pH 7.2 to obtain better staining of thin and thick films.

In emergencies the concentration of the Giemsa stain can be raised to 10% and the staining time reduced to 5–10 minutes.

Technique of staining thick films with Field's stain (Fig. 6.7)

This rapid method gives excellent results when the technique is carefully followed. It is used preferably for thick films on single slides.

1. The Field's stain consists of two solutions:

Solution A

Methylene blue (medicinal)	0.8 g
Azure I	0.5 g
Disodium hydrogen phosphate (anhydrous)	5.0 g
Potassium dihydrogen phosphate	6.25 g
Distilled water	500 ml

Solution B

Eosin	1.0 g
Disodium hydrogen phosphate (anhydrous)	5.0 g
Potassium dihydrogen phosphate	6.25 g
Distilled water	500 ml

If the anhydrous salt is not available, then crystallized sodium phosphate, $Na_2HPO_4 + 12H_2O$ can be used, at 12.6 g.

2. The phosphate salts are dissolved first in separate containers and the stain is added to each container. Leave the appropriate solutions for 24 hours and filter. Keep in separate bottles for subsequent use.
3. The Field's method of staining requires the use of three wide-mouth staining jars, about 40 mm in diameter and 100 mm long. Jar No. 1 is filled with staining solution A, jar No. 2 is filled with distilled and buffered water, jar No. 3 is filled with staining solution B.
4. The technique of staining individual slides is as follows:
   (a) Dip the slide for 2–3 seconds in solution A.
   (b) Wash off the stain from the back of the slide with a stream of tap water.
   (c) Dip the slide in the buffer solution in jar No. 2 until the excess of the blue stain has left the film.
   (d) Dip the slide for 1 second in solution B.
   (e) Wash off the stain with a gentle stream of tap water.
   (f) Stand the slide upright to dry.

Examination of blood films

The thick film method, which concentrates by a factor of 20–30 the layers of red blood cells on a small surface, is, in practised hands, by far the best for general clinical use.

The parasites are easily detected in the thick film but they may be more difficult to identify than in a thin film. This is due to the fact that the red blood cells are not visible, as a result of haemolysis subsequent to staining an unfixed film. The only elements that are seen in the film are leucocytes and the parasites. However, the appearance of the latter is somewhat altered because of dehaemoglobinization and slow drying in the course of preparation of the film. Thus, the young trophozoites appear as incomplete rings or spots of blue cytoplasm with a detached red chromatin dot. In the late trophozoites of *P. vivax* the cytoplasm may be fragmented and Schüffner's stippling may be less obvious; the band forms of *P. malariae* are less characteristic. However, the schizonts and gametocytes of these species retain their usual appearance and the same goes for the crescents of *P. falciparum* (see Plate 25).

It appears that the dehaemoglobinization of the thick film may cause some loss of parasites detached from the unfixed blood layer, but this depends on the processing of the blood slide and is difficult to assess. Pigment granules undergo little change in the thick film. The interpretation of the parasites seen in a thick film requires some experience, which can be easily acquired by studying first the morphology of parasites in a thin film and then searching for corresponding forms in a thick film. As mentioned before, the thick film is a time-saving method which reveals even scanty infections within a short period (Fig. 6.8).

Although the thick film is recommended as a routine method, most experienced microscopists supplement it by taking a thin film on the same slide. This could be of value when the correct identification of some parasite species (e.g. *P. ovale*) is of importance. For staining these double films Giemsa is the best method. The thin film must be fixed with methyl alcohol, but care should be taken to leave the thick film untouched by this fixing agent. Standard practice requires that the thick film should be examined for at least 5 minutes (corresponding to approximately 100 microscopic fields under oil immersion) (Table 6.1).

Some authors advise that the standard duration of examination of the thick film should be extended to 200 oil immersion fields, as this may allow for detection of very low parasitaemia which would not be seen on the examination of 100 fields. This is a valuable suggestion, achieving some compromise between the need for greater sensitivity of the microscopic examination and the time that is allowable in field practice. An absence of malaria parasites ('negative slide') should not be reported

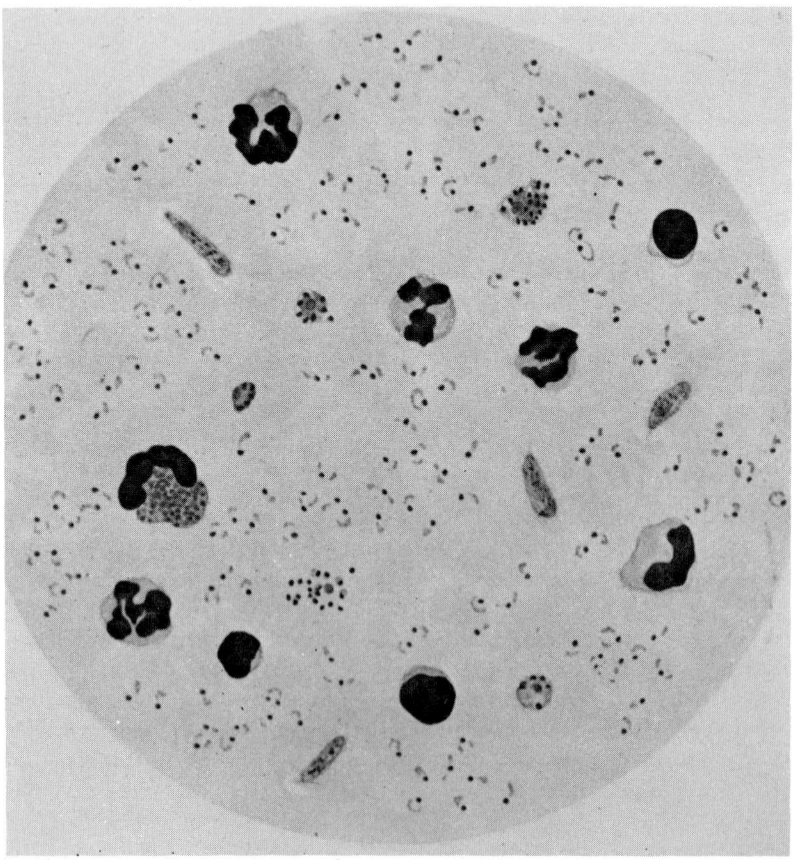

Fig. 6.8 Heavy infection with *P. falciparum* in a thick blood film stained by Giemsa–Romanowsky. × 460. *Note*: Four 'crescents' of *P. falciparum* and several developing and fully grown schizonts. Also one eosinophil, four polynuclear leucocytes, one large and three small leucocytes. The field is studded with hundreds of trophozoites of *P. falciparum*. (Wellcome Museum of Medical Science.)

Table 6.1 Quantitative aspects of thick and thin blood films for examination of malaria parasites

	Thin film	Thick film
Area on slide	250–450 mm²	50–90 mm²
Blood volume	1 µl	3–5 µl
Mean thickness	0.0025 mm	0.06–0.09 mm
Mean difference in concentration	1	20–30
Volume in 100 microscope fields (obj. ×100; ocul. ×6)	0.005–0.007 µl	0.1–0.25 µl
Time for examination (approximate)	200–300 fields/20–25 minutes	100 fields/5 minutes
Loss of leucocytes or parasites during staining	None	Leucocytes up to 8% Parasites up to 20%
Red blood cells	Fixed	Haemolysed
Parasite morphology	Not distorted	Distorted
Parasite transfer during mass staining	Impossible	Likely
Artefacts	Uncommon	More common

before at least 200 fields of a thick film are examined. In doubtful cases repeated blood films must be taken every 4 hours and examined. In severe infection with *P. falciparum* such repeated examinations are necessary to assess the response of the parasite to treatment. It is advisable to have some indication of the density of parasitaemia by counting in a thin blood film the mean number of parasitized erythrocytes in relation to an arbitrary (such as 10 000) number of red blood cells (there are on average between 300 and 500 red blood cells in a microscope field under oil immersion, but this depends largely on the optical system used and its magnification) or the average number of parasites per microscope field. A more precise method consists of counting the number of parasites and leucocytes in a thick film until several hundred of the latter have been enumerated. If a total white blood cell count of the patient's blood is made the ratio of parasites to leucocytes will give the number of parasites per µl of blood. This is known as the *parasite count*. (A few authors have recently taken to the presentation of the parasite count per litre of blood, by multiplying the number of parasites seen in a microlitre (µl) by 1 million. This is unsound, cumbersome and should not be followed.)

For designation of the relative parasite count a simple code from one to four crosses is often used by laboratory technicians. For the usual magnification between 500 and 600 times this is as follows:

+	1–10 parasites per 100 thick film fields
++	11–100 parasites per 100 thick film fields
+++	1–10 parasites per one thick film field
++++	more than 10 parasites per one thick film field

However, such counts are highly susceptible to subjective bias over time and are not recommended for research-related studies.

For all parasite counts the use of a hand operated tally counter is necessary. It should always be remembered that examination of 100 thick film fields corresponds to the average volume of only about 0.2 µl of blood. Thus, the part played by chance factors in the microscopic diagnosis of malaria infection must be recognized. The chance factor rises as the true number of parasites in a unit of blood decreases. Thus, in doubtful cases it is desirable to increase the time devoted to the examination of a single blood slide and if necessary to take several blood slides at proper intervals of time.

Based on the examination of 100 microscopic fields under oil immersion, with a magnification of ×500–600, the numerical threshold at which malaria parasites can be detected by an experienced technician in well-stained blood films is about 100 parasites per µl if a thin film technique is used; for a thick film the threshold is lower – about 10–20 parasites per µl of blood – but here the experience of the microscopist is an important factor. The examination of smears from the bone marrow, obtained by sternal puncture as a supplementary diagnostic method, has no advantage over the usual blood examination. For *postmortem* examinations, if death from malaria is suspected and no full autopsy can be carried out, a specimen can be obtained from a puncture of the spleen or brain. For the latter specimen a large-bore needle can be pushed through the supra-orbital plate into the brain and a smear, obtained by suction, should be spread on the slide, fixed, and stained in the usual way.

Some reports, stating that parasites of *P. falciparum* could be found in bloodless exudate from scarified skin of African children, have been consistently disproved by competent parasitologists. In China, however, late trophozoites and schizonts are significantly more commonly seen in intradermal smears than in peripheral blood; than in patients with cerebral malaria.

Technical details for microscopical examination of blood films are outside the scope of this book and can easily be found elsewhere. The best illustrated guides for staining and identification of human malaria parasites in thick and thin blood films are undoubtedly those of Aimée Wilcox, *Manual for the Microscopical Diagnosis of Malaria in Man* (1960) and the *Bench Aids for Malaria Diagnosis* available from the Distribution and Sales Unit of the World Health Organization, Geneva, Switzerland, or its authorized country agents worldwide (see Selected References). Whenever possible a binocular microscope with a substage illumination should be used in preference to a monocular instrument. Nevertheless, in experienced hands a good monocular microscope is perfectly adequate for routine work. The use of a wide angle eye-piece to obtain a better coverage of the microscopic field of an oil immersion is of great value and thoroughly recommended providing adequate illumination is available. Ideally, such lens combinations should not be used with total magnifications as high as ×1000 or more; unfortunately these unnecessarily high magnifications are often provided as standard on many field microscopes. The optimum definition/magnification for malaria diagnosis with most standard microscopes is ×600–700, i.e. ×6 or ×7 eyepieces and ×100 oil immersion lens (spring loaded for protection).

Care should be taken, when examining the thick film, not to confuse artefacts or blood platelets with malaria parasites. Only a few of these errors can be mentioned here:

1. Ghosts of haemolysed immature erythrocytes (reticulocytes) may be mistaken for Schüffner's stippling of *P. vivax*.
2. Clusters of blood platelets may also simulate *P. vivax*; in thin films when several platelets are superimposed and stain differently with Giemsa they may be mistaken for malaria parasites outside the red blood cell.
3. Vegetable spores, yeast, pollen or algae in buffer solution may look like various blood parasites, especially haemogregarines.
4. Bacteria can contaminate aqueous solutions of Giemsa stain and may interfere with the identification of plasmodia.
5. In patients with a degree of anaemia the nuclear residues of erythrocytes, such as Howell–Jolly bodies, on a background of reticulum of ghosts of immature cells may be easily mistaken for malaria parasites.

In doubtful cases blood films should be sent to the nearest competent laboratory for confirmation of diagnosis. Human infections with *Babesia* (piroplasmosis or babesiosis) may be easily mistaken for *P. falciparum*. Fortunately, human babesiosis is a rare occurrence.

Diagnostic characters of human malaria parasites as seen in a well-stained thick or thin film are given in Tables 6.2 and 6.3.

Various more or less refined methods have been used to improve and facilitate the conventional ways of examining stained blood slides under the microscope. These methods vary: centrifugation of heparinized blood specimen, staining of the blood slide with fluorescent stains (fluorochromes), density gradient centrifuge methods or selective magnetic separation techniques have been used, but the results were only moderately good in relation to the complexity of techniques involved, particularly when fluorescence microscopy is required.

Several variations of the centrifugation/fluorochrome technique have been developed for the rapid diagnosis of malaria. One commercially available application – the quantified Buffy coat (QBC) technique – employs a patented heparinized tube, precoated with acridine and an anticoagulant, containing a separatory plastic float. Another uses a hinged cover-slipped microscope slide which has been pre-coated with an RNA-specific fluorochrome – benzothiocarboxypurine (BPC). In both techniques, wet blood preparations are used and examination of the blood sample can be made in several minutes. Examination times are also much shorter than the standard light microscope/Giemsa-stained blood slide. Accordingly, there are significant reductions in both the staining and examination times. Unfortunately, the reliability of species diagnosis and parasite enumeration remains problematic. Because of the high cost of the standard fluorescence microscope which is seven, or more, times that of the standard light micro-

Table 6.2 Appearance of malaria parasites in a thick blood film (mainly after Russell *et al.*, 1963)

Stage	*Plasmodium vivax* (and *ovale*)	*Plasmodium malariae*	*Plasmodium falciparum*
Early trophozoite	Fairly numerous; irregular cytoplasm; fairly large single chromatin bead; often mixed with later stages	Few; more regular cytoplasm; medium size single chromatin bead; segmenters present occasionally	Often very numerous; delicate cytoplasm; small, sometimes double chromatin bead; no other forms usually present except perhaps crescents
Half-grown trophozoite	Great irregularity of cytoplasm which tends to scatter away from single chromatin bead; few small granules of pigment	Regular compact deep blue cytoplasm around single chromatin bead; pigment forms early and tends to concentrate	Not common in peripheral blood; regular cytoplasmic ring, broken ring, and comma patterns; single and double chromatin bead
Late trophozoite	Considerable cytoplasmic scatter and irregularity; chromatin bead often isolated; fine granular pigment with moderate dispersion and often isolated from cytoplasm; other stages usually present; Schüffner's stippling sometimes seen as a pink halo	Numbers generally few, older stages present; round compact cytoplasm often obscuring chromatin; scattered pigment relatively abundant	Not in peripheral blood except in very heavy infections; solid, irregularly rounded; chromatin indistinct; pigment concentrated
Early schizont or pre-segmenter	Large amount of cytoplasm loosely covering abundant chromatin which is beginning to segment; pigment granules discrete and lightly concentrated in one or two areas; Schüffner's stippling often seen as a pink granular halo, more prominent in *ovale*	Smaller and not so numerous; some scatter of cytoplasm and segmentation of chromatin; pigment in small separate granules	Seldom in peripheral blood, but if so will be associated with numerous typical ring forms; irregular, fairly compact, dark staining; pigment fused in a single mass
Mature schizont (segmenter)	8–24, usually 12–16 merozoites; relatively large size, early vacuole formation; pigment granular and loose: other stages often present	6–12, usually eight merozoites, each with vivid purple, ovoid head of chromatin; early vacuole formation; pigment compact clump of granules	Very rare in peripheral blood; 12–24 or more merozoites, fairly uniform ovoid or round chromatin beads; merozoites grouped or scattered; pigment a single dark mass
Gametocyte	Round or oval, relatively large, with fairly uniform cytoplasm somewhat frayed at edges, small rodlet-shaped pigment, irregularly scattered, abundant chromatin, more diffuse in males	Rounded, compact, with abundant peripheral pigment in round granules; single chromatin mass often obscured and more diffuse in males	When mature and normal has distinctive crescentic shape, females longer and more slender with central pigment and chromatin; males fatter and paler, with scattered pigment and diffuse chromatin, coarse grains of pigment

Note: In properly stained thick films the erythrocytes are lysed and invisible, except for a cloudy, bluish background. Nuclei of white blood cells stain deep mauve, while clumps of platelets are pink. The parasites show a dull red or magenta-coloured nucleus and light blue cytoplasm. Species differentiation of very young forms of parasites is often impossible. In *P. vivax* and *P. ovale* infections stippling is usually present. Gametocytes of *P. falciparum* ('crescents') are distinctive but in slowly dried films they are rounded up and can be then confused with schizonts or gametocytes of *P. malariae*.

While in vivax, quartan and ovale malaria all stages of development of malaria parasites can be usually found in the peripheral blood, in falciparum malaria the schizogony takes place in the internal organs and normally only early trophozoites ('rings') appear in the blood. In very severe infections with *P. falciparum*, the appearance of schizonts is a danger signal.

scope, special fluorescence objectives and adaptors have been developed which convert standard light microscopes to fluorescence microscopy at comparatively low cost. Rugged portable centrifuges have also been developed to facilitate the use of centrifugation where this is required.

While the thick film is usually the standard method for examination of blood for the presence of malaria parasites the thin film may be needed for identification of *P. ovale* or some infections in which scanty parasites in early stages of development cannot provide the diagnostic clues. Moreover, the thin film method routinely used in hospital laboratories for differential counts of various types of white blood cells may occasionally and surprisingly reveal the presence of malaria parasites in the erythrocytes. The diagnostic criteria of malaria parasites of the four species are essentially the same in thin as in thick blood films, although at times the distortion of *Plasmodia* in the unfixed thick film adds to the difficulties faced by the beginners. Although the examination of the thin film may be much slower, especially if the parasites are scanty, it has one advantage, namely, the preservation of the shape and details of the infected red blood cell, and this may be of value in doubtful cases when the identification of the species of the *Plasmodium* causes some difficulty (Fig. 6.8 and Plate 25).

In view of this an additional table indicating the characteristic changes of the infected red blood cells may be of value. (Table 6.4).

Serological tests

Serological methods of diagnosis of malaria have become of practical value since 1962 when the indirect fluorescent antibody test (IFAT) was introduced.

Generally speaking, serological tests are of value in providing a retrospective confirmation of malaria infection or a history thereof. They are also useful for epidemiological purposes when infections are few and/or parasites scanty. However, due to the acute nature of *P. falciparum* infections they are of limited value in diagnosis as a guide to treatment and management of the disease.

Other applications of serological techniques are the diagnosis of hyperactive malaria splenomegaly and the screening of blood collected for blood banks.

Homologous antigens used in the IFAT consist of a film of human malaria parasites of a given plasmodial species and preferably erythrocytic schizonts obtained from humans, from an infected Aotus monkey or from an *in vitro* blood culture. The use of cultured parasites of *P. falciparum* offers a most convenient and stable source of antigens from different strains of this plasmodial species without the previous laborious adaptation to susceptible monkeys. *Heterologous antigens* of lesser specificity are malaria parasites of monkeys (*P. brazilianum*, *P. cynomolgi*, *P. fieldi*) which have a wider range of antigenic determinants.

In the IFAT procedure the antigen consists of a

Table 6.3 Differential characteristics of infected erythrocytes and human *Plasmodia* in stained thin films

Characteristics	*P. falciparum*	*P. vivax*	*P. ovale*	*P. malariae*
Infected erythrocyte enlarged	–	+	±	–
Infected erythrocyte not enlarged	+	–	±	+
Infected erythrocyte oval, crenated margin*	–	–	+	–
Infected erythrocyte decolorized	–	+	+	–
Infected erythrocyte, Schüffner's dots* *(stippling)*	–	+	+	–
Infected erythrocyte, Maurer's dots*	+	–	–	–
Multiple infections in erythrocytes*	+	Rare	–	–
Parasite, all forms in peripheral blood	–	+	+	+
Parasite, large coarse rings	–	+	+	+
Parasite, double chromatin dots*	+	Rare	–	–
Parasite, accolé forms*	+	Rare	–	–
Parasite, band forms*	–	–	–	+
Parasite, crescentic gametocytes	+	–	–	–
Number of merozoites	8–24	12–24	8–12	6–12

*Not invariable but suggestive when seen.

Table 6.4 Changes in the red blood cells infected with human malaria parasites as seen in the thin blood film

	P. vivax	*P. malariae*	*P. falciparum*	*P. ovale*
Infected cell	Larger than normal, paler, often slightly distorted. Schüffner's dots present in nearly all infected cells except for very young rings. Multiple infection by several parasites not uncommon. Pigment brownish in short scattered rods	About normal size or slightly smaller. Stippling not seen by normal staining. No multiple infection of erythrocyte, as a rule. Pigment seen even in early stages, dark granules rather than rods, often seen at the periphery of the cell	Normal in size. Multiple infections of erythrocyte very frequent. Some cells yellowish, seem to have a thicker rim (brassy cells). No Schüffner's stippling but irregular clefts (Maurer's dots) may be seen in overstained films. Pigment granular with tendency to coalesce. In gametocytes (crescents) the outline of erythrocyte barely seen	Many infected erythrocytes enlarged and definitely oval in shape while the parasite is round or elongated. The outline of infected cells often ragged (fimbriated). Schüffner's dots prominent at all stages of the parasite. Pigment brownish similar to that of *P. vivax*

film of infected blood on a microscope slide. The slide is covered first with one of the serial dilutions of the test serum; then it receives a solution of antihuman globulin labelled with fluorescein isothiocyanate; after washing and drying the slides are examined in a fluorescence microscope. Antibody in the test serum reacts with antigen of the malaria parasites and the antiglobulin reaction with the antibody is indicated by the fluorescence of the parasites. Fluorescence of the last serial dilution is given as a 'titre' of the antibody present (Fig. 6.9).

The antihuman sera may be polyvalent (for all immunoglobulins) or monovalent (for IgG or IgM only); these sera must be conjugated with fluorescein isothiocyanate as a marker. The blood can be collected after a finger prick in a capillary tube, for subsequent separation of serum, or it can be collected on filter paper and dried before an eventual elution using physiological saline. There are a number of modifications of the test itself, which indicates the presence of an immune response to a malaria infection and not necessarily the synchronous presence of malaria parasites. The test is of particular value for epidemiological studies and for tracing asymptomatic infections in blood donors. High titres (1:200 and over) point to a recent infection and the use of an appropriate human antigen points to an infection with one of the species of human *Plasmodia*. Generally fluorescence at a dilution of serum of over 1:20 is regarded as a positive test (Table 6.5).

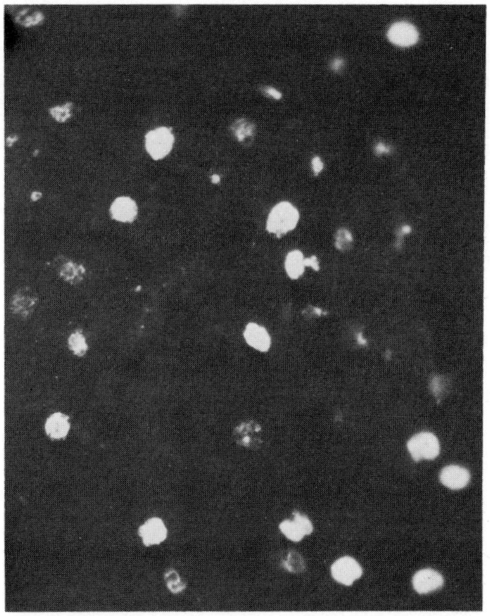

Fig. 6.9 Indirect fluorescence antibody test using a 14-day culture of *P. falciparum* as antigen. Note different degree of fluorescence of malaria parasites; fully grown schizonts have the brightest fluorescence when reacting with the homologous antibody. × 1000. (Dr A. J. Sulzer, Centres for Disease Control, Atlanta.)

This method has the advantage of giving a visual

Table 6.5 Serological tests commonly used for detection and measurement of malaria antibodies

Test	Current application	Source of antigens	Antibodies identified	Remarks
Immunoprecipitation	Epidemiological studies and research	Erythrocytic schizonts and soluble antigens	IgG, IgM	1
Immunofluorescence (IFAT)	Epidemiological studies, research and aid to diagnosis	Erythrocytic schizonts	IgG, IgM and IgA	2
Indirect haemagglutination (HA)	Epidemiological surveys	Antigen-coated erythrocytes	IgG	3
Enzyme-linked immunosorbent assay (ELISA)	Epidemiological studies and aid to diagnosis	Soluble antigens	IgG, (IgM)	4
Radioimmunoassay	Research	Soluble antigens (or antibodies)	IgG, IgM	5
Merozoite inhibition in culture	Research	Merozoites from erythrocytic schizonts	IgG, IgM	6

Note: Complement fixation tests are obsolete and have not been included in this table.
1 Good test for study of multiple antigen–antibody responses in a community. Low sensitivity and slowness make it less suitable for immunodiagnosis in single subjects. Nevertheless, a method of immuno-electrodiffusion on cellulose acetate seems to be satisfactory for detection of malaria antibodies in prospective blood donors.
2 Widely used. More sensitive with homologous antigens. Suitable for individual diagnosis but proper laboratory equipment necessary. Fairly specific.
3 Can be performed with simple equipment and suitable for the study of large number of sera under field conditions. Moderate sensitivity, since false positives, and even more false negatives, occur. Antigens difficult to standardize. Antibodies detected some time after parasitaemia becomes patent.
4 Requires small quantities of antigen, and is easy to carry out without expensive equipment. Antigens at times difficult to standardize. Highly specific but moderately sensitive.
5 Very sensitive for identification of antigens or antibodies at low concentration, but expensive and not suitable for field use.
6 Research method used mainly for detection of protective antibodies.

picture of parasites used as an antigen. Moreover, the slides with the antigen film can be easily prepared and stored at −70°C for long periods. (Complete kits, including prepared slides with *P. falciparum* antigen from blood culture, anti-human globulin conjugated with fluorescein, phosphate buffer saline, Evans blue and mounting medium are now commercially available from the Institute Mérieux, Lyon, France.)

The indirect haemagglutination (IHA) test is also used and lends itself more as a field method since it does not require the special fluorescent microscope. In this test glutaraldehyde stabilized tanned sheep cells are sensitized with the specific soluble antigen obtained from an Aotus monkey infected with *P. falciparum* or another human *Plasmodium.*

Dilutions of test sera are then added to the sensitized erythrocytes; the presence and amount of malaria antibody are indicated by the serum dilution leading to agglutination. While this test can be used on a large scale for sero-epidemiological surveys its sensitivity and specificity are less satisfactory.

Immuno-precipitation techniques (double gel diffusion tests) have been used mainly for identification of antigens formed in the course of infection, although the study of the antibody response was also investigated by this method. The test is highly sensitive but is used more as a research tool than as a diagnostic method.

In this method the test sera are allowed to diffuse against soluble malaria antigen in agar gel. Such antigens prepared from highly parasitized blood, from infected placentae or from *in vitro* cultures of *P. falciparum* react with the antibody by forming a number of precipitin bands reflecting the individual level of immunity or the exposure of the community the amount of transmission.

The *enzyme-linked immunosorbent assay* (ELISA)

test is similar in concept to the IFAT. A base of a plastic tube or plate is coated with a soluble antigen. The serum containing antibody is incubated in the coated tube and the excess of antibody is removed. The anti-antibody specific globulin labelled with the appropriate enzyme is then added to the tube, and the excess of it removed. The enzyme substrate is then added and its change of colour is proportional to the antibody concentration in the test serum. The enzyme widely used was alkaline phosphatase conjugated with anti-human globulin; paranitrophenyl phosphate serves as an indicator of the enzyme reaction. This technique lends itself particularly well to processing large numbers of samples on microplates and the results can be read visually or more accurately with a photometer. A disadvantage of this method is that the antigen is difficult to standardize and the detection of low levels of antibodies is less accurate than with the IFAT.

The ELISA test has also been employed in antigen detection.

Antigen detection

Solid-phase inhibition radioimmunoassays have been used to demonstrate parasite antigens. These assays use solubilized erythrocytes infected with *P. falciparum* and are based on the ability of washed infected red blood cells to inhibit the binding capability of radio- or enzyme-labelled antibody on a plastic microtitre plate precoated with crude extracts of malaria antigen obtained from *in vitro* cultures of *P. falciparum*. Such test systems are useful where low parasitaemias in the range 5–50 asexual parasites/μl blood are found. An inhibition radioimmunoassay test based on a monoclonal antibody labelled with a radioisotope, iodine-125, and used in an antibody 'sandwich', has also been described. In field trials it produced a detection level of >1 asexual parasites of *P. falciparum*/μl blood; better than one would expect from routine light microscopy. More details of these developments in serology can be obtained from the publications in the Selected References with the *Bulletin of the World Health Organization* (1988) Vol. 66(5) giving a particularly useful review of the subject.

However, it is important to note that the use of radioisotopes in any test system inevitably limits its use to institutions with trained personnel and the facilities to handle and transport them safely. This requirement seriously limits the use of radioisotopes in the field.

Developments of the ELISA system (the so-called dot-ELISA), which uses the inhibition of antibody binding, have also given reportedly high sensitivity with detection levels as low as 50 asexual parasites of *P. falciparum*/μl blood; close to that obtainable with standard light microscopy.

Progress has also been made towards the development of an antigen detection system based on monoclonal or polyclonal antibodies against specific circulating antigens of *P. falciparum*, but no clear correlation could be obtained between parasitaemia and the amount of circulating antigen. This would indicate that these antigens persist in the circulating blood after the parasitaemia has cleared, or has been greatly reduced, which would compromise their value in the detection of active infection. Studies are continuing to discover easily identified target proteins (ideally, by non-isotopic, i.e. visual, means) which would relate more closely to the status of the parasitaemia in the patient.

Tests of immunofluorescence, immunohaemagglutination, immunoprecipitation and the enzyme-linked immunosorbent method have been used widely for the detection and measurement of antibodies in response to the erythrocytic stages of malaria infection. However, antibodies against sporozoites have been detected experimentally and in the field. Each of these tests has its advantages and limitations; not one of them is able to distinguish the protective from non-protective antibody. Recently, other tests using *in vitro* growth of malaria parasites have been developed and these are of promise for the detection of true protective antibodies; the methods employed are based either on the uptake of labelled amino acids by the growing parasites or they measure the capacity of merozoites to reinvade erythrocytes.

Appraisal of the value of serological tests

As mentioned previously, the serological tests are of limited use for the diagnosis of acute malaria, since they become positive only several days after the appearance of malaria parasites in the blood (Fig. 6.10). Thus, these tests cannot replace the simple and yet reliable technique of examination of the blood by an alert and experienced microscopist. Nevertheless, serological testing for malaria has now been recognized as an invaluable method in epidemiological studies. For this purpose it is best to use the most practical and sensitive test available, because it will yield much information, providing that the possible disadvantages of non-specific positive reactions are recognized and assessed. In general, the level and duration of the antibody wave following the infection depends on the severity of the parasitaemia, and any re-infection. Thus, early treatment of malaria in a non-immune patient will produce a low level of antibody for a few weeks or months. On the other hand, in residents in endemic malarious areas there is a high level of long-lasting antibodies with a wide spectrum of reactivity to various strains and species of the parasite antigen. It should be remembered that high sensitivity is sometimes obtained at a cost of low specificity of the test. In areas where malaria is or has been endemic, serology will be particularly useful for the following aims: (1) establishment of age-specific indices of malarial endemicity; (2) assessment of changes in the degree of malaria transmission; (3) delineation of malarious areas and of foci of transmission. Whenever possible the serological and parasitological information should be collected and evaluated together. In areas where malaria is not endemic serological tests can be of use for the following purposes: (1) screening of blood donors; (2) exclusion of diagnosis of malaria in patients with symptoms such as pyrexia, anaemia, hepatosplenomegaly or nephrotic syndrome and with negative results of blood examination for plasmodia; (3) case detection and identification of

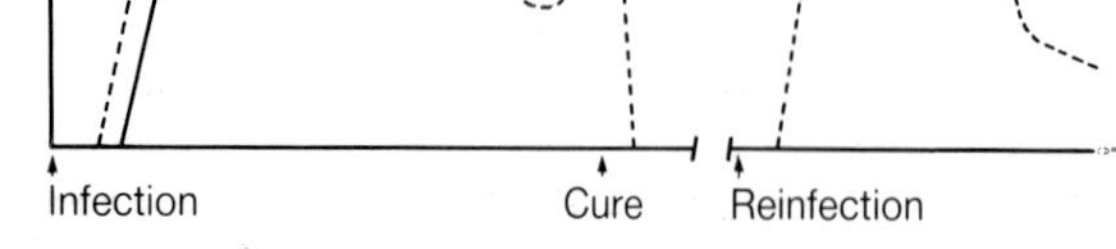

Fig. 6.10 Evolution of parasitaemia and antibodies in malaria as measured by immunofluorescence. (Amended from Voller and Draper, 1982.)

the species of malaria parasites when other methods failed. The present serological tests suffer from the general disadvantage that the methods of collection of serum or plasma, as well as the selection of antigens and techniques of various tests, are not standardized, so that comparison of results between them is subject to caution.

After the first attack of malaria it is usually possible to detect antibodies for about 6 months; with the IFAT, serum titres of 1/256 and higher indicate recent plasmodial infection. Titres below 1/20 are of doubtful significance. It is always advisable to use as antigens homologous species such as *P. falciparum*, *P. vivax* and *P. malariae*. Since the latter two are not often available the simian *P. cynomolgi* (for *P. vivax*), *P. brazilianum* (for *P. malariae*) or *P. fieldi* can be employed.

The simple technique of collection of blood on filter paper for the IFAT is described below.

Collection of capillary blood on paper for serology

The instructions given below are those according to the technique used by Dr C. C. Draper of the Ross Institute, London School of Hygiene and Tropical Medicine.

1. Whatman No. 3 chromatography paper cut into strips of about 14 × 9 cm should be stored in self-sealing polythene bags, each containing up to ten pieces. For use in humid climates it is preferable, before cutting them into strips, to soak the sheets of paper in 1/10 000 thiomersal (Merthiolate), to act as a fungicide, and to allow them to dry thoroughly.
2. A finger or ear lobe is cleaned. Ensure that cleaning fluid, if used, has dried. A *deep* prick is made and drops of blood are allowed to fall onto the paper, so that the skin does not touch the paper. Collect a minimum of two to three spots of *not less than* 50 μl each, from every subject. If necessary several drops of blood may be allowed to fall on top of each other on the same spot of the paper and to soak in until this is about 1 cm in diameter. Let each of the drops spread out on its own. Up to five sets of blood samples from different subjects can be put on one piece of paper. Ensure that each set is clearly marked with a reference number.

3. Papers should be protected from dirt and flies, e.g. by standing on their sides inside a covered bowl. Allow to dry thoroughly at room temperature or by holding in *gentle* heat – not more than 37°C. Under field conditions this is often not practicable. The partially dried papers are then taken back to the laboratory, preferably within a few hours, where they are thoroughly dried and then sealed in the polythene bags. The bags are stored as soon as possible in a refrigerator (4°C) or preferably deep freeze (−20°C or less). Under these conditions specific immunoglobulins are probably stable for at least several months. So long as the papers are *well dried* the bags can probably be kept at ambient temperature for several weeks without serious degradation of the immunoglobulins.
4. At the serological laboratory, a calibrated paper punch is used to cut out circles of paper containing the equivalent of 50 µl of blood. When eluted in 0.4 ml of diluent this will given an approximate 1/16 dilution of serum.
5. Slightly greater precision, of doubtful value for most survey work and taking more time, may be obtained by taking up measured amounts of 50 µl of blood in a pipette or capillary tube and expelling these on to a paper. (This obviates the need for a calibrated punch when the processing of the blood samples takes place in the laboratory.)

Molecular biological detection tests

The burgeoning development of molecular biological technology has already provided the basis for several new test systems for the diagnosis of malaria in humans.

DNA and RNA probes

All organisms possess genes which contain deoxyribonucleic acid (DNA). Some sequences of the genomic DNA base pairs which make up the double-stranded DNA helix are unique to a particular species and if these can be isolated from the respective organism and reliably detected, this provides an infallible system of species diagnosis. The technology which can achieve this is known as the DNA probe and is based on hybridization of the DNA whereby the two complementary strands of the DNA helix are separated (denatured) by chemical means, or heat treatment, and separately bound to a solid surface. These separated strands of DNA are then put into contact with a DNA probe. This probe has been obtained using recombinant DNA techniques, or produced synthetically, to contain hundreds of copies of a specified nucleotide sequence of a family of 21-base pairs of tandem repeats unique to a species of human malaria, for example, *P. falciparum*. This target sequence is naturally repeated many times in the genomic DNA of the target *Plasmodium* spp. A second treatment allows the individual pieces of DNA probe to join up (hybridize) with the matching nucleotide sequence of the test sample and again form the normal status of a double strand helix of DNA. If the DNA probe has been labelled with an indicator, such as radioisotope or a colorimetric indicator enzyme, the presence of the specific nucleotide sequence can be detected by photographic or optical means and the species diagnosis confirmed. Thus DNA probes can be made specific to a single species of *Plasmodium*. Most of the available DNA probes are specific to *P. falciparum* and sensitivities as low as 5 asexual parasites/µl blood have been reported but, unfortunately, these results have only so far been obtained with radioisotopic methods using iodine-125 or phosphorus-32. Enzyme-based systems with biotin and others are rather less sensitive although new probes specifically designed for enzyme detection may improve these levels considerably.

Ribonucleic acid (RNA) probes have also been evaluated with promising results. RNA polymerase functions in nature to copy genes for translation into protein. The product of RNA polymerase is an RNA copy of DNA which has the same unique sequence of bases as the DNA and, when separated into single strands, can hybridize with it. Accordingly, a detection system can be produced by incorporating into the RNA copy radioactive ribonucleotide triphosphates. Ribosomal RNA is, moreover, much more abundant with between 10 and 50 times as much RNA as DNA in a cell; despite this dominance RNA gives lower background signals. Unfortunately, RNA is less stable and cross-species reactivity could occur. RNA probes have been developed for all four human malarias and show an increased sensitivity due to the high number of target sequences which occur in RNA. Detection techniques using 12-hour autoradiography exposure have reportedly produced detection levels as low as 10 parasites/μl blood. No effective non-radioactive label has as yet been reported but chemiluminescence appears to offer potential for direct visual detection. A further approach to improving the sensitivity of DNA and RNA probes is that of the amplication of a defined region of DNA or RNA. Currently, this amplification process has been achieved by one, or a combination of, three amplification methods: (1) target amplification – polymerase chain reaction (PCR) or transcript amplification system (TAS); (2) probe amplification ring Q-beta replicase and (3) signal amplification using enzyme-linked probes or compound 'Christmas Tree' probes.

The PCR and TAS techniques have already had dramatic impact and have found wide applications in the laboratory, particularly in the diagnosis of viral infections, as well as in industry. The PCR technique has the ability to amplify selected regions of DNA and RNA rapidly and specifically from a small number of starting copies. The principle of the reaction is that: (1) short oligonucleotides comprising 15 to 25 bases can be hybridized rapidly and specifically to complementary DNA sequences, even when a large amount of non-complementary (contaminated) DNA is present, and (2) DNA polymerase needs a primer bound to a template for the synthesis of DNA/RNA. By the presentation of suitable primers DNA synthesis can be initiated and two new strands of complementary DNA produced. When these strands are denatured (separated) and reannealed (rejoined) all the new individual strands will act as substrates for more and more cycles of DNA synthesis with an exponential increase in the numbers of the specific DNA target. The whole cyclic process is controlled by temperature changes effected by a microprocessor-controlled thermal cycling unit. Visualization can be obtained by ultraviolet fluorescence produced by agarose gel electrophoresis, or by the detection of immobilized amplified nucleic acids (DIANA). DIANA captures the specific DNA sequences produced by PCR onto a solid support (magnetic beads) by the use of a recombinant fusion protein. The immobilized material is detected by means of a colorimetric indicator system – biotin and streptavin. The TAS technique also uses DNA and RNA as starting material and consists of several steps of DNA synthesis each followed by an *in vitro* transcription step using the DNA as the template. This produces, by reverse transcription, one molecule of DNA for each DNA or RNA target molecule. In addition a promoter sequence for DNA-dependent RNA polymerase is incorporated into the newly synthesized strand of DNA. The end result of this reaction is a DNA copy of the DNA or RNA target molecule with a phage RNA polymerase promoter at one end which serves as the template for the next cycle of amplification. Four such cycles can produce a million-fold amplification of the target molecule. However, there are considerable drawbacks to the TAS, the principal of which appears to be an increased possibility of non-specific hybridization.

Q-beta replicase, which is an RNA-directed RNA polymerase, replicates genomic RNA of the bacteriophage recognizing the unique folded RNA structure of the base pairs of the Q-beta RNA genome. This characteristic has been used to amplify recombinant molecules of probes which are specific for *P. falciparum* to give an increase of one billion-fold in 30 minutes. But here again, there are potential problems of the amplification of molecules other than the intended target.

Compound, or 'Christmas Tree', probes aim at increasing the hybridization signal of the probe molecule itself by means of the simultaneous use of primary and secondary probes which provide a network (Christmas Tree) of cross-binding DNA sequences. The probe in this case is a sequence of DNA or RNA complementary to the target which has been labelled with a radioisotope and detected on photographic film. Non-isotopic probes have also been developed for this system using the biotin –avidin technique to produce the colorimetric reaction which can be visually read and in this application fluorescent or chemiluminescent probes have shown considerable potential.

Obviously the application of these new technologies to routine field use is still some way off unless a really simple visually read colorimetric detection system is developed and a cheap, portable and reliable thermal recycling device made available for the amplification procedures.

For more details on these techniques see Selected References.

Future prospects

Past experience shows that it would be foolhardy to attempt to predict the fantastic rate of evolution of modern technology, or to underestimate the ability of modern science to develop as yet unimagined new diagnostic tools. But it seems probable that none of the current individual new diagnostic techniques have the potential to replace entirely, in the immediate future, the combination of the trained human eye and the light microscope for the routine diagnosis of human malaria; particularly so at the peripheral level of the health services of the malaria endemic countries where the need for rapid and accurate diagnosis is often greatest and their sources are the least. However, these new techniques are already finding a place in research as epidemiological tools, in specific applications where the necessary resources of trained personnel and equipment are available and where the limitations of cost, specificity/sensitivity, and a general reliance on radioactive detection methods, are not as crucial as in the routine diagnosis for the treatment and management of the malaria patient.

Nonetheless, there are already on the horizon indications of an application of the available technology which could be adapted to meet the needs of routine malaria diagnosis at the peripheral levels of the health services. Generically called 'dipstick technology', it is based on the application of high technology in the manufacturing process to produce at the end of a dipstick device, or on the surface of a card, the detection system (e.g. monoclonals of parasite antigens or unique molecular sequences) for the human malaria parasite species or even antimalarial drugs. The active principle is bound to a plastic strip which is located at the tip of the dipstick, or to zoned areas of the test card. The sample, which could be blood, urine or saliva, is put into contact with the active area and the detection system is activated to produce a positive or negative reaction which is demonstrated by a visually observable colour change. A single dipstick or card, or a series of them, could be processed to provide the diagnosis of all the four species of human malaria, the degree of parasitaemia and even the resistance status of the parasite to a range of antimalarial drugs. Such test systems are already employed in the diagnosis of viral infections, notably HIV, some tropical parasites other than malaria, and in the food industry for the detection of bacterial contamination. If these diagnostic tools can be produced cheaply and reliably, and the necssary technology transferred to the industrial base of the endemic countries to provide the required degree of self-sufficiency, the diagnostic capability of all levels of the health service could be transformed and, incidentally, the light microscope relegated to the back-up role for which it is more eminently suited.

Chapter 7

The *Anopheles* vector

M. W. Service

Human malaria can be transmitted only by anopheline mosquitos. In addition to transmitting malaria, anophelines also transmit filariasis and some arboviral diseases, but other mosquitos are more important as vectors of the two latter infections.

The genus *Anopheles* belongs to the order Diptera, sub-order Nematocera, family Culicidae, subfamily Culicinae and tribe Anophelini in the zoological classification. Within the tribe Anophelini the genus *Anopheles* has six sub-genera (Fig. 7.1).

There are about 422 species of *Anopheles* mosquitos throughout the world, but only some 70 species are vectors of malaria under natural conditions; of these some 40 species are of major importance. Natural susceptibility or resistance of *Anopheles* to infection with a defined species of malaria parasite is still only partially understood, although it is certainly related to biochemical processes in the body of the mosquito. Among the main factors determining whether a particular species of *Anopheles* is an important vector, the frequency of its feeding on humans (in preference to animals) is of particular relevance. The other factors are the mean longevity of the local population of an anopheline species and its density in relation to humans. Thus, a particular species of *Anopheles* may be an important vector in one area of the world and of little or no importance in another area.

Although *Anopheles* mosquitos are most frequent in tropical or subtropical regions they are also found in temperate climates and even in the Arctic during the summer. As a rule *Anopheles* are not found at altitudes above 2000–2500 m.

A large area of the Pacific Ocean roughly bounded by and including New Zealand, the Galapagos Islands, Hawaii, Midway Island, Palau Island, the Caroline Islands, the Gilbert Islands, Samoa, Fiji and New Caledonia is free from *Anopheles* mosquitos and there is no indigenous malaria within this area. There are, however, *Anopheles* on Guam.

Anatomy and physiology of *Anopheles*

The external morphology of both female and male *Anopheles* provides the main criteria for recognizing both the genus and the species of these mosquitos. The successive stages of growth and metamorphosis of the mosquito are the egg, larva, pupa and finally the adult or imago (Fig. 7.2).

Anopheline egg

Eggs are about 0.5 mm in length, boat-shaped and nearly all species are provided with tiny air-filled floats that allow them to remain on the water surface. The frill, separating the upper 'deck' of the egg from the rest of it, is more or less continuous. Eggs are laid singly by the female *Anopheles* on the type of water preferred by a particular species. The pattern of grey exochorion on the surface of the blackish egg, its shape and size are useful for species differentiation. The site chosen by the *Anopheles* for egg laying and subsequent development of the larvae is known as the breeding place, or more accurately the *larval habitat*.

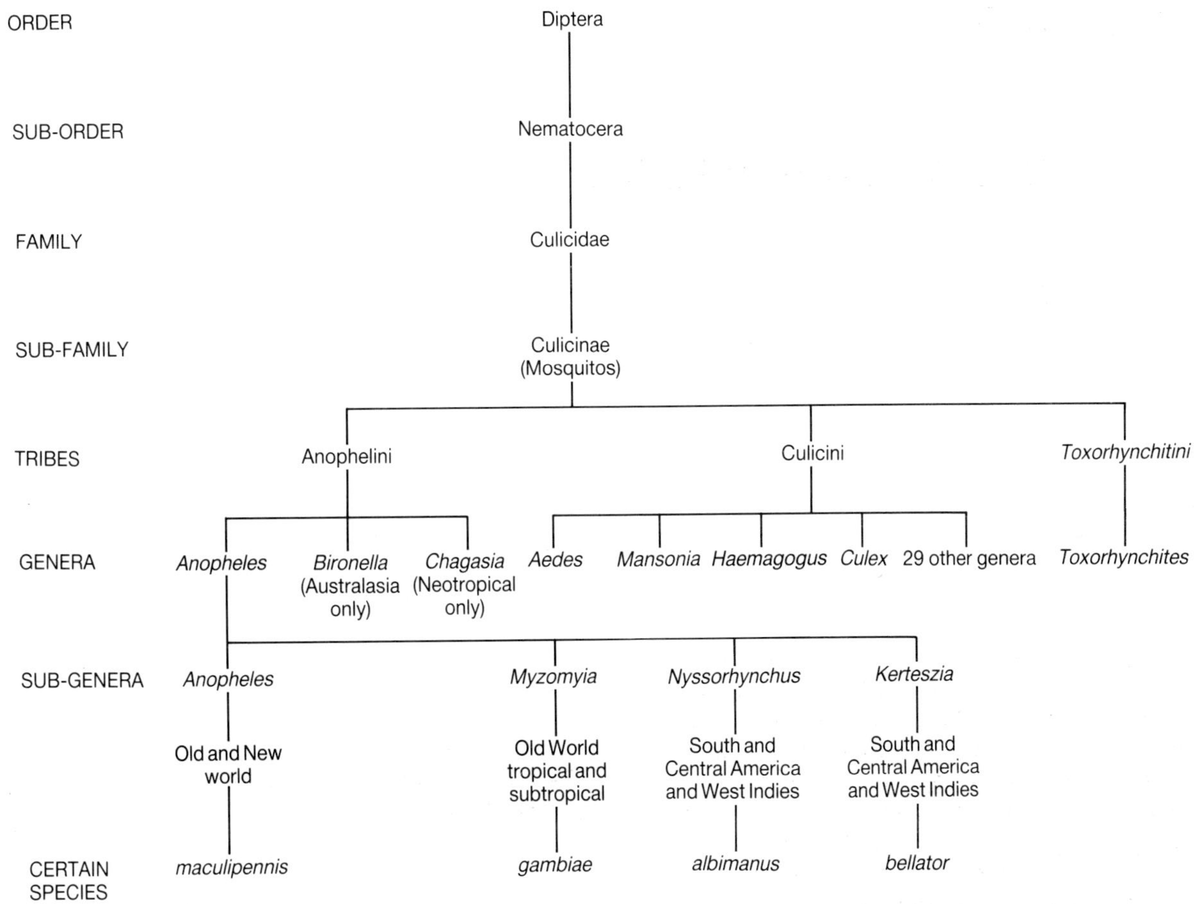

Fig. 7.1 Classification of mosquitos, naming just four of the six sub-genera of the genus *Anopheles*. *Note*: It is customary to omit the sub-generic name when referring to a species, e.g. *Anopheles maculipennis* and *Anopheles gambiae* except in strictly systematic work.

Anopheline larva

The larvae hatch from the eggs as small 'wrigglers' and have a distinct head and thorax and an abdomen composed of nine segments (Fig. 7.3).

The globular thorax is broader than the head or abdomen and somewhat flattened. It has several groups of hairs that are useful in identifying the species.

The abdomen is long, subcylindrical and segmented. Its first seven segments are similar, but the eighth and ninth are considerably modified. The eighth segment bears the respiratory apparatus, which in anophelines consists of paired spiracular openings. All other groups of mosquitos (toxorhynchitines and culicines) have a prominent air tube called the siphon, but this is absent in all *Anopheles*. The ninth segment is out of line with the other segments and bears four tapering membranous structures called anal papillae or gills. Each abdominal segment is provided with hairs, which are useful for distinguishing different species of *Anopheles*. Larvae have conspicuous mouth brushes which sweep food particles into the mouth. In feeding at the surface the head of the larva turns through 180°. The body of an anopheline larva lies parallel to the water surface; on the upper side of the abdomen it has two rows of conspicuous *palmate* or *float hairs*. Like all mosquito larvae those of *Anopheles* undergo three successive moultings (*ec-*

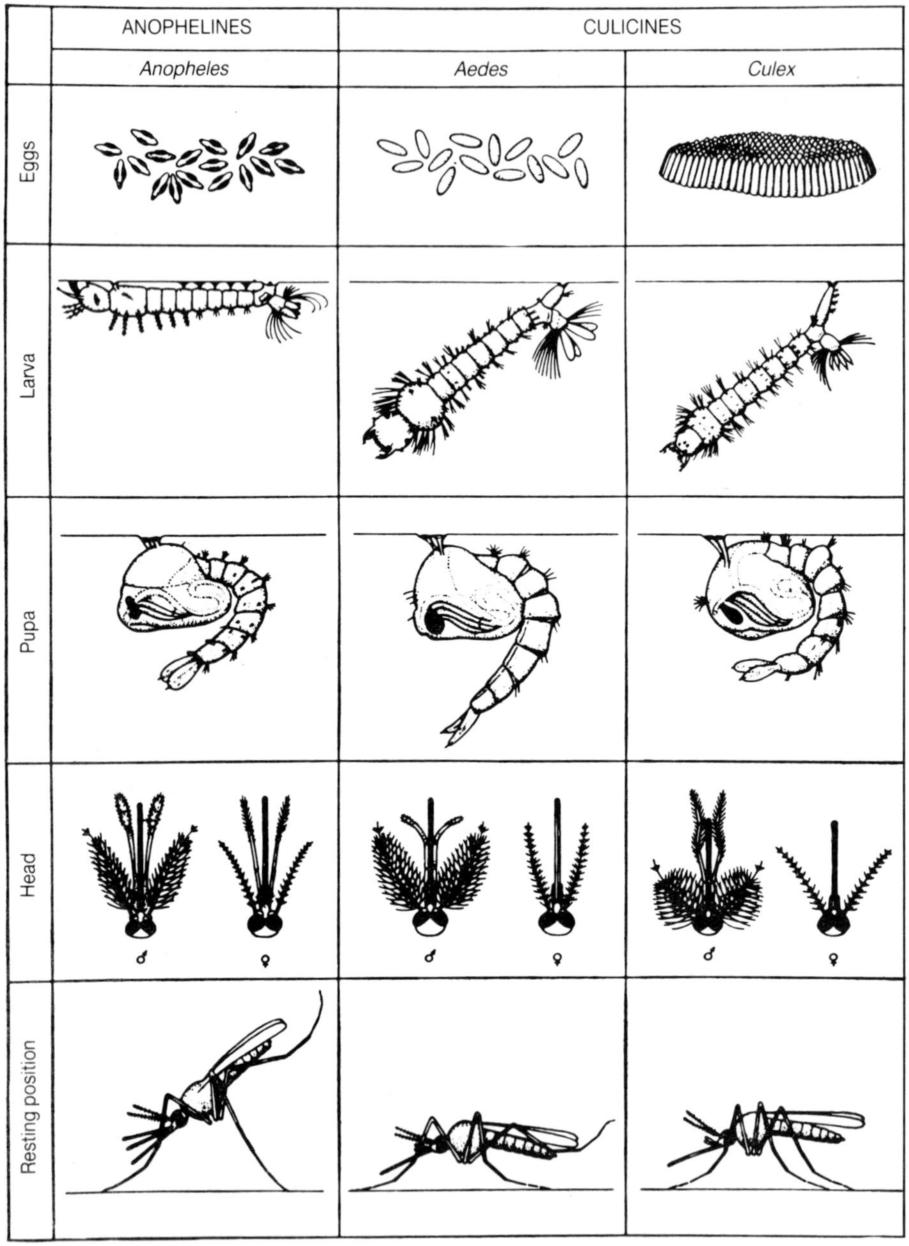

Fig. 7.2 Differentiation of *Anopheles*, *Aedes* and *Culex* mosquitos at various stages of their development. Note the length of the palps in female *Anopheles* in comparison with other genera of mosquito. (Wellcome Museum of Medical Science.)

dyses) during their growth, when they shed their chitinous skins. These successive moults separate the life of the larva into four stages or instars. At the end of the fourth stage the larva changes into a pupa.

Anopheline pupa

This has a superficial similarity to that of other mosquitos although it differs from them in several details, such as having a peg-like seta on posterior

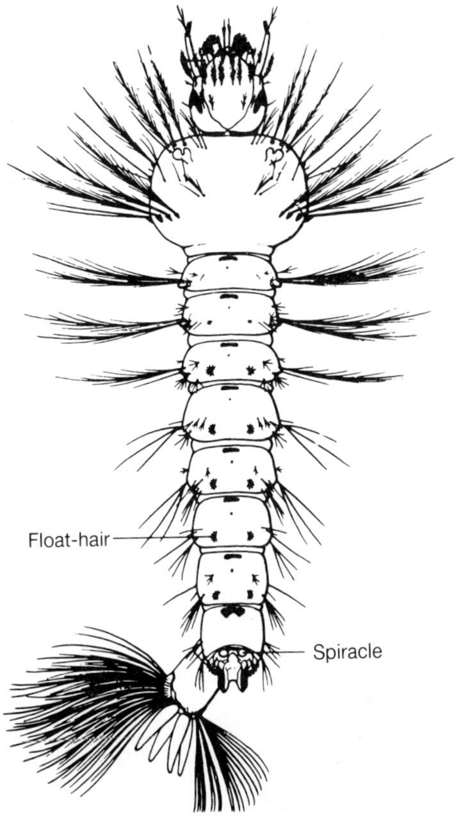

Fig. 7.3 Larva of *Anopheles* mosquito. (Wellcome Museum of Medical Science.)

corners of the abdominal segments (usually 3–7). The pupa is comma-shaped and differs greatly from the larva in appearance. The front part consists of the head and thorax which are combined into a large cephalothorax, on the upper surface of which is a pair of respiratory trumpets. The abdomen comprises eight freely movable segments with a pair of paddles at the tip. Pupae do not feed during their aquatic existence, but come to the water surface to breathe through their short paired respiratory trumpets (Fig. 7.2).

Anopheline adult

The head, thorax and abdomen of an adult (*imago*) *Anopheles* are shown in Fig. 7.4. The head with its prominent compound eyes has a pair of *antennae* which are plumose in the male and sparsely feathered in the female. The *maxillary palps* situated on

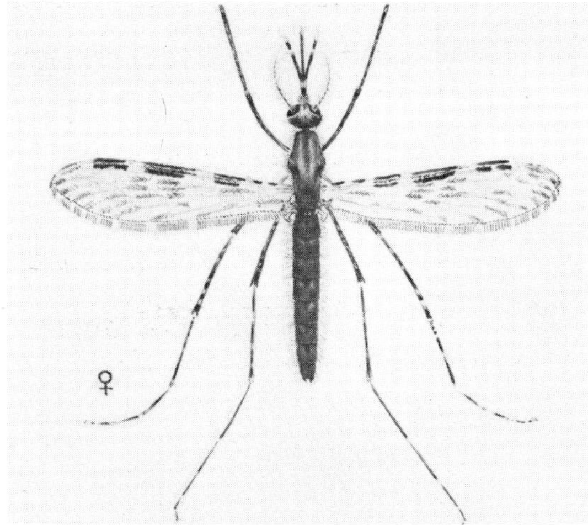

Fig. 7.4 Female specimen of *Anopheles gambiae*, the most important vector of malaria in the African tropical areas. (Wellcome Museum of Medical Science.)

both sides of the *proboscis* are about as long as the latter in both male and female *Anopheles*, whereas in culicine mosquitos the female palps are short. The proboscis in the female is a composite structure that includes a *labium* terminating in paired *labella*, a *labrum-epipharynx*, a *hypopharynx* (leading to the pharyngeal pump), and two pairs of toothed *mandibles* and *maxillae*. All components of the proboscis, except the labium, penetrate the skin of the animal on whose blood the female *Anopheles* feeds (Fig. 7.5). The thorax with its rounded *scutellum* carries a pair of *wings* and a pair of *halteres*. The wings of *Anopheles*, and also culicines, have a characteristic venation. Each of the six legs has a *femur*, a *tibia* and a five-segmented *tarsus* (Fig. 7.6). The arrangement and colour of the scales on the wing veins, the palps and legs of *Anopheles* are important for the identification of species.

The abdomen has eight similar segments each with a dorsal plate or *tergite* and a ventral plate – *sternite*; the last terminal segment is modified into *terminalia* (*genitalia*) for mating, and in the female also for oviposition. Most anophelines rest at an angle, while culicines usually rest with the abdomen parallel to the resting surface.

Internal anatomy of *Anopheles*

Certain internal structures of the adult anopheline mosquito are important for a study of malaria transmission (Fig. 7.7).

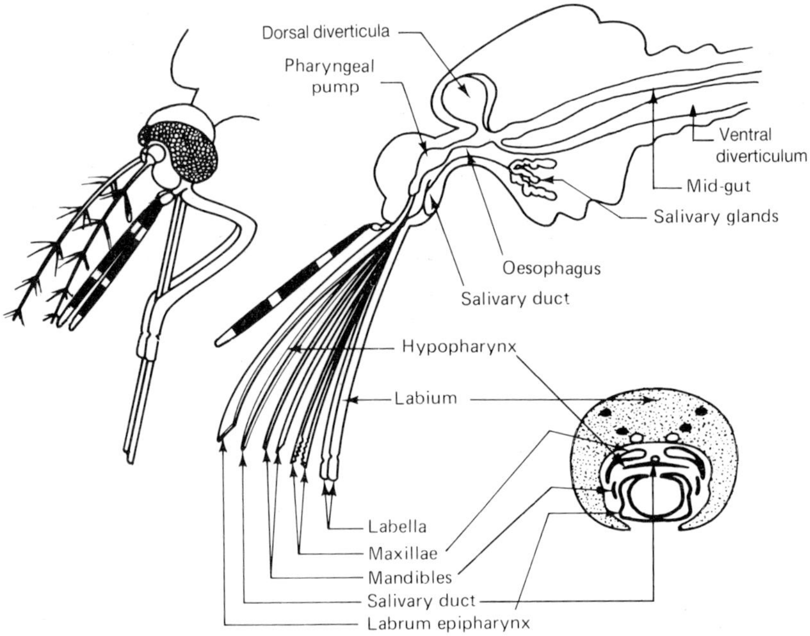

Fig. 7.5 Anatomy of the proboscis of a female *Anopheles* mosquito. Left: Position on blood feeding. Right: Cross-section through the proboscis showing component parts.

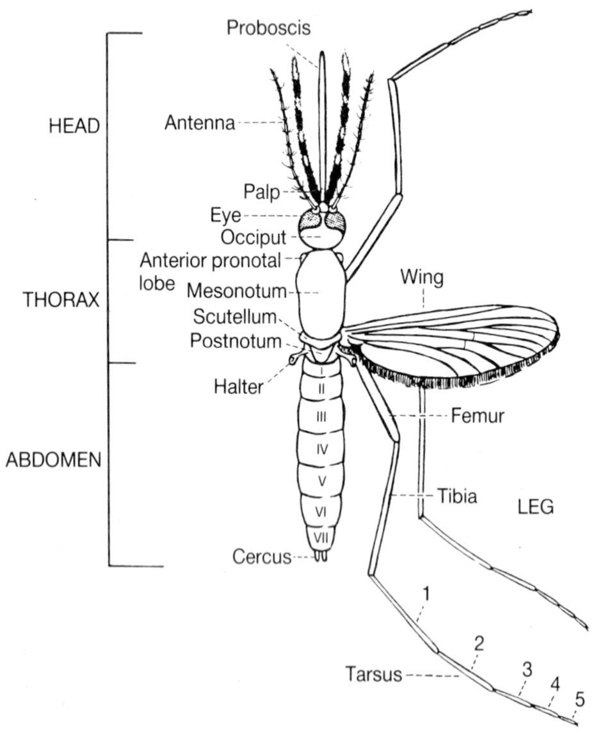

Fig. 7.6 General anatomy of a female *Anopheles* mosquito. (Modified from WHO, 1972, *Vector Control in International Health.*)

There are two *salivary glands* situated in the fore-part of the thorax above the forelegs. Each gland consists of three lobes; the two outer ones are long while the central one is short. A duct from each lobe immediately unites with the others to form the right and left ducts; these in turn unite to make one main salivary duct. Near the base of the hypopharynx there is a *salivary pump*.

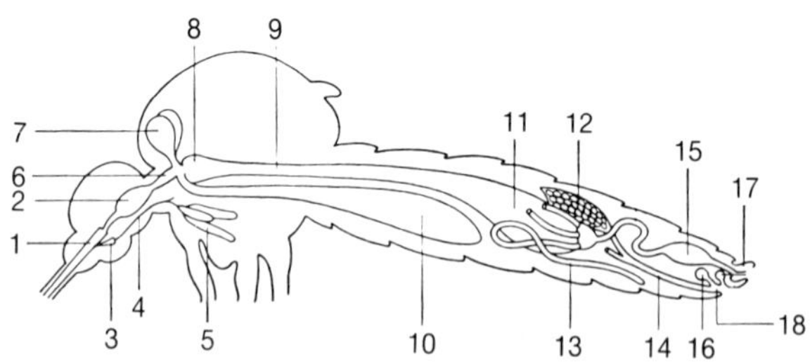

Fig. 7.7 Schematic diagram of the internal anatomy of a female mosquito: 1. pharynx; 2. pharyngeal pump; 3. salivary pump; 4. salivary duct; 5. salivary glands; 6. oesophagus; 7. dorsal diverticula; 8. proventriculus; 9. midgut; 10. ventral diverticulum (crop); 11. stomach; 12. ovary; 13. Malpighian tubules; 14. oviduct; 15. rectum; 16. spermatheca; 17. cercus; 18. atrium. (Redrawn from Marshall, 1938, *The British Mosquitoes*, British Museum (Nat. Hist.) London.)

The *alimentary canal* consists of three main parts: the fore-, mid- and hindgut. Inside the head are the pharynx and oesophagus, which form the foregut. The *pharyngeal pump* causes liquid food to be sucked through the food channel, formed by the juxtaposition of the mouthparts, through the oesophagus into the midgut. Near the posterior end of the oesophagus two tubes lead off to a pair of *dorsal diverticula*. At about the same place a ventral tube leads to a *ventral diverticulum* or *crop*. When fed on liquids other than blood the liquids pass to the diverticula, particularly the crop; when fed on blood the food passes directly to the midgut and stomach. Digestion of the blood meal takes place in the expanded portion of the *midgut*, the 'stomach', where important changes in the malaria parasite also occur. Five *Malpighian tubules* open into the hindgut at the junction with the midgut; these have an excretory function. At the distal extremity of the hindgut is the *rectum*, the inner walls of which are furnished with six rectal papillae. In the female the anus lies between the *cerci* and the postgenital lobe.

In the male *Anopheles* a pair of testes occupy the posterior part of the abdomen; each testis has a short duct which leads to a central ejaculatory duct and on to a complex structure of external genitalia with its central *phallosome* and two prominent *claspers*.

In a newly emerged female the *ovaries* lie under the fourth and fifth tergites, but in a gravid one they occupy a large part of the abdominal cavity. An *oviduct* from each ovary leads to a *common oviduct*, the distal portion of which is expanded to form the *atrium* into which the sperm duct opens. This duct comes from a single round *spermatheca* (Fig. 7.8) in which are stored the spermatozoa introduced by the male during copulation.

Several stages of blood digestion and of the development of ovaries of female *Anopheles* are of value for entomological studies. These stages, recognized in 1910 by Sella, have been widely used in research and field work (Fig. 7.9). Moreover, the nurse cells in the ovaries of half-gravid females contain polytene chromosomes, the banding pattern of which often makes possible the identification of some closely related species within a species complex. This method opened new ways for the science of cytotaxonomy and mosquito genetics.

Determination of the age of female mosquitos is of importance for a full understanding of the

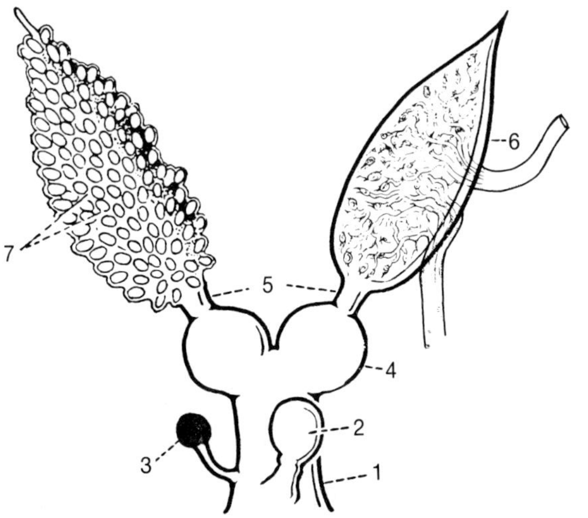

Fig. 7.8 Diagram of the reproductive system of female *Anopheles*: 1. common oviduct; 2. accessary gland; 3. spermatheca; 4. paired ovarian ampullae; 5. paired ovarian ducts; 6. ovary showing on its surface the tracheal system of a nulliparous female with closely wound terminal tracheoles; 7. ovary with developing follicles. (Amended from Russell *et al.*, 1963.)

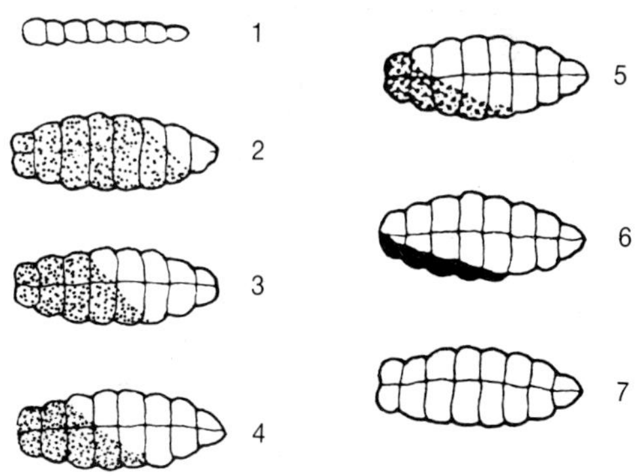

Fig. 7.9 Stages of blood digestion and ovary development in female *Anopheles* according to Sella's classification. 1. empty female, ovaries not developed; 2. freshly blood-fed female, ovaries not developed; 3. blood meal darker, area of 2–2.5 sternites and 4–5 tergites free of blood; 4. blood very dark, area of 2.5–3.5 sternites and 6.5–7.5 tergites free of blood; 6. remaining blood black, only on the ventral side, the rest of the abdomen occupied by developing white ovaries; 7. no blood visible, eggs fully developed. *Note*: the drawings represent the lateral view of the abdomen. (From Detinova, 1962.)

epidemiology of malaria and for assessment of the efficacy of antianopheline measures, most of which aim at shortening the average life-span of the population of the malaria vector. Physiological age is determined from the structure of the ovaries and indicates whether a female has, or has not, laid eggs and sometimes the number of gonotrophic cycles it has undergone. By means of age-grading it is possible to determine the age composition of the mosquito population and to find out the proportion of females which lives long enough to transmit malaria. A number of age-grading methods were formerly used. The earliest one classified the age of the mosquito by the degree of wear of the wing; later methods were based on such physiological characteristics as the presence of a 'mating plug', fertilization and enlargement of the ampullae of the oviducts. At present two methods, developed by Soviet entomologists, are mainly used:

1. A simple technique for distinguishing between parous (females already having laid at least one batch of eggs) and nulliparous (females which as yet have not laid eggs) is the examination of the tracheoles of the ovaries of unfed females. Each ovary has two main tracheal trunks which sub-divide into several branches and cover the ovary. In newly emerged females the fine tracheoles are closely wound at the terminal ends forming tight skeins or coils (Fig. 7.8). After the first blood meal and growth of the ovaries, the loops and coils of the terminal tracheoles stretch out and unwind. This process is irreversible and distinguishes the ovary of a parous female from that of a nulliparous one. This therefore permits an assessment of the nulliparous-to-parous ratio. From knowledge of the proportion parous and the duration of the gonotrophic cycle, the probability of daily survival of mosquitos can be calculated and their average longevity estimated.
2. A more elaborate technique is based on the dissection of the ovaries to count the number of dilatations left in the ovariole stalks subsequent to each ovulation and oviposition. The number of dilatations corresponds to the number of gonotrophic cycles, and this gives more detailed information on the physiological age of females. Thus females can be classified as 1-parous, 2-parous, 3-parous etc.

The larva of *Anopheles* has a dorsal heart, an aorta, tracheae, a simple alimentary canal and a ventral nerve cord. Two salivary glands situated in the thorax are of importance since their cells contain polytene chromosomes.

Systematic classification of genera and species of *Anopheles* mosquitos is based on their morphological characters at all stages of their development, but mostly on adults and fourth instar larvae. Various, but usually dichotomous, keys for the identification of species have been prepared, usually for a well-defined geographical area. Simple pictorial keys are illustrated in Figs 7.10 and 7.11.

Distribution of *Anopheles*

The following six zoogeographical regions of the world have been generally recognized:

1. *Palaearctic region*: comprising the whole of Europe and North Africa, Asia north of 30°N including China, the Japanese islands, northern Arabia including Iraq, Iran and Afghanistan.
2. *Oriental region*: all of southern Asia, the Indonesia islands, the Philippines and Taiwan.
3. *Australasian region*: comprising Australia, Tasmania, New Zealand, Papua New Guinea, the islands of Micronesia and Polynesia, and the Hawaiian islands.
4. *Afrotropical region* (formerly known as '*Ethiopian*'): all of Africa south of the Sahara including Madagascar, the Seychelles, the Comoro islands, Mauritius and Réunion.
5. *Nearctic region*: northern Mexico and North America.
6. *Neotropical region*: from central Mexico to southern Argentina, and the Caribbean islands.

Table 7.1 gives the most important species of *Anopheles* vectors of human malaria. The former classification of *Anopheles* into primary and secondary vectors is uncertain and arbitrary. 'Secondary' vectors are supposed to be species of *Anopheles* in the relevant area which, after the elimination of the 'primary' species responsible for endemic malaria, are able to maintain a degree of transmission of the infection, at least in a part of the area. A better terminology is to classify vectors as main and subsidiary, the latter comprising incidental vectors which are localized but may never-

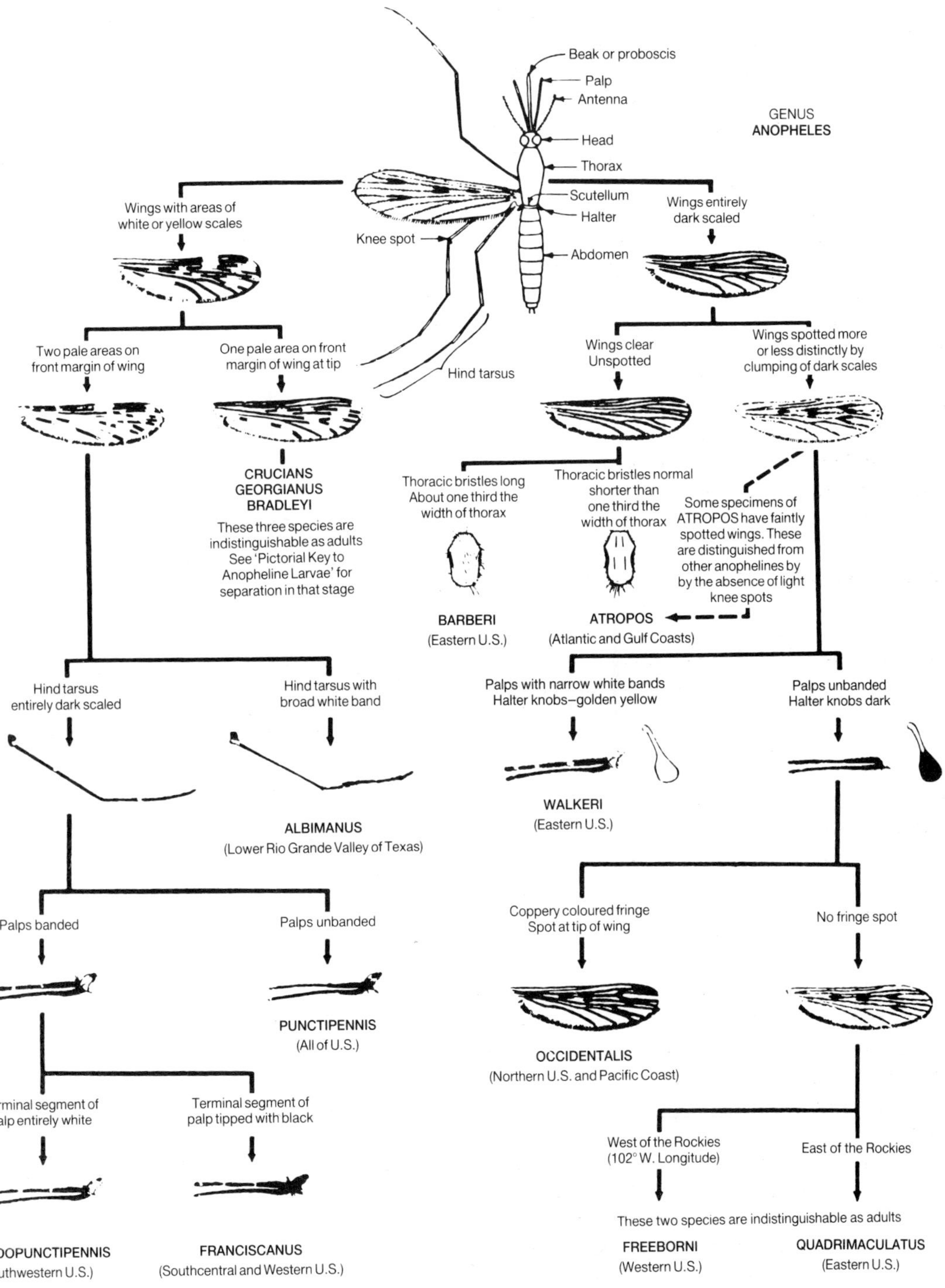

Fig. 7.10 Example of the use of a taxonomic key for identification of a species of adult female *Anopheles*, according to a pictorial guide valid for the USA. (From *Malaria Control in Impounded Waters*, 1945, by courtesy of the Superintendent of Documents, US Government Printing Office, Washington DC.)

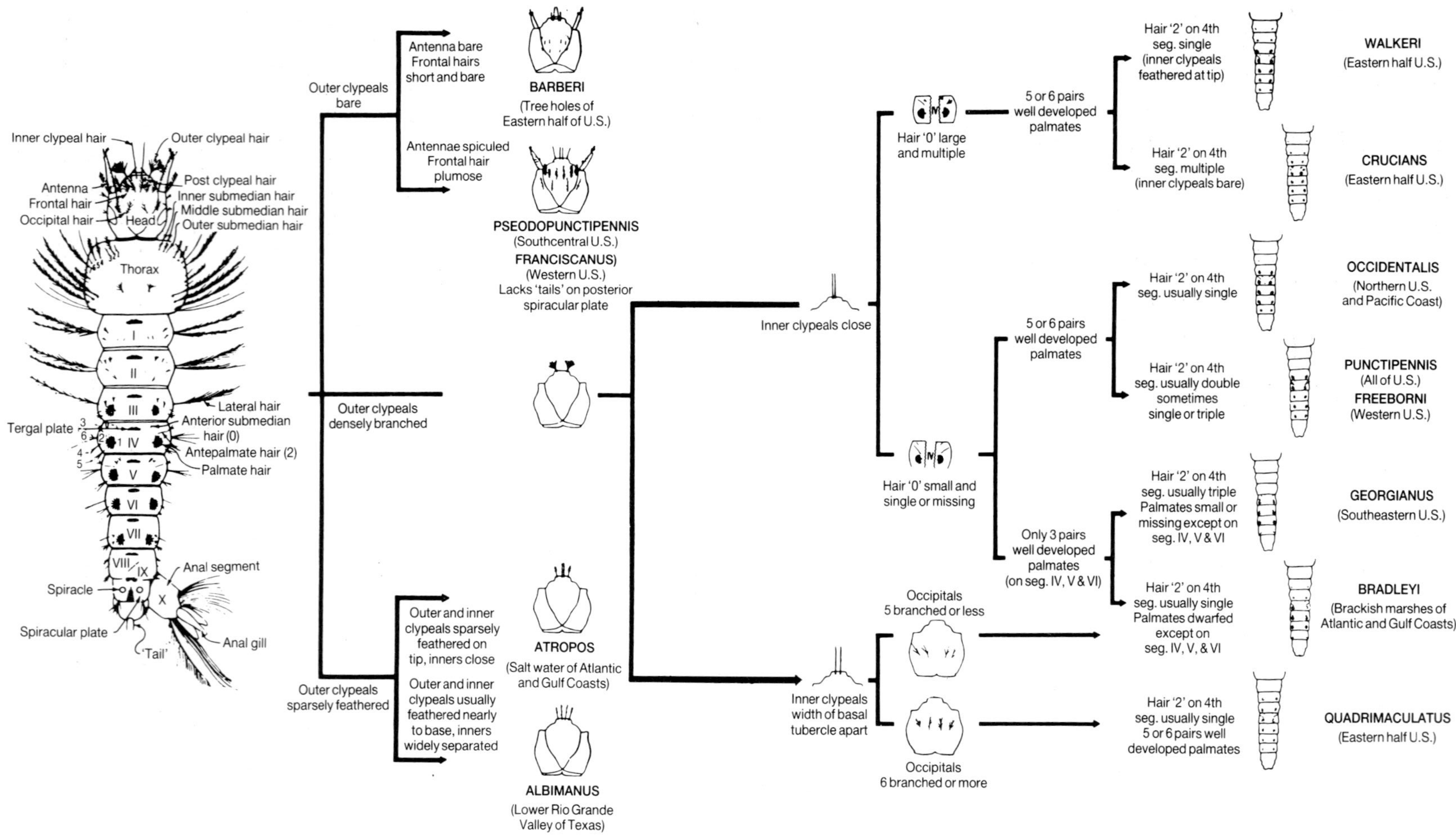

Fig. 7.11 Example of the use of a taxonomic key for identification of a species of anopheline larva, according to a pictorial guide valid for the USA. (From *Malaria Control in Impounded Waters*, 1945, by courtesy of the Superintendent of Documents, US Government Printing Office, Washington DC.)

Table 7.1 Species of *Anopheles* vectors of importance in the transmission of malaria (after Service, 1993)

A. aconitus Dönitz, 1902	*A. culicifacies* Giles, 1901	*A. maculatus* Theobald, 1901	*A. pulcherrimus* Theobald, 1902
A. albimanus Wiedemann, 1821	*A. darlingi* Root, 1926	*A. mangyanus* (Banks), 1906	*A. punctimacula* Dyar & Knab, 1906
A. albitarsis Lynch Arribalzaga, 1878	*A. donaldi* Reid, 1962	*A. melas* Theobald, 1903	*A. punctulatus* Dönitz, 1901
A. annularis van der Wulp, 1884	*A. dirus* Peyton & Harrison, 1979	*A. messeae* Falleroni, 1926	*A. quadrimaculatus* Say, 1824
A. anthropophagus Xu & Feng, 1975	*A. farauti* Laveran, 1902	*A. merus* Dönitz, 1902	*A. sacharovi* Favre, 1903
A. arabiensis Patton, 1905	*A. flavirostris* (Ludlow), 1914	*A. minimus* Theobald, 1901	*A. sergentii* (Theobald), 1907
A. argyritarsis Robineau-Desvoidy, 1827	*A. fluviatilis* James, 1902	*A. moucheti* Evans, 1901	*A. sinensis* Wiedemann, 1828
A. aquasalis Curry, 1932	*A. freeborni* Aitken, 1939	*A. multicolor* Cambouliou, 1902	*A. stephensi* Liston, 1901
A. atroparvus van Thiel, 1927	*A. funestus* Giles, 1902	*A. neivai* Howard, Dyar & Knab, 1917	*A. subpictus* (Grassi, 1899)
A. aztecus Hoffman, 1935	*A. gambiae* Giles, 1902	*A. nigerrimus* Giles, 1900	*A. sundaicus* (Rodenwaldt), 1926
A. balabacensis Baisas, 1936	*A. hilli* Woodhill & Lee, 1944	*A. nili* (Theobald), 1904	*A. superpictus* (Grassi, 1899)
A. bancroftii Giles, 1902	*A. hispaniola* (Theobald), 1903	*A. nuneztovari* Gabaldon, 1940	*A. tessellatus* Theobald, 1901
A. bellator Dyar & Knab, 1908	*A. jeyporiensis* James, 1902	*A. pattoni* Christophers, 1926	*A. triannulatus* (Neiva & Pinto), 1922
A. braziliensis (Chagas), 1907	*A. karwari* James, 1903	*A. pharoensis* Theobald, 1901	*A. varuna* Iyengar, 1924
A. campestris Reid, 1962	*A. koliensis* Owen, 1942	*A. philippinensis* Ludlow, 1902	*A. whartoni* Reid, 1963
A. claviger (Meigen), 1804	*A. labranchiae* Falleroni, 1926	*A. pseudopunctipennis* Theobald, 1901	
A. cruzii Dyar & Knab, 1908	*A. letifer* Sandosham, 1944		
	A. leucosphyrus Dönitz, 1901		
	A. ludlowae (Theobald), 1903		

Note: In writing the full scientific name of a mosquito the genus may be abbreviated to one or two letters, but should always start with a capital letter. The name of the species must not be capitalized, even if it is derived from an author's surname. In precise description the surname of the author who first described and named the species is added without an intervening comma; the year of the publication is separated from the previous word by a comma. If the species was originally described as being in a different genus, or the name of the genus is changed, then the author's name is given in brackets.

theless be 'main' in their area. In the incrimination of the main vectors of human malaria the dissection of wild caught *Anopheles* for the presence of plasmodial infection (with oöcysts or sporozoites) is important. However, it is known that some anopheline species not normally associated with human habitations might be vectors of *Plasmodia* of monkeys, rodents and other animals. Thus, detection of sporozoites in the salivary glands does not necessarily identify the species as a vector of human malaria. Knowledge of the biology and feeding preferences of mosquitos and the presence or otherwise in the area of animal *Plasmodia* has to be taken into consideration. However, modern immunological techniques such as enzyme-linked immunosorbent assay (ELISA) identify sporozoites to species, e.g. as sporozoites of *Plasmodium falciparum* or *Plasmodium vivax*, and so animal infections are excluded.

The concept of species complexes has introduced an additional difficulty into the classification of *Anopheles* species considered as main vectors of malaria, but the list given in Table 7.1 is not greatly different from the one given by Russell (1952) or Russell *et al.* (1963). The new trends in systematics of *Anopheles* attach importance to biological as well as to morphological concepts of a species. This is of relevance to malariologists, as it helps them to understand the vagaries of the relationships between some anopheline populations within a species complex and malaria transmission. Nevertheless, the existence of sibling or isomorphic species, the behaviour pattern of which influences their role as a vector, complicates what formerly appeared to be a simple problem.

Few of the species listed in Table 7.1 are vectors of human malaria over the whole area of their geographical distribution. Certain external factors

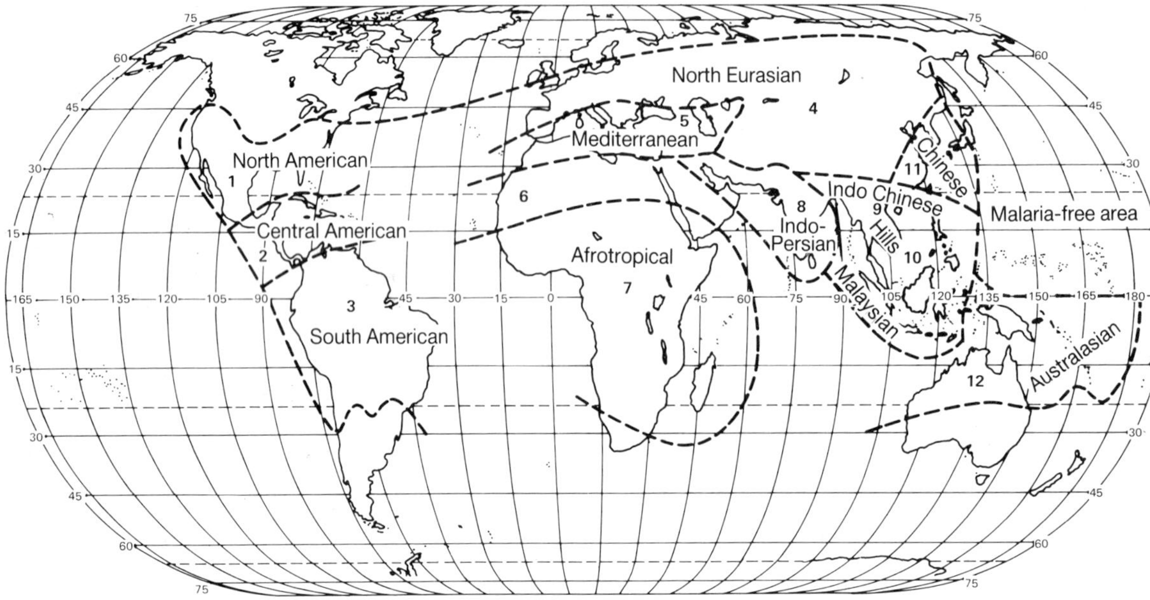

Fig. 7.12 Twelve epidemiological zones of malaria according to the classification by Macdonald (1957) and modernized terminology.

such as temperature and humidity influence the development of the mosquito and its protozoan parasite. In addition to this the inherent susceptibility of *Anopheles* to infection with human *Plasmodia* varies somewhat in relation to the species of malaria parasite and its strain. The physiological and biochemical reasons for such susceptibility or refractoriness to malaria infection are still not fully understood.

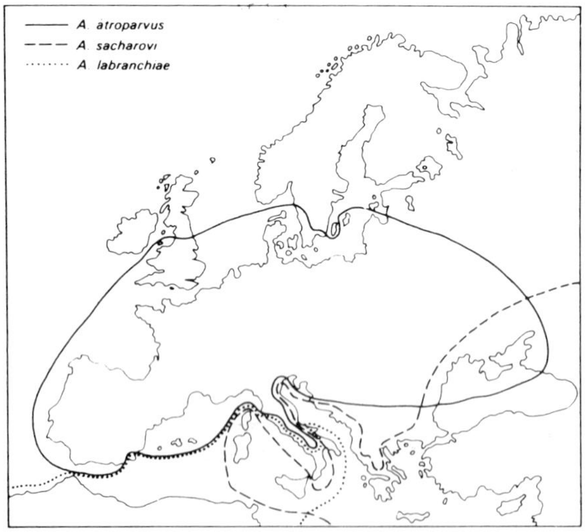

Fig. 7.13 Geographic distribution over the continent of Europe of three important species of the *Anopheles maculipennis* complex. (From Bruce-Chwatt and de Zulueta, 1980.)

Various species of *Anopheles* have well-defined behaviour characteristics and these often determine the distribution of malaria. Thus, in addition to climatic conditions, other factors affecting the breeding, feeding and survival of *Anopheles* must be taken into consideration in any control programme based on antimosquito measures.

The natural distribution of main vectors of malaria can be given broadly for the 12 epidemiological zones of malaria according to the classification by Macdonald (1957). These are shown, together with the main vector species in Table 7.2 and Fig. 7.12.

Some important vectors of malaria have a very definite pattern of distribution over large areas (Fig. 7.13). This is also shown by the example from the Indian sub-continent in Fig. 7.14. The close relationship between various ecological zones within a relatively small area and the prevalence of certain species of *Anopheles* of West Malaysia is indicated in Fig. 7.15.

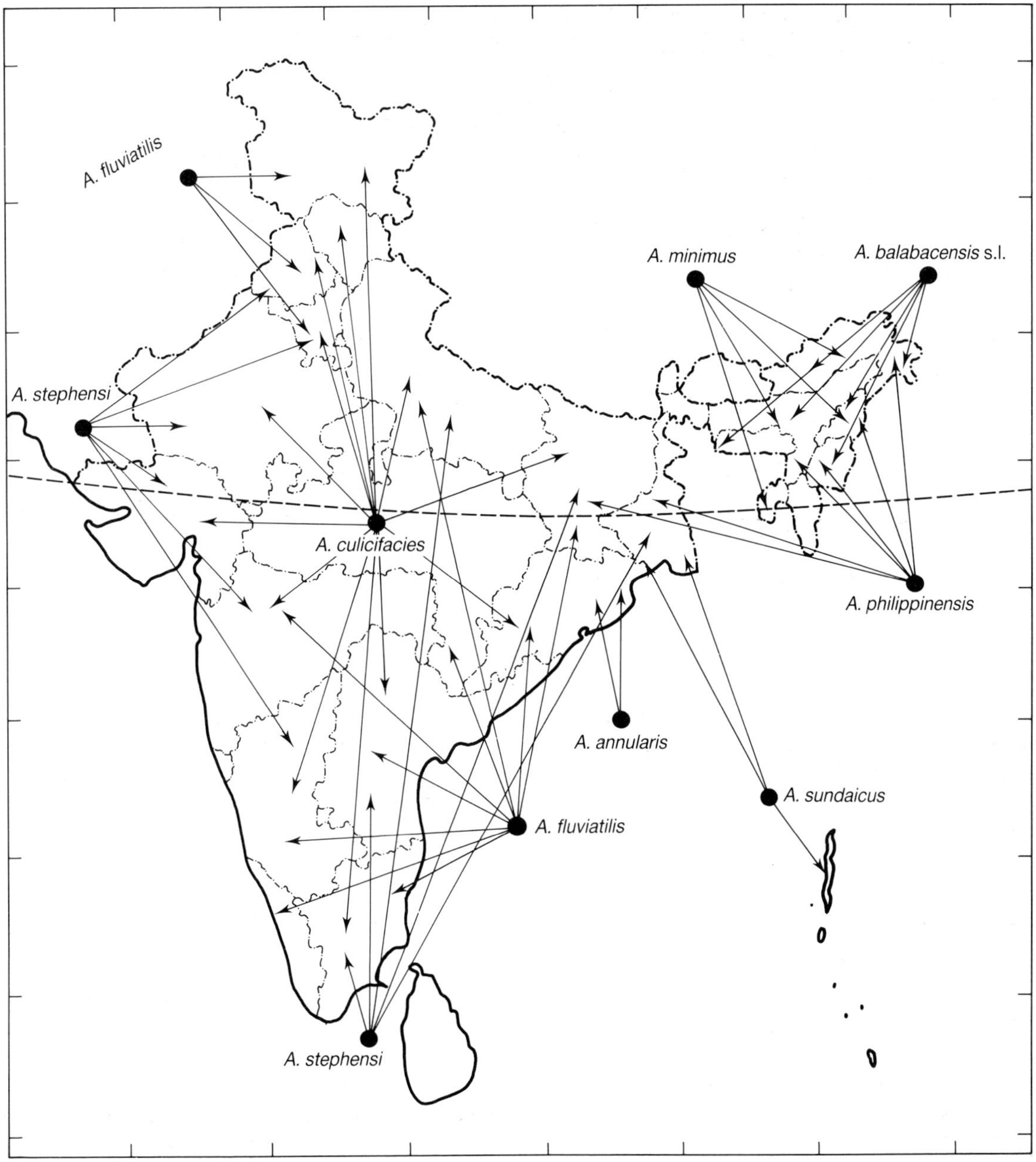

Fig. 7.14 Geographical distribution of main *Anopheles* species, vectors of malaria in the Indian sub-continent. Note that in some parts of North-east India *A. dirus*, a cryptic species of the *A. balabacensis* complex has been identified. (Reproduced with permission from S. K. Subbarao and incorporating additional data from R. Reuben.)

Table 7.2 Twelve epidemiological zones of malaria and some of the main (primary) and subsidiary (incidental and local) vectors* (after Service, 1993)

Zone	Extension	Vectors†
1. North American	From the Great Lakes to southern Mexico	***A. (A.) freeborni*** ***A. (A.) quadrimaculatus*** *A. (N.) albimanus*
2. Central American	Southern Mexico, the Caribbean islands, the fringe of the South American coast	*A. (A.) aztecus* *A. (A.) punctimacula* ***A. (N.) albimanus*** *A. (N.) albitarsis* ***A. (N.) aquasalis*** ***A. (N.) argyritarsis*** ***A. (N.) darlingi***
3. South American	Most of the South American continent irregularly beyond the Tropic of Capricorn	***A. (A.) pseudopunctipennis*** ***A. (A.) punctimacula*** *A. (K.) bellator* *A. (K.) cruzii* *A. (K.) neivai* ***A. (N.) albimanus*** ***A. (N.) albitarsis*** ***A. (N.) aquasalis*** *A. (N.) argyritarsis* *A. (N.) braziliensis* ***A. (N.) darlingi*** *A. (N.) nuneztovari* *A. (N.) triannulatus*
4. North Eurasian	Within the Palaearctic region excluding the Mediterranean coast of Europe	***A. (A.) atroparvus*** *A. (A.) messeae* *A. (A.) sacharovi* *A. (A.) sinensis* *A. (C.) pattoni*
5. Mediterranean	Southern coast of Europe, north-western part of Africa, Asia Minor and east beyond the Arabian sea	***A. (A.) atroparvus*** *A. (A.) claviger* ***A. (A.) labranchiae*** *A. (A.) messeae* ***A. (A.) sacharovi*** *A. (C.) hispaniola* ***A. (C.) superpictus***
6. Afro-Arabian	Africa north and south of the Tropic of Cancer including the central part of the Arabian peninsula	*A. (C.) culicifacies* *A. (C.) fluviatilis* *A. (C.) hispaniola* *A. (C.) multicolor* ***A. (C.) pharoensis*** ***A. (C.) sergentii***
7. Afrotropical (formerly 'Ethiopian')	Southern Arabia, most of the African continent, Madagascar and the islands south and north of it	***A. (C.) arabiensis*** ***A. (C.) funestus*** ***A. (C.) gambiae*** *A. (C.) melas* *A. (C.) merus* *A. (C.) moucheti* *A. (C.) nili* *A. (C.) pharoensis*
8. Indo-Iranian	North-west of the Persian gulf and east of it including the Indian sub-continent	*A. (A.) sacharovi* *A. (C.) aconitus* *A. (C.) annularis*

Table 7.2 *cont.*

Zone	Extension	Vectors†
		A. (C.) culicifacies ***A. (C.) fluviatilis*** *A. (C.) jeyporiensis* *A. (C.) minimus* *A. (C.) philippinensis* *A. (C.) pulcherrimus* *A. (C.) stephensi* *A. (C.) sundaicus* *A. (C.) superpictus* *A. (C.) tessellatus* *A. (C.) varuna*
9. Indo-Chinese Hills	A triangular area including the Indo-Chinese peninsula, the north-western fringe beyond the Tropic of Cancer	*A. (A.) nigerrimus* *A. (C.) annularis* *A. (C.) culicifacies* ***A. (C.) dirus*** ***A. (C.) fluviatilis*** *A. (C.) jeyporiensis* *A. (C.) maculatus* ***A. (C.) minimus***
10. Malaysian	Most of Indonesia, Malaysian peninsula, Philippines and Timor	***A. (A.) campestris*** ***A. (A.) donaldi*** ***A. (A.) letifer*** ***A. (A.) nigerrimus*** *A. (A.) whartoni* ***A. (C.) aconitus*** ***A. (C.) balabacensis*** ***A. (C.) dirus*** ***A. (C.) flavirostris*** *A. (C.) jeyporiensis* ***A. (C.) leucosphyrus*** ***A. (C.) ludlowae*** ***A. (C.) maculatus*** *A. (C.) mangyanus* ***A. (C.) minimus*** *A. (C.) philippinensis* ***A. (C.) subpictus*** ***A. (C.) sundaicus***
11. Chinese	Largely the coast of mainland China, Korea, Taiwan and Japan	***A. (A.) anthropophagus*** ***A. (A.) sinensis*** *A. (C.) balabacensis* *A. (C.) jeyporiensis* *A. (C.) pattoni*
12. Australasian	Northern Australia, Papua New Guinea and the islands east of it to about 175° east of Greenwich, but excepting the malaria-free zone of the south-central Pacific‡	*A. (A.) bancroftii* ***A. (C.) farauti type 1*** ***A. (C.) farauti type 2*** *A. (C.) hilli* *A. (C.) karwari* ***A. (C.) koliensis*** ***A. (C.) punctulatus*** *A. (C.) subpictus*

*Names in **bold** denote main vectors, subsidiary vectors not in bold.
†Subgenera are indicated as follows: *A* = *Anopheles*, *C* = *Cellia*, *K* = *Kerteszia*, *N* = *Nyssorhynchus*.
‡The malaria-free zone of the south-central Pacific includes New Caledonia, New Zealand, the Caroline Islands, Marianas, up to the Hawaiian islands, east to Galapagos and Juan Fernandez and rejoining the southern tip of New Zealand.

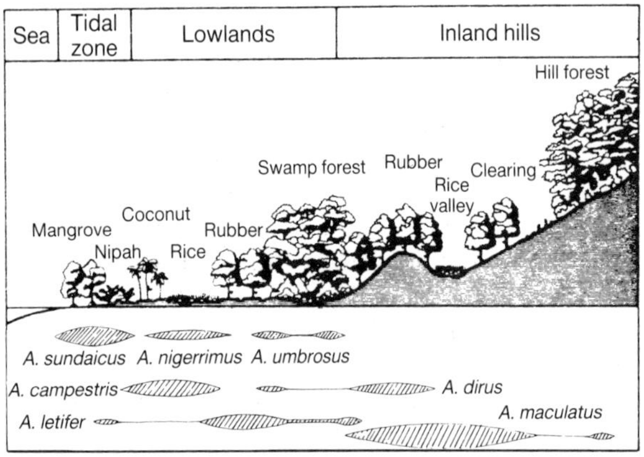

Fig. 7.15 Ecological distribution of habitats of several species of *Anopheles* vectors in a coastal area of West Malaysia. (Sandosham and Thomas, 1983.)

Natural history of *Anopheles*

The male *Anopheles* feeds exclusively on nectar and fruit juices while the female feeds primarily upon blood. The mating of many species is preceded by the formation of male swarms which occur during twilight, and often at a certain light incidence. Males are apparently attracted to the females by their higher wing-beat frequencies. Copulation is usually initiated in flight. It is probable that the females of most species receive sufficient sperm for all subsequent egg batches from a single mating. In temperate regions the sperm has to remain viable in the spermatheca of overwintering females for several months. Immediately after copulation a mating plug is produced in the genital chamber, at least in some species. This is formed by a secretion from the male accessory glands. Females of many species may require two blood meals before the first batch of eggs can develop. Females usually lay their first batch of eggs 3 to 6 days after emergence, the time depending on the duration of the gonotrophic cycle, which can be defined as the period from one egg-laying to the next one. In subsequent cycles a batch of eggs produced by the ovaries develops after each blood meal. At temperatures above 23°C the gonotrophic cycle is completed within about 48 hours, so that oviposition (egg laying) and host-seeking for the next blood meal are repeated every 2 to 3 nights.

Female *Anopheles* of most species feed on warm-blooded animals, with some preferences for humans or certain animal hosts. Adult female *Anopheles* respond to various stimuli in foraging for food such as carbon dioxide, host odours, moisture and warmth, and also show some discrimination in finding a suitable host. Having located a source of a blood meal the mosquito uses her labrum-epipharynx, maxillae and mandibles, supported by a bent labium, to pierce the skin (Fig. 7.16). When a capillary vessel has been ruptured blood is sucked up through the food channel by the action of the pharyngeal pump. Saliva from the salivary glands is injected down the hypopharynx during the process of blood sucking and serves as an irritant, to increase the flow of blood to the capillary vessel. Some individuals are particularly attractive to mosquitos while others are much less so.

The amount of blood ingested by the female mosquito depends largely on her own size and ranges

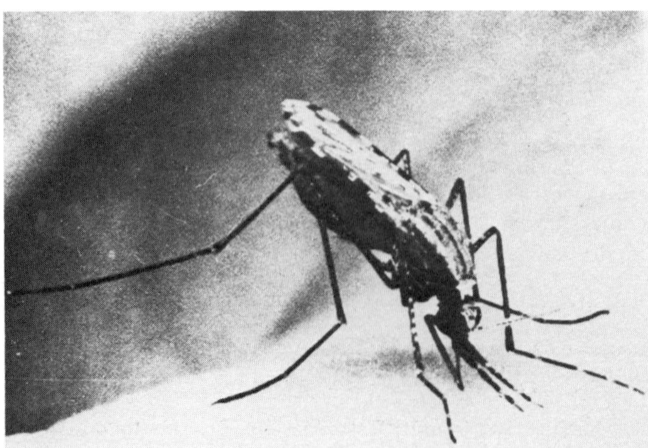

Fig. 7.16 Female of *Anopheles gambiae* in the act of feeding on a person. (Wellcome Museum of Medical Science.)

between 1.3 and 3.0 µl, and approximates to the weight of the mosquito. Blood contained in the stomach undergoes some concentration through excretion of plasma and is digested in one to a few days, depending on the environmental temperature. When the environmental temperature drops below a certain threshold, females of some species of *Anopheles* undergo a process of hibernation during which they develop fat bodies, and cease producing eggs. This process, known under the name of *gonotrophic dissociation*, may also occur in tropical *Anopheles* during the period of drought. The period of reproductive inactivity is termed *diapause* (see also aestivation, p. 114).

Eggs are always deposited in or near water, the number per batch varying between 70 and 200. Successive egg batches tend to decrease in size and may also show a seasonal variation. Newly laid eggs usually require a period of 2 to 3 days for completion of embryonic development before they can hatch. In some species of *Anopheles* eggs can remain alive for 16 days or even longer on wet mud; when flooded, such eggs hatch within 3 to 4 minutes. However, anopheline eggs cannot survive after desiccation, though some species are more resistant to partial drying.

Anopheline larvae are easily recognized by their appearance, as they float horizontally on the surface of the water and feed by means of their mouth brushes which sweep floating particles towards the mouth. The larva moves by sharp jerks and if disturbed sinks below the surface.

After the third moult the fourth instar *Anopheles* larva develops into a comma-shaped, still aquatic, pupa. Pupae do not feed but are nevertheless extremely active and respond quickly to all external stimuli, by diving to the bottom of the water, but they soon rise again to the surface where they breathe through their paired respiratory trumpets. After 2 to 4 days, depending on the temperature and other factors, the pupal skin splits dorsally and the adult insect (or *imago*) emerges. The process of emergence (or *eclosion*) takes a few minutes, and if its outcome is successful the mosquito may rest for some time on the pupal case to harden its wings before flying away.

The duration of the cycle from the egg to the adult *Anopheles* may vary between 7 days at 31°C and 20 days at 20°C. Each species has its own optimum range of temperature.

The length of life of adult *Anopheles* varies somewhat between species, but even more so on external factors among which temperature, humidity and presence of natural enemies are the most important. When the mean temperature is over 35°C or the humidity less than 50% the longevity of *Anopheles* is drastically reduced, unless they find more favourable conditions in the microclimate of their resting places. The *average* duration of life of a female *Anopheles* under favourable climatic conditions is often about 10–14 days, but occasionally much longer, and some females in a population will live for 3 to 4 weeks. Males live less long than the females.

The longevity of the local anopheline population has a direct bearing on its transmission potential of malaria. If the mean daily mortality of a population is 35% then less than 1% of them will survive the 10 days necessary for the development of *P. falciparum*, up to the infective stage (sporozoites) in the salivary glands. The importance of this concept is fully explained in the next chapter.

Larval habitats

Collections of water which provide habitats for anopheline larvae may be temporary or permanent, natural or man-made. There is great diversity in the types of habitat utilized by the various species. This is due to the number of factors involved in the selection of sites by ovipositing females. The factors concerned include exposure to sunlight, temperature, salinity and organic content. No classification of larval habitats is completely satisfactory but the following is a simplified but useful one.

Permanent or semi-permanent standing fresh water

- Large open marshes or marshy parts of lakes
- Small ponds, pools, borrow-pits, stagnant canals and ditches
- Spring fed pools, springs and seepages from higher contours
- Standing water in fields (rice fields, plantations)
- Open wells
- Swamps and pools in the forest

Transient fresh-water collections

- Open pools in the fields or stagnant stream beds
- Cattle hoof prints, pools in car tracks etc.

Permanent or semi-permanent running fresh water
- Open stream beds with vegetation
- Stream beds running over gravel
- Flowing water in canals and ditches
- Streams in forests or plantations

Container habitats
- Rock holes
- Tree holes
- Plant axils and epiphytic water-bearing plants, e.g. bromeliads
- Discarded containers, natural and artificial (coconut husks, tins, tyres etc.)
- Crab holes and cracks in the mud (fresh or brackish water)

Brackish water
- Marshes, ponds and swamps (not tidal)
- Tidal swamps
- Small collections of brackish water

Larval habitats of many species are found in association with floating or emergent vegetation (Fig. 7.17). However, the larval habitat is usually well-defined for any particular species. The majority of them are found in fresh-water pools or marshes; some species (*A. nili*, *A. rivulorum* of Africa) show preference for floating vegetation; others (*A. plumbeus* of Europe) prefer rain-filled tree holes; certain species of the *Kerteszia* group (*A. bellator*, *A. cruzii*) in Central and South America select water-containing axils of bromeliad plants (Fig. 7.18); a number of species are found mainly in brackish water (*A. atroparvus* of Europe, *A. aquasalis* of Latin America, *A. sundaicus* and *A. litoralis* of South-east Asia, *A. melas* and *A. merus* of West and East Africa, respectively). Some species are more catholic and may adapt their habits to various existing conditions.

Artificial containers, such as pots or tubs, are generally unsuitable for most anopheline species, although *A. stephensi* in India is often found in overhead water tanks and cisterns, wells, tin cans, earthenware pots and other man-made receptacles. Some species readily breed in temporary rain pools and in small puddles of water, such as those formed in the imprints of animals' hooves (Fig. 7.19). Large expanses of open water, free from vegetation, seldom support anopheline larvae, although breeding may occur in more or less isolated pools and pockets of relatively still water along the grassy margins of lakes, streams and rivers.

Man-made malaria is a term applied to many human activities which produce breeding places suitable for malaria-carrying mosquitos and so favour increased incidence of the disease. Untouched mangrove swamps are often innocuous until man fells the trees and interferes with the natural line of drainage by constructing roads and railways. Riverine deltas are also often harmless until man creates breeding places and alters the water table by erecting embankments to reclaim land for agriculture, or building, without providing proper drainage.

Irrigation projects are frequently to blame in this matter, chiefly by a failure to provide adequate drainage facilities, thus predisposing to water-logging. Other causes of 'irrigation malaria' are defective sluice-gates, badly maintained irrigation ditches, seepage from canal banks and beds, and

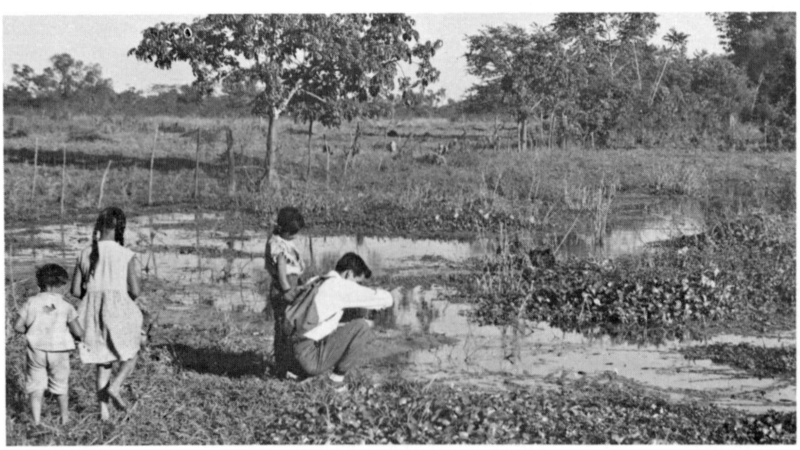

Fig. 7.17 A typical larval habitat (breeding place) of *Anopheles albimanus*, one of the main vectors of malaria in Mexico and Central America. (WHO photograph by M. Rude.)

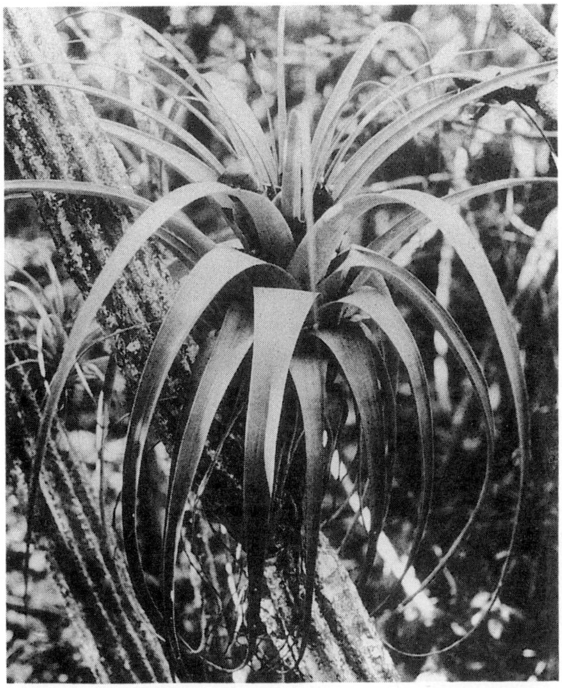

Fig. 7.18 A typical South American bromeliad shown growing on a cactus, although more usually they are epiphytes of forest trees. Water accumulating in their leaf axils provides larval habitats for vectors such as *Anopheles bellator* and *Anopheles cruzii*. (Photograph by M. W. Service.)

lack of a planned or controlled system of field channels. However, with a crop like rice most breeding often occurs in the water standing in the rice fields. One of the commonest faults in road and rail construction is the improper placement of culverts. They tend to be either too high, so that water is held up on the upper side of the embankment; or too low, so that water remains in the bed of the culvert itself. Another common source of mosquito breeding is the line of borrow-pits commonly dug alongside roads and railways. Breeding places are also often produced during the course of building construction, especially in connection with docks and other large works in urban areas of the tropics.

Seasonal fluctuations

At the onset of the cold season some species are killed off. They may then be found only at lower altitudes where temperatures are still suitable. In other species the males only die, the females seeking shelter in protected sites from the cold (*hibernation*). Before such mosquitos hibernate a last blood meal is taken which, instead of resulting in the formation of eggs, goes to make fat on which the females live while hanging immobile in their winter quarters. Before the females arrive at a hibernation place some species, in subtropical areas, may indulge in

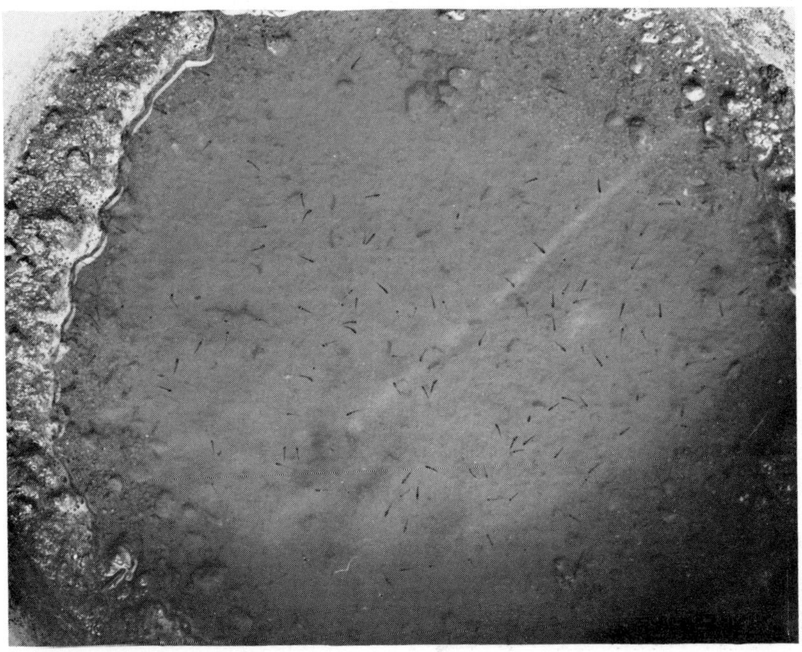

Fig. 7.19 A typical habitat (breeding place) of *Anopheles gambiae*, the major vector of malaria in tropical Africa. Note the hundreds of larvae on the surface. (WHO photograph by D. Henrioud.)

a long prehibernation flight, which is much longer than their normal one, extending to as much as 19 km, e.g. *A. sacharovi* in Syria. In complete hibernation the female mosquitos remain torpid until the arrival of the warm season. In some species only a partial hibernation occurs, and the females emerge occasionally from their winter quarters to take another feed in order to renew their store of fat, after which they return. Such occasional blood feeding of the European *A. atroparvus* was the cause of cases of transmission of malaria during the winter in the Netherlands, Germany and England in the 1930s. In other species the winter is passed in the larval stage, for example, *A. claviger* (northern Europe). Another seasonal effect is *aestivation*, seen in the hot dry season of some countries, where the female seeks to avoid the intensely dry atmosphere by remaining inactive in a cool damp place until the dry spell is over.

Seasonal changes such as temperature, rainfall and humidity have an obvious effect on anopheline populations and thus also on the incidence of malaria. In most tropical countries breeding continues throughout the year, but in the dry season the population is very small due to paucity of breeding places; with the onset of the rainy season or monsoon, numerous breeding places are created and the anopheline population increases explosively. Some unusual events may give rise to major effects. Thus, in 1958 in Ethiopia an excessive rainfall combined with high temperatures resulted in high breeding activity of *A. gambiae* s.l. followed by an epidemic of malaria with 3 million cases and 150 000 deaths. On the other hand, a severe drought in south-western areas of Sri Lanka contributed to excessive breeding of *A. culicifacies* in small pools formed by half-dry streams; this resulted in a severe epidemic of falciparum malaria in 1934–35.

Behaviour pattern of adult *Anopheles*

The adult female takes her first blood meal the night after she emerges from the pupal stage. Feeding occurs, almost without exception, between dusk and dawn, but anophelines may feed during the day-light hours in densely shaded woodland or dark interiors of shelters and houses. Some species have early peaks of biting at night such as *A. albimanus* (1900–2100 hours), whereas others such as *A. gambiae* are late feeders (2400–0300 hours). Times of biting can be epidemiologically important. The readiness of *Anopheles* mosquitos to feed at a particular time of night depends to some extent on environmental conditions, but the biting cycles of many species of mosquitos are so constant in different and yet comparable conditions that they reflect in-built circadian rhythms of biting.

The feeding habits vary greatly. Some species prefer a non-human host and will feed on animals even if humans are readily available, and the converse may be true of other species. The terms '*anthropophilic*' and '*zoophilic*' are used to indicate, respectively, a supposed preference for feeding on humans or on animals, often domestic ones such as cattle. It must be understood, however, that such terms are relative, since many *Anopheles* species are ready to feed on alternative hosts when the favourite one is not available.

The origin of the ingested blood in the stomach of a freshly engorged mosquito can be determined by immunological techniques such as ELISA, or less frequently these days by the earlier interfacial precipitin ring test. In practice the important answer that the results of such tests give is whether the blood was human or of animal origin. The proportion of *Anopheles* giving a positive reaction for human blood is '*the human blood index*'; such an index is a valuable pointer to the importance of an *Anopheles* species to act as a vector of human malaria.

Resting places are frequently inside houses. Female mosquitos commonly enter a house after dark, take a blood meal, and then, being heavily engorged with blood, fly to a nearby wall or ceiling where they normally rest until all blood is digested and they are gravid and thus ready to fly outside to lay eggs. Mosquitos may rest on clothing hanging on a wall, on the back or underside of pieces of furniture or pictures etc. The females frequently prefer the lower portions of the interiors of houses where temperatures are lower and the humidity is higher.

Some species seek secluded natural out-of-doors resting places such as clumps of vegetation, hollow trees and logs, buttress roots of trees, and holes or crevices in rocks and soil. Other times females can be found in man-made structures such as in thatched granaries, empty and abandoned buildings, in culverts and under bridges.

It is obvious that house-resting is of special importance in relation to control methods using residual insecticides. Generally speaking the daytime resting place is dark and with a degree of humidity that provides a tolerable microclimate for the mosquito. Natural resting places outside houses are important as they may yield samples of the mosquito population for determination of their feeding patterns that are less biased than collections from human habitations or animal shelters. This is the reason why entomologists often use artificial resting places for collecting mosquitos.

The behaviour characteristics of *Anopheles* species may be artificially grouped, according to their feeding habits and their relationship to humans into three kinds: *domestic*, those which come into houses to feed and rest there afterwards; *wild*, those which will only feed outside and never enter houses; and an *intermediate group*, those which may feed in houses but leave soon afterwards. The feeding and resting habits of adult anopheline mosquitos have been intensely studied and special terms are used in relation to their pattern of behaviour. They are: (a) *endophily*, the habit of remaining within a man-made shelter throughout the whole or a definite part of the gonotrophic cycle (food may be sought within or without a man-made structure); (b) *exophily*, the habit of spending the greater part of the gonotrophic cycle out of doors (food may be sought within or without a man-made structure); (c) *endophagy*, the habit of obtaining the blood meal within a man-made structure; (d) *exophagy*, the habit of seeking the blood meal out of doors. There can be all combinations of these behavioural traits. For instance, *A. aquasalis* (Latin America) may feed outside (exophagy) or inside a house (endophagy) but nearly always rests outside afterwards (exophily). *A. fluviatilis* (India) feeds indoors, rests indoors until it is about half-gravid then rests outside houses.

Since all these characteristics are of great importance in control programmes, the habits of the vector species must be well understood by teams engaged in malaria control.

Flight range

Anopheles mosquitos are not usually found more than 2 or 3 km from their breeding places in any large number. However, strong seasonal winds may carry *Anopheles* up to 30 km or more from their main breeding place, and various other factors may greatly influence the average flight range of some species. Generally, tropical *Anopheles* have a shorter flight range than mosquitos present in temperate climates. Normally females disperse further than males.

Dispersal by flying is known as *active dispersal*, whereas *passive dispersal* means carriage by any means other than the insects' own wings; this may be wind, aeroplane, train, truck and ship, and may result in *Anopheles* being found very far from their place of origin. The carriage of exotic *Anopheles* by aircraft arriving into temperate areas from endemic parts of the world has recently caused a series of cases of imported malaria in Europe. Concern about this problem has been expressed in several countries.

Generally speaking, the control of anophelines within 2 km of docks, parking bays for aircraft or other systems of transportation, and storage areas where migrating mosquitos may rest, should provide adequate protection.

For the study of *Anopheles* dispersal or flight range, adult mosquitos may be marked with different coloured paints or fluorescent powders. Adults can also be made radioactive by dosing larval water with radioisotopes of phosphorous or strontium. Radioactive adults can be detected by Geiger and scintillation counters, or by their 'fogging' of photographic film.

Anopheles species complexes

Early in the present century it was recognized that within a species group of some *Anopheles* there are forms with some biologically and morphologically different characteristics. The practical implications of this phenomenon became more obvious at the end of the First World War when the return of troops to Europe from some extremely malarious areas resulted in highly localized outbreaks of the indigenous malaria instead of widespread epidemics that could be expected from the known distribution of potential mosquitos vectors. This situation of '*anophelism without malaria*' remained puzzling until the discovery of some subtle differences in groups of *Anopheles* within one apparently single species.

The detection of 'long-winged' and 'short-winged' forms of *Anopheles maculipennis* in the

Netherlands and their association with fresh and brackish water of their breeding places provided the first clue. Other studies in Italy resulted in the discovery of forms of *A. maculipennis* that could be separated on the basis of their egg markings. Further studies of behaviour patterns of these groups and their reproductive compatibility showed that within the *A. maculipennis* species there are at least five sibling species. It is now known that in the Palaearctic region there are ten species within the *A. maculipennis* complex, and another five Nearctic species.

The practical importance of this work was the clear evidence that the different species within the *A. maculipennis* complex differ in their feeding and other habits and thus in their ability to transmit malaria. It follows that those which are not involved in the transmission of the infection can be largely ignored in control activities.

The pioneering work by Guido Frizzi in Italy demonstrated the value of studying the structure and the banding patterns of chromosomes in the salivary glands of *Anopheles* for identification of such sibling species. These cytotaxonomic methods were concentrated on the polytene or giant chromosomes found in various tissues, but most clearly seen in the larval salivary glands. The banding pattern of polytene chromosomes is constant, corresponding to the gene sequence. Later it was found that *Anopheles* had good polytene chromosomes in the ovarian nurse cells of half-gravid adults.

Further studies by George Davidson were based on crossing experiments to determine the genetic compatibility of various groups and the sterility or otherwise of hybrids. For this purpose it is necessary to colonize separate groups of *Anopheles* in cages in laboratory conditions. Where mass cage mating between separate groups is impossible crossing can be obtained by an artificial forced mating technique. This involves the presentation of the genitalia of an anaesthetized female to those of a male *Anopheles* whose head is cut off just before, thus inducing the reflex action of copulation and fertilization. Using this technique it has been possible to cross species which will not mate in cages.

Thus, the former concept of morphological species based on distinctive external characters has now been replaced by the genetic species concept, where the criterion is the presence or absence of a barrier of interbreeding between two or more populations of mosquitos. It is evident that the number of such biologically distinct species is greater than the number of species recognizable by their external characters. Such groups of species are known as *species complexes*; species within a complex may show more or less marked differences in feeding, resting and other types of behaviour.

Over 100 species of mosquitos have been studied with regard to their biological characters and their karyotypes (namely, chromosome patterns) as well as their fertility on intermating. The study of genetics of mosquitos, including *Anopheles*, assumed greater importance (and complexity) with the use of electrophoresis for determination of enzyme variations. This technique can be applied to any developmental stage of the mosquitos, and it is often useful for identification of sibling species within a species complex. Of great interest is the fact that some enzyme differences are related to the susceptibility or refractoriness to plasmodial infections (as in *A. stephensi*), and to the development of insecticide resistance, and also to some behaviour characteristics. More recently species within several complexes have been shown to differ in their cuticular hydrocarbon pattern as shown by gas chromatography of hexane washes of adult mosquitos, and even larvae. Finally, advances in molecular biology have allowed DNA and RNA probes to be used for species identification, such as for members of the *A. gambiae* complex. These methods, however, necessitate the use of radiolabelled probes, but non-radioactive probes using a colour marker have recently been developed, and it is hoped that this will eventually become a simple field technique – much as the ELISA method is used to identify blood meals of mosquitos.

Anopheles gambiae, the most important malaria vector in Africa, has been studied more than any other species complex. Until 1956 *A. gambiae* was considered a single species with some dark or light varieties breeding in fresh and salt water. A vast amount of research has now shown that it is a complex of at least six sibling species exhibiting differences in behaviour and each with a specific polytene chromosome pattern. Crosses between the members of these sibling species produce sterile hybrid males but all hybrid female mosquitos are fertile, although in certain crosses few or no females are produced. Three of these sibling species are adapted to fresh-water breeding sites; *A. gambiae* s.s. (sensu stricto), formerly named species A, predominates in humid areas, is highly anthropophilic and is an important vector of malaria; *A. arabiensis* (formerly species B) extends more into savannah areas, is in many areas more zoophilic and exophilic but nevertheless can be an efficient malaria vector. In contrast *A. quadriannulatus* (species C) is zoophilic and consequently is not a vector. The last fresh-water species *A. bwambae* (formerly species D) has a very restricted distribution in a small area of the Rift Valley, west of Ruwenzori, where it breeds in geothermal waters. It is a very localized and minor malaria vector. The two salt-water species, *A. melas* of West Africa and *A. merus* of East Africa, are local malaria vectors, but they are generally more exophagic and zoophilic and thus poorer vectors than *A. gambiae*. In many parts of Africa the *A. gambiae* complex occurs as mixed populations, of two or even three species, without interbreeding. They respond unequally to insecticidal spraying, because some are more exophilic, and good knowledge of their different behaviour patterns is of value in assessing the results of vector control campaigns.

Among other *Anopheles* species complexes in which cross-breeding and hybrid sterility have been investigated are the *A. maculipennis* complex (comprising ten recognized Palaearctic species, namely, *A. atroparvus*, *A. beklemishevi*, *A. labranchiae*, *A. maculipennis*, *A. martinus*, *A. melanoon*, *A. messeae*, *A. sacharovi*, *A. sicaulti* and *A. subalpinus*), the *A. punctulatus* complex (*A. punctulatus*, *A. koliensis* and *A. farauti* species 1, 2 and 3), the Oriental *A. balabacensis* complex (11 species) and the *A. culicifacies* complex (species A, B, C and D). It may be of interest to point out that *A. beklemishevi* was the first mosquito species ever named and described primarily from cytotaxonomic studies carried out in 1976 in the former USSR.

The taxonomy of the *A. leucosphyrus* group is particularly difficult, comprising three species complexes, namely, the *A. leucosphyrus* complex, the *A. balabacensis* complex and the *A. dirus* complex. *Anopheles leucosphyrus* s.s. is a malaria vector in Sarawak. *Anopheles balabacensis* s.s. is also a malaria vector but is found only in Sabah, a small area of Sarawak, Balabac island, Palawan island in the Philippines, and North Kalimantan. *Anopheles dirus* is the most important vector and has a much wider distribution being found in Thailand, Hainan island, Vietnam, Kampuchea, Laos, the Union of Myanmar, Sumatra and Java.

Among the neotropical sub-genus *Nyssorhynchus*, many sibling groups have been described in the medically important species, for example, chromosomal evidence of speciation exists in *A. nuneztovari*, *A. darlingi*, *A. albitarsis* and *A. evansae*. The Colombian and Venezuelan populations of *A. nuneztovari* are known to be vectors of malaria, whereas the species is not a vector in Brazil. Similarly, three chromosomal types of *A. albitarsis* have recently been identified from southern and eastern Brazil and from Colombia and Venezuela.

It must be said that although such genetic studies have proved valuable for the discovery of sibling species within *Anopheles* complexes, they have greatly complicated the field work of entomologists not experienced in the use of cytogenetic techniques.

Entomological methods

There are a number of techniques, either simple or elaborate, for collection of *Anopheles* in their aquatic stages or as adults. The main practical indications for these methods are mentioned in the section describing the purpose of a malaria survey, and only a few of these methods can be described here (Fig. 7.20).

For the collection of mosquito eggs, larvae or pupae, various scoops, ladles and dishes, having a white bottom, are used in the field. Aquatic nets are useful in detecting breeding when larval density is low. The proper technique of dipping for anopheline larvae and pupae demands a fairly good knowledge of the type of water and aquatic vegetation preferred by malaria vectors (Fig. 7.21). Perseverence is just as important as proper clothing and footwear for muddy conditions.

Sketch-maps indicating the distribution of streams, swamps and other sources of flowing or standing water are needed to pin-point the location of larval habitats producing dangerous species of malaria vectors.

Particulars of the type of larval habitat, type of vegetation, conditions of water (clear, muddy, fresh, brackish) should be entered into the notebook, together with the number of the sample. It is best to record the numbers of larvae per dip

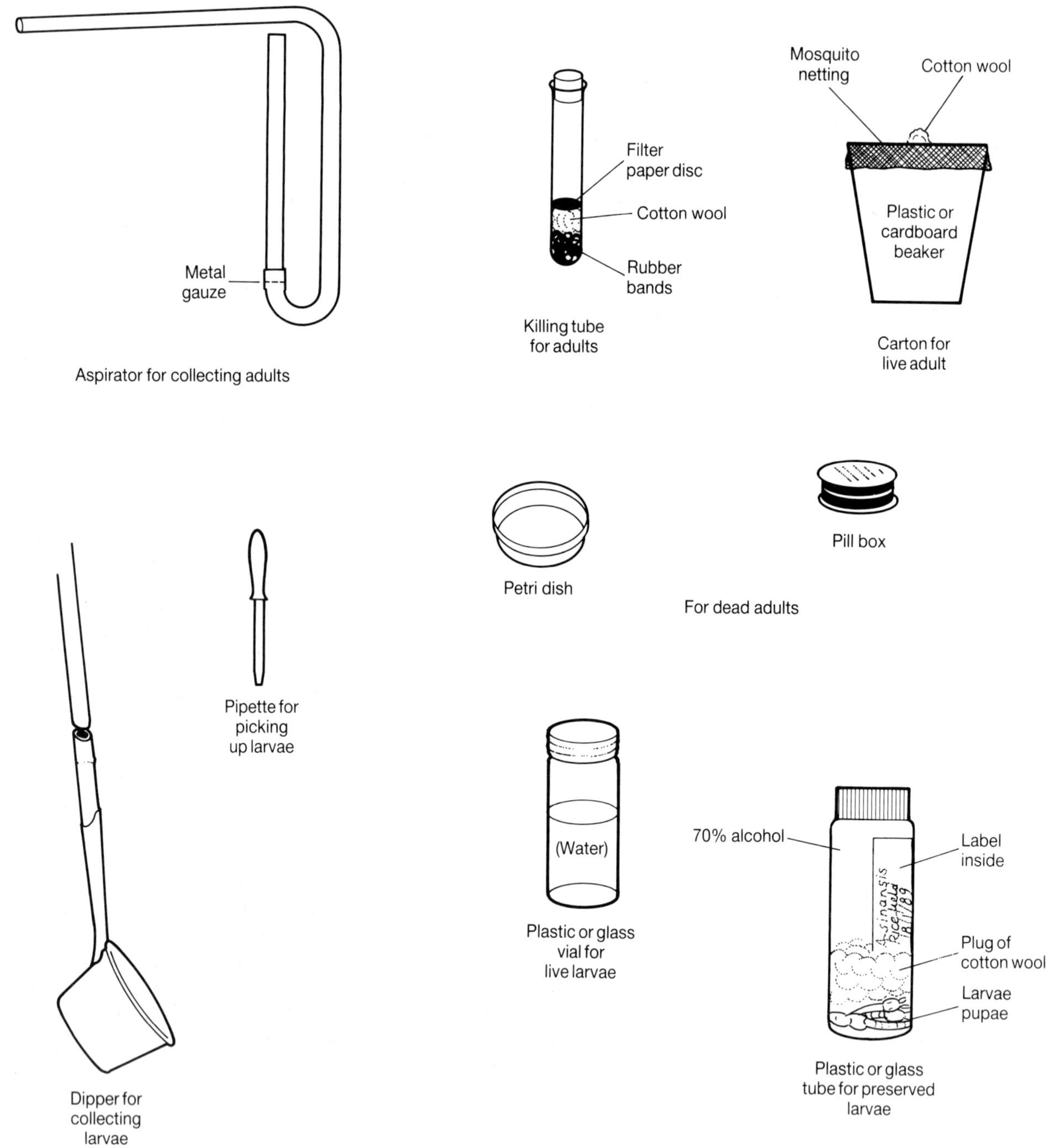

Fig. 7.20 Basic equipment for collection of larvae and adults of mosquitos in the field. (Modified from WHO, 1972, *Vector Control in International Health.*)

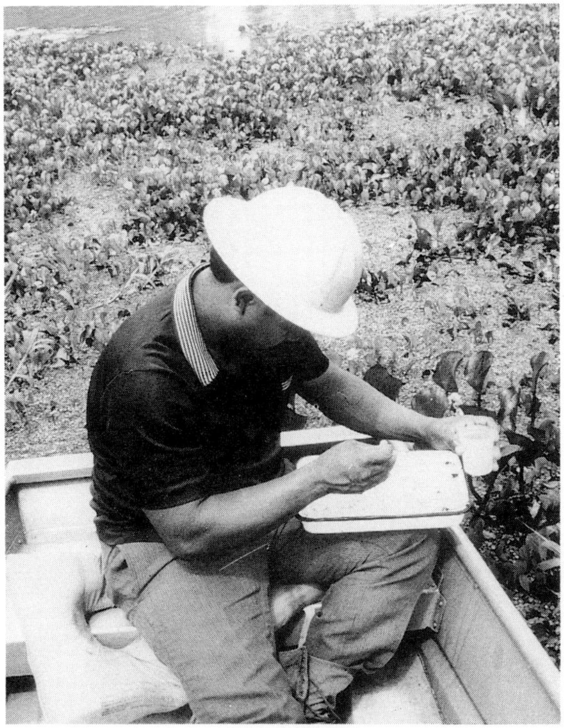

Fig. 7.21 A collector on a boat amongst vegetation on a lake pipetting *Anopheles* larvae into a small container. (Photograph by M. W. Service.)

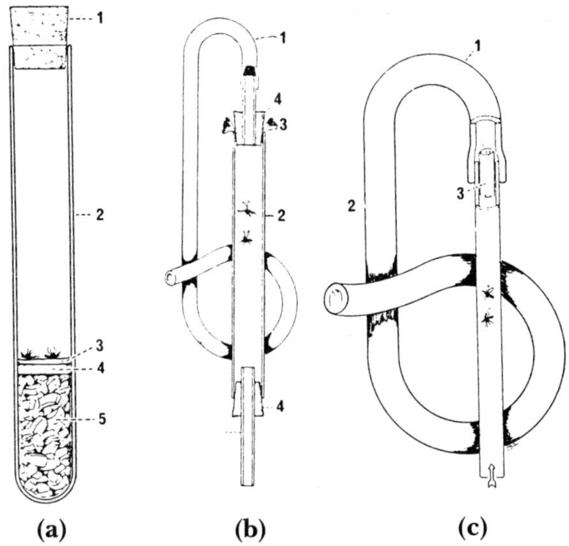

Fig. 7.22 Three types of simple equipment for collection of adult mosquitos. (a) Killing test-tube: 1. cork stopper; 2. glass (or plastic) tube; 3. filter or blotting paper; 4. cotton wool, cork disc or gauze; 5. fragments of rubber bands. For collecting live mosquitos. (b) Reservoir-type aspirator: 1. rubber or plastic tubing; 2. glass or plastic reservoir; 3. fine gauze netting; 4. perforated corks. (c) Non-reservoir-type aspirator ('suction tube'): 1. rubber or plastic tubing; 2. glass or plastic tube; 3. narrow glass or plastic tube covered with fine gauze.

separately so that a standard error can be attached to the mean number per dip. Larvae placed in collecting bottles half-filled with water must not be unduly shaken or exposed to the hot sun. If the identification of the species from the larval characters presents difficulties, they may be reared through the pupal stage to allow the emergence of adult mosquitos. The pupae should be transferred to a plugged test-tube with some water and a blade of grass for the adult mosquito to rest on after emergence.

It may be pertinent here to quote P. F. Russell's dictum that 'sun-loving *Anopheles* are not effectively sampled by shade-loving personnel; nor can aquatic larvae be adequately scouted by dry-footed collectors'.

Live adult *Anopheles* are collected by simple 'tube catching' or by suction tubes (aspirators). Various types of suction tubes are used (Fig. 7.22). Figure 7.20 shows the type of collecting equipment which is simple and generally adequate. It consists of an aspirator, a killing tube, Petri dishes with wet cotton wool covered with filter paper, netting-covered paper cups or cages (if live mosquitos are collected), field record forms, a pencil, a torch and a map. The killing bottle is made from a glass or suitable plastic tube about 2.5 cm in diameter and 16.5–18 cm in length. The tube is filled to a depth of about 2.5 cm with finely chopped rubber bands or plaster of Paris; a sufficient quantity of chloroform is added to saturate the rubber. Cotton wool or fine gauze is placed over the rubber, and covered with a disc of filter or blotting paper. The tube is closed with a cork stopper. Such a tube remains effective for several weeks and can be recharged with chloroform when necessary.

Obviously this simple method of collecting adult *Anopheles* sheltering in houses or animal quarters suffers from many errors and depends not only on the time of day when the collection is made but also on the skill and reliability of the collector (Fig. 7.23). An alternative, widely used and very convenient method of collecting dead *Anopheles* from

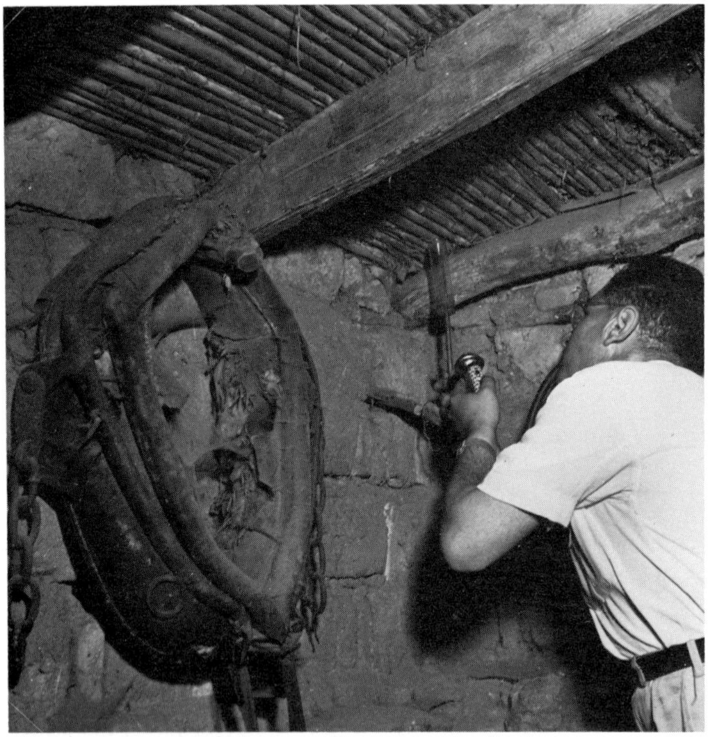

Fig. 7.23 Collecting adult *Anopheles* in a stable, during the malaria eradication programme in Greece. (WHO photograph.)

houses and animal shelters consists of using simple 'flit-guns' to spray inside closed rooms with 0.1% pyrethrum in kerosene. Some pyrethrum formulations are sold as emulsion concentrates and can be diluted with water not kerosene. After spraying, the sprayers leave the rooms. Dead and dying mosquitos fall onto white sheets that have been spread over the floor of the room or house. Ten minutes should be allowed before closed rooms are re-entered and the mosquitos collected from the floor sheets.

A large variety of other techniques have been developed for sampling mosquito populations. Captures at night of mosquitos attracted to human volunteers is one of the best methods of measuring human–vector contact. Other methods use special traps with animal or human 'baits' (Fig. 7.24); while Communicable Disease Center (CDC) type battery-operated light-traps are often used for collecting mosquitos from houses and cattle sheds. Naturally, none of these sampling techniques has a direct relationship to the actual mosquito population in the locality. Nevertheless, each of these methods, if used properly, gives some idea of the relative trends of population size, and enables appropriate baseline data to be established. Thus, the mean number of *Anopheles* females in relation to a dwelling unit such as a house or a room is known as the '*anopheline density*'. Such sampling indicates

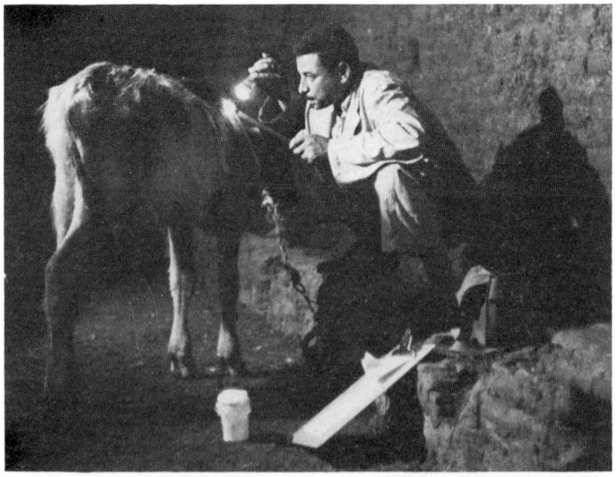

Fig. 7.24 Night collection of mosquitos on animal bait in Egypt to establish the feeding preferences of some malaria vectors. (WHO photograph by Ph. Boucas.)

which species of mosquitos are present in the locality and, by the number of specimens collected in proportion to the number of houses or rooms visited, it provides information on whether the control operations are effective. Regular sampling over long periods gives a meaningful set of data. Thus, it is important to establish sampling stations in the early part of a control programme and select them so that they reveal the situation over the whole area. In addition to the collection of adult mosquitos, regular sampling for larvae in known larval habitats is helpful for monitoring the control operations.

Identification of *Anopheles* species collected in the field is of obvious importance since it permits the separation of harmless species from those that are important malaria vectors. Some knowledge of mosquito anatomy is necessary for the use of taxonomic keys for species identification. Most adult characters mentioned in the keys can be observed with the aid of a good magnifying glass, or a simple binocular microscope. Identification of larval mosquitos requires a compound microscope. The principle of the use of binary entomological keys is explained in Figs 7.10 and 7.11.

Maintenance of laboratory colonies of some *Anopheles* for subsequent studies of the pattern of insecticide resistance is not difficult with some species such as *A. stephensi* and *A. albimanus*, but other species may not mate or lay eggs in cages, in spite of feeding on guinea pigs, rabbits or other small animals. Artificial mating, already briefly described, may be needed with some species.

Malaria infection in *Anopheles*

The presence of an infection in *Anopheles* may confirm the importance of a given species as a vector of malaria. In relation to the cycle of development of *Plasmodia* in mosquitos it is important to recognize the relevant parasite stages in the stomach (oöcysts) of the *Anopheles* and in the salivary glands (sporozoites).

Dissection of the midgut of the female mosquito is not difficult, although it requires some practice (Fig. 7.25). The sequence of operations is as follows:

1. Identify the species of the killed *Anopheles* and record its source of collection.
2. Remove the wings and legs.
3. Place a drop of normal (0.85%) saline on the glass slide and place the trimmed insect close to the drop, with the abdomen pointing towards the observer.
4. Under a low-power magnification of a dissecting microscope, using a dissecting cutting needle (e.g. Shute's needle) nick the chitinous skin at the sides of the abdomen between segments 6 and 7.
5. Holding the thorax with one needle, place the other needle across the tip of the abdomen and draw the abdominal contents out with a steady gentle traction, so that they touch the drop of saline.
6. When the contents, including the midgut, come out cut off and remove the tip of the abdomen, the ovaries and the Malpighian tubules.
7. Transfer the loosened midgut into a fresh, larger drop of saline on the same slide.
8. Gently place a small coverslip on the isolated midgut and examine under a compound microscope for the presence of oöcysts. Transferring the midgut to 0.5% mercurochrome for staining helps identify oöcysts, and is recommended for beginners. Use low power first and confirm under higher magnification. The oöcysts lie on the outer surface of the midgut and appear as clear round or oval bodies, containing distinct granules. Larger, more mature oöcysts are 30–60 μm in diameter, they have lost the pigment are are filled with hundreds of sickle-shaped sporozoites, which escape from the oöcysts when the latter are ruptured by gentle pressure on the coverslip.

Occasionally, on dissecting a female *Anopheles* for oöcysts one may observe clusters of dark, round or oval bodies on the gut wall or on the ovaries. These 'black spores of Ross' are degenerated and chitinized oöcysts.

Dissection of salivary glands of the female mosquito is more difficult and needs practice (Fig. 7.25).

1 & 2. As for gut dissections.

3. Cleanly cut off the head. Place the neck end of the thorax into a drop of saline.
4. Gently press with a blunt needle (e.g. side of a Shute's needle), the glands should pop out of the thorax.
5. Cut off the glands and after removing other

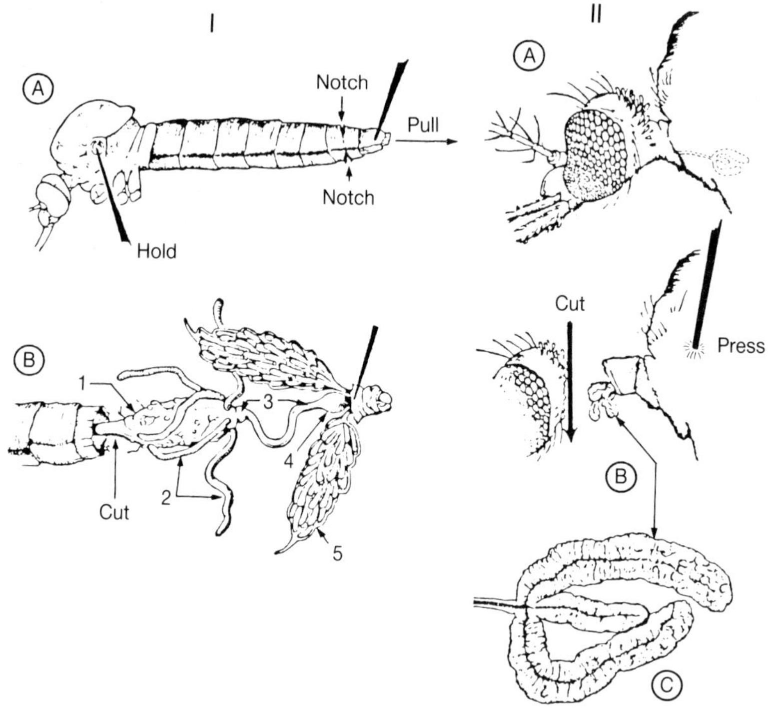

Fig. 7.25 Dissections of female *Anopheles* for presence of plasmodial infection. I. Dissection of midgut. (A) After making two small notches on the ventral and dorsal seventh segment of the exoskeleton of the mosquito pull the terminal segment away from the abdomen until the whole of the midgut emerges. (B) Cut off the midgut from the oesophagus, remove the Malpighian tubules (2), the hindgut (3 and 4) and the ovaries (5), and examine the midgut in a drop of saline under a coverslip. II. Dissection of salivary glands. (A) Cut off head. (B) Press the thorax until the glands emerge from it. (C) Cut off the glands, and examine under coverslip, using the high power of the microscope.

debris of the dissection place a small coverslip on the glands.

6. Rupture the glands by a gentle pressure and examine under the high power of a compound microscope for sporozoites.
7. The presence of sporozoites can be confirmed by removing the coverslip, inverting it on the slide, then securing it with a drop of Canada balsam DPX or other suitable mountant and, after fixing with absolute methyl alcohol, staining it with Giemsa stain.

An *Anopheles* which on dissection shows oöcysts on the stomach wall is *infected*; when it shows sporozoites in the salivary glands, it is *infective*. This is the more important parameter because it shows the vector has lived sufficiently long to be capable of transmitting malaria. The percentage of female *Anopheles* caught in nature showing sporozoites in the glands is the *sporozoite rate*. The percentage showing oöcysts on dissection of the midgut is the *oöcyst rate*. These rates should be related to specific *Anopheles* species, and the number of mosquitos dissected should be indicated. Information as to the source of capture (e.g. houses, stables, natural shelters) is important. In highly endemic areas, considerable variation in the sporozoite rate may be due to seasonal increase or decrease of the mosquito population. An important parameter is the inoculation rate which is the sporozoite rate multiplied by the average number of a species biting a person per night. This allows a better comparison between the importance of different mosquito species in transmitting malaria. Sporozoite rates of around 5% are not uncommon in *A. gambiae* in Africa, but much lower rates (0.01 or 0.1%) are usually encountered in the Neotropical region and in Asia. Hundreds, or even thousands, of mosquitos may be dissected before a positive gland is found. To reduce this onerous task methods have been developed involving the maceration of batches of mosquitos followed by density gradient centrifugation and then microscopic detection of sporozoites.

Although gland dissections are still routine in many laboratories, microscopical detection of sporozoites does not indicate which human malarial parasite is involved. Furthermore, in areas such as South-east Asia many anopheline species will be transmitting rodent or simian malaria, and it is impossible to differentiate the sporozoites from those of human malaria. However, immunological tests will differentiate between human and the non-important malarias. For example, the ELISA test, using monoclonal antibodies to the circumsporozite antigen, can be performed on fresh or old dry mosquitos. Such a test for *P. falciparum* is specific for that species, other tests allow the identification of *P. vivax*, *P. malariae* and *P. ovale*, although as yet tests for the latter two species have not been well tested in the field.

Chapter 8

Epidemiology of malaria

H. M. Gilles

> Everything about malaria is so moulded by local conditions that it becomes a thousand epidemiological puzzles. Like chess, it is played with a few pieces but is capable of an infinite variety of situations.
>
> Hackett (1937)

Geographical distribution

Indigenous malaria has been recorded as far north as 64°N latitude (Archangel in the former USSR) and as far south as 32°S latitude (Cordoba in Argentina). It has occurred in the Dead Sea area at 400 m below sea level and at Londiani (Kenya) at 2600 m above sea level or at 2800 m in Cochabamba (Bolivia).

Within these limits of latitude and altitude there are large areas free of malaria, which is essentially a focal disease, since the transmission of malaria depends greatly on local environmental and other conditions.

Malaria has a major place among the endemic tropical diseases. It has been estimated in the 1950s that the annual incidence of the disease was of the order of 250 million cases, with 2.5 million people dying of malaria every year. The extent of endemic malaria has now decreased as a result of eradication and control programmes carried out during the past 35 years.

Epidemics of malaria, so common in the past, are now less frequent. One of the greatest epidemics of malaria in modern times struck the former USSR after the First World War; more than 10 million cases were reported in 1923–26, and there were at least 60 000 deaths. The Sri Lankan or Ceylon epidemic of 1934–35 caused nearly 3 million cases of malaria and 82 000 deaths; in 1938 the invasion of Brazil by *A. gambiae* was followed by an epidemic with over 100 000 cases and at least 14 000 deaths; in 1942–44 the same mosquito invaded lower Egypt and caused about 160 000 malaria cases and more than 12 000 deaths; in 1958 an epidemic of malaria in Ethiopia caused more than 3 million cases and 150 000 deaths; in 1963 there was an epidemic of malaria in Haiti, in the wake of the typhoon Flora, with 75 000 cases. In 1967 a serious resurgence of malaria in Sri Lanka greatly handicapped the progress of eradication of this disease from the island. Since 1973 there has been a marked resurgence of malaria in several countries of southern Asia. In 1976 alone, well over 7 million cases of malaria were reported from the Indian subcontinent. In the Asian part of Turkey some 270 000 cases of *P. vivax* malaria occurred during the period 1977–80 alone. In Madagascar in 1988, an epidemic of *P. falciparum* malaria is estimated to have killed over 25 000 people; and a number of other countries in Africa have faced severe, sometimes unprecedented, epidemics during the last decade. These include Botswana, Burundi, Ethiopia, Namibia, Rwanda, Sudan, Swaziland, Zaire and Zambia.

Plasmodium vivax has the widest geographical range; it is prevalent in many temperate zones, but also in the subtropics and tropics. *Plasmodium falciparum* is the commonest species throughout the tropics and subtropics, although it may occur in some areas with a temperate climate. *Plasmodium malariae* is patchily present over the same range as *P. falciparum* but much less common. *Plasmodium ovale* is found chiefly in tropical Africa, but also occasionally in the West Pacific.

Natural transmission of malaria infection occurs

through exposure to the bites of infective female *Anopheles* mosquitos. The source of human malaria infection is nearly always a human subject, whether a sick person or a symptomless carrier of the parasite.

With the possible exception of chimpanzees in tropical Africa, which may carry the infection with *P. malariae*, no other animal reservoir of human *Plasmodia* is known to exist. However, there have been a few cases of natural or accidental infection of humans with some *Plasmodia* of simian origin.

The alternation between the human and the mosquito host represents the biological *cycle* of transmission of the malaria parasite. The transmission of the infection by the mosquito from the human carrier (donor) to the human victim (recipient) represents the *chain* of transmission.

However, the infection may also be transmitted *accidentally*; this occurs not infrequently as a result of blood transfusion when the donor harbours malaria parasites. Drug addicts using the same hypodermic needle have been known to infect one another. *Congenital* infection of the newborn from an infected mother also occurs, but is comparatively rare.

Deliberate transmission of malaria was common during the first half of this century for malaria therapy of neurosyphilis. Other instances of deliberate infection refer to experimental trials of antimalarial drugs or vaccines when the disease is transmitted to volunteers. In both cases the transmission may be carried out either by injection of infected blood or by bites of intentionally infected mosquitos.

Natural transmission of malaria depends on the presence of and relationship between the three basic epidemiological factors: the *host*, the *agent*, and the *environment*. Human beings are the vertebrate host of human *Plasmodia*; the *Anopheles* mosquito is the invertebrate host. However, the latter may also be considered as the agent of transmission while the malaria parasite is the true agent of the infection. The environment should be considered from its three aspects: physical, biological and socio-economic (Fig. 8.1).

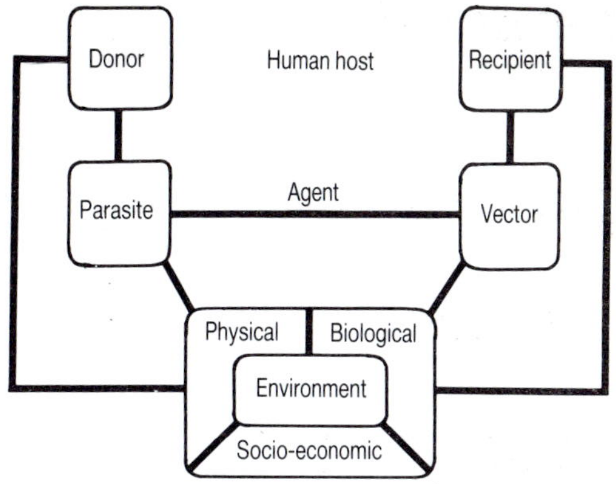

Fig. 8.1 Epidemiological factors of host, agent and environment involved in the transmission of malaria.

Host factors

Sex and age are not important factors with regard to the malaria infection, but children have generally a higher degree of susceptibility than adults. There are factors involved in the immune response; persons of African origin seem to have a greater innate immunity to some types of malaria than other races.

There are many epidemiological variables in the response of the human victim to the infection. There is evidence that in certain parts of the world the high frequency of haemoglobin S in the population is due to the evolutionary selection related to the fact that the presence of this haemoglobin has a mitigating effect on the severity of *P. falciparum* infections.

It seems that persons with red blood cells negative to Duffy blood group determinants are relatively unsusceptible to infections with *P. vivax*. There is also some evidence of the protective action of genetic deficiency of an enzyme (glucose-6-phosphate dehydrogenase) normally present in the erythrocytes (see Chapter 5).

Generally speaking, populations exposed continually to intense malaria in highly endemic areas develop a degree of immunity to the infection. Mosquitos derive the infection from an individual with parasites in the blood, but not necessarily from an individual with fever or other manifest signs of disease. When malaria is endemic a proportion of the population is usually a carrier of gametocytes and this may be particularly the case amongst young children. In endemic malarious areas the prevalence of gametocytaemia decreases with rising age, until it reaches low levels in adults.

Agent

Within each of the four species of human *Plasmodia*, there are a number of strains which have different epidemiological and other features, although they are indistinguishable morphologically. Thus, the European strains of *P. falciparum* are readily carried by *A. atroparvus*.

Studies on the susceptibility of various species of *Anopheles* to imported species and strains of human *Plasmodia* revealed that *A. atroparvus*, *A. messeae* and *A. sacharovi* present in Europe can be easily infected with *P. vivax* from Africa, Asia and South America. On the other hand, *A. atroparvus* and *A. messeae* could not be infected with tropical strains of *P. falciparum*. However, *A. sacharovi* while not very susceptible to *P. falciparum* has been infected experimentally in a few such trials, thus indicating a degree of heterogeneity of this plasmodial species. The pattern of relapses in West Pacific strains of *P. vivax* is different from the relapse pattern of vivax malaria occurring in other parts of the world. There are also considerable differences between the long incubation period of the disease caused by some North European strains of *P. vivax*, and the short incubation period seen in infections by other strains of this plasmodial species. Finally, several geographical strains of *P. falciparum* and *P. vivax* show different types and degrees of resistance to antimalarial drugs.

There are nearly 400 species of *Anopheles* of which some 60 are proven vectors of human malaria. However, in each geographical area there are usually not more than three or four anopheline species that can be regarded as important vectors. To be an effective vector a species must be present in adequate numbers in or near human habitations. A species with a marked preference for human blood rather than for animal blood is a better vector. Finally, the length of life of a mosquito is a paramount factor in malaria transmission; the latter varies in different places in relation to temperature and humidity. Thus, the development of *Plasmodia* in the *Anopheles* depends on a minimum temperature below which it does not occur, and above which the amount of transmission is dependent on this and other environmental factors.

There is a condition known under the term *anophelism without malaria*; this generally means the presence of *Anopheles* which cannot transmit the infection either because they are non-vectors, or because they do not normally feed on humans, preferring animal blood. In areas where malaria eradication has been achieved and there is no reservoir of infection in the local population, no transmission should occur unless it is imported from elsewhere.

Environment

Variation in climatic conditions has a profound effect on the life of a mosquito and on the development of malaria parasites. Hence its influence on the transmission of the disease and on its seasonal incidence. The most important factors are temperature and humidity. Malaria parasites cease to develop in the mosquito when the temperature is below 16°C. The best conditions for the development of *Plasmodia* in the *Anopheles* and the transmission of the infection are when the mean temperature is within the range 20–30°C, while the mean relative humidity is at least 60% (Fig. 8.2). A high relative humidity lengthens the life of the mosquito and enables it to live long enough to transmit the infection to several persons.

Strong winds affect the flight of *Anopheles* and may prevent their egglaying; however, in some cases, they may extend their flight range well beyond the normal limits. Building of dams and man-made lakes raises the ground water-table and often causes seepages and flooding, thus contributing to the creation of new larval habitats.

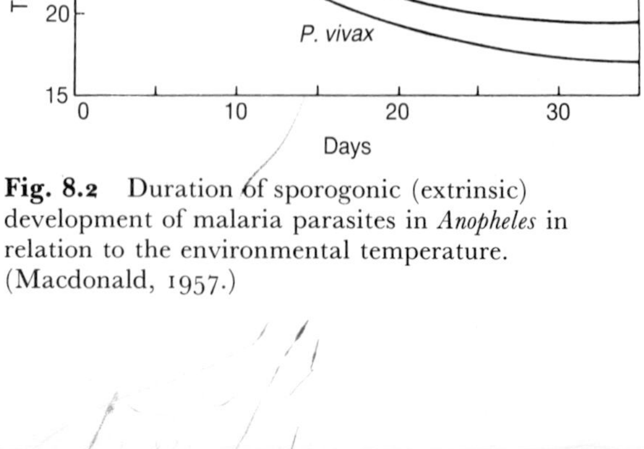

Fig. 8.2 Duration of sporogonic (extrinsic) development of malaria parasites in *Anopheles* in relation to the environmental temperature. (Macdonald, 1957.)

The association of malaria with rainfall in parts of the world where the latter is seasonal is due not only to greater breeding activity of mosquitos, but also to the rise in relative humidity and higher probability of survival of female *Anopheles*. Excessive rainfall or drought play an important part in the production of regional epidemics of malaria.

Rainfall, which normally increases the amount of surface water, may have, at times, a negative effect on the amount of transmission of malaria. Excessive rainfall may transform small streams into rapid torrents and thus strand many larvae and pupae on the edges of the water channel. Conversely, deficient rains in other parts of the world change many rivers into a string of pools in which certain *Anopheles* would breed in profusion. The latter occurrence was often observed in a north-west zone of Sri Lanka where during the years of relative drought greatly increased breeding of *A. culicifacies* took place and was followed by severe epidemics of malaria. It is not only the total amount of rainfall which is important but also its distribution over the month of the year. Russell proposed a formula for the distribution of rainfall:

$$\frac{\text{Total rainfall} \times \text{Number of rainy days}}{\text{Number of days in the month}}$$

The presence of waterbearing plants (which favour the breeding of *Anopheles*) or the presence of cattle (on which some *Anopheles* feed) constitutes a biological factor of the environment (Fig. 7.18, p. 113).

Finally, social and economic factors, such as sanitation, housing, occupation, poverty etc. have an important effect since malaria is more prevalent in underdeveloped countries. The evidence concerning the susceptibility to malaria infection in relation to human malnutrition is inconclusive.

Various human activities may be conducive to dispersal of *Plasmodia* or dangerous vectors of malaria to new areas of the world. In 1930 Brazil was invaded by *A. gambiae* from Africa probably transported by ships plying between Dakar and Natal in connection with the new sea route. This resulted in a serious epidemic of malaria in north-eastern Brazil but an antimosquito campaign resulted in the eradication of *A. gambiae* from South America. In 1966 *A. stephensi* was recorded for the first time in Africa, having been probably carried by aircraft from Saudi Arabia to Egypt. The incidental importation by passenger or cargo aircraft of *Anopheles* infected in certain tropical countries is dealt with on p. 162.

Wars and large-scale population movements, whether of pilgrims or labour forces from endemic areas, have often been a factor in the spread of malaria. The return of troops from malarious war areas to England during the First World War resulted not only in a high number of cases of imported malaria, but also in an outbreak of local disease which caused nearly 500 cases of 'introduced' malaria among the civilian population. In the USA, nearly 20 000 cases of imported malaria were reported during the period 1969–74 in soldiers returning from South-east Asia.

During the past decade the greatly increased speed and volume of human travel has resulted in large numbers of imported malaria in many countries. Problems of malaria imported or introduced into non-endemic countries by persons infected elsewhere are dealt with on p. 161.

Malaria in the human community

The term *endemicity* refers to a general statement indicating the amount or severity of malaria in an area or community. Any precise information on the degree of endemicity must be based on quantitative and statistical concepts.

Malaria is described as *endemic* when there is a constant incidence of cases over a period of many successive years. *Epidemic malaria* is a term which indicates a periodic or occasional sharp increase in the amount of malaria in a given indigenous community.

A more general classification into *stable* or *unstable* malaria has been introduced. In *stable* malaria the amount of transmission is high without any marked fluctuations over the years, although seasonal fluctuations may exist. In *unstable* malaria the amount of transmission varies from year-to-year. In the first case the collective immunity is high and epidemics are unlikely; in the second case the collective immunity of the population is low and epidemics are possible (Table 8.1).

These two terms represent extremes of a very wide range of situations. The first indicates an almost perennial transmission, little affected by climatic changes, caused by highly infective vectors,

Table 8.1 Some characteristics of unstable and stable malaria (after Macdonald, 1957)

Characteristics	Unstable	Stable
Type of vector	Vector with infrequent human biting habit and/or low daily survival rate	Vector with frequent human biting habit and high daily survival rate
Environmental conditions	Not favourable for a rapid sporogonic cycle	Favourable for a rapid sporogonic cycle
Endemicity	Usually low to moderate; high endemicity may occur	Very high endemicity common; low to moderate may occur
Determining causes	Vector of low anthropophily and low to moderate longevity. Climatic conditions favourable for short priods of transmission	Vector of high anthropophily and moderate to high longevity. Climatic conditions favourable for long periods of transmission
Anopheline density (needed to maintain transmission)	High (1–10 or more bites per person/night)	Low (as low as 0.025 bites per person/night)
Seasonal changes of incidence	Pronounced	Not very pronounced, except for short dry season
Fluctuations in incidence and predominant parasite	Very marked and uneven. Most often *P. vivax* as main parasite	Not marked and related to seasons. *Plasmodium falciparum* prevalent parasite
Immunity of the population	Variable with some groups of low immunity	High, though varying in degree in different age groups
Epidemic outbreaks	Likely when climatic or other conditions suitable	Unlikely to occur in the indigenous population
Amenability to control or eradication	Not unduly difficult by imagicides and larvicides combined with chemotherapy. Daily anopheline mortality of 20–25% may be adequate for control of transmission	Very difficult to control, especially in rural areas. Eradication unlikely unless socio-economic conditions favourable. Daily anopheline mortality of at least 50% needed for a degree of control

with a high prevalence of *P. falciparum*, and high level of collective immunity in the human population. Within a degree of stability the intensity of individual infection varies in different age groups, but epidemics are not likely. The feature of unstable malaria is the variability of its incidence from place-to-place, from month-to-month and from year-to-year, with an occasional cyclic pattern. *Plasmodium vivax* is predominant, but sharp outbreaks of severe *P. falciparum* occur and can be devastating.

Malaria is *autochthonous* when contracted locally; it is *indigenous* when natural to an area or country. Malaria is *imported* when the infection was acquired outside the specified area. Secondary cases contracted locally but derived from imported cases are referred to as *introduced* malaria. Infections deliberately produced for the purpose of malaria therapy or caused accidentally (by blood transfusion or otherwise) are known as *induced* malaria.

Two types of measurement are commonly used for the assessment of the impact of the malaria infection on the community and are described below.

The terms *index* and *rate* express the relationships between various frequencies or counts. The word 'rate' usually carries the idea of some simple form of proportion such as percentage. The word 'index' is applied to a measurement of one type of value indicating its relationship to another. Thus, the proportion of enlarged spleens is the 'spleen rate' of a group but it provides an index of the endemicity of malaria in the relevant population. This semantic difference between the 'index' and 'rate' exists only in the English language. In other languages the term 'rate' is generally expressed as a percentage and only the expression index (or 'indice') is commonly used.

Incidence describes the frequency of illnesses *commencing* during a defined period; it refers to the number of cases of disease or infection occurring per unit of population during a given time interval. *Prevalence* refers to the number of cases of disease or infection *existing* in a population at any given time. Usually in morbidity statistics one should distinguish between 'period prevalence' (over a stated time) and 'point prevalence' (at a particular point in time). However, the difficulty of distinguishing between a new malaria infection and a recrudescence or relapse has resulted in the conventional acceptance of the term prevalence as being synonymous with 'point prevalence', while incidence means always the frequency of cases of malaria over the period, irrespective of whether the disease resulted from a new infection or not. The difference between the two concepts is shown in Fig. 8.3.

The *morbidity rate* (or morbidity) is the proportion of the number of cases of malaria in a unit of time in the population in which they occur. It is closely related if not identical to the incidence of malaria and usually expressed with regard to 1000 or 10 000 population. Except in conditions when the diagnosis and reporting of each case is carried to perfection the morbidity rate is based on recorded admissions or attendances at hospitals and dispensaries. Naturally, in areas of high endemicity with a large proportion of asymptomatic carriers of malaria parasites the morbidity rate refers only to clinical cases and represents only a small proportion of the total amount of malaria.

Malaria mortality represents the number of deaths from malaria, usually per 100 000 of the population per year. In practice, the true mortality rate from malaria is equally if not more difficult to determine than the morbidity rate for similar reasons. The often quoted average mortality rate due to malaria (1%) is not more than an estimate, since the fatality varies considerably in relation to the infecting species of *Plasmodium* and according to the provision of medical facilities, which depend on socio-economic conditions of the country or area concerned.

It should be distinguished from the *fatality rate*, which is the number of deaths in relation to all cases of malaria; however, since infections other than *P. falciparum* are rarely fatal it is advisable to indicate the fatality rate as a proportion of deaths out of the number of cases of *P. falciparum*.

Epidemic malaria

The term *epidemic* may be applied to a sharp rise of the incidence of malaria among a population in which the disease was unknown. Conversely, it may refer to a seasonal or other increase of clinical malaria in an area with moderately endemic malaria.

According to Russell (1952) in the genesis of malaria epidemics the following major points should be considered: (1) increased susceptibility of the human population, often due to introduction of non-immune individuals into an endemic area; (2) increased infective reservoir in the population; (3) increased contact between humans and the *Anopheles* vector; (4) greater effectiveness of local *Anopheles* in transmitting the malaria parasite.

The exact causes of an epidemic of malaria are often difficult to determine. The increased suscepti-

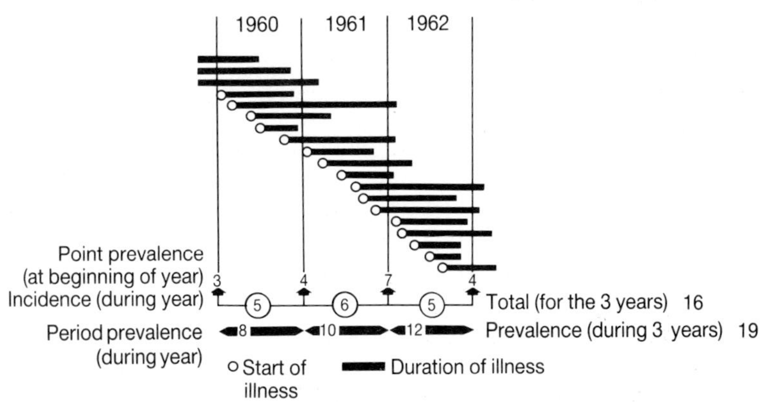

Fig. 8.3 Diagram of epidemiological concepts of prevalence and incidence. (WHO, 1966.)

bility of the local population may be due to some social or other upheavals such as war or a natural disaster, both of them resulting in poor housing, poor sanitary facilities and malnutrition. However, the relationship between susceptibility to malaria and the state of nutrition is not clear. In areas where malaria is unstable, any previous epidemic would produce a proportion of people partly immune to the infection; but the gradual decline of this immunity would eventually create a large number of people without any protective response. However, the most common factor in the increased susceptibility of a community is the introduction of a large number of non-immune persons, as often happens in large-scale development projects in the tropics.

The increase of the infective reservoir in the community is most commonly due to the introduction of newcomers from an area with a species or strain of malaria parasite unknown or rare in the main locality. Some carriers of the new infection may be asymptomatic but, nevertheless, the gametocytes circulating in their blood may be highly infective to local *Anopheles*. A sudden wave of gametocyte production in a proportion of the population as a cause for an epidemic of malaria has also been postulated. A surge of seasonal relapses of a former infection has been incriminated.

The third and probably most important cause of epidemic outbreaks is due to the sudden increase of the number of vectors, and to greater mean longevity of the female *Anopheles* of the species responsible for transmission. Climatic conditions are usually involved in this phenomenon but often a sharp decrease of animals, in areas where zoophilic *Anopheles* predominate, compels those mosquitos to seek alternative sources of blood, namely, the human population. Other incidental causes such as greater accessibility of vectors to humans because of defective housing have also been postulated but are less easy to prove. Finally, epidemics have occurred in the past, and will occur in the future as a result of introduction into a potential or actual malarious area of a new vector species with high susceptibility to plasmodial infection and with marked tendency of feeding on humans.

Malaria epidemics may be seasonal, generally related to climatic factors which increase the breeding activity of *Anopheles* and their longer survival in summer and early autumn. However, some epidemics may occur in the early spring and are due to relapses of *P. vivax* malaria, from infections received during the previous summer. This was the pattern of seasonal outbreaks of malaria in northern Europe. In some seasonal epidemics where *P. vivax* and *P. falciparum* are both involved the former starts earlier and reaches a peak, to be followed by a seasonal peak of *P. falciparum* infections.

In an epidemic of malaria three periods can be distinguished, although they cannot be easily separated from one another. Following on the pre-epidemic increase of transmission due to the higher gametocyte rate and the greater density and infectivity of the *Anopheles* population, there is a sharp rise in the incidence of the disease. This is the *epidemic wave* which is also accompanied by an increase of mortality, directly due not only to malaria but also to the other intercurrent diseases. The severity of an epidemic of malaria cannot be easily related to the increase of transmission which has caused it; even small increases of transmission may produce quite dramatic epidemics. The rise of the epidemic wave is usually faster in *P. vivax* outbreaks than in those due to *P. falciparum*, although the severity of the latter is far greater. During the *post-epidemic* period the incidence of malaria falls to its usual low endemic levels but the spleen rates in the population remain high for some time.

The extent of malaria epidemics varies. Localized epidemics occur in an area where unprotected groups of non-immune workers or soldiers are moved into an endemic zone, especially where human activities have increased the breeding potential of mosquitos by interference with the environment.

When the incidence of malaria increases sharply over a vast geographical area one refers to *regional epidemics* which are often severe with a high mortality and due to unusual climatic conditions as one of the main factors.

Finally, some epidemics may exceed the natural geographical limits of endemic malari and are loosely called pandemics. This was the case of the widespread epidemic of malaria in Russia after the First World War.

Malaria epidemics occur mainly in hypo- and mesoendemic areas. One of the characteristics of these epidemics was their occurrence in cycles of 5–8 years; however, it is difficult to forecast a cyclical epidemic as the cycles are far from regular. The most obvious pointers to a possible epidemic are meteorological and environmental factors, but a reasonably good collection of vital statistical data may detect it at an early stage and facilitate the initiation of appropriate measures. Christophers's method of mapping geographical points of excessive mortality (ratio of mortality in the epidemic months to normal mortality) permitted the early prediction of incipient epidemics in the Punjab in 1908. This method may still be of value in areas where no other ways for the early detection of increasing incidence exist. In countries where the disease has been eradicated or its endemicity reduced, there is now a risk of malaria epidemics occurring in non-immune populations if the density of local vectors shows a marked rise and if there is a large influx of cases imported from abroad.

Endemic malaria

This term is applied to malaria when there is a constant measurable incidence both of cases of the disease and of its natural transmission in an area over a succession of years. Conventionally, if the disease ceased to be transmitted over at least 3 years one may presume that malaria is no longer endemic in the area, although the *Anopheles* vectors responsible for the previous transmission may remain. In these conditions, potential endemicity may still exist and if there is a probability of importation of cases of malaria from other parts of the world the *malariogenic potential* is said to be high.

The two factors which determine the level of the malariogenic potential are *receptivity* of the area and its *vulnerability*. The first refers to the number of new cases of malaria that could theoretically originate from one single imported case; the second factor is related to the actual numbers of imported cases entering the area in a unit of time.

Endemic malaria may be present in various degrees and the following classification of it is commonly used.

Hypoendemicity denotes areas where there is little transmission and the effects of malaria on the general population are unimportant.

Mesoendemicity is found typically among small rural communities in the subtropical zones with varying intensity of transmission depending on local circumstances.

Hyperendemicity is seen in areas with intense but seasonal transmission where the immunity is insufficient to prevent the effects of malaria on all age groups.

Holoendemicity denotes a perennial transmission of high degree resulting in a considerable degree of immune response in all age groups, but particularly in the adults.

This classification is based on epidemiological data obtained in the field usually in the course of a study known as a *malaria survey*, and described in the following section.

The presence and degree of both the endemic and epidemic malaria depend on a number of factors which can be divided into three groups, namely, humans, malaria parasites and the mosquito vector. The relationship between these main factors will be the subject of the following few pages. However, a simple qualitative interdependence between the various elements of malaria transmission could be expressed, according to Russell (1952), as a formula:

$$(X\ Y\ Z)\ pibect$$

in which X is the human carrier of the *Plasmodium*, Y the *Anopheles* vector, Z the human recipient of the infection. The single letters of the acronym 'pibect' refer to *p*–the *Plasmodium*, *i*–immunity, *b*–bionomics (habits – of both the individual and of the mosquito), *e*–the environment, *c*–control of malaria in the locality, and *t*–treatment.

Malaria survey

Any attempt at control of malaria in a locality or a larger area should be preceded by an evaluation of the amount and conditions of transmission of the disease. This is called a *malaria survey* and it should extend not only to the area to be protected but also to the contiguous unprotected area. The differences noted between the amount of malaria in the two areas following the application of control measures will indicate their effectiveness. The quantitative methods involved in a malaria survey are often referred to as *malariometry*.

The degree of malaria transmission in any region is determined by a number of interrelated factors. These include:

1. The prevalence of malaria infection in humans and its seasonal incidence.
2. The species of *Anopheles* mosquitos, their relative abundance, feeding and resting habits and infectivity.
3. The presence of susceptible human population.
4. Climatic conditions, such as rainfall, temperature, humidity and environmental features which affect the breeding of *Anopheles*.

The *malaria survey* proper involves investigations under the following headings:

1. Collection of existing environment and epidemiological data.
2. Investigations relating to the human host.
3. Investigations relating to the insect vector.

For a general knowledge of the epidemiological situation, information is required regarding malaria morbidity and mortality, vital statistics, meteorological, topographical and other relevant features. This involves the examination of hospital and dispensary returns, records maintained by health services, and interviews with medical officers of health, private practitioners and auxiliary medical personnel.

Investigations relating to the human host require:

Spleen examination. The *spleen rate* is the proportion of enlarged spleens in the indigenous population.

Blood examination. The *parasite rate* is the proportion of blood films showing malaria parasites in the indigenous population.

Investigations relating to the *Anopheles* vectors are based on the collection of four groups of data:

Estimation of mosquito density. This is given in relation to the human population and is determined by the result of mosquito collections, indicating the number of *Anopheles* entering dwellings, or feeding on inhabitants.

Estimation of natural infection. The *sporozoite rate* is the percentage incidence of sporozoite infection in the salivary glands of *Anopheles*. The *oöcyst rate* is the percentage incidence of oöcyst formation on the stomach wall of *Anopheles*.

Estimation of biting habits. This is determined by the results of the precipitin test of mosquito blood meals, indicating whether the *Anopheles* had fed on human or animal blood. It is therefore a means of distinguishing between anthropophilic and zoophilic species.

Estimation of longevity. Various entomological techniques used for this purpose include comparison of the sporozoite rate and total infection rate, comparison of the immediate and delayed sporozoite rate, measurement of the ampulla of the oviduct, and estimation of daily survival rate from the proportion of parous *Anopheles* females.

Spleen examination

One of the earliest methods used for estimation of the amount of malaria in a given locality is that of determining the proportion of persons with a palpable enlargement of the spleen. This method introduced by Dempster in India in 1848 is still commonly used, although it is admittedly a crude measure.

The object of palpation of the spleen is to determine not only the percentage of individuals with demonstrable enlargement of the organ but also the approximate degree of splenomegaly.

Two techniques of spleen palpation are used. In one the individual is examined lying down, with the examiner seated on the subject's right, so that the right hand can explore the splenic region below the left costal margin. The second method, less cumbersome in the field, has the subject standing, with the examiner sitting on a low stool in front of the examined person. The examiner's right hand gently explores the left side of the abdomen from below the umbilicus towards the coastal border. If no spleen is palpable, the subject is requested to breathe deeply, while the exploring hand attempts to feel the tip of the spleen by pressing the abdomen under the costal border (Figs 8.4 and 8.5).

Palpation of the spleen in children is relatively easy, but in adults with greater muscular development more experience is necessary. The main errors, made usually by non-medical examiners, are to mistake the outer end of the left rib or a hard faecal bolus in the large intestine for the enlarged spleen. On the other hand, very large spleens may be missed if only the upper part of the abdomen is palpated. It should be remembered that occasionally large spleens are due to kala-azar (visceral leishmaniasis) or intestinal schistosomiasis, but generally the proportion of splenomegaly over 10% is due to malaria.

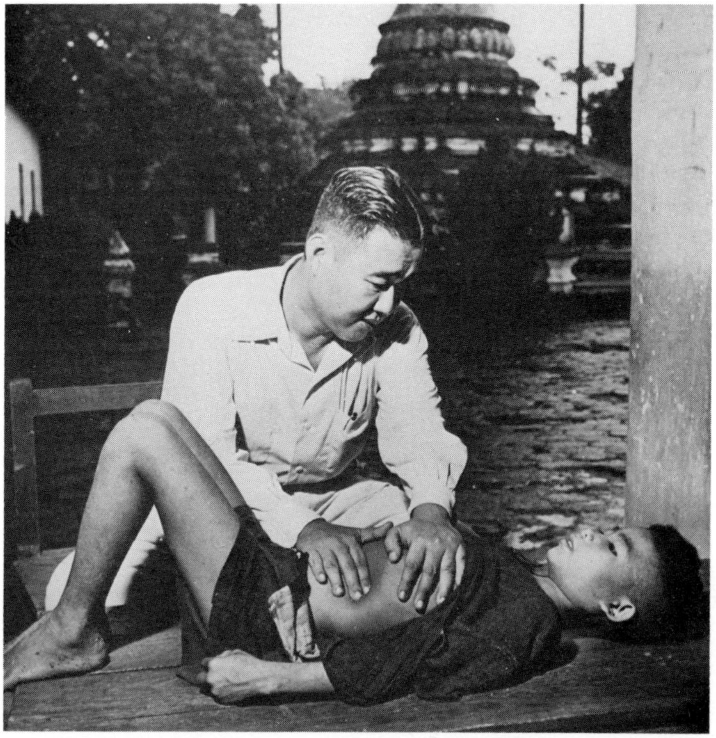

Fig. 8.4 Spleen palpation method used for malaria surveys in Thailand. (WHO photograph.)

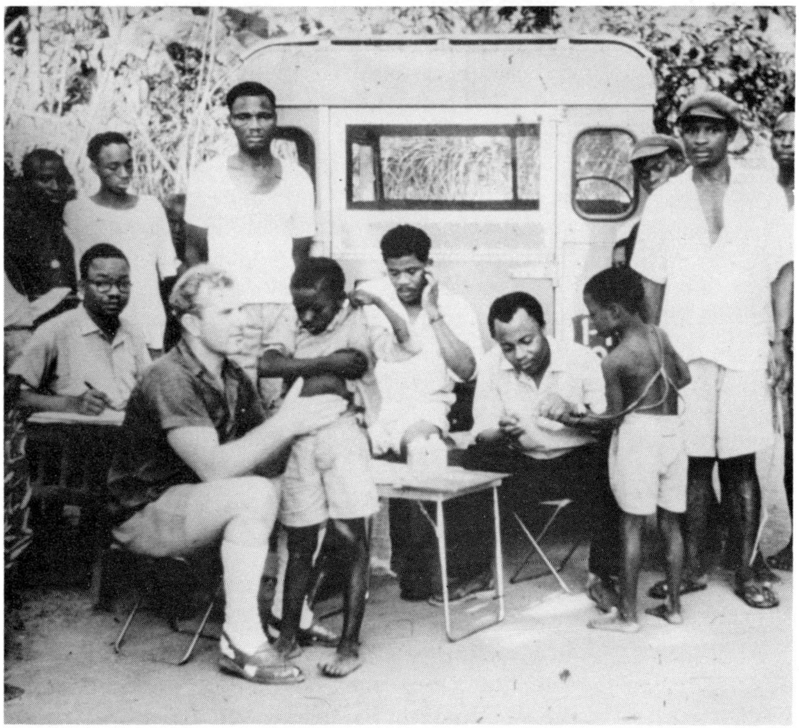

Fig. 8.5 Procedure adopted for malaria surveys in Nigeria. The malariologist palpating the spleen of the child sits on a low stool, which allows him to feel the spleen, even when slightly enlarged. The technician who takes the blood slide and the clerk who keeps the records are in the background.

The proportion (expressed as a percentage) of enlarged spleens in a sample of the population is known as the *spleen rate* and is a crude but nevertheless valuable measure of endemic malaria. Usually the spleen rate is determined in children 2–10 years of age; this is because the enlargement of the spleen is greatest when the immune response is building up. However, for a complete picture of the amount of malaria in a locality the prevalence of enlarged spleens in adults should also be known.

An important refinement of the method of spleen rate determination is the evaluation of the degree of splenic enlargement. This can be done by classifying the size of the enlarged spleen and determining the proportion of various classes of splenomegaly.

For the determination of the degree of enlarged spleens Hackett's method of arbitrary classification of the size of the palpated spleen is now generally accepted according to criteria given in Table 8.2 and Fig. 8.6.

Table 8.2 Classification* of sizes of the spleen according to Hackett

Class of spleen	Description
0	Normal spleen not palpable even on deep inspiration
1	Spleen palpable below the costal margin, usually on deep inspiration
2	Spleen palpable below the costal margin, but not projected beyond a horizontal line half way between the costal margin and the umbilicus, measured along a line dropped vertically from the left nipple
3	Spleen with lowest palpable point projected more than half way to the umbilicus but not below a line drawn horizontally through it
4	Spleen with lowest palpable point below the umbilical level but not projected beyond a horizontal line situated half way between the umbilicus and the symphysis pubis
5	Spleen with lowest point palpable beyond the lower limit of class 4

*This classification obviously does not apply to children with a very distended abdomen or with a pronounced umbilical hernia. The error in classifying the spleen size in these children will be largely eliminated if the child is examined in recumbent position and not standing. The horizontal midline in the case of a large umbilical hernia cannot be more than approximate.

A useful malariometric index is that of *average enlarged spleen* (AES) which can be easily calculated from the frequency distribution of various classes of spleens recorded in the way shown by the following example:

Class of spleen	**Age group 2–9 years Numbers of various classes found**	
0 (not palpable)	14	
1	25	41 (classes 1–5)
2	10	
3	3	
4	2	
5	1	
	Total 55	

The AES index is calculated by multiplying the number of individuals in each class of enlarged spleen by the class of spleen and dividing this figure by the total number of individuals with splenomegaly. In the example above, the spleen rate is 41 out of 55, or 75%. *The average enlarged spleen* will be $25 + 20 + 9 + 8 + 5 = 67/41 = 1.63$.

Blood examination

The other important measure of the prevalence of malaria in an area is the evaluation of the proportion of persons in a given community who harbour the parasites of malaria in their blood. This epidemiological index is known as *parasite rate*. To be precise the parasite rate must be determined for a relatively narrow range of age groups from infants, through toddlers, small children, school children, adolescents and adults.

The following age grouping is recommended by the WHO (1963):

Group	**Description**
0–11 months	Infants, babies
12–23 months	Toddlers
2–4 years	Small children
5–9 years	Juveniles
10–14 years	Adolescents
15 years and over	Adults

The technique of blood examination was indicated in a section of Chapter 6. The proportion (as a percentage) of the sample of the population showing malaria parasites in the blood is the *para-*

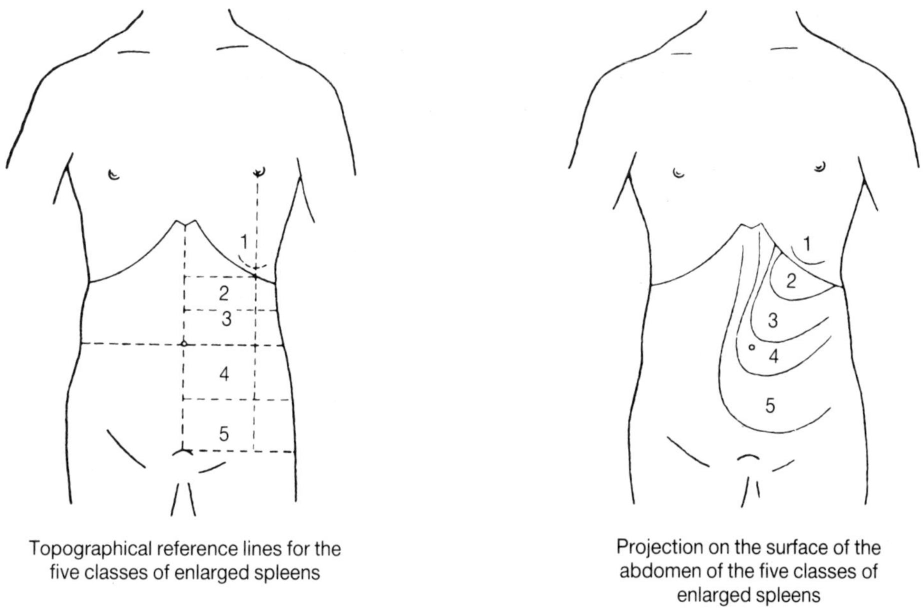

Fig. 8.6 Classification of spleen sizes according to Hackett's method. (WHO, 1963, *Terminology of Malaria.*)

site rate, which should be related to one of the age groups of the population sample as shown above. The infant parasite rate is of special importance as it is a good indicator of a recent transmission of malaria.

It should be remembered that the reliability of results of blood examination depends on the standardized technique of the collection of blood slides and their examination by competent technical staff. For field surveys, only the thick film method is normally used. The average microscopist can examine 100 thick film fields in 5 minutes. This represents about 0.1–0.25 μl of blood and some very scanty infections may escape detection.

In some surveys (as indeed in cases of individual infections) it may be useful to know the degree of malarial infection. The term *parasite count* is the number of malaria parasites seen on an average in a number (such as 100) of blood film fields, or in relation to the number (such as 5000 or 10 000) of red blood cells. Usually the parasite count is given in relation to 1 μl of blood, after a suitable conversion. The parasite count may also be calculated in relation to the number (400–500) of white blood cells seen in 100 fields of the blood film when the number of those cells per μl is known.

As in the case of the average enlarged spleen it may be useful to know the average degree of parasitaemia in a sample of a well-defined group of the population. Since the range of individual counts per μl of malaria parasites in the blood is very wide, to obtain the *parasite density index* the individual counts are divided into ten classes as follows:

Class	Parasite count per μl
1	Less than 100
2	101–200
3	201–400
4	401–800
5	801–1600
6	1601–3200
7	3201–6400
8	6401–12 800
9	12 801–25 600
10	25 601–and over

The *parasite density index* for a given group can be calculated in the same way as the average enlarged spleen. Only the positive slides are included in the denominator.

Example: Out of 120 slides 90 are positive; they are composed of the following classes:

Class	1	2	3	4	5	6	7	8	9	10	**Total**
Fre-	15	30	13	12	8	6	3	2	0	1	90
quency	15	60	39	48	40	36	21	16	0	10	285

$$\textit{Parasite rate } \frac{90}{120} \times 100 = 75\%$$

$$\textit{Parasite density index } \frac{285}{90} = 3.17$$

In the above calculation of the parasite rate and parasite density index all species of parasites are lumped together and mixed infections are counted as one. This is the *crude parasite rate* or *crude parasite density index*.

If infections with different *Plasmodia* are counted separately one refers to a *species infection rate* or *species parasite density index*.

The determination of the species density index is not always necessary but the indication of the frequency of the individual species of malaria parasites is of importance. This can be given either as the *species infection rate*, namely, percentage of subjects found with infections of one particular species of *Plasmodium* or as the parasite formula. The latter indicates the relative prevalence of the various species in the total of positive slides. Thus, if in a series of slides from 100 children there are 62 positive (parasite rate 62%) of which 40 show *P. vivax* ($^{40}/_{62}$), 20 *P. falciparum* ($^{20}/_{62}$) and two *P. malariae* ($^{2}/_{62}$) the *parasite formula is*: V 64.5, F 32.3, M 3.2. But the *species infection rate* of the examined group will be $^{40}/_{100}$ = 40% for *P. vivax*, 20% for *P. falciparum* and 2% for *P. malariae*.

Classification of endemicity of malaria

The degrees of endemicity of malaria mentioned before have been adopted by the WHO on the basis of spleen rates determined on a statistically sgnificant sample of the population involved. These degrees are as follows:

1. *Hypoendemic malaria*: Spleen rate in children (2–9 years) not exceeding 10%.
2. *Mesoendemic malaria*: Spleen rate in children (2–9 years) between 11% and 50%.
3. *Hyperendemic malaria*: Spleen rate in children (2–9 years) constantly over 50%. Spleen rates in adults also high (over 25%).
4. *Holoendemic malaria*: Spleen rate in children (2–9 years) constantly over 75%, but spleen rates in adults low.

The reason for the reference to the adult spleen rate in the last two types of endemic malaria is the presence of a considerable immunity acquired in the areas, where the population is exposed to an intense transmission.

An alternative method of classification of endemicity has been proposed using the same ranges of parasite rates (less than 10%, 11–50%, 51–75%, and over 75%) as parameters of the four classes of endemic malaria. There is no fully satisfactory method of expressing in an arbitrary way the dynamics of malaria transmission. Quantitative methods, which estimate the vectorial capacity and the subsequent risk of infection, come closest to such an appraisal.

Recording of data and their statistical significance

For proper recording of data obtained in the course of malariometric surveys the use of standard forms is convenient.

Two such forms are shown in Fig. 8.7. The first is used in the field while the second is more useful for the consolidation of all results obtained. The number of subjects to be examined within the locality selected on epidemiological grounds is chiefly determined by statistical considerations. The adequacy of a sample size can be determined either in advance of the survey or when reporting on its results. The size of the sample required depends on the general prevalence of the phenomenon that is being investigated. It is obvious that for valid comparisons a smaller sample is sufficient when the spleen or parasite rate is high in the investigated areas; on the other hand, a large sample is needed for the statistical validity of the results.

The range of chance variation of the results that must be considered in relation to the magnitude of the percentage observed in the sample is given in Table 8.3. If, for example, in a sample of 100 children parasites are found in 40, then the parasite rate in the total population of children of the same age group lies between 30 and 50%, and this may be assumed with a 95% probability.

INDIVIDUAL SPLEEN/BLOOD RECORDS

Place:				Project:		
Date:				Investigator:		
Serial No. of slide	Name	Age	Sex	Spleen class	Result of blood examination	Remarks

CONSOLIDATED SPLEEN/BLOOD RECORD

Age group	No. of spleens examined	Spleen class						No. of blood films examined	No. of positive blood films	*P. falciparum* trophozoites	*P. falciparum* gametocytes	*P. vivax* or *P. ovale*	*P. malariae*	Mixed infections	Class of parasite count										
		0	1	2	3	4	5								Neg. 0	1	2	3	4	5	6	7	8	9	10

Fig. 8.7 Individual and consolidated spleen/blood records as used for malariometric surveys.

The appraisal of the statistical significance of the difference between two rates should be done according to the well-known methods, in relation to the standard error of the difference. However, the use of a convenient nomogram, reproduced in Fig. 8.8, will dispense with the need for calculation. In this nomogram, the left-hand scale, M, refers to the combined numbers of the two samples that are to be tested; and the right-hand scale, P, refers to the combined percentages in the two samples that have a specified characteristic.

The value of M is marked on the left-hand scale, and the value of P on the right-hand scale. A straight-edge is then placed to connect the two points, and the value is read where it intersects the 5% side of the centre scale. If the difference in the two rates exceeds the scale value, then it may be considered to be significant at the 5% probability level. Similarly, significance at the 1% probability level can be found by using the 1% side of the centre scale.

Serological epidemiology

Serological methods are of particular value to epidemiological studies of malaria, as they indicate the period prevalence of the infection in a population where the fluctuating nature of parasitaemia and the uncertainty of splenic indices are the major obstacles for the assessment of the true situation. During the early studies these methods confirmed the transfer of maternal antibodies to the newborn in highly endemic areas. The age-related increase of the specific serological profile reflects the degree of malaria transmission experienced by the whole community in such areas. This is particularly valuable where the use of antimalarial drugs is widespread, although not regular enough to influence the transmission; in this condition the results of parasite rates, reflecting an uneven drug distribution may be misleading.

Mathematical analysis applied to serological data, in order to assess the transmission rate,

Table 8.3 Confidence intervals at 95% probability level corresponding to varying sample sizes and sample percentages from 5% to 95%

Sample size	Percentage observed in sample					
	5%	10%	20%	30%	40%	50%
50		3–22	10–34	18–45	26–55	36–64
60	1–14	3–20	11–32	19–43	28–54	37–63
80	1–12	4–19	12–30	20–41	29–51	39–61
100	2–11	5–18	13–29	21–40	30–50	40–60
200	2–9	6–14	16–26	24–38	33–47	43–57
300	3–8	7–14	16–25	25–36	35–46	44–56
400	3–8	7–13	16–24	26–35	35–45	45–55
500	3–7	8–13	17–24	26–34	36–44	46–54
1000	4–7	8–12	18–23	27–33	37–43	47–53
	60%	70%	80%	90%	95%	
50	45–74	55–82	66–90	78–97		
60	46–72	57–81	68–89	80–97	86–99	
80	49–71	59–80	70–88	81–96	88–99	
100	50–70	60–79	71–87	82–95	89–98	
200	53–67	62–76	74–84	86–94	91–98	
300	54–65	64–75	75–84	86–93	92–97	
400	55–65	65–74	76–84	87–93	92–97	
500	56–64	66–74	76–83	87–92	93–97	
1000	57–63	67–73	77–82	88–92	93–96	

should take into account the sensitivity and specificity of the serological tests involved, and also the possible fading of antibodies in a proportion of the population (Fig. 6.10, p. 92).

In the Garki malaria control project in northern Nigeria a positive association was found between the lesser exposure to infection and lower immune response, following the withdrawal of control measures.

When, after chemotherapeutic control measures, the standard malariometric methods lose some of their value, and yet there is indirect evidence of some remaining foci of transmission, the serological methods may be of considerable value by indicating areas of recent transmission in children and immigrants. Practical application of these detection methods was successful in Tunisia, Mauritius, Greece and Guyana. An excellent example of the value of serology in pointing out the area of recent transmission was seen in Grenada, where an outbreak of *P. malariae* was thus localized and dealt with. New procedures based on the use of monoclonal antibodies are of much promise in this field.

In serological surveys employing IFAT, two parameters are important. The first is that of the ratio (expressed as a percentage) of positives, with a clear indication of the lowest dilution of the serum at which the test is accepted as positive. The second parameter is the highest dilution of each individual serum giving positive reaction, this 'titre' being regarded as a measure of the concentration of antibody in the given serum. For convenience, the latter figure is expressed as a reciprocal (1/titre) and the series of particular tests are presented as a geometric mean titre (GMT). Naturally, as was the case for the parasite rate, the GMT should be stated for the defined age groups of the investigated population.

For large-scale surveys the indirect ELISA is more suitable, as it allows for processing very many samples and the results can be read visually. However, it seems that low levels of antibodies are less well detected by this method.

An important development of the sero-epidemiology of malaria concerns antibodies to sporozoites. It seems that the age-specific rise in seropositivity and in antibody titres is much slower against sporozoites than against blood stages.

In parallel with and in part as a by-product of malaria vaccine research new and improved immu-

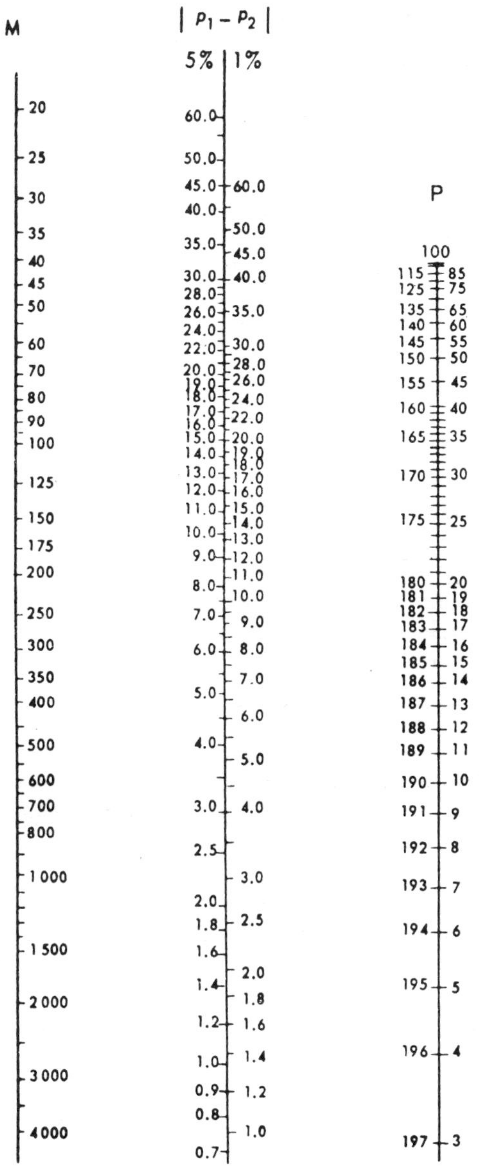

Fig. 8.8 Nomogram for rapid testing of the degree of statistical significance of the difference between two rates. (WHO, 1966.)

nodiagnostic tests have been developed. Their use specifically for epidemiological purposes is, however, still limited by logistical problems. Some of these tests are reviewed in Chapter 6.

Quantitative epidemiology of malaria

Many aspects of a malaria survey require some quantitative data, the collection and interpretation of which depends on the use of elementary mathematical principles. In answering the usual epidemiological questions: 'Who? When? Where? Why?' some degree of precision is needed and here the well-known statement of J. J. Thomson should be remembered:

> When you can measure what you are speaking about and express it in numbers, you know something about it, but when you cannot measure it or express it in numbers, your knowledge is of a meagre and unsatisfactory kind.

It may be worthwhile to quote Ronald Ross's opinion which has been used as the leading maxim of George Macdonald's book, *The Epidemiology and Control of Malaria* (1957).

> To say that a disease depends upon certain factors is not to say much, until we can also form an estimate as to how largely each factor influences the whole result. And the mathematical method is really nothing but the application of careful reasoning to the problems at issue.

There is no other tropical communicable disease to which a mathematical approach has been applied more widely or thoroughly. The first and most inspired attempt at formulating the quantitative laws of epidemiology of malaria and its transmission and control was made by Ronald Ross at the beginning of this century. A number of other studies followed, but the interest in this subject died down until the 1950s, when Moshkowsky in the former USSR and George Macdonald in Britain revived it in a series of remarkable investigations. The reader interested in this aspect of epidemiology of malaria should study the original works quoted in the list of references.

In the basic outline of the principles of a malaria survey, several of the quantitative factors of malaria transmission have already been pointed out. Some of these factors are so obvious that they do not require any additional explanation, others need a few comments.

Anopheles vary greatly in their infectivity, some being likely to carry malaria while others rarely do so. Certain species have characteristics which exclude them from the role of important vectors, such as a marked preference for animal blood or a very short life.

The female *Anopheles* take a blood feed once in every 2 to 4 days, the length of the intervals depending mainly on temperature. They are by no means invariable feeders on humans; some have a marked preference for human blood, choosing it whenever possible; others have a strong preference for animals and rarely feed on humans, so that it is very unusual for them to transmit malaria. Between these two extremes there are large groups less set in their habits. The final choice depends to a considerable extent on the availability of blood, so that under some circumstances they feed predominantly on humans and under others only rarely so. The degree of variation within one species may be wide; in the instance of *A. culicifacies* in India the percentage of human blood feeds may vary between 2 and 80%. This variation in feeding habit may have a great effect on the incidence of disease.

An adult female mosquito acquires malaria parasites by receiving them in a blood feed from a malarious person. She has no prospect of transmitting the disease unless she lives through the time taken for the sporogonic development of the malaria parasite; this is estimated at between 8 and 25 days, according to temperature and parasite species. Even if the *Anopheles* survives through this time the number of people whom she will bite and so to whom she will transmit the parasite depends on the length of her survival after that time. The length of life of a mosquito in nature is very difficult to measure, but some general indication of the range may be helpful. Under certain situations some anophelines can live for several months, especially if they hibernate or aestivate during winter or adverse climatic conditions. However, most adults live much shorter periods and die not so much from old age but from hazards such as predators and adverse environmental conditions such as desiccation during dry periods. It seems probable that most species live about 20–25 days, some individuals being more and some less lucky; this corresponds to a daily death rate of 4 or 5%. At the other end of the scale, the expectation may be as little as 2 or 3 days, but even among these short-livers a few may live long enough to maintain transmission of malaria. Under such adverse conditions it is clear that only a very small minority of all mosquitos can live long enough to carry the disease from one person to another, and that one mosquito is not likely to infect many people. As a consequence, large numbers of mosquitos are often needed to maintain the disease in a community when these conditions prevail, and if the numbers fall below the requisite figure transmission will become rare and the disease will tend to disappear.

The average number of adult female *Anopheles* of a defined species, caught sheltering in human habitations or biting exposed individuals indoors or outdoors, is the *anopheles density*. It can be expressed as a relative proportion per room, per person, per day etc.

The proportion of freshly fed female *Anopheles* whose midgut (stomach) contains human blood is the *human blood index*. Following the blood feed (on humans or on animals) the ovarian development of the female *Anopheles* begins and ends with egg-laying. This period is known as the *gonotrophic cycle* and averages 2–4 days.

The period necessary for the development of the *Plasmodium* in the mosquito from the fertilization of the female gamete by the male, through the subsequent stages of oökinete, oöcyst and finally sporozoite is the *sporogonic cycle*. Its duration depends on the species of the *Plasmodium* and on the environmental temperature.

The percentage of female *Anopheles* of a defined species caught in nature and showing oöcysts in the midgut on dissection is the *oöcyst rate*. Conversely, the percentage of female *Anopheles* with sporozoites in their salivary glands is the *sporozoite rate*.

The risk of getting malaria clearly depends on the sporozoite rate and the biting rate on a person. The product of these two is the *entomological inoculation rate*. So the number of *Anopheles* caught biting a single person per night times the sporozoite rate is an estimate of the inoculation rate. Another approach is to divide the numbers of freshly blood-fed mosquitos caught in a bedroom by the numbers of sleepers to obtain the biting rate, which can then be multiplied by the sporozoite rate. However, checks should be made that all engorged adults have in fact fed on people and not on animals and then entered the bedroom to rest. Also this approach will underestimate human–vector contact if the species exhibits *exophily*, that is, if a number of mosquitos leave the bedroom after feeding and are consequently not available for capture in the morning. It should be noted that the reciprocal of the entomological inoculation rate is the theoretical number of days for a person to be bitten by an infective mosquito and so acquire malaria.

The mosquito/human contact can be defined as the *man biting rate*, namely, the average incidence of anopheline bites per day per person. It may be expressed as *ma* where *m* represents the relative density of female *Anopheles* to humans and *a* is the human *biting habit*, or the probability that a mosquito will feed on a person during a day. The incidence of bites per day of an individual female mosquito on the human population is composed of the feeding frequency per mosquito per day (24 hours) multiplied by the proportion of such bites on a person. This is the *human blood index* obtained from the results of immunological (ELISA) tests. A different approach has been used by Macdonald (1957) who calculated the inoculation rate in a community from the known parasite rate of infants. Details of this investigation are beyond the scope of this book, but it may be pointed out that generally the inoculation rate estimated by this method is 20 to 100 times less than the inoculation rate derived from entomological data. This discrepancy is pronounced when the endemicity of malaria is high, and indicates the effect of immunity transmitted by the mother as well as other factors such as the difficulty of accurately measuring the biting rate that is experienced by an ordinary member of the community.

The key factor in the mathematical analysis of transmission of malaria is the *longevity of the vector*, in other words, the survival rate. The duration of the sporogonic period of the development is at least 9 days for *P. vivax* and 12 days for *P. falciparum* at 26°C. Obviously, any mosquito that lives less than this period will not be able to transmit the infection through sporozoites.

The direct estimation of the average age of mosquitos may be obtained if we know the mean duration of each gonotrophic cycle (from blood meal to oviposition) and the mean number of such cycles in female *Anopheles*. Such a direct estimation of the physiological age of mosquitos is possible by intricate dissection methods that show the number of dilatations in the ovaries, each dilation in an ovariole usually taken to represent one successful oviposition. So, a female may be age-graded as having undergone one, two, three etc. ovipositions, the more ovipositions the older the mosquito. But these dissections, pioneered by Russian entomologists, are both time-consuming and difficult. An easier method is to classify mosquitos as either just *nulliparous*, that is, females which have not as yet oviposited or *parous*, that is, those which have laid one or more batches of eggs. For this, ovaries of *unfed* females are dissected in water, not saline, and are allowed to dry out. Examination under a compound microscope shows that nulliparous mosquitos have their ovaries covered with tightly coiled tracheole skeins, whereas in parous females the skeins are unravelled. The proportion of parous mosquitos, the *parity rate*, can therefore readily be determined. From this proportion, the probability of survival through 1 day can be derived and from that the calculation of the *mean expectation of life* of the vector population is simple enough. Conventionally, the probability of survival through 1 day (p) is equivalent to the square root of the proportion of gravid females in the sample if the blood meal is taken once in 2 days; p is equivalent to the cube root of this proportion if the female feeds on blood every 3 days. The validity of this technique is not absolute but depends on a number of assumptions.

Finally the expectation of life of *Anopheles* surviving long enough to become infective to humans, after having fed previously on blood containing gametocytes, presents no great difficulty for estimation.

The *expectation of infective life* of a vector population can be defined as their mean number of days of life in the infective condition. It is a function of the daily survival rate of the female mosquito and of the sporogonic period of a given species of the malaria parasite. This is the most important factor in the transmission of malaria, and any decrease of it is the key to malaria control by use of insecticides.

The concept of *vectorial capacity* is a convenient way of expressing the malaria transmission risk, or, in other words, the 'receptivity' to malaria of a defined area. Vectorial capacity can be expressed mathematically as:

$$C = \left(\frac{ma^2 p^n}{-\log_e p} \right)$$

In epidemiological terms this equation may be translated as follows: when a person is bitten ma times per day and a proportion p^n of the vector population survives the incubation period of the malaria parasite in the mosquito, and if this proportion is expected to live for another ($1/-\log_e p$) days, during which they bite another person *a* times a day, then we may estimate the rate of potentially infective bites. This is the measure of transmission, which determines the endemic level of malaria in given conditions and, indirectly, the impact of eventual control activity. Vector control by larvicids or other measures will reduce *m*, screening of houses will reduce *a*, while residual spraying will also greatly reduce the factor *p*.

The importance of the probability of daily survival of vectors for efficient transmission of infection is obvious; it must be not less than 60% and preferably higher. If the survival rate is less than 50% per day then less than 1% of the females are likely to survive the minimum of 8 days needed for completion of the sporogonic cycle of *P. vivax*; for *P. falciparum* (which needs 10–12 days for the completion of this cycle) the minimum span of daily survival of vectors is 65%.

The most important factors of the complex epidemiological picture resulting from the vectorial capacity of an anopheline population are: the *vectorial capacity* of the anopheline population and the *basic reproduction rate*, which is the estimated number of secondary malaria infections potentially transmitted within a susceptible population from a single non-immune individual.

The mathematical relationship and derivation of these factors from a series of quantitative indices was presented by Black (1968) and is shown in Table 8.4.

Although the basic reproduction rate is an important cumulative epidemiological factor, it represents the theoretical estimate of the intensity of transmission. In practice, the *net reproduction rate* is much closer to real conditions. The *net reproduction rate*, namely, the actual number of secondary infections, is always much lower than the basic reproduction rate and can be estimated from the equation:

$$\frac{p^n}{p^n - s}$$

where p^n is the probability of survival of *Anopheles* through *n* days of the duration of sporogonic period and *s* is the sporozoite rate.

Another valuable epidemiological factor is the *index of stability* of transmission of malaria. It depends on the human biting habit of the main vector (*a*) and its probability of survival through 1 day (*p*), and can be derived from the expression:

$$\frac{a}{-\log_e p}$$

The higher the frequency of vector bites on humans the higher the stability index; on the other hand, the high daily mosquito mortality lowers the index. Values of over 2.5 indicate stability, values of 0.5–2.5 are intermediate, values below 0.5 indicate unstable conditions of transmission. A good account of vectorial capacity is given by Dye (1992).

In summary it can be said that epidemiological features of malaria in a community depend on the amount and duration of transmission and on the diversity of the parasite species involved. The frequency of transmission depends on the density and infectivity of anopheline vectors and also on the fluctuations of the source of infections, namely, gametocyte carriers. The transmission rate of malaria within the community produces a collective immune response, which at high level decreases the severity of the infection of older age groups, while the burden of the disease falls on infants and children. The rate of transmission can be estimated by the parasite rates of young age groups, while the level of endemicity is indicated by the proportion of acute cases and the age-group distribution of enlarged spleens, parasite densities and gametocyte rates.

Mathematical models of malaria transmission and its control

A mathematical model is the expression in mathematical terms of a system or a set of phenomena. The aim of such a model is to gain insight into the relationship of the elements of the system, and of effects of any changes between them. There are two types of such models: deterministic models refer to the use of rates to express changes in a system as a function of time; stochastic models use the probability distribution to express such changes.

Macdonald's early model based on data obtained from East Africa discussed the role of immunity as a regulating mechanism of transmission. His theory of control, aiming at the reduction of the basic reproduction rate below 1, is relevant to

Table 8.4 Factors composing the vectorial capacity of a mosquito population and the basic reproduction rate of malaria (after Black, 1968)

Factor	Definition of index	Common name of index	Method of obtaining the index	Macdonald's (1957) expressions
1	Bites *per person* per night by vector population	Human biting rate	Night-biting captures on human baits (e.g. 10 bites per person)	ma
2	Bites *per mosquito* per night	Human biting habit	Composed of: (i) the feeding frequency based on the observed gonotrophic cycle in nature (e.g. 0.4 where the female oviposits and feeds once in 2.5 days on an average); and (ii) the human blood index, assessed by the precipitin test applied to daytime resting samples (e.g. 0.5): $a = 0.4 \times 0.5 = 0.2$	a
3	Proportion of bites on a person ('Human blood index')			
4	Probability of vector's survival through sporogonic period of parasite	Expectation of infective life of the vector population	Based on age-grading or proportion parous, and knowledge of gonotrophic cycle duration (e.g. 0.60 days)*	p^n
5	Expectation of life of female vectors			$\frac{1}{-\log_e p}$
6	Expected inoculations of man per infective case per day	Vectorial capacity of vector population	Multiplication of factors 1 × 2 × 3 × 4 × 5. (e.g. 10 × 0.2 × 0.6 = 1.2). (When this value descends below 0.01, basic reproduction rate is 1 for *P. falciparum*)	$\frac{ma^2 p^n}{-\log_e p}$
To obtain the basic reproduction rate:				
7	Proportion of vector females developing parasite normally following ingestion of gametes	Mosquito's receptivity (susceptibility) to infection	Only assessable by infections of captive samples on malaria cases (e.g. 0.9)	b
8	Days of infectivity per case (i.e. reciprocal of proportion of cases recovering in 1 day)	Reciprocal of recovery rate	Longitudinal observations of local cases of malaria in the absence of transmission (e.g. 100 days)	$\frac{1}{r}$
9	Expected new infections per case in the absence of immunity	Basic reproduction rate of parasite	Multiplication of factors 6 × 7 × 8 (e.g. 1.2 × 0.9 × 100 = 108)	$\frac{ma^2 bp^n}{-r(\log_e p)}$

*To compute the factors from the proportion parous it is necessary to know also the mean difference in age between the nulliparous and the youngest parous females in the sample, and the sporogonic period of the parasite. Graphs are available to enable the field worker, who has observed these parameters, to read off from the data the proportion surviving 1 day, the expectation of infective life and the expectation of life.

Note: e is the base of natural logarithms (2.718).

the interruption of transmission, as the first step to eradication. An expanded model which indicates the relationship of a number of endemic levels in relation to the whole range of 'vectorial capacity' involved in transmitting *P. falciparum* was developed as a result of the Garki project in northern Nigeria, carried out in 1973–80 with the support of the WHO.

The model's main output variable was the prevalence of *P. falciparum* parasitaemia as a function of season, and of the age group of the population. It was fitted to the data obtained after 1 year of baseline observation in the field and after 2 years of insecticidal spraying with propoxur; other data obtained in East Africa were also used. The model can be used to indicate the relationship between the prevalence of *P. falciparum* and vectorial capacity, when the latter undergoes natural or man-made changes (e.g. under the impact of antivector or antiplasmodial measures). It confirmed that the daily rate of the survival of the vector is the most crucial component of vectorial capacity. The practical measurement of vectorial capacity in the field is still fraught with difficulties due to variable sampling methods of collection and age-grading of vectors and also of the determination of their infectivity, but the Garki model simulates reasonably well the transmission of falciparum malaria under African conditions. Consequently, it could be used tentatively for planning malaria control and seeking answers to such questions as: (1) to what extent can malaria be controlled by available measures; (2) what pilot trials are needed; and (3) what could be expected from additional measures?

Mathematical models have not claimed to provide a comprehensive representation of reality, nonetheless, indirectly they have contributed considerably to our understanding of the epidemiology of malaria. An excellent synopsis and review of basic models is given by Dietz (1988).

Synopsis of the quantitative approach to the transmission of malaria and its control

In the development of quantitative epidemiology the study of malaria occupied an important place from the beginning of this century, when Ronald Ross defined the basic approach to the 'theory of happenings' relevant to the transmission of this infection. Malaria has not only the usual numerical features applicable to morbidity or mortality of human groups exposed to a specific disease. Infection of an individual and of the population also has the quantitative characteristics of the incubation period, proportion and size of enlarged spleens, rate, count and density of parasite, gametocyte rate, duration of infection and the frequency of relapses, to mention only the main elements.

The infection is carried by mosquitos which have the characteristics of relative numbers, range of flight, proportion and frequency of female *Anopheles* feeding on humans, their oviposition interval and mean duration of life. In the host/parasite relationship there are the factors of ambient temperature relevant to the duration of sporogony, proportion of infective *Anopheles* and numbers of their oöcysts and sporozoites.

In the series of factors of the epidemiology of malaria some of the most important relate to the vector. The proportion of the population of mosquitos which live long enough for the development of malaria parasites in them depends on the mortality to which they are exposed. Next comes the question of how long the mosquitos may be expected to survive before they transmit the infection to another person.

The curve of the longevity of an *Anopheles* population decreases exponentially in relation to their daily mortality, and this has an important bearing on the probability of transmission. The concept of the mean expectation of life of mosquitos which depends on the environmental conditions, runs like a red thread through the weave of the pattern of epidemiology of malaria.

The keystone of the understanding of the dynamics of transmission of the infection is the *basic reproduction rate* or the number of secondary infections that would originate from a single primary case of malaria if there had been no suppressive effect of the immune response of the human host enhanced by the possibility of superinfection.

The probability of survival of a proportion of the anopheline vector population through 1 day and through the extrinsic period of the development of the parasite, forms an important element in the expression of the reproduction rate. Other factors related to the behaviour pattern of the mosquito are also of significance since they govern the degree of contact between the human host and the vector.

The mean daily number of infective bites inflicted on the human victim is the *inoculation rate* which has usually been estimated from the entomological data. An alternative method of assessing this index *a posteriori* from the infant parasite rate shows the difference between the results obtained by the two methods and is due to the effect of immunity which rises with the increasing exposure to infection.

The antiparasitic and antitoxic effects of immunity protecting the individual received much attention but another manifestation, namely the restriction of the gametocyte output (thus lessening the infectivity of humans to the mosquito) has a protective effect on the community. This is one of the facets of the biological system by which transmission in an endemic area may be stabilized at a tenable level.

Together with the behaviour characteristics of the vector, the expectation of life of the *Anopheles* population enters into the components of the *index of stability* of the disease and determines why malaria should be in some places apparently static and in others almost unpredictably epidemic. It explains the dependence of the chain of transmission on the environmental conditions and defines quantitatively the features of the environment which influence the pathogen and the two types of host. It also denotes the amenability of the control of transmission through the decrease of the reproduction rate, so that each successive number of cases will be progressively smaller until the disease eventually fades out.

The aim of malaria eradication is to reduce the reproduction rate below one and to maintain it consistently below this critical level. The attack on the vector using residual insecticides has normally a rapid effect on transmission because it drastically reduces the probability of anopheline survival. The degree of this impact can be estimated by various entomological methods. Its overall effect on the vector can now be assessed by measuring the 'vectorial capacity' – a term that expresses the mean number of probable inoculations transmitted from one case of malaria in a unit of time. The periodic regional epidemics of malaria have often revealed the constant menace of this disease. Such events are due either to the sudden increase of the density of the vector and its enhanced longevity, or to the change of the behaviour pattern of the vector or to the introduction of the new sources of infection into the receptive area.

This brief account of the principles of quantitative epidemiology of malaria gives only a rudimentary idea of the complexity of theoretical and practical field work connected with it. For those who are interested in this approach, the sources quoted in Selected References will be of value for future reading.

Epidemiological prototypes related to ecological and socio-economic conditions

A more pragmatic approach to the epidemiological stratification of malaria has been developed. The determinants which to a greater or lesser extent influence the *eight* malaria prototypes are:

(a) The characteristic of the population, e.g. immune status; population movement, occupations, socio-economic status
(b) The level of transmission
(c) The species of malaria parasites and their susceptibility to antimalarial drugs
(d) The species and behaviour of vectors and their resistance to insecticides
(e) The nature of development projects, e.g. dams, deforestation, road construction
(f) The structure of the existing health services

The major malaria prototypes and their salient characteristics are:

1. *African savannah*

Eighty per cent of the world's malaria and 90% of mortality occurs in Africa south of the Sahara and is associated with this prototype. The burden of disease occurs in young children and pregnant women, particularly primigravidae. Asymptomatic infections are common in older children and adults because of a high level of acquired immunity resulting from a high level of transmission. African health authorities report that in the last few years cerebral malaria is being seen increasingly more often in older children and young adults. It has been suggested that this may be a result of greater availability of antimalarial drugs from a variety of sources and personal protection, both of which reduce the risk of infection and delay the development of immunity. Seasonal variations are related to latitude, altitude and aridity. The spread of drug resistance across the content has aggravated the situation.

2. *Plains and valleys outside Africa* (traditional agriculture)

As in the African savannah transmission ranges from continuous to seasonal depending on latitude, altitude and aridity. Development of health services and vector control have resulted in low levels of endemicity in many of these areas which exemplify the classical descriptions of malaria as a rural disease of poor communities.

3. *Forest and forest fringe*

Intensified exploitation of forest resources in South America, South-east Asia and Africa has increased the importance of this prototype. Forests and forest fringe areas are inhabited by nomadic tribal groups as well as sedentary populations who utilize the forest for hunting and collecting firewood. Agricultural activities in the deforested areas are mostly associated with *P. vivax* infection while in the forest or forest fringe the risk of acquiring *P. falciparum* is high. On the Colombian–Venezuelan and the Thai–Kampuchean borders chloroquine resistance originated in this prototype. Gold and gem miners frequently migrate between mining areas in remote forests and towns or villages. Forest malaria transmission in South-east Asia is discussed in depth in a recent monograph by Sharma and Kondrashin (1991).

4. *Desert fringe and highland fringe*

In desert fringe areas, the long dry season, low population density and its nomadic nature severely limit the potential for malaria transmission. Communal immunity is low and epidemics occur in years of exceptional rainfall or changed patterns of agriculture, e.g. irrigation.

In the fringes of highland areas, the combination of high population density, regular migration to the valleys and increased mean temperatures in the rainy season can all result in serious epidemics.

5. *Coastal and marshland*

Mosquitos which breed in brackish water are responsible for this prototype of malaria. In South-east Asia and the Pacific islands intense transmission occurs in this way.

6. *Urban slums*

Malaria is uncommon in well-planned densely populated urban areas; except in some cities in southern Asia where *Anopheles stephensi* has adapted to breeding domestically and peridomestically. Uncontrolled urbanization resulting in an ever increasing number of slums simulating a rural environment has led to increased malaria transmission in these periurban areas.

7. *Agricultural developments*

Agricultural colonization of jungle areas and irrigation for large-scale cultivation of crops such as rice, sugar and cotton are related to a large influx of temporary non-immune workers who live in crowded unsanitary camps where malaria vectors abound.

8. *Sociopolitical disturbances*

Wars, revolutions, political unrest and famines may cause epidemic outbreaks even in areas previously well under control because of the displacement of populations and general disruption of basic and health services.

The natural history of malaria parasitaemia in an holoendemic area

Cohort studies on the natural history of malaria parasitaemia in an holoendemic area are becoming increasingly difficult to carry out because of the frequency with which antimalarial drugs are now given to all age groups of the population but especially during pregnancy and childhood. The observations given below were collected in the Gambia between 1956 and 1958, at a time when self-treatment was virtually unheard of and the basic health services were at a rudimentary stage of development. The detailed evolution of malaria parasitaemia in one infant from day 15 after birth until the child was 2 years of age are presented, together with a summary of the findings in another 25 children similarly studied. Thick and thin blood films and temperature were taken *daily* except on Sundays or if the child was away from the village.

BJ was born on 24 October 1955, the first blood film was taken on 8 November 1955. Parasitaemia appeared for the first time on 11 July 1956, 8½ months after birth. Malaria transmission in the Gambia was markedly affected by seasonal changes. Throughout the dry months, December to May, it declined rapidly, but with the onset of the rains it began to rise until it reached its peak in October and November. The pattern of parasitaemia and fever for the month of July is given in Fig. 8.9a. The highest recorded parasitaemia was 1600/100 fields and the total number of days of parasitaemia was 8.

In *August* 1956, the infant had no parasitaemia. The pattern of parasitaemia in *September* is given in Fig. 8.9b; the total number of days of parasitaemia

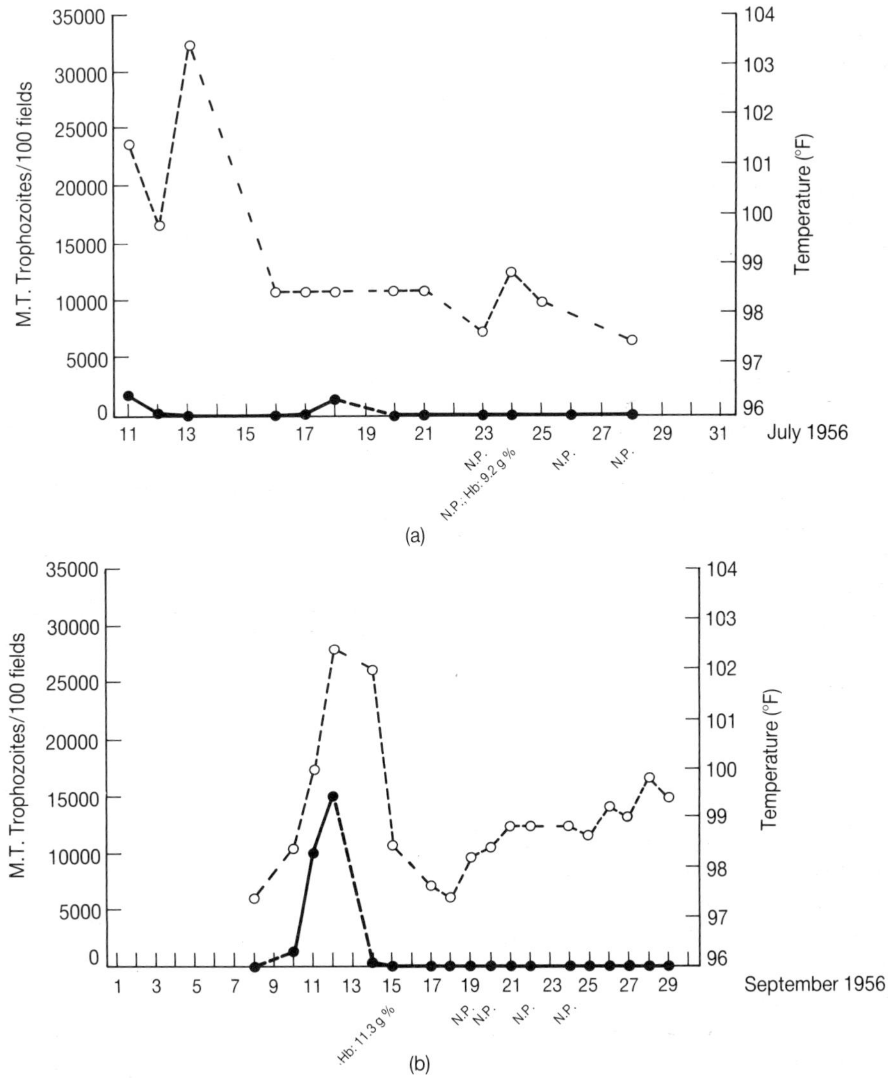

Fig. 8.9 Natural history of malarial parasitaemia. (a) July 1956, (b) September 1956, Malignant tertian (M.T.) trophozoites/100 fields = *P. falciparum* trophozoites in 100 oil-immersion fields of a thick blood film. Vertical axis = density of parasitaemia: arithmetical scale (●); Temperature = Fahrenheit scale (○). Horizontal axis = days of the month; ● = Parasitaemias below 500/100 fields. N. P. = blood film taken but no parasites seen. – – – = Child not examined on intervening days. Blank space = blood film not taken on that day. Species differentiation was confirmed by examining thin fields.

was 14 and the highest density recorded was 15 000/100 fields. In *October* the infant was parasitaemic for 26 days; *P. malariae* appeared for the first time in the middle of the month. On the day the infant looked unwell for the first time; he had a temperature of 101.8°F and one wondered whether the advent of *P. malariae* on top of *P. falciparum* may not have been responsible for this clinical observation. The highest recorded *P. falciparum* parasitaemia was 7000/100 fields (Fig. 8.9c). In *November* once again parasitaemia was frequently encountered (20 days); a triple infection of falciparum, malariae and ovale was recorded and the highest density of *P. falciparum* was 8000/100 fields (Fig. 8.9d).

In *December*, and up to 17 *January* 1957, the infant

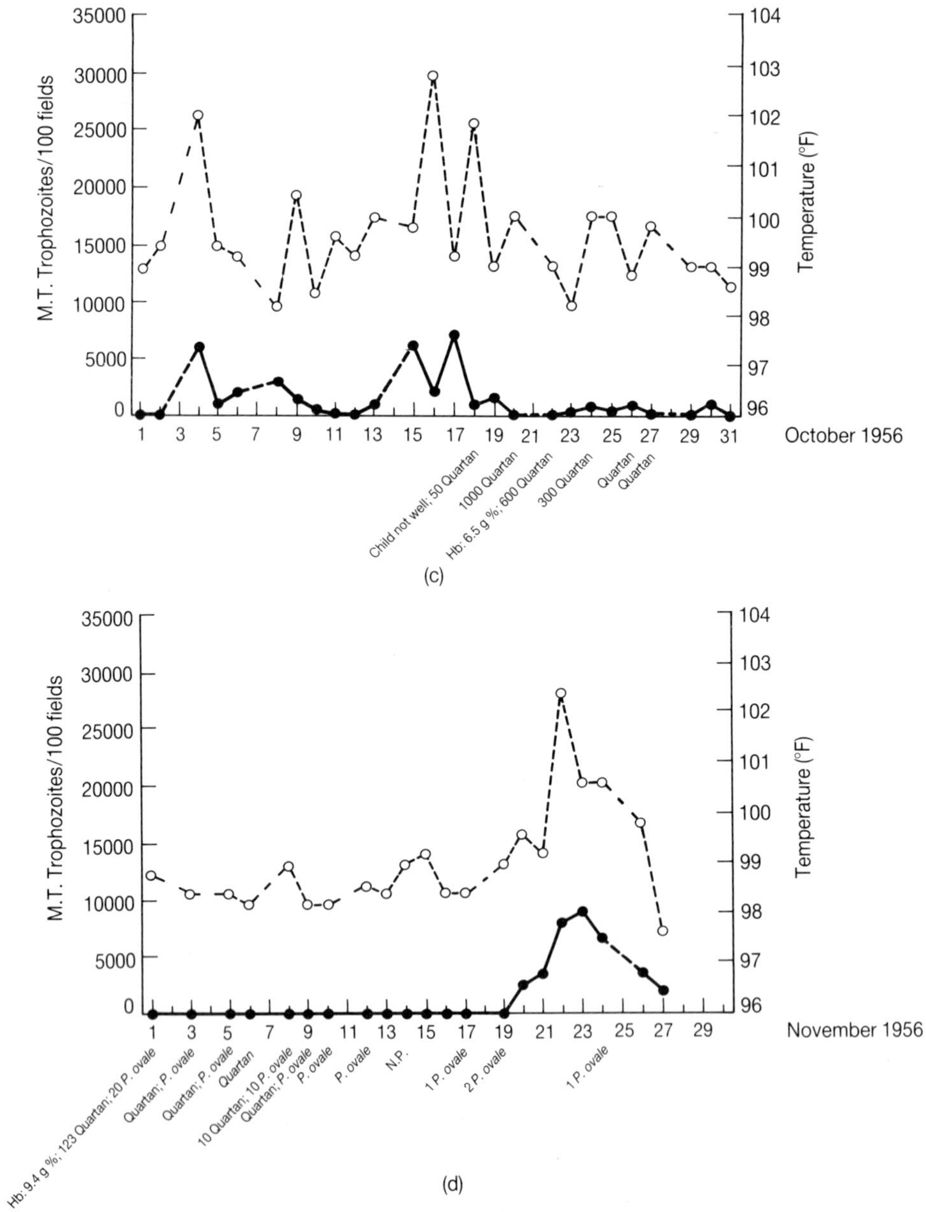

Fig. 8.9 (c) October 1956, (d) November 1956,

experienced 24 days of parasitaemia, the highest recorded being 10 000/100 fields. After this, no parasitaemia was detected for nearly 6 months (18 January–mid-July). To-date the child had received no antimalarial treatment either from us or from any other source. The pattern of parasitaemia for the month of *July* 1957 is given in Fig. 8.9e. On 19 July the child looked ill; his temperature was 102°F; he had hepatosplenomegaly; the density of parasitaemia was 25 000/100 fields and he was treated

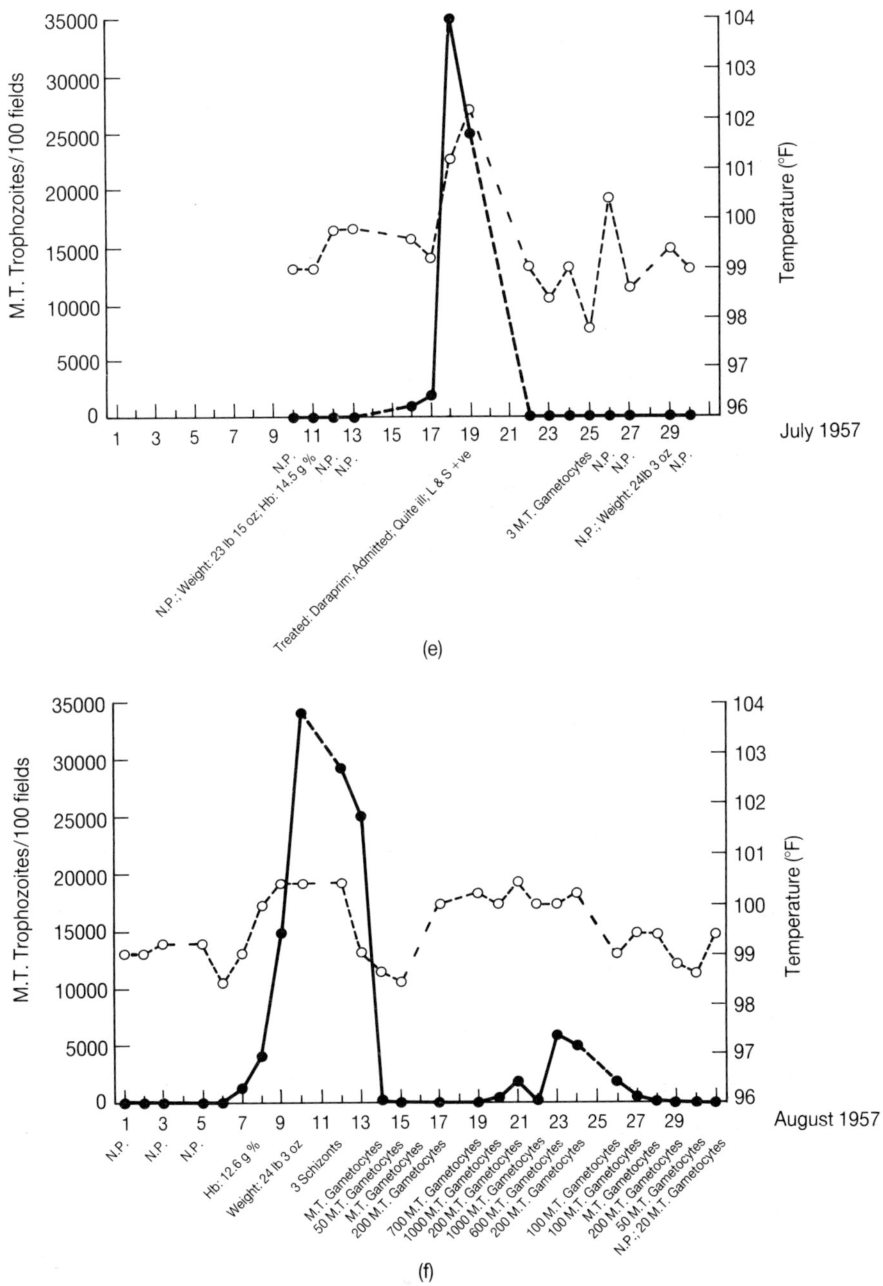

Fig. 8.9 (f) July 1957, (d) August 1957,

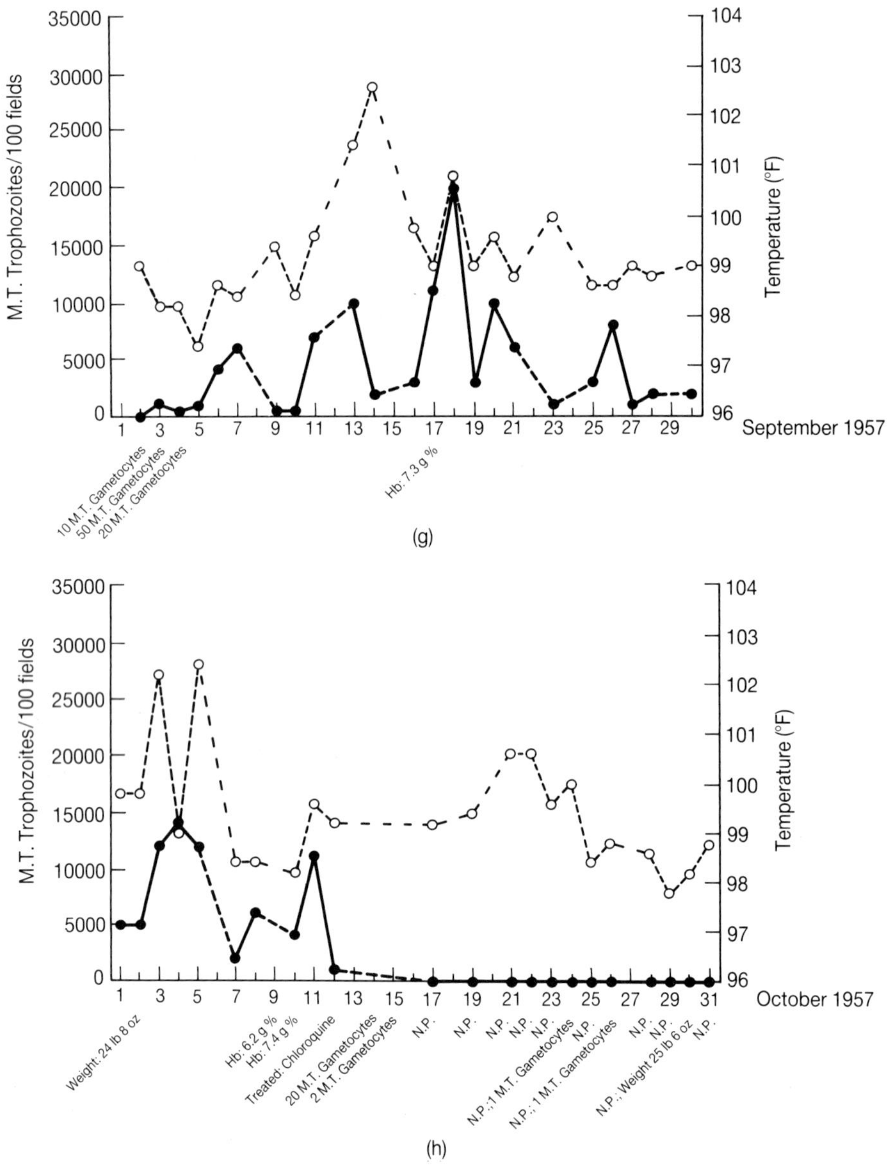

Fig. 8.9 (g) September 1957, (h) October 1957,

with pyrimethamine (Daraprim). Figure 8.9f shows that the child had parasitaemia for 23 days in *August*. The highest parasitaemia was 34 000/100 fields. Three peripheral falciparum schizonts were seen, yet the child did not look ill and his temperature was 100.4°F on the day. M.T. gametocytes were detected for 16 days. Figure 8.9g gives the pattern for *September*, the highest recorded density of parasitaemia was 20 000/100 fields; Fig. 8.9h that for *October* when the child was treated for the second time because he looked ill despite a low grade parasitaemia (1000/100 fields) and temperature (99.2°F). In *November* 1957, when the child was just over 2 years old, he experienced parasitaemia for

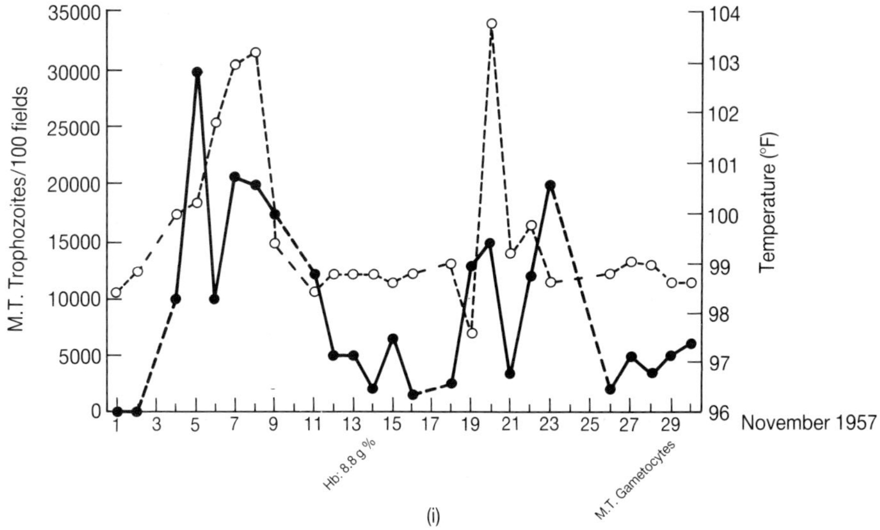

Fig. 8.9 (i) November 1957.

25 days with the highest density recorded 30 000/100 fields (Fig. 8.9i).

In summary, this Gambian child experienced 185 days of parasitaemia in his first two years of life; he was treated on two occasions, once with pyrimethamine and the second time with cloroquine; the lowest haemoglobin recorded was 6.2 g%. With this degree of parasite challenge it was not surprising that by the age of 5 years surviving children in the Gambia had developed enough immunity to make severe manifestations a great rarity after this age.

Study in 25 Gambian children

a. *Primary parasitaemia*

A summary of data in the first year of life of 25 children similarly studied revealed that the first appearance of parasitaemia after birth was very variable; it ranged from as early as 3½ months after birth to as late as 14½ months. The date of birth in relation to the transmission season may be partially responsible for this variation; but other factors, e.g. genetic, may well play a part. The range of density of the primary parasitaemia was also very variable being as low as 1/100 fields in an infant and as high as 40 000/100 fields in another. Irrespective of when the primary parasitaemia occurred, only one child was deemed ill enough to require antimalarial treatment during this period. The longest primary parasitaemia occurred in an infant born in April 1956; *P. falciparum* parasites appeared for the first time in August (i.e. 4 months later) and continued unabated for 50 days until early October (Fig. 8.10). (The occasional day when no blood film was taken has been ignored, on the assumption that parasitaemia was likely to have been present.) At no time did the child look ill and the density of parasitaemia was generally low ranging from as little as 1/100 to 1600/100 fields.

b. *Natural history of parasitaemia in the first year of life*

A summary of the data in the first year of life of the 25 children studied including the period of primary parasitaemia revealed the following information.

The range of duration of parasitaemia was very variable. One child experienced only 2 days of parasitaemia while another experienced 89 days with a mean for the group of 25 days. Mixed infections with *P. falciparum* (94.7%), *P. ovale* (26.3%) and *P. malariae* (5.3%) occurred. Nine out of the 25

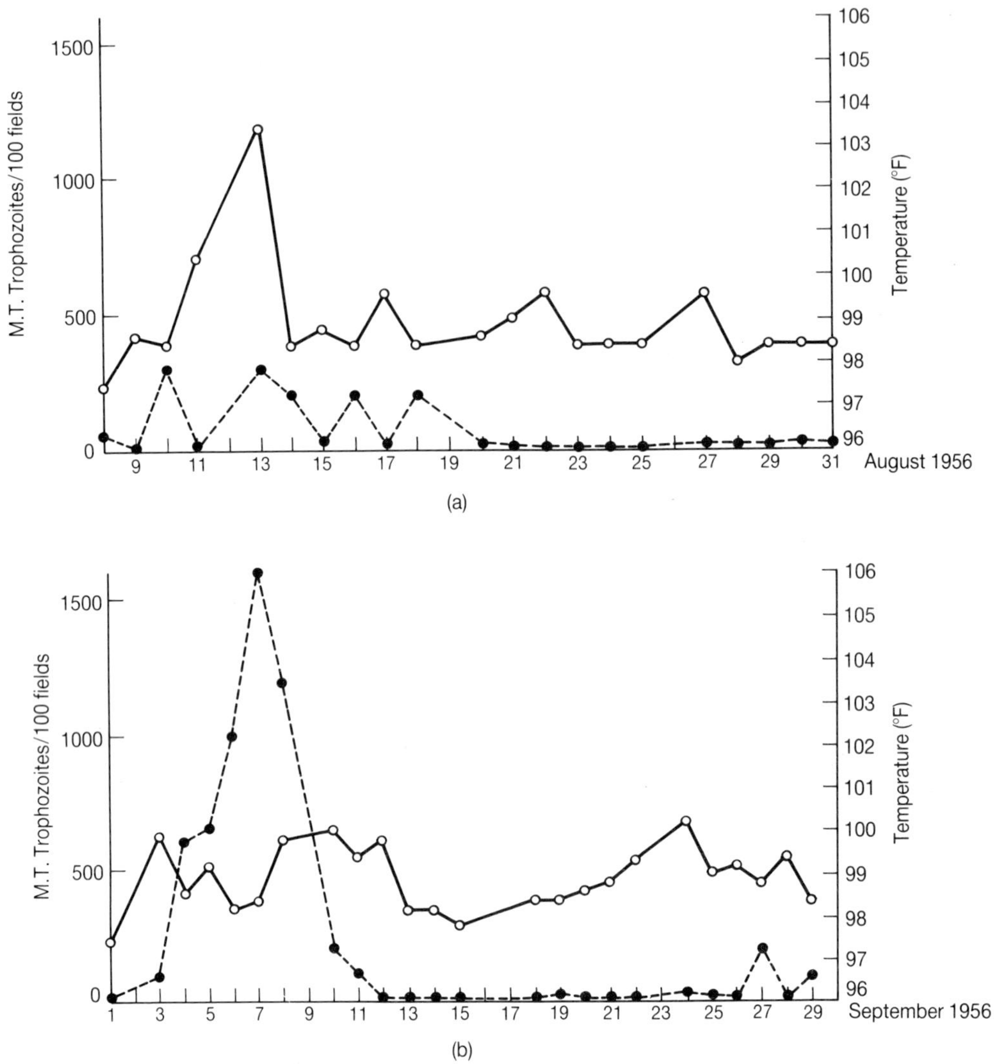

Fig. 8.10 Natural history of primary parasitaemia. (a) August 1956. (b) September 1956. Vertical axis = left arithmetical scale for density of parasitaemia (●). Temperature = Fahrenheit scale (○). Horizontal axis = days of the month.

children were considered ill enough to require antimalarial treatment.

c. *Natural history of parasitaemia in the second year of life*

The mean duration of parasitaemia for the group in the second year of life was over three times longer – 87 days instead of 25. Mixed infections continued to occur with *P. falciparum* predominating at 100% with *P. ovale* at 47.6% and *P. malariae* at 28.6%. In general, densities of parasitaemias were higher than in the first year, the children looked more ill and 17 required antimalarial treatment as opposed to nine in the first year. The longest *continuous* parasitaemia occurred in a child born in May 1956; it started in July with a density of parasitaemia of 25 000/100 fields and continued unabated until mid-October (109 days). The child was anaemic

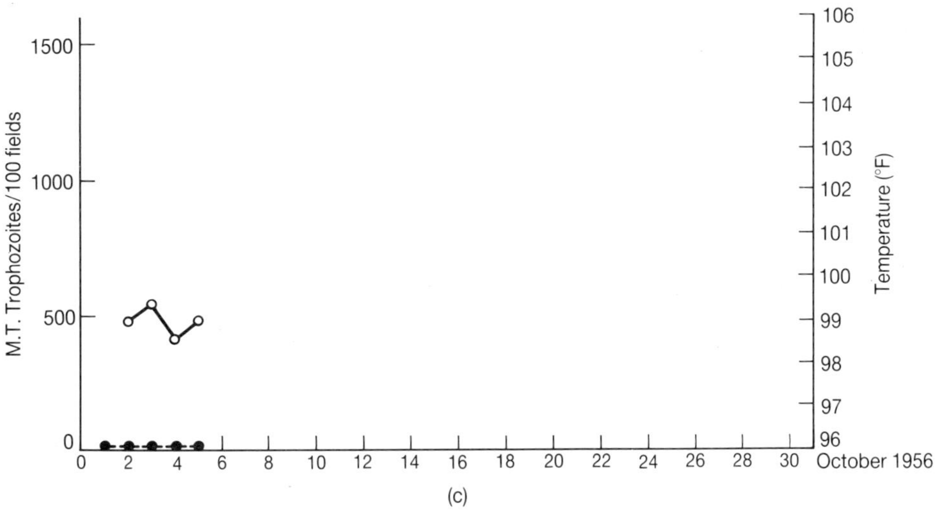

Fig. 8.10 (c) October 1956.

and the parasitaemia was terminated by treatment with chloroquine. The parasitaemia had ranged from 2/100 to 25 000/100 fields (Fig. 8.11).

Recent studies from the Gambia indicate that the natural history of malaria now bears little resemblance to the above due to a variety of possible factors, e.g. Sahelian drought, greatly increased drug usage, etc.

Although no statistical analysis of the data has been done I formed the following impressions:

(1) During the rainy season parasitaemia frequently occurred without fever.
(2) When fever did occur it was frequently associated with parasitaemia.
(3) During the dry season the association of fever with parasitaemia was weak.
(4) Morbidity and mortality from malaria had a marked seasonal distribution. This observation has been reported in several previous publications by McGregor and recently reconfirmed.

Why, in holo-hyperendemic areas of malaria, some develop severe disease and die while others do not, has yet to be established. A recent study in 42 Cameroonian families, using segregation analysis, provides evidence for the presence of a recessive major gene controlling the intensity of infection in human malaria.

Epidemiological characteristics of malaria in some selected areas

Northern and Central Europe

Here malaria slowly disappeared during the nineteenth century thanks to improved agriculture and draining of marshy areas. The brackish water breeding *A. atroparvus* was the main vector of indigenous malaria in coastal areas. *Anopheles messeae*, the fresh-water breeding member of the *A. maculipennis* complex, was responsible for outbreaks of malaria in exceptional circumstances when its numbers were very high and there was a shortage of domestic animals on which this mosquito usually fed.

The Mediterranean area and the Middle East

Throughout much of this area malaria has been effectively eradicated, but in some parts of it a considerable degree of endemic malaria still persists. The disease was seasonal throughout the whole of the area and severe regional epidemics were well known in countries on both shores of the Mediterranean. Several vectors are involved. The two most widespread are *A. labranchiae* in the western parts and *A. sacharovi* in the eastern parts. Both of them

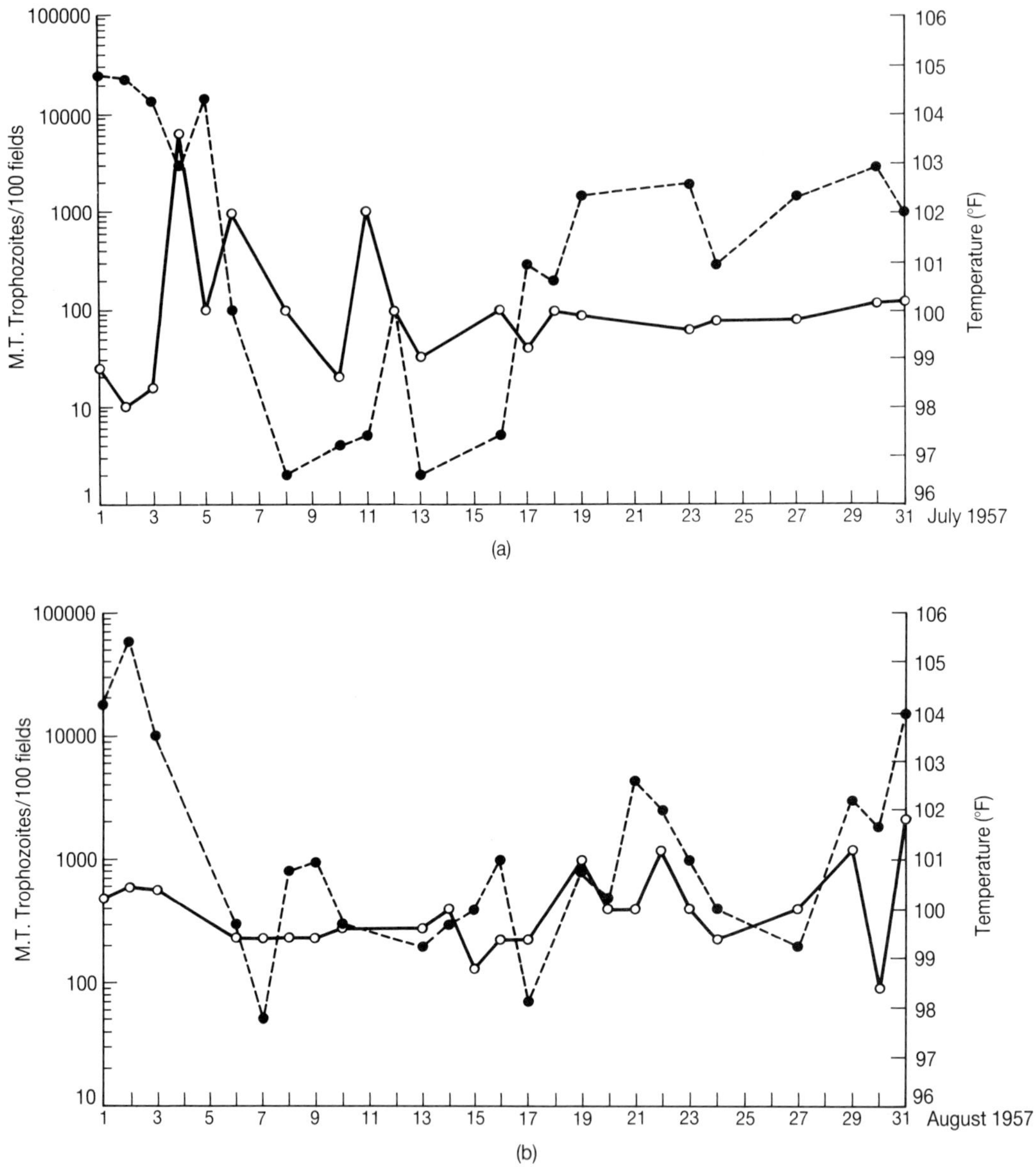

Fig. 8.11 Longest continuous parasitaemia. (a) July 1957, (b) August 1957, Vertical axis = density of parasitaemia: log scale (●). Temperature = Fahrenheit scale (○). Horizontal axis = days of the month.

are preferentially grassy pool breeders, and hence malaria was especially associated with swamp formation. One vector prevalent in the eastern parts, *A. superpictus*, bred in clear sunlit water, usually without vegetation, and typically in shingly streams, a fact which made many river valleys extremely unhealthy. There were also other vectors of local significance, such as *A. claviger* which was notorious as a result of its habit of breeding in domestic water cisterns in the Middle East, and *A. sergentii* which from time to time caused severe epidemics often in the neighbourhood of springs and irrigation systems of date palm groves.

Much of this has, however, gone and there is no indigenous malaria in Mediterranean countries of southern Europe, while in those of northern Africa

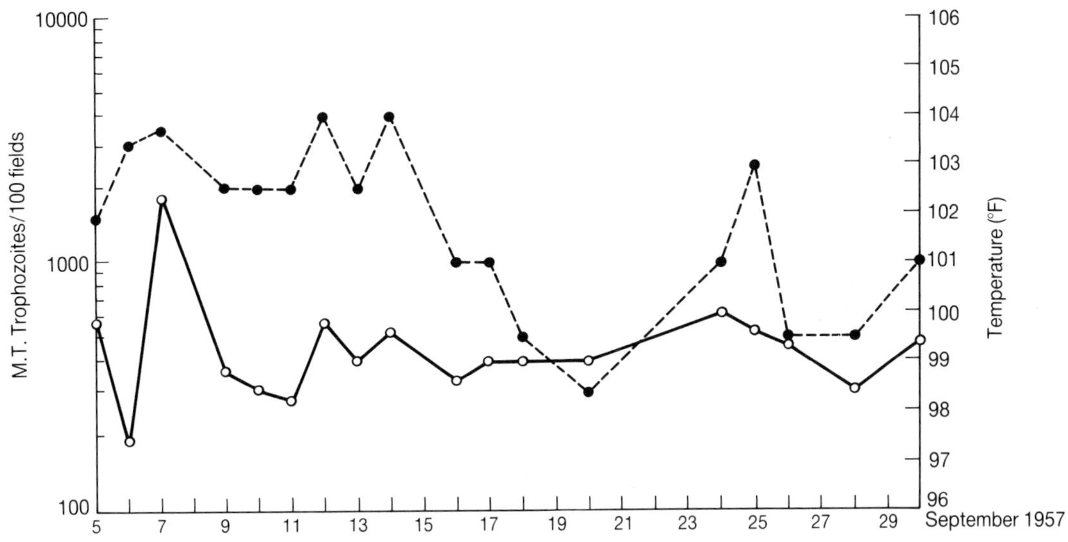

(c)

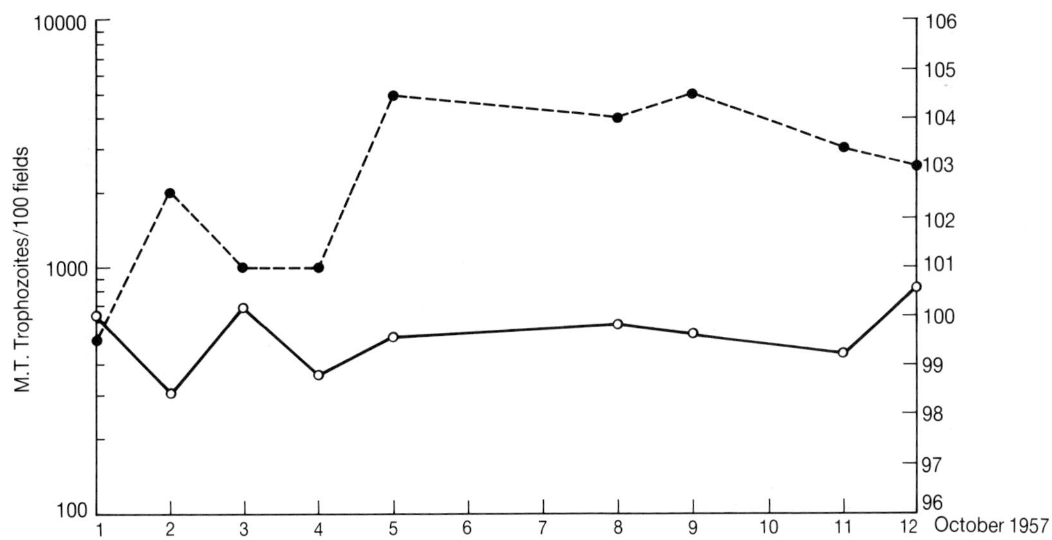

(d)

Fig. 8.11 (c) September 1957, (d) October 1957.

the amount of malaria has greatly decreased. The same applies to some countries of the eastern Mediterranean. There have been setbacks to malaria eradication or control in Asian Turkey, Afghanistan, Iran and Iraq where anopheline resistance to insecticides has occurred.

North-east India, Assam, Northern Bengal

Formerly, malaria was seasonal and highly endemic and large areas of this part of the subcontinent were uninhabited on account of their insalubrity. *Anopheles minimus* is by far the most important carrier in these areas. It seems to be more dependent on humans for its food than many other species, and is relatively long-lived and susceptible to infection. It bites mainly in the second half of the night, shelters in houses and cattle sheds, and breeds in cool water. This preference for relatively cool water determines the type of breeding place which varies with the season. In winter, larvae are found along the grassy banks of major rivers, in grassy pools and other places; in the summer, breeding becomes confined, occurring particularly in running water and in exposed subsoil water, as in primitive wells and seepages. Larvae can only persist in the presence of some vegetation such as grass along the edge, but they do not occur where the overhanging vegetation is dense; therefore the typical breeding place is an exposed sunlit drain or stream with grassy banks.

Anopheles leucosphyrus species complex is now known to be of great importance in limited areas where it occurs. It is much attracted to humans but rests in houses for only a short period after feeding; in consequence it is rarely found in daytime catches. It breeds in small pools in the forest, and since it does not seem to fly far, it is important only in the neighbourhood of heavily overgrown land.

Other mosquitos may be of local importance. Thus, *A. annularis* has been incriminated, and *A. maculatus* is apparently a vector in the hills near Shillong, India. *Anopheles philippinensis* is not a carrier in Assam, but is important in parts of Bengal; the dividing line is not exactly drawn. *Anopheles sundaicus* is a coastal mosquito which breeds exclusively in brackish water, and is sometimes important in some coastal areas.

The transmission season is well over 6 months and perennial in parts of the area. Clearing of forests increased the prevalence of malaria, and *P. falciparum* is the main parasite species, with *P. vivax* a close second.

The plains of India and Pakistan

Malaria throughout the plains is seasonal and shows a marked tendency to epidemics over large areas, particularly in the Punjab and Sind, and in some coastal areas of Tamil Nadu and Kerala. Early and prolonged monsoons are responsible for intensive transmission of both *P. vivax* and *P. falciparum*.

Anopheles culicifacies is by far the most important vector; it prefers feeding on cattle rather than on humans and its life is relatively short. Malaria is maintained by force of numbers of the vector and where they are insufficient to keep the disease going, one may find quite healthy areas. Where, however, they are numerous the malaria they carry may be severe and subject to extreme fluctuations in amount from year to year. *Anopheles culicifacies* is a pool breeder, occurring in natural and artificial pools exposed to the sun and often in those without vegetation, rarely in permanent swamps. Roadside pools, borrow-pits and such like are much favoured, as are rock-pools and sand-pools in the beds of dry rivers. This last preference explains why malaria in some places, particularly in the extreme south, is closely linked with dry weather; failure of the rains is more likely to precipitate epidemics than excess rain. Excess irrigation which raises the subsoil water and makes pooling common is a frequent cause of high endemicity. In the Punjab, pools of these types are rare; most breeding occurs during the monsoon, an excess of rain causing epidemics.

Anopheles stephensi is a vector of malaria in Bombay, Delhi, and in Karachi, as also in other towns where larvae are found in wells, cisterns, rooftop water tanks and in a variety of other man-made habitats. It is responsible for most transmission of urban malaria in the Indian subcontinent. *Anopheles stephensi* is also found in rural areas, but is generally not such an important vector because it frequently feeds on cattle.

There are other vectors of local importance. *Anopheles annularis* is important in some parts of Orissa and Bengal; it breeds in pools, swamps and rice fields. *Anopheles varuna* is a local vector of some importance. *Anopheles philippinensis* is the common carrier in the plains of Bengal; it breeds in ponds and tanks with much surface vegetation. *Anopheles sundaicus* is a carrier in the coastal areas of Bengal and Orissa and perhaps in a part of Andhra Pradesh; it breeds in brackish water only, and occurs near the sea (Rao, 1983).

The Western Ghats and hills of Peninsular India

These hills were notorious for their severity of malaria and there were many areas which were not populated for this reason. Control was first achieved by the application of the knowledge of the habits of *A. fluviatilis*, largely in the form of straightening and flushing streams. Later the full efficacy of the residual insecticides has been realized. Malaria is now greatly reduced in these areas.

Anopheles fluviatilis, which is a close relative of *A. minimus*, is the principal vector. Much attracted to humans and feeding very largely on them, it rests in houses and breeds in places similar to those favoured by *A. minimus*, except that it does not demand the presence of vegetation, occurring in rocky streams in which *A. minimus* could not maintain itself. It also occurs in rice fields fed by seepage water, from any part of which the total output may be insignificant, although the gross output from the entire area may be much more than enough to keep malaria transmission going (Rao, 1983).

Sri Lanka

There are very great variations in the incidence of malaria in different parts of the island, depending on the climate. Generally speaking, it is absent at heights over 1000 m and in areas where the annual rainfall is heavy, but highly endemic in those areas where it is low. As a result of the monsoon distribution the disease was very prevalent in the north and east, extending in its severity round a part of the south coast. In the south-west corner, where the south-west monsoon occurs in full force, it was absent. Between these two areas is an intermediate one where the incidence of malaria varied greatly from year to year; period epidemics of disastrous severity occurred.

Although recently several anophelines have been suspected in the transmission of malaria in Sri Lanka, by far the most important vector is *A. culicifacies*. An account of which has been given above in describing malaria of the plains of central and north India and Pakistan. The type of pool preferred as a breeding place is associated with slight rain rather than continuous downpours, a fact which causes the spatial and seasonal distribution of malaria. In the areas of highest malaria incidence breeding may be found in almost any type of pool, but in the epidemic areas it occurs more particularly in pools of river beds during the dry season. Monsoon failure is therefore related to epidemics.

The history of control included long and energetic efforts at prevention of breeding, with local success which did not amount to general control. Residual insecticides were brought into use soon after the war, their application became general, and in 1947 a campaign throughout malarious areas of the entire country was started. Soon malaria as a serious public health problem ceased to exist. In 1960 a further expansion was made and the objective has been changed, from control to eradication of the disease. However, since 1967 adverse climatic conditions and a certain slackening of the rigorous search for remaining cases have caused a considerable increase of malaria incidence amounting to cyclical epidemics of vivax malaria at intervals of 5 to 6 years. During the last malaria epidemic which occurred in 1986, *P. falciparum* constituted 30% of the total malaria.

South-east Asia and the Philippines

Malaya (West Malaysia) had a history of disastrous outbreaks of malaria. This phase came to an end largely as a result of the introduction of rational methods of control; there was a marked exacerbation during the Second World War but since then there has been a marked reduction in general incidence. It seems that the main anopheline carrier, *A. maculatus*, is attracted more to cattle than to humans, and may not always be an important vector. Development of the country provides favourable conditions for it through the multiplication of breeding places by estate clearance, the introduction of non-immune labourers, and the growth of groups of people without domestic animals. These three factors working together caused the epidemics, and as each of them is now coming to an end the incidence of malaria is correspondingly in decline. Extensive clearing or the aggregation of new labour forces could, however, easily precipitate a recurrence of past conditions.

Over the whole area the climatic conditions are such that transmission is generally perennial. There are very many species of *Anopheles* of which some act as secondary vectors of *P. falciparum*, *P. vivax*, *P. malariae* and of monkey malaria.

There are many malaria vectors in the general area, their importance often differing regionally. Among the more important vectors are *A. balabacensis*, *A. dirus*, *A. campestris* (formerly known as the dark-winged form of *A. barbirostris*), *A. donaldi*, *A. flavirostris*, *A. letifer*, *A. leucosphyrus*, and *A. sundaicus*, but one of the most important is undoubtedly *A. maculatus*. This species occurs in streams, rock pools, and seepages of hilly areas when they are exposed to broad daylight. Clearance of forests can expose such places and make them highly dangerous or can be selective and do no harm. *Anopheles sundaicus* is a strictly coastal mosquito as it breeds in saline water, usually between high neap tide level and spring tide level. Its control was for long based exclusively in the construction of embankments with controlled internal drainage which prevented the access of saline water to this area and removed fresh water from it. *Anopheles letifer* breeds in brown peaty water pools and stagnant agricultural drains, with and without vegetation, in the low country. *Anopheles campestris* breeds in rice fields and pools, often containing decaying vegetation, in the lowlands near the coast. The *A. leucosphyrus* group of mosquitos contains three species complexes, namely the *A. balabacensis* complex, the *A. dirus* complex and the *A. leucosphyrus* complex, and there has been much confusion concerning the identity of species within these complexes and consequently their role in malaria transmission. In Malaysia *A. balabancensis* s.s. is confined to the states of Sabah and Sarawak and is an important vector in forested areas; *A. dirus*, previously confused with the former species, is also a forest species and vector in the northern parts of peninsular Malaysia. Both *A. balabacensis* and *A. dirus* are important vectors in Burma, Thailand, Sabah, Vietnam and the north-eastern borders of Myanmar, Bangladesh and India. Chloroquine resistant strains of *P. falciparum* are common in areas where these two forms are prevalent.

In Vietnam and Kampuchea where *A. minimus* and *A. sundaicus* are the main endophilic vectors, both responded well to residual insecticide spraying, but the exophilic *A. dirus*, which does not commonly feed in human habitations, has not been affected. The same is largely true in Thailand, where the increase of human activities in forested areas exposed the population to these *Anopheles*. In the Philippines the main vectors are *A. flavirostris*, which breeds in clear, slow-flowing streams; another vector *A. litoralis*, a brackish water breeder, is of local importance.

Indonesia and Borneo (Kalimantan)

Conditions in Indonesia resemble those in Malaysia, both in past history and in the nature of the common carriers, the chief of which are *A. maculatus* and *A. sundaicus*. A number of other mosquitos have, however, been incriminated in different places. Two of these, *A. hyrcanus* and *A. aconitus*, breed in extensive exposed sheets of water such as rice fields during some part of the cultivation cycle. *Anopheles aconitus* has been successfully discouraged by ensuring that all rice fields in one locality were in the same stage of cultivation, so that a common off-season occurred when no suitable harbourage presented itself. However, the association of these species with agriculture, and that of *A. sundaicus* with the fish industry, made control very difficult until the arrival of the new residual insecticides. Extensive schemes of control have been initiated with the objective of general control throughout the country. These schemes are in progress, covering large areas in Java and Bali. Full success has not been achieved partly because of resistance to both DDT and dieldrin in *A. sundaicus* and *A. aconitus* in some areas.

Malaria is widely distributed in Borneo, and commonly of the low epidemic type. The most important are *A. leucosphyrus* and *A. balabacensis*, groups of mosquitos with the habit of resting for only a short time in houses after having fed in them. They breed in the forest, in seepages and pools often under tangled undergrowth surrounded by swampy areas, and in places which are inaccessible for any routine weekly antilarval measures. The shade afforded by the forest is apparently essential to the survival of larvae in the water. *Anopheles leucosphyrus* is not a strong flier; it carries malaria only within a short range of dense bush. Other carriers of local importance are *A. sundaicus* and *A. umbrosus*.

China

The immense territory of the Peoples Republic of China, with its population of 1.15 billion, has been covered during the past three decades by a number of extensive epidemiological surveys. The country can be divided into four large zones.

Zone I is the area south of latitude 24°N, where *A. minimus* is the main vector in the tropical and subtropical parts of the country, including the southern part of Yunnan province, most of the Guandong province, Guangxi region, the south-east part of Fujian province and geographically the whole of Taiwan. In this zone, malaria has a long transmission season of 9–12 months but it has been eradicated in Taiwan.

Plasmodium falciparum is the predominant species of the parasite, but mixed infections with *P. vivax* are very common; *P. malariae* has a patchy distribution, and it is possible that rare cases of *P. ovale* were diagnosed along the south-west border of Yunnan province. In mountainous and hilly districts malaria is of the stable type.

The main vector is *A. minimus*, with *A. jeyporiensis* as a secondary vector. In the jungle areas of Hainan island *A. dirus* is an important vector. In the plains, where the prevalent malaria is of an unstable type, *A. sinensis* is a vector wherever its numbers are large. On Hainan island the peak incidence of malaria is between April and May, before the rainy season; on the mainland, the bulk of cases occur between August and October.

Zone II lies between latitudes 25°N and 33°N and includs the provinces of Guizhou, Hunan, Jiangxi, Hubei and Zhejiang; it also covers the greater part of Sichuan, Fukian, Anhui and Jiangsu as also other provinces. This zone of unstable malaria is inhabited by about one-half of the whole population of China. The transmission season lasts for 6–8 months, with a peak from August to October. Although *P. vivax* predominates occasional severe outbreaks of malaria occur, with *P. vivax* and *P. falciparum* playing an equal role. *Anopheles sinensis* and *A. anthropophagus* are the usual vectors, although at times *A. minimus* may be involved.

Zone III is the area north of 33°N latitude; it covers the northern part of China, including the provinces of Shandong, Liaoning, Jilin, Heilongjiang and parts of other adjoining provinces and also the Xinjiang region. *Anopheles sinensis* is the vector of malaria of unstable type, with *P. vivax* as virtually the only parasite, and outbreaks occurring between August and October.

Zone IV is the malaria-free zones of the cold, high altitudes of the south-west, the dry desert of the north and north-west, and the mountainous districts of the north-east.

The China malaria control programme, including the use of pyrethroid treated mosquito nets, has met with considerable success.

Australasia and the South Pacific

The South Pacific includes a very large area which is free from malaria; the disease does not extend east of 170°E or south of 20°S. In continental Australia, malaria had in the past a restricted distribution in the more extreme north, chiefly in coastal areas in the east to north-western Australia.

Very high incidences occur in New Guinea, particularly in coastal areas, and in the neighbouring islands. Incidence is also high in the Solomon Islands and in Vanuatu, although these two are of lower grades than New Guinea, typically with seasonal epidemic malaria. Experience of the war showed that extremely serious outbreaks may be expected in any imported human groups.

The most important vectors in the region are species of the *A. punctulatus* complex, which includes *A. punctulatus* s.s., *A. koliensis* and *A. farauti*. In addition to biting humans adults often feed on cattle. These species are mainly pool breeders, but *A. koliensis* seems to prefer marshy areas or pools at the edges of forest streams, and some forms of *A. farauti* breed in brackish waters. Adults enter houses to feed, but tend to rest out of doors.

Tropical Africa

Throughout most of Africa south of the Sahara, malaria shows a high endemicity, but has a low epidemic potential. Exceptions to this last statement are to be found on the slopes of mountains in Kenya, at the periphery of the distribution of malaria in Zimbabwe and the Republic of South Africa, and formerly in Mauritius, in all of which places epidemics were well known. In the centre of the continental area, transmission is nearly perennial, although there are seasonal exacerbations, and very high endemicities are common in the coastlands and other places at a low altitude. Endemicity is reduced, though still high, on the plateau of East Africa which is at an average altitude of 1400 m; the disease occurs up to a height of 2500 m on some mountains, although rather as occasional outbreaks than as a continuous endemicity. Epidemics in the lowlands of the central region are rare unless precipitated by obvious causes such as the importation of labour from non-malarious places or construction work producing many new breeding places.

There are three main vectors in sub-Saharan Africa, *A. gambiae* s.s., its sibling species *A. arabiensis*, and *A. funestus*. In coastal areas of West Africa, *A. melas* can be an important though local vector. In East Africa its salt-water breeding counterpart is *A. merus* and, although unlike *A. melas* this species can sometimes be found inland, it is not such an important malaria vector as *A. melas*.

Anopheles gambiae s.s. is without question the most important vector. It is widely distributed and feeds predominantly on humans, biting and resting mainly indoors, although it will also feed out of doors and may rest out of doors. *Anopheles arabiensis*, which is morphologically indistinguishable from *A. gambiae* and has to be separated chromosomally or by DNA technology, is often found together with *A. gambiae* (that is, it has a sympatric distribution) but has a greater tendency to feed on cattle and to rest outside, and is often a less important vector. However, when there are large populations it can be responsible for considerable transmission. This species is also more common in the drier savannah areas, where *A. gambiae* may be absent.

Larvae of *A. gambiae* and *A. arabiensis* are commonly found in pools, usually exposed to the sun. Although they occur in all types of pools they are more common in temporary ones than in those of long standing. Breeding in rice fields and in swamps may occur. Owing to the nature of the breeding places, the species tends to be more numerous in the rainy season than in dry weather.

Anopheles melas and *A. merus* are both species within the *A. gambiae* complex but are distinguished by breeding in salt water. The former is confined to coastal localities, but *A. merus* often extends its distribution inland. In their general behaviour they resemble *A. gambiae*. Because of the nature of their breeding places, for example, mangrove swamps, the control of these species requires special methods.

Anopheles funestus is a very widely distributed carrier, second in importance only to *A. gambiae*. It feeds predominantly on humans, is relatively long-lived, shelters almost exclusively in houses, and is readily susceptible to infection.

The larvae are commonly found in streams, and particularly under shade; swamps, seepages, fallow rice fields, and the grassy edges of rivers may be important breeding places. Owing to the nature of its breeding places its season is often different from that of *A. gambiae* and in many places the one species takes over from the other as chief vector when the season changes. It has a relatively long flight range, but has not demonstrated the invasive tendency shown by *A. gambiae*. Moreover, it responds more readily to residual insecticides.

Some anophelines in equatorial Africa which are important in limited localities include:

A. moucheti: This is found in parts of West and Central Africa, and can be a secondary vector in riverine forest tracts.

A. nili: This is seen in West Africa and may be an important secondary carrier in some places; it breeds in streams.

A. pharoensis: A common carrier in Egypt; it may play a minor role in the drier parts of West Africa, the Sudan, Uganda and Kenya.

The Caribbean area

In this area, eradication programmes have made great progress (except for Haiti). Formerly, the general incidence of malaria on the islands of the Caribbean was much less than in most of the areas already described, although there were localities with high prevalence. Throughout the area the disease was of the high epidemic potential type, liable to marked fluctuations from time to time and from place to place.

The Bahamas are free from malaria, but all the other islands were to some extent malarious, the disease having a very patchy distribution. Malaria eradication has been achieved in Jamaica, Dominica, Grenada and Carriacou, Barbados, Trinidad and Tobago, Puerto Rico and Cuba. In the Greater Antilles (Cuba, Jamaica, Puerto Rico and Hispaniola) the chief carrier is *A. albimanus*, a mosquito of the plains, very prevalent in irrigated areas where it breeds in cane fields, rice fields and other places with stagnant water. It is a relatively poor carrier, possibly being normally short lived, and is important only by reason of large numbers.

In the Lesser Antilles, notably in Trinidad and neighbouring islands, *A. aquasalis* is the common carrier. It is always coastal in its distribution, but as the islands are mostly small this is little restriction. It breeds in brackish water, in drainage channels, slow streams, mangrove swamps, borrow-pits, and a great variety of waters within 5 or 6 miles of the coast. It feeds on cattle in strong preference to humans, and is very short lived, characteristics which would have made it a very poor carrier if it had not been present in enormous numbers. It is apparently diverted by cattle and the amount of malaria may be in inverse proportion to their numbers in some places.

Another vector in some areas is *A. bellator*, an unusual vector. It breeds high above the ground in bromeliads and epihytic plants growing on trees. It bites mainly out of doors and in the hours of daylight. It has proved susceptible to control by the use of residual insecticides in houses. An additional method used is the destruction of the bromeliad by spraying them with copper solutions, or the cutting down of the parent trees (Fig. 7.18, p. 113).

The Americas

On the mainland, there are areas in which *A. aquasalis* is the vector, but the most important is *A. darlingi*, which breeds profusely in irrigation channels, irrigated fields and swamps. It is strongly attracted to humans, shelters exclusively in houses, and may be short lived. It is a fairly potent carrier, and its ubiquity has made severe malaria a feature of several countries. The first large-scale control by residual insecticides was started in Venezuela and Guyana, and resulted in the actual elimination of the mosquito from the main areas and eradication of endemic disease.

Anopheles darlingi is also the vector in the hills of the interior, where it is not universally distributed but can readily establish itself near human settlements. Fortunately its susceptibility to control is likely to be as marked as in the lowlands.

Other vectors of malaria in South America include *A. punctimacula* (in Peru and Colombia), *A. aquasalis*, *A. pseudopunctipennis*, *A. albitarsis* (in Brazil) and *A. albimanus* in coastal lowlands. Special attention has been given recently to *A. nuneztovari*, a forest dwelling mosquito with elusive habits, which maintains a degree of transmission in the border areas of Venezuela and Colombia.

In parts of Brazil *A. cruzii*, with peculiar breeding habitats in water-containing bromeliad plants, deserves mention (Fig. 7.18, p. 113).

In Central America the list of vectors include *A. darlingi*, *A. argyritarsis*, *A. aquasalis* and *A. punctimacula*, but the most important of all is *A. albimanus*, which breeds in pools, puddles, ponds, marshes and artificial containers and has gained much notoriety because it has become resistant to nearly every insecticide available at present.

In the USA, *A. quadrimaculatus* was the major vector of malaria in the past, although in some localities *A. freeborni* was incriminated. Today there is no more transmission of endemic malaria in that country, even though isolated cases of infection from imported carriers may occur. In the southern part of North America *A. albimanus* is the main vector in the lowlands adjacent to the Pacific Ocean.

Imported malaria

Importation of malaria into countries from which it has been eliminated (or where it is very rare) is a relatively new public health problem, due to the tremendous increase of human mobility and particularly to air travel. It was estimated that in 1985 the number of passengers carried by all scheduled and charter airlines was in excess of 900 million and growing at the rate of 6% per annum. About one-quarter of air passengers are tourists or businessmen but a large proportion of people travelling by air and land are workers, immigrants and refugees. The problem of imported malaria has become serious since 1970, especially in Europe, North America and Australia. In the USA in 1991, 1170 cases of malaria were reported to CDC; while in Australia 939 cases were reported in 1991.

In Europe alone the number of cases of malaria imported from the tropics reached nearly 8000 in 1989. For Great Britain the numbers were as follows for the years 1988–92.

	Total	***P. falciparum***	***P. vivax***	**Others or species unknown**
1988	1674	1026	507	141
1989	1987	992	733	262
1990	2096	1059	831	206
1991	2332	1268	863	201
1992	1629	935	512	182

In recent years, there has been a notable shift in parasite species with *P. falciparum* now the predominant type of 'imported malaria'. In 1992 it was responsible for 11 deaths.

Most of the cases of vivax malaria originate in Asia, while nearly all cases of falciparum malaria come from Africa. In Australia, most of the cases come from Papua New Guinea, where *P. falciparum* resistance to chloroquine is widespread and resistance to *P. vivax* has recently been reported.

Airport malaria

Several cases of malaria have occurred in persons working at large European airports or living near them. These infections were transmitted by infected *Anopheles*, brought by large aircraft from tropical airports and able to survive the flight.

One of the weirdest examples of malaria transmission outside the endemic area occurred when two passengers boarded an aircraft emanating from the tropics at Heathrow Airport, alighted in Rome, and developed malaria on their return to the UK, having obviously been infected while on board the aircraft – 'commuter malaria'.

It is obvious that cases of malaria imported into countries where the local *Anopheles* are abundant and climatic conditions are suitable for transmission, may become sources of new infections for people who never travelled abroad. The high fatality rate of *P. falciparum* malaria in non-immune individuals is disturbing. The list of wrong diagnoses of malaria includes dysentery, dengue, influenza, hepatitis, heat stroke, nephritis and many other diseases. It is not uncommon that a patient, after first seeing his or her doctor and being given a palliative drug, develops within a few days, and with dramatic suddenness, signs of cerebral involvement, hyperpyrexia or renal failure. An emergency admission to the hospital may lead to a correct diagnosis of cerebral malaria but such severe infections with *P. falciparum* may not always respond to belated treatment.

The interval between the infection contracted abroad, usually in Africa or Asia, and the onset of symptoms, may be as long as 1 month or more in cases of falciparum malaria. This adds to the probability of overlooking malaria in a febrile patient, especially when gastrointestinal symptoms, myalgia, arthralgia and jaundice complicate the clinical picture. Attacks of vivax or quartan malaria may be seen in some patients up to 9 months or longer after their return from the tropics. One should bear in mind that the usual prophylactic drugs taken by the traveller while in the tropics and for 1 month after his return may not protect him from true relapsing infections with vivax and ovale; nor from quartan malaria. The suppressive action of antimalarial drugs on the primary attack may not extend to the secondary relapse after the latent period. Moreover, some strains of *P. vivax* have an inherently long incubation period.

Thus, malaria must be suspected in any patient with fever of unknown or doubtful origin who has been to a malarious tropical area during the previous 1 or 2 years or who has had a blood transfusion up to about 3 months before the start of his febrile illness. Simple questioning of the patient about his recent visits abroad will often lead to the correct diagnosis and treatment.

Information on malaria risk for international travellers is collected and published annually by the World Health Organization. This may be of considerable assistance to the medical practitioner or medical adviser of any organized group or agency in assessing the need for personal protection of prospective travellers and in evaluating the probability of malaria infection on their return.* (See Annex V.)

Transfusion malaria

While natural malaria infection takes place through the bite of an infective *Anopheles* mosquito, direct transfer of erythrocytes containing *Plasmodia* may also be responsible for the infection. This may occur accidentally by usage of syringes or needles contaminated by blood, as happens among a group of drug addicts or among hospital staff. Transmission of malaria by plasmapheresis, erythrocyte concentrates or *organ transplantation* has also been recorded. However, the most common occurrence is accidental infection of a recipient by blood transfusion from an infected blood donor.

Estimates of the total number of cases of malaria related to blood transfusion are approximate. Only a proportion of such episodes has been reported

***The latest information on malaria risk for international travellers is given in a pamphlet published by WHO entitled *International Travel and Health. Vaccination Requirements and Health Advice, 1992*.**

and the information ranges from a brief mention of malaria as a complication of surgery to a comprehensive analysis of a series of cases, reported singly by different authors.

During the past 65 years not less than 3500 cases of transfusion malaria were recorded. Transfusion malaria is particularly common in countries where blood donation has become a commercial transaction and where the blood donors come from the less affluent social classes. *Plasmodium vivax* infections are most commonly incriminated in accidental infections following blood transfusion; however *P. falciparum* infections occur not infrequently and more recently *P. malariae* was reported with increasing frequency, because of the asymptomatic, long-term carrier state of donors infected with this *Plasmodium*.

While the longevity of *P. falciparum* in humans seldom exceeds 1 year and *P. vivax* or *P. ovale* usually die out within 3 years, *P. malariae* which is prone to long persistence, with or without febrile symptoms, may remain in the infected host for 10, 20, 30 or over 40 years. In fact, one may say that in some cases a quiescent infection with *P. malariae* may be maintained for life and the epidemiological implications of this special position of *P. malariae* with regard to its human host are considerable.

The viability of malaria parasites depends on that of their erythrocyte hosts. A series of studies carried out during the 1940s showed that malaria parasites of all species can remain viable in the blood destined for transfusion for at least 1 week. Further studies revealed that both *P. falciparum* and *P. malariae* remain viable for well over 10 days in blood stored at 4°C, especially when the anticoagulant contains dextrose.

The time of appearance of symptoms of blood-induced infection depends on the number of parasites introduced, on the method of inoculation, and on the susceptibility of the recipient. Much information on this subject has been gathered in the course of malaria therapy.

Generally speaking, the main symptoms of accidental infection with *P. falciparum* develop within 10 days after transfusion, *P. vivax* takes 16 days, while *P. malariae* takes 40 days or longer. The interval between the onset of symptoms and diagnosis depends also on the degree of awareness of the possibility of transfusion malaria, but it can vary from 1 week to 1 month or considerably longer; in one case, the disease was finally diagnosed 6 months later, in another one – after a year.

When any patient who has received a blood transfusion up to 3 months previously shows an unexplained fever, the possibility of malaria must be considered, and microscopic examination of the blood and, if necessary, serological tests should be carried out.

The prevention of transfusion malaria depends on the screening of possibly infected blood donors and the elimination of actual or possible plasmodial infection in the donor and in the recipient of the blood. Screening of blood donors is primarily based on their history of malaria or exposure to the infection. Regulations governing the acceptance of donors of whole blood for transfusion vary considerably from one country to another and it would be desirable for some internationally acceptable criteria to be established.

The detection of a malaria infection in a blood donor who is suspected on circumstantial evidence may prove very difficult. Microscopic examination of a blood film is of little value for the detection of asymptomatic parasitaemia, since the parasites are usually very few in number. On the other hand, modern serological techniques and particularly the indirect fluorescent antibody test (IFAT) are very useful for detection of persons who have had malaria in the past, although the test does not always indicate the actual presence of infection. The recent introduction of commercially available and ready for use homologous antigens has greatly simplified such testing.

Pre-medication of donors suspected of having had malaria is impracticable as a rule though it may be possible in exceptional cases. The general consensus of authoritative opinion is that a curative dose of an appropriate antimalarial drug, given to a recipient of infected blood 24 hours before transfusion or immediately after it, protects from induced malaria. It seems that this is the best solution where there are unusual risks of accidentally induced infection and no other source of 'malaria safe' blood is available; providing of course that the parasites are not resistant to the antimalarial given.

Chapter 9

Treatment and prevention of malaria*

D. A. Warrell

Chemotherapy and chemoprophylaxis

Antimalarial drugs have a selective action on the different phases of the parasite life cycle and may be divided into *causal prophylactic drugs* which prevent the establishment of the parasite in the liver and *blood schizontocidal drugs* which attack the parasite in the red blood cell, preventing or terminating the clinical attack.

The term *tissue schizontocide* refers to compounds acting on pre-erythrocytic forms in the liver. The *gametocytocidal drugs* destroy the sexual forms of the parasite in the blood; some of these drugs are *hypnozoitocidal*, they will kill the dormant hypnozoites in the liver (responsible for relapses in *Plasmodium vivax* and *Plasmodium ovale*) and are extensively used as antirelapse drugs. Finally, *sporontocidal drugs* inhibit the development of oöcysts on the stomach wall of the mosquito which has fed on the gametocyte carrier so that the mosquito cannot transmit the infection. The relationship between the phases of development and the action of the drug is shown diagrammatically in Fig. 9.1. Certain drugs bring about the rapid cure of falciparum and malariae malarias, but for complete and permanent cure of vivax and ovale malarias, use of hypnozoitocides is necessary.

In addition to these clearly definable differences between the action of drugs on the four species of malaria parasites, there are differences between strains of the same species, so that generalizations which are true about malaria in one part of the world may be quite incorrect in other parts.

The state of immunity has a bearing on the use of drugs since people who have, by a prolonged exposure to the infection, acquired a degree of immunity can be cured or protected much more easily than those who have not. Evidence obtained from treatment or prevention of the partially immune groups cannot be applied to non-immune groups or to other groups whose immunity may be less, and much confusion has resulted from efforts to do so.

Ideally a drug used for antimalarial therapy should be effective in a single dose so as to be practicable in developing countries where rural health services may be inadequate. In addition, an activity on all stages of the parasite would be a feature of the ideal drug. Not surprisingly, such an ideal drug has not yet been developed. In addition, the resistance of the malaria parasite, especially *Plasmodium falciparum*, to existing drugs is a serious problem in many parts of the world.

Uses of antimalarial drugs

A drug may be put to several uses, in each of which its efficacy may be determined by several factors such as the species of malaria parasite concerned, its sensitivity to the drug, the presence of partial immunity in the human host, the risks of toxic effects, as well as by other simpler ones such as availability, preference, acceptability to the patient (compliance) and cost. The main uses of antimalarial drugs are:

***We are grateful to Dr David Warhurst for his helpful contributions to this chapter.**

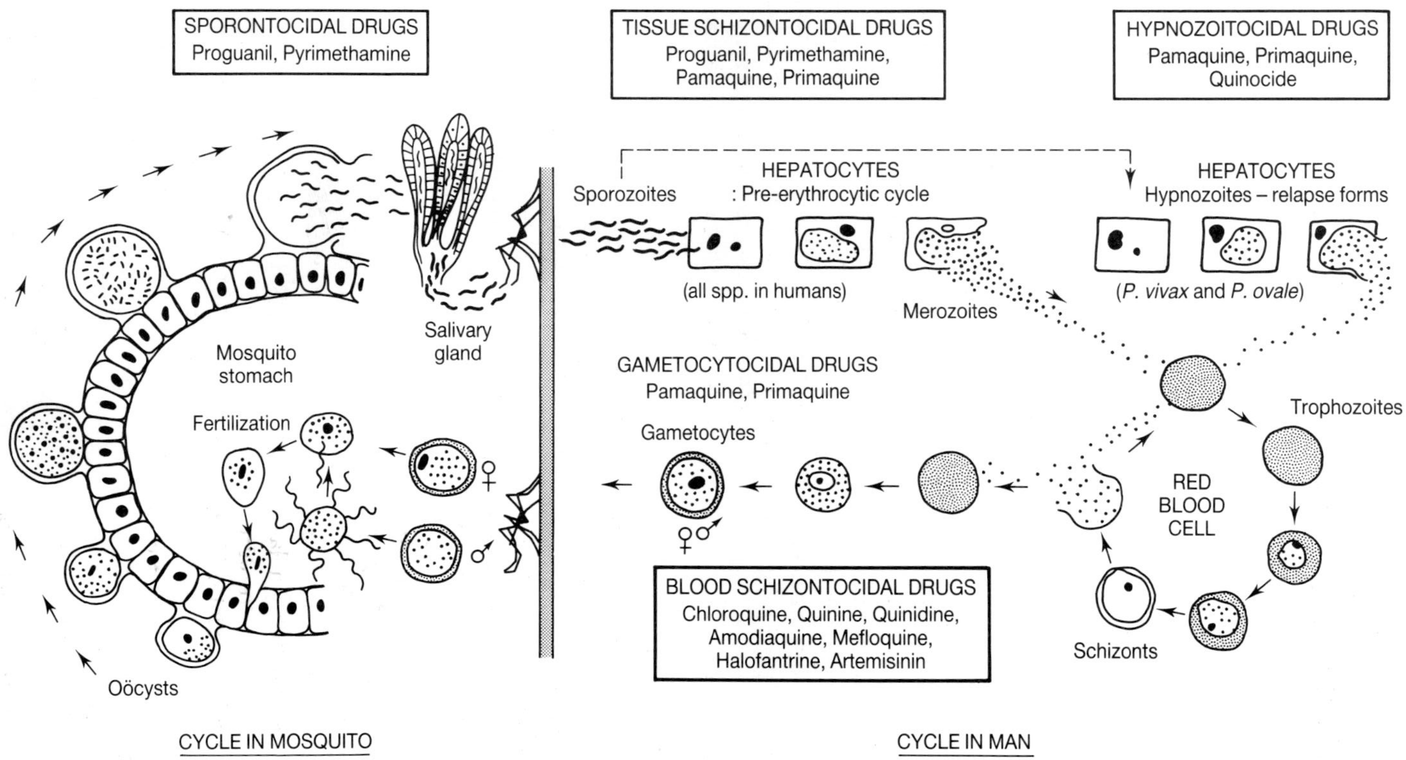

Fig. 9.1 Diagram of action of antimalarial compounds at different stages of the development of the malaria parasite in *Anopheles* mosquitos and in the human host. (Redrawn by David Warhurst after David Payne.)

1. Protective (prophylactic)
2. Curative (therapeutic)
3. Prevention of transmission

Protective (prophylactic) use

This implies that the drugs are used before infection occurs or before it becomes evident, with the aim of preventing either the occurrence of the infection or any of its symptoms.

Absolute prevention of infection implies destruction of sporozoites soon after they have been inoculated by the bite of an infected *Anopheles*. There is no drug that can achieve this at present.

On the other hand, there are drugs that act on the early growing stages of the parasite, while it is still confined to the liver tissue, and destroy these stages before merozoites are liberated into the bloodstream. These are causal (or true) prophylactics. A blood schizontocidal drug may have minimal effects on the growing liver stages, but if it is still present in the blood when the merozoites leave the liver and invade erythrocytes for the first time, it will effectively prevent symptomatic malaria. Such an effect is termed suppressive (or clinical) prophylaxis. Where the malaria parasite has dormant liver stages (hypnozoites of vivax or ovale) these will remain unaffected in the liver and may give rise to a symptomatic blood infection at a later stage if prophylaxis has been discontinued.

Curative (therapeutic) use

This refers to action on the established infection, and consists of treatment of the acute attack usually with blood schizontocidal drugs and, in the case of relapsing malarias, radical treatment of the dormant liver forms.

Prevention of transmission

This refers to the prevention of infection of mosquitos and implies an action on gametocytes in the peripheral blood of the human host or interruption of the development of the sporogonic phase in the mosquito, when the latter feeds on the blood of an infected person who has been given the appropriate sporontocidal compound.

Use of drugs in malaria control

This subject is dealt with in Chapter 10.

Available antimalarial drugs: their structure and relationships

There are several chemical groups of antimalarial compounds in general use. The international nonproprietary names are given here in bold type, and the structures and chemical names in Fig. 9.2. Their proprietary names are given in Appendix I.

1. The arylaminoalcohols (including the quinoline methanols **quinine** and **mefloquine** and the phenanthrene methanol **halofantrine**). Quinine and its diastereomer, **quinidine**, are alkaloids extracted from the bark of the Cinchona tree. The arylaminoalcohols are blood schizontocides effective only on the blood stages of the malaria parasite engaged in digesting haemoglobin. In view of their rapid effect on the blood stages they are used for treatment of the acute disease, but mefloquine can also be used for suppressive prophylaxis.
2. The 4-aminoquinolines (**chloroquine** and **amodiaquine**) are blood schizontocides like the arylaminoalcohols. Blood schizontocides are thought to act by being concentrated in the parasite's lysosomes were haemoglobin is being digested, and by inhibiting the polymerization of toxic haemin into insoluble haemozoin (malaria pigment). Where the malaria parasite concerned is susceptible to these drugs, they are invaluable for treatment as they act rapidly, and chloroquine is used for suppressive prophylaxis. (The acridine **mepacrine** and the benzonaphthyridine **pyronaridine** are blood schizontocides similar to chloroquine, and the latter has activity in strains of falciparum malaria resistant to chloroquine.)
3. Sulfones (**diaminodiphenyl sulfone**) and sulfonamides (**sulfadoxine**, **sulfalene** and **co-trimoxazole**). These drugs, known as type 1 antifolate drugs, compete for the enzyme dihydropteroate synthase found only in microorganisms (see below). They are used for causal prophylaxis and treatment.
4. The biguanides (**proguanil** [**chlorguanide**] and **chlorproguanil**), have triazine active metabolites (**cycloguanil** and **chlorcycloguanil**) similar to the diamino-pyrimidine **pyrimethamine**. They are known as type 2 antifolate drugs since they specifically inhibit

malarial dihydrofolate reductase (see Fig. 9.3) which is used by the parasites to make folinic acid cofactors for use in synthesis. Since they inhibit all growing stages of the malaria parasite, these drugs are used as causal prophylactics and are effective in preventing the growth of sporogonic stages in the mosquito (sporontocides). Potentiating mixtures of type 1 and type 2 antifolates (for example, sulfadoxine–pyrimethamine) are used in the treatment of infections resistant to blood schizontocides and especially to consolidate clinical cure produced by quinine in quinine-refractory strains of falciparum malaria. Some combinations are also valuable as causal prophylactics, although there may be problems with sulfonamide toxicity. The antibacterial combination sulfamethoxazole–trimethoprim also has significant antimalarial activity.

5. 8-Aminoquinolines (**primaquine** and **WR-238,605**) are believed to be converted in the liver to quinone active metabolites. These are particularly active against the non-growing stages (hypnozoites and gametocytes) in the human host. At concentrations effective against the growing stages they show toxicity to the host. These drugs are used as gametocytocidal drugs for falciparum and hypnozoitocidal (antirelapse) drugs for vivax and ovale malaria.
6. The antibiotics (**tetracycline**, **doxycycline**, **clindamycin** and **fluoroquinolones**) have little action on the pre-erythrocytic stages and a slow but marked action on the blood stages. They are all inhibitors of ribosomal protein synthesis, probably directed at the mitochondrion of the parasite. The use of these drugs in treatment is to consolidate a clinical cure achieved using quinine upon strains of malaria refractory to this drug. Doxycycline is also used as a suppressive prophylactic, but may have a photosensitizing effect in some individuals.
7. The peroxide antimalarial drugs [**artemisinin**, derived from the Chinese medicinal plant *Artemisia annua* and semi-synthetic analogues such as **artemether** and **arteether** (soluble in oil like **artemisinin**), **artesunate** and **artelinic acid** (water soluble)]. These are blood schizontocides with characteristics (such as concentration within infected erythrocytes and possible interactions with haemin) resembling groups 1 and 2 (above), but effective against parasites resistant to chloroquine and quinine. Prophylactic use of these, as yet, experimental drugs is considered to be unwise, because of their embryotoxic effects, but they are particularly promising in the treatment of severe and complicated falciparum malaria where rapid effects on the parasites are required. There is a marked potentiation between these drugs and arylaminoalcohols which has been useful clinically.
8. The naphthoquinones (**atovaquone** previously designated BW566C80) are slow-acting but potentially valuable experimental drugs which act upon the electron transport chain in the malarial mitochondrion by virtue of their structural similarity to coenzyme Q. They are potentially active on all growing stages of the parasite, and so have prophylactic potential. When used for treatment of falciparum malaria, recrudescence due to selection of resistant clones is a common problem, but observations of potentiation with other antimitochondrial drugs such as tetracycline and with proguanil are encouraging.

Clinical uses of common antimalarial compounds

Quinine

For more than three centuries cinchona and its alkaloids, especially quinine, were the only effective drugs available for the relief of malaria. Within recent times, however, the new substances described below were synthesized and were believed to be not only superior to quinine but also less toxic. However, strains of *P. falciparum* resistant to chloroquine and other synthetic antimalarial drugs are now widespread and quinine is again the treatment of choice for severe falciparum malaria and is widely used in uncomplicated falciparum malaria.

After oral administration to healthy subjects or patients with uncomplicated malaria, quinine is almost completely absorbed by the intestinal tract. Twenty per cent is excreted in the urine and the rest by hepatic biotransformation, first to 3- and 2-hydroxyquinine and then to a series of more polar water-soluble metabolites. Peak plasma concentrations are reached in 1–3 hours. The mean elimination half-time is approximately 11 hours in

Arylaminoalcohols

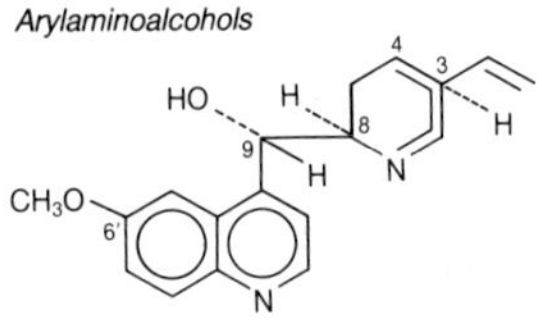

1. **Quinine**
(8S,9R)-6′-methoxycinchonan-9-ol

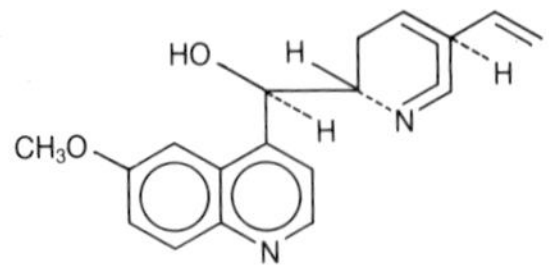

2. **Quinidine**
(8R,9S)-6′-methoxycinchonan-9-ol

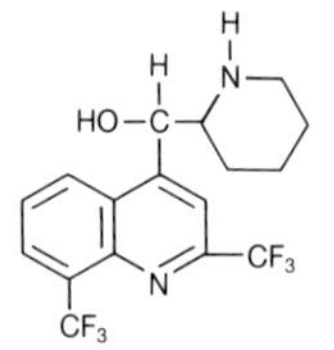

3. **Mefloquine (WR 142,490)**
α-(2-piperidyl)-2,8-bis(trifluoromethyl)-4-quinolinemethanol

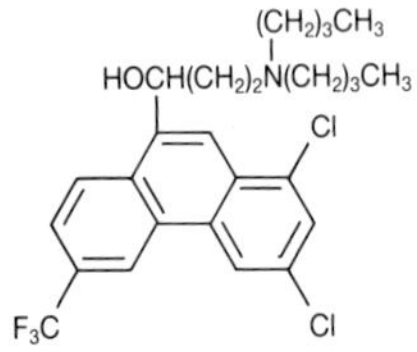

4. **Halofantrine**
1,3-dichloro-α-[2-(dibutylamino)-ethyl]-6-(trifluoromethyl)-9-phenanthrenemethanol

4-Aminoquinolines

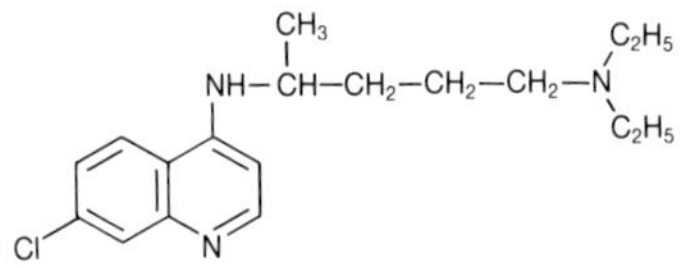

5. **Chloroquine**
7-chloro-4-(4′-diethylamino-1′-methylbutylamino)quinoline

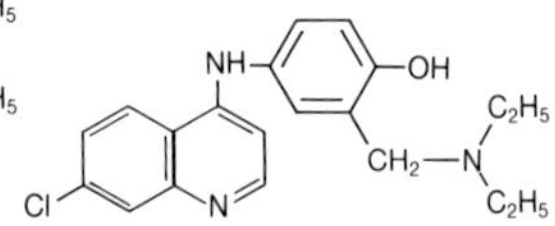

6. **Amodiaquine**
7-chloro-4-(3′-diethylaminomethyl-4′-hydroxyanilino)-quinoline

Acridines

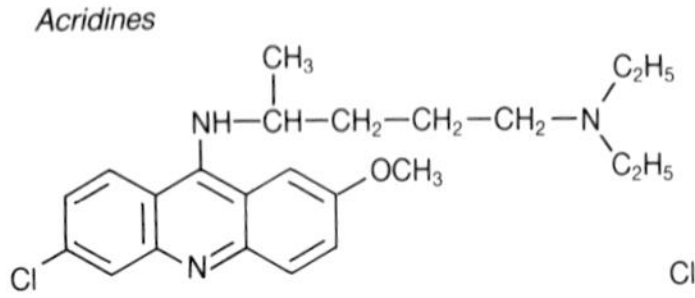

7. **Mepacrine**
2-methoxy-6-chloro-9-(4′-diethylamino-1′-methylbutylamino)-acridine

Benzonaphthyridines

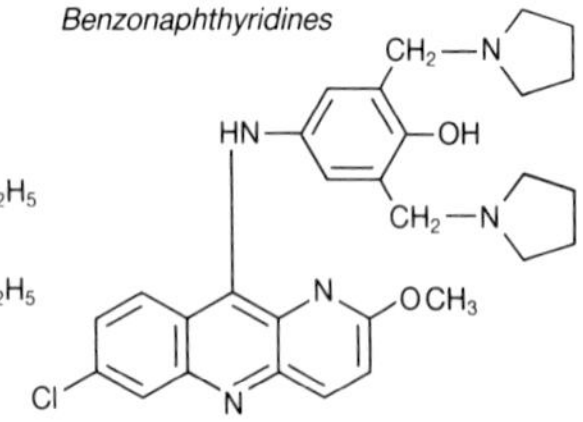

8. **Pyronaridine** (7351)
2-methoxy-6-chloro-9[3,5-bis(1-pyrrolidinylmethyl)-4-hydroxy]anilino-1-aza-acridine

Sulfonamides

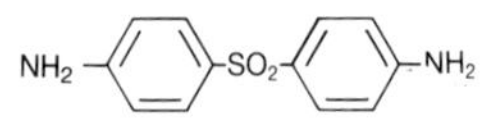

9. **Dapsone**
4,4′-diaminodiphenylsulfone

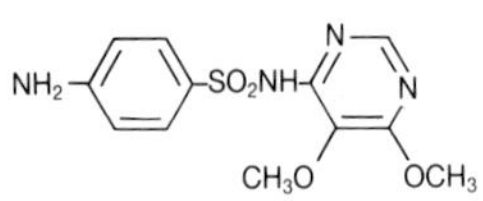

10. **Sulfadoxine**
N′-(5,6-dimethoxy-4-pyrimidinyl)-sulfanilamide

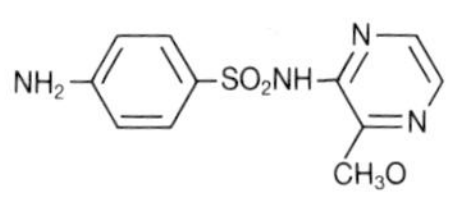

11. **Sulfalene**
N′-(3-methoxy-2-pyrazinyl)-sulfanilamide

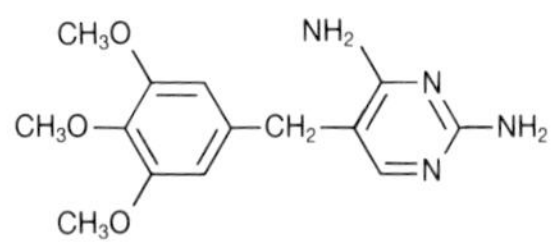

12. **Trimethoprim**
2,4-diamino-5-(3′,4′,5′-trimethoxybenzyl)pyrimidine

Dihydrofolate reductase inhibitors

Biguanides

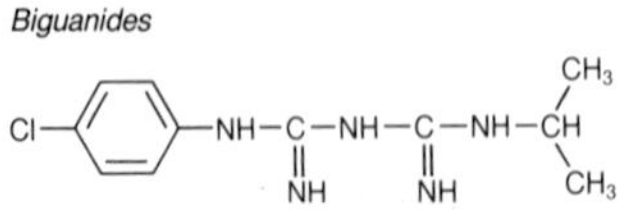

13. **Proguanil**
N[1](*p*-chlorophenyl)-*N*[5]-isopropyldiguanide

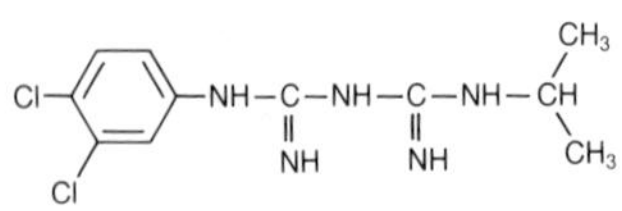

14. **Chlorproguanil**
N[1]-(3,4-dichlorophenyl)-*N*[5]-isopropyldiguanide

Diaminopyrimidines

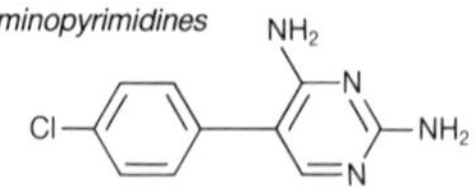

15. **Pyrimethamine**
2,4-diamino-5-*p*-chlorophenyl-6-ethylpyrimidine

8-Aminoquinolines

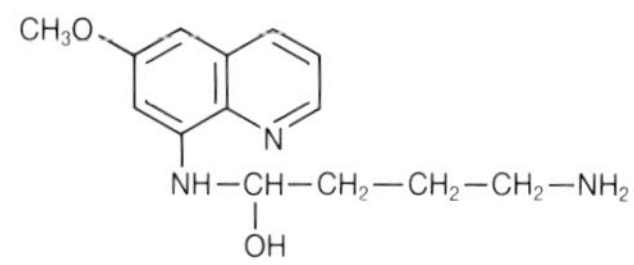

16. **Primaquine**
6-methoxy-8-(4′-amino-1′-methylbutylamino)quinoline

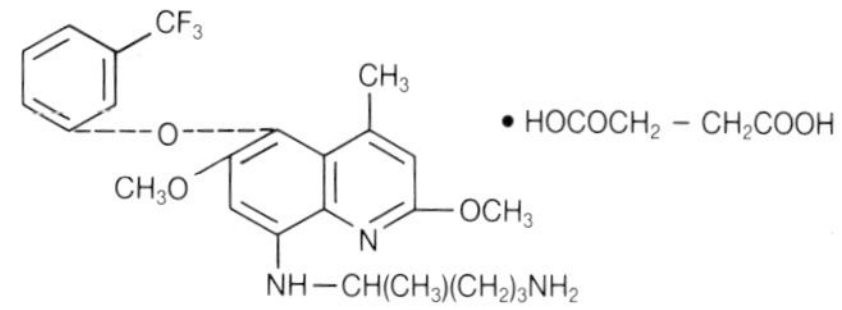

17. **WR 238,605**
2,6-dimethoxy-4-methyl-5-(3-trifluoromethyl)-phenoxy-8-(4-amino-1-methylbutyl-amino)quinoline

Antibiotics

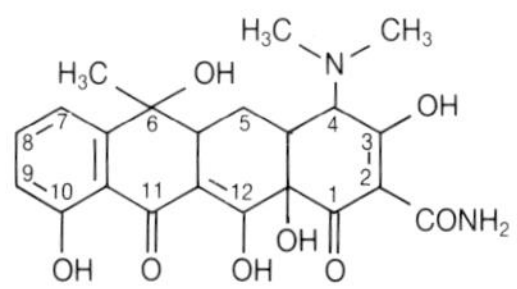

18. **Tetracycline**
4-dimethylamino-1,4,4a,5,5a,6,11,12a-octahydro-3,6,10,12,12a-pentahydroxy-6-methyl-1,11-di-oxo-2-naphthacenecarboxamide

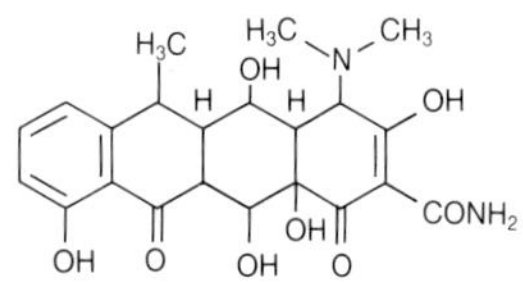

19. **Doxycycline**
4-dimethylamino-1,4,4a,5,5a,6,11,12a-octahydro-3,5,10,12,12a-pentahydroxy-6-methyl-1,11-di-oxo-2-naphthecenecarboxamide

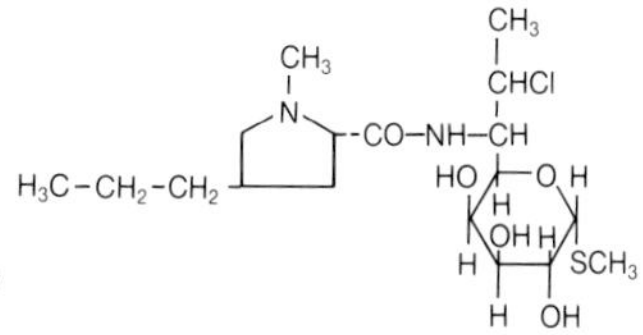

20. **Clindamycin**
methyl 7-chloro-6,7,8-tri-dioxy-6-*trans*-(1-methyl-4-propyl-L-2-pyrrolidine-carboxamido)-1-thio-L-*threo*-α-D-*galacto*-octo-pyranoside or: 7-(5)-chloro-7-desoxylinco-mycin)

Fluoroquinolones

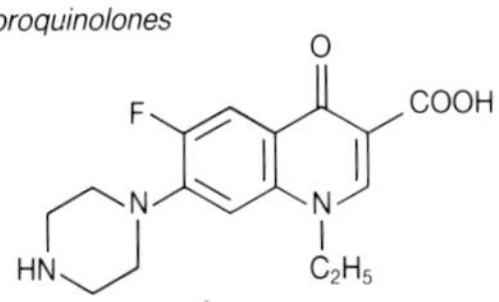

21. **Norfloxacin**
1-ethyl-6-fluoro-1,4-dihydro-4-oxo-7-(piperazin-1-yl) quinoline-3-carboxylic acid

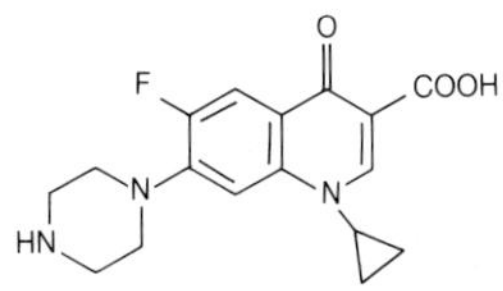

22. **Ciprofloxacin**
1-cyclopropyl-6-fluoro-1,4-dihydro-4-oxo-7-piperazin-1-yl quinoline-3-carboxylic acid

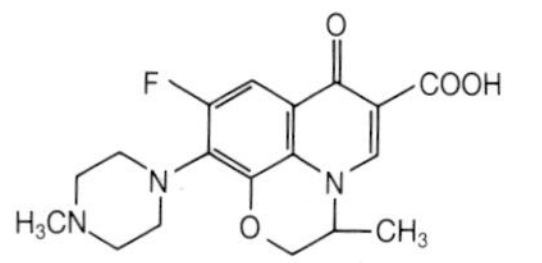

23. **Ofloxacin**
(+−)-9-fluoro-2,3-dihydro-3-methyl-10-(4-methyl-1-piperazinyl)-7-oxo-7H-pyrido[1,2,3-de]-1,4-benzoxacine-6-carboxylic acid

Sesquiterpene lactones

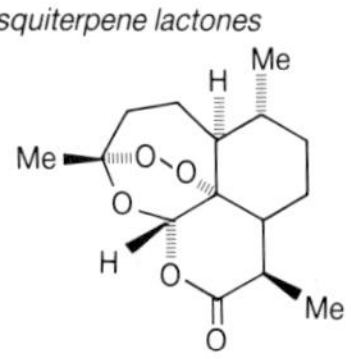

24. **Artemisinin**
(3R,5aS,6R,8aS,9R,12S,12aR) octahydro-3,6,9-trimethyl-3,12-epoxy-12*H*-pyrano[4,3-j]-1,2-benzodioxepin-10(3*H*)-one

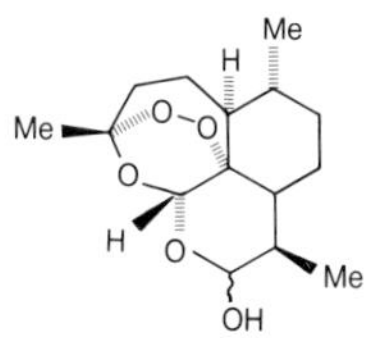

25. **Dihydroartemisinin**
3α, 12α-epoxy-3,4,5,5aα,6,7,8,8aα,9,10,12β,12a-dodecahydro-10β-hydroxy-3β,6α,9β-trimethylpyrano[4,3-j][1,2] benzodioxepin

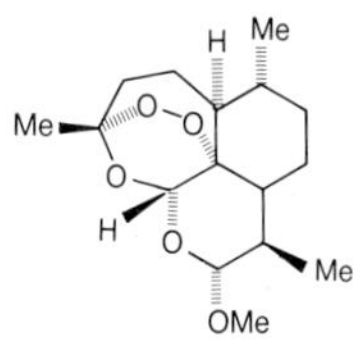

26. **10β artemether (crystalline)**
3α,12α-epoxy-3,4,5,5aα,6,7,8,8aα,9,10,12β,12a-dodecahydro-10β-methoxy-3β,6α,9β-trimethylpyrano[4,3-j][1,2] benzodioxepin

10α artemether is an oil

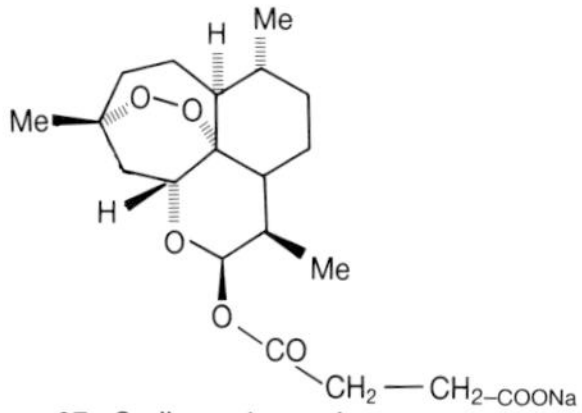

27. **Sodium artesunate**
3α,12α-epoxy-3,4,5,5aα,6,7,8,8aα,9,10,12β,12a-dodecahydro-3β,6α,9β-trimethylpyrano[4,3-j] [1,2]benzodioxepin-10α-yl sodium butanedioate

Naphthoquinones

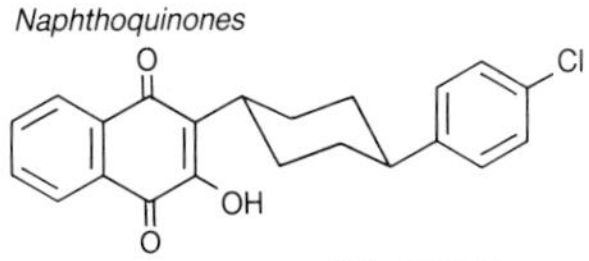

28. **Atovaquone (BW 566 C80)**
2-[*trans*-4-(4-chlorophenyl) cyclohexyl]-3-hydroxy-1, 4 naphthoquinone

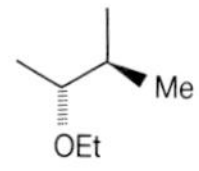

Arteether, as prepared by the method recommended by Brossi *et al.* is composed of the crystalline beta isomer only

3α,12α-epoxy-3,4,5,5aα,6,7,8,8aα,9,10,12β,12a-dodecahydro-10β-ethoxy-3β,6α,9β-trimethylpyrano[4,3-j][1,2] benzodioxepin

Fig. 9.2 Structures, chemical formulae and chemical names of principle antimalarial drugs.

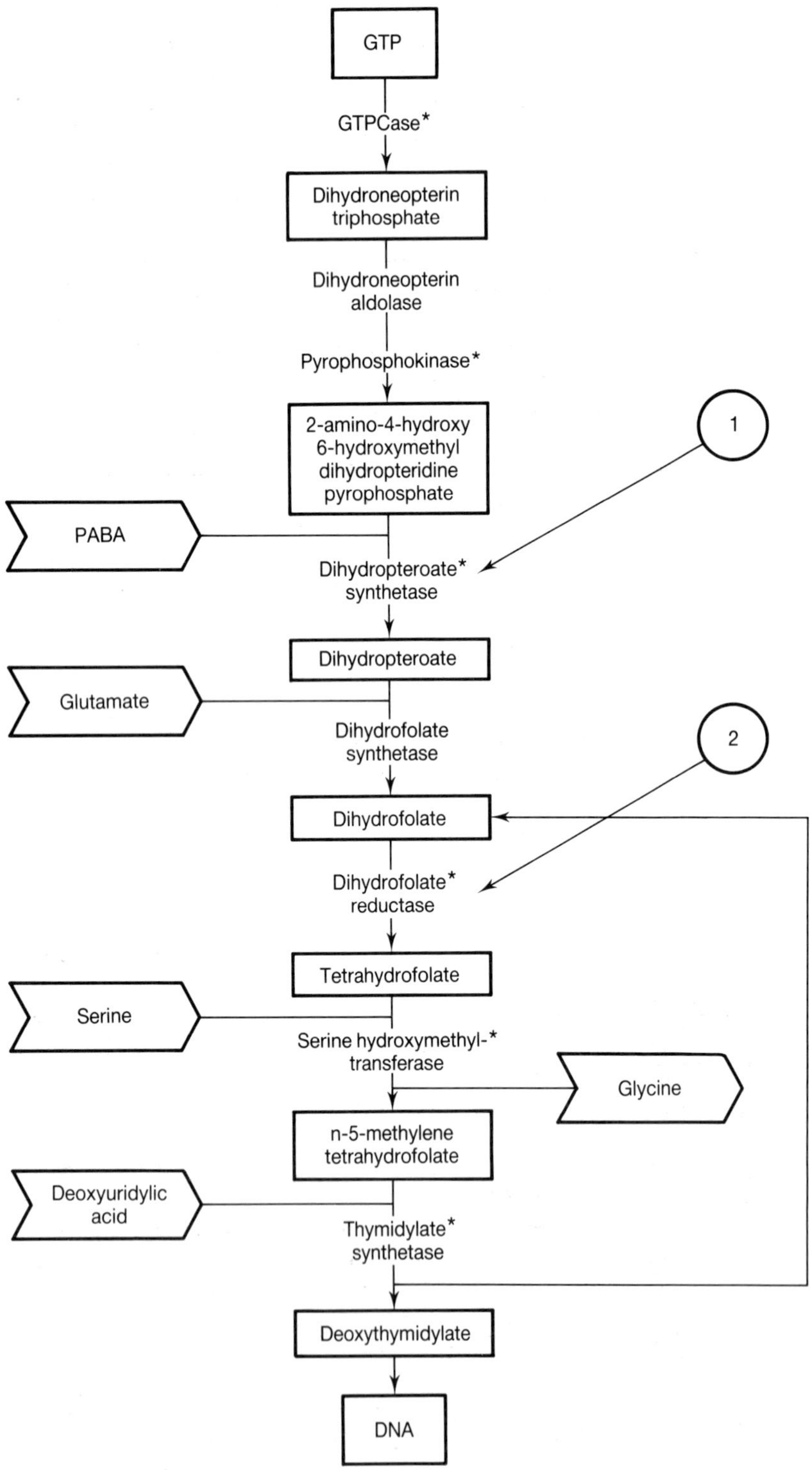

Fig. 9.3 Synthesis of DNA from guanosine triphosphate (GTP) by malaria parasites. Starred enzymes have been detected in malaria parasites, others are presumptive. 1 indicates site of action of sulfonamides such as sulfadoxine. 2 indicates site of action of pyrimethamine and cycloguanil. (Reproduced from Warhurst, *Parasitology Today* 1986, Vol. 2 (3), p. 58.)

healthy subjects, 16 hours in patients with uncomplicated malaria and 18 hours in those with severe disease. Quinine is most valuable in the treatment of severe falciparum malaria when it must be administered parenterally. Intravenous injection is dangerous as high plasma concentrations may result during the distribution phase causing potentially fatal hypotension or cardiac arrhythmias. However, quinine can be given safely if it is diluted and infused intravenously over 4 hours. When intravenous infusion is impossible because of lack of nursing supervision or facilities (Fig. 9.4), quinine may be given by intramuscular injection into the anterior part of the thigh. It is well absorbed from this site in adults and children including those with severe disease. Since most deaths from severe falciparum malaria occur within the first few days of starting treatment, parasiticidal plasma concentrations of quinine must be achieved as quickly as possible by giving an initial loading dose of twice the maintenance dose, provided that the patient has not received quinine, quinidine or mefloquine within the preceding 24 hours. In adults, the loading dose of quinine dihydrochloride is 20 mg of the salt/kg body weight followed by a maintenance dose of 10 mg/kg every 8–12 hours. Recent studies in Kenya indicate that in children rather lower and less frequent doses would achieve optimal plasma concentration profiles: a loading dose of 15 mg of the salt/kg body weight, followed by a maintenance dose of 10 mg/kg every 12 hours (all infusions given over 2 hours). In patients requiring more than 48 hours of parenteral treatment, the maintenance dose should be reduced by one-half to one-third (i.e. 5–7 mg/kg). The initial dose of quinine should not be reduced in patients who are severely ill with renal or hepatic impairment. Administration should be changed to the oral route as soon as patients can swallow and retain tablets. Resistance to quinine is beginning to develop in some parts of the world such as South-east Asia, where RIII resistance has been suspected. In countries such as Thailand and Vietnam, 7 days of quinine must be given together with a 1-week course of tetracycline (250 mg four times a day) except in children under 8 years of age and pregnant women. A recent report indicates that although 7 days of quinine and tetracycline is still effective treatment for multidrug-resistant falciparum malaria in Thailand, there is a gradually increasing recrudescence rate and decreased *in vitro* sensitivity. However, in some areas a shorter course of quinine (3–5 days) followed by a single dose of pyrimethamine–sulfonamide (e.g. 'Fansidar') or a course of tetracyline is effective. Quinine, in conventional doses, has proved safe in pregnancy, even in the final trimester. In patients with evidence of intravascular haemolysis quinine should not be withheld as the evidence that it causes 'Blackwater fever' is not convincing. Quinine is effective for the treatment of benign malarias but would not normally be used for this purpose. In the treatment of uncomplicated falciparum malaria 10 mg of quinine salt per kilogram body weight (or 600 mg for most adults) is given three times a day for periods of up to 10 days. However, unsupervised patients are unlikely to complete long courses of quinine because of an unpleasant group of symptoms ('cinchonism') associated with therapeutic plasma quinine concentrations of above 5 mg/litre. This consists of transient high tone deafness, tinnitus, nausea, vomiting, dizziness, blurring of vision and malaise. Rarely, quinine may cause haemolysis, severe thrombocytopenia associated with quinine-dependent antiplatelet antibodies, disseminated intravascular coagulation, hypersensitivity reactions, cutaneous neutrophilic vasculitis, photosensitization and granulomatous hepatitis. Quinine overdose can cause severe central nervous system and cardiovascular toxicity including blindness, coma, convulsions, hypotension

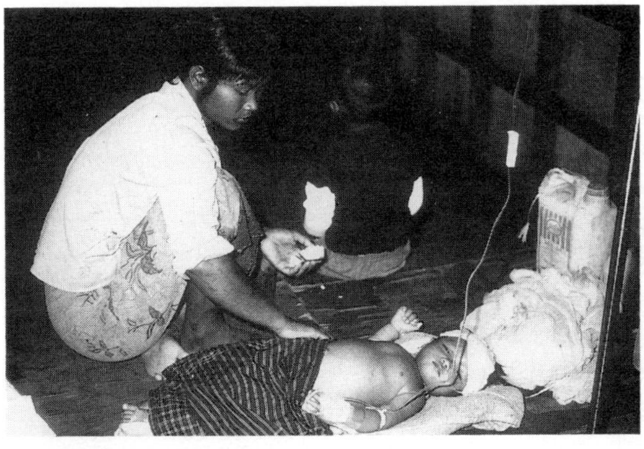

Fig. 9.4 Rural hospital in South-east Asia. Under these conditions the administration of quinine by intravenous infusion may be difficult or impossible, but the drug can be given by intramuscular injection (© D. A. Warrell.)

and myocardial conduction disturbances. These features are rare in patients being treated for malaria even though their total plasma quinine concentration may exceed 20 mg/litre. This may be explained by the increased binding of quinine to α-1 acid glycoprotein (orosomucoid) and other acute phase reactive serum proteins, the plasma concentrations of which may be more than doubled in patients with acute malaria.

The most common severe side effect of quinine during the treatment of malaria is hyperinsulinaemic hypoglycaemia (see above).

Quinine overdose should be treated with repeated oral charcoal (50 g four hourly). Quinine amblyopia and deafness has been treated with bilateral stellate ganglia block and the selective calcium antagonist, flunarizine.

Quinidine

Quinidine, the dextrorotatory diastereomer of quinine, is more effective than quinine against *P. falciparum* but is more cardiotoxic. In Europe and North America, parenteral quinidine gluconate injection is often stocked by hospitals for the treatment of cardiac tachyarrhythmias and may be a valuable alternative treatment for severe falciparum malaria if parenteral quinine is not available. It must be given by slow infusion while the ECG and blood pressure are monitored. It is as likely as quinine to cause hypoglycaemia.

Mefloquine ('Lariam')

This quinoline methanol which is structurally very similar to quinine is a potent long-acting blood schizontocide effective against all malarial species including *P. falciparum* parasites resistant to 4-aminoquinolines, pyrimethamine–sulfonamide combinations and quinine. It is too irritant to be given parenterally, but is well absorbed when given by mouth. Peak plasma/blood concentrations are achieved in 11–48 hours, the elimination half-time is 6–33 days. In patients with cerebral malaria, mefloquine suspension is absorbed rapidly but bioavailability is reduced so that plasma concentrations are only ½ to ⅓ of those in healthy subjects. The great advantage of mefloquine is that it can be given as a single dose of 15–25 mg base/kg body weight in adults and children. To reduce the risk of vomiting and other gastrointestinal side effects, the dose can be divided into two halves, given 6–8 hours apart. Mefloquine proved very effective in the first line treatment of slide-positive falciparum malaria when used in clinics of the Malaria Division throughout Thailand (Fig. 9.5). Recently, however, there has been a dramatic decline in efficacy especially along the Thai–Cambodian border, probably as a result of indiscriminate and intermittent use of the drug for prophylaxis among itinerant gem miners.

Toxic effects include dose-related dizziness, nausea, vomiting and abdominal colic, sinus bradycardia, sinus arrhythmia and postural hypotension. An 'acute brain syndrome', consisting of fatigue, asthenia, seizures and psychosis, has been observed in 0.2–1% of patients treated with mefloquine and in up to 1 in 10 000 Europeans given mefloquine for malarial prophylaxis. There has been a suggestion that mefloquine taken during the first trimester of pregnancy may be responsible for

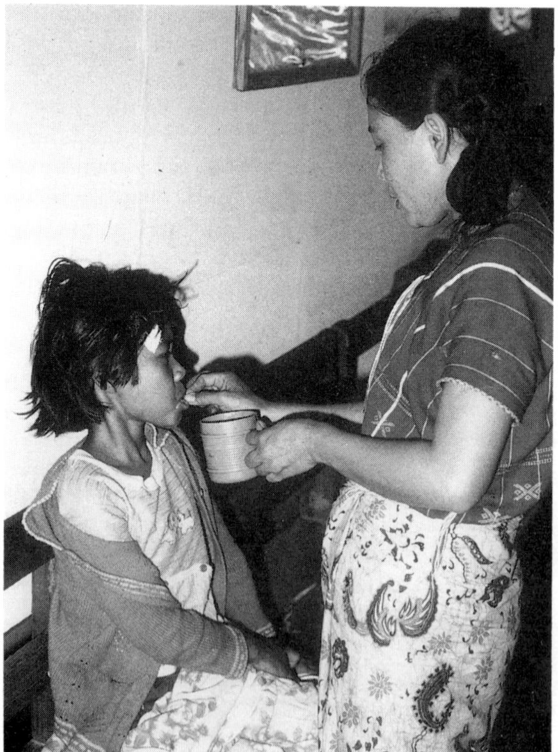

Fig. 9.5 Thai child receiving a single dose of mefloquine treatment for slide-positive falciparum malaria in the Malaria Division clinic at Mae Sod, Thailand in 1984 (© D. H. Warrell).

foetal abnormalities. At present, mefloquine treatment and prophylaxis should be avoided in those whose work demands fine coordination and spatial discrimination (such as airline pilots), those with known hypersensitivity to mefloquine, pregnant women, people taking beta-blockers and those with a past history of epilepsy or psychiatric illness.

Mefloquine has proved safe and effective as prophylaxis against malaria in an adult dose of 250 mg per week (see below).

The theoretical basis, efficacy and safety of combining mefloquine with sulfadoxine–pyrimethamine (in the form of 'Fansimef' or 'MSP') is questionable and this combination should not be used.

Halofantrine ('Halfan')

Halofantrine, a phenanthrene methanol, is another synthetic antimalarial drug active against multiresistant, including mefloquine-resistant, falciparum malaria.

Parenteral preparations are not yet available. Bioavailability is low, variable, but perhaps doubled if the drug is taken with a fatty meal. The recommended dose for adults and children weighing more than 37 kg is 500 mg of the salt (two tablets) taken every 6 hours for three doses (total 24 mg/kg body weight); in non-immune patients the manufacturers recommend that this dose should be repeated 1 week later. Maximum plasma concentrations are reached 6 hours after a single dose or 3 hours after the last of three divided doses. Halofantrine is almost entirely eliminated by hepatic biotransformation. The principal metabolite mono-N-desbutyl halofantrine has antimalarial activity equal to that of the parent drug but is more slowly cleared (terminal elimination half-life 3–5 days compared with 1–3 days for halofantrine itself). There is some evidence of cross-resistance with mefloquine and decreasing *in vitro* sensitivity. RI resistance has been observed in Africa, South America and South-east Asia. The drug is embryotoxic in animals and should not be given to pregnant or lactating women. Side effects are generally less than with mefloquine and consist only of abdominal pain and diarrhoea, but there is some concern about prolongation of the electrocardiographic QT_c interval in patients taking this drug.

Chloroquine

No other antimalarial drug has matched the speed of action, safety and breadth of activity exhibited by chloroquine when it was first introduced in the 1940s. Despite the very extensive spread of chloroquine-resistant strains of *P. falciparum* and the recent emergence of chloroquine-resistant *P. vivax* in New Guinea, chloroquine is still by far the most widely used antimalarial drug in the world. Chloroquine is so widely and readily available as a treatment for fevers and suspected malaria that in many parts of Africa more than half the patients presenting to hospital with malaria are found to have chloroquine in their blood. Chloroquine remains effective treatment for benign malarias worldwide and for uncomplicated and even severe falciparum malaria in restricted areas such as Central America west of the Panama Canal, Haiti, the Dominican Republic and parts of the Middle East and West Africa (Plate 28). Against sensitive strains it is a highly effective and rapid blood schizontocide and is gametocytocidal against *P. vivax*, *P. malariae* and *P. ovale*.

In healthy adults and in patients with uncomplicated malaria it is rapidly absorbed, peak plasma concentrations being reached in 2 hours. The bioavailability is 70–75%. Absorption after intramuscular or subcutaneous injection is very rapid which can produce transient dangerously high plasma concentrations unless small doses are given frequently (for example, 3.5 mg *base*/kg 6-hourly or 2.5 mg base/kg 4-hourly, rather than the more conventional 5 mg base/kg 12-hourly). Cases of children dying soon after intramuscular injection of chloroquine are probably explained by its rapid absorption and the resulting hypotension. About half of the absorbed chloroquine is cleared unchanged by the kidney and the remainder is biotransformed by the liver, mainly to desethyl- and bisdesethyl-chloroquine. Therapeutic blood concentrations persist for 6–10 days after a single dose but the terminal elimination half-time is 1–2 months.

The total dose of chloroquine for the treatment of malaria is 25 mg *base*/kg body weight. The simplest regimen is 10 mg base/kg on the first and second days and 5 mg/kg on the third day. Another commonly used regimen is 10 mg base/kg followed by 5 mg/kg 6–8 hours later and 5 mg/kg on the second and third days.

Chloroquine is generally very well tolerated but when plasma concentrations exceed 250 μg/ml unpleasant symptoms such as dizziness, headache, diplopia, disturbed visual accommodation, dysphagia, nausea and malaise may develop. These symptoms are most likely to occur when the drug is administered intravenously. Systolic hypotension and ECG abnormalities have been observed during the initial distribution phase. In Africans, Haitians and dark-skinned Asians, pruritus of the palms, soles and scalp is a tiresome problem. Rare toxic effects include photoallergic dermatitis, skin pigmentation, leucopenia, bleaching of the hair and aplastic anaemia.

For the treatment of chloroquine-sensitive severe falciparum malaria chloroquine is best administered by continuous intravenous infusion of the total dose of 25 mg base/kg over 30 hours (for example, split up into 5 × 6-hour infusions of 5 mg base/kg). Infusion of 10 mg base/kg over 8 hours, followed immediately by 15 mg base/kg 8-hourly continuously over the next 24 hours gives an even better plasma concentration profile.

Chloroquine has proved more rapidly effective than quinine in chloroquine-sensitive falciparum malaria. Some caution should be exercised in giving chloroquine to patients with epilepsy and psoriasis.

Chloroquine overdose* (ingestion of 20 mg base/kg or more at one time) produces symptoms within 30 minutes to 6 hours: these include nausea, headache, drowsiness, blurring of vision, malaise, vomiting, speech abnormalities, jaw contractions, hypokalaemia, thrombocytopenia, increased fibrin/fibrinogen degradation products (FDPs), coma, convulsions, hypotension, respiratory paralysis and cardiac arrest. Fatal cardiac arrest may occur only 1 hour after ingestion. Electrocardiographic changes include sinus tachycardia, bradycardia, prolongation of the QT interval, ectopic beats, ventricular tachycardia and fibrillation, idioventricular rhythm, torsade de pointes and asystole.

Blood chloroquine concentrations of more than 7 μmol/l and certainly of more than 25 μmol/l were fatal before the introduction of the modern treatment for chloroquine overdose which consists of diazepam, adrenaline and mechanical ventilation. Diazepam competes with chloroquine for binding at benzodiazepine receptors in heart muscle and adrenaline counteracts the effects of chloroquine on the myocardium and blood vessels.

Chloroquine remains the most widely used chemoprophylactic drug (see below). The usual adult dose is 300 mg base taken once a week. A cumulative dose of 50–100 g taken over several years can cause irreversible neuroretinitis. Chloroquine is safe in pregnancy.

Amodiaquine

This 4-aminoquinoline is similar to chloroquine in many respects but appears to retain some activity against chloroquine-resistant strains of *P. falciparum*. However, this advantage is usually short-lived and, unlike chloroquine, one of its metabolites, a quinoneimine, produces toxic hepatitis and potentially lethal agranulocytosis (occurring in 1 in 2000 of people taking amodiaquine prophylactically). Amodiaquine is still used in some countries such as Papua New Guinea and Myanmar, but because of its risks and the limited therapeutic advantage over chloroquine, its use for prophylaxis and repeated treatment is now discouraged.

Mepacrine (quinacrine, atabrine)

Mepacrine was introduced for the treatment of malaria in 1930 and, at one time, was thought to be superior to quinine. Mepacrine is deposited in the skin (causing a bright yellow colour) and also causes skin eruptions and mental disturbances, while intramuscular mepacrine may produce fatal collapse or brain damage. In the 1950s it was superseded by chloroquine and is now obsolete for the treatment of malaria although it is still widely used for the treatment of giardiasis and occasionally for diphillobothriasis and taeniasis.

Pyronaridine

Pyronaridine is a naphthyridin derivative and mannich base synthesized in China. Its structure is reminiscent of mepacrine and amodiaquine but it is effective against multiple-resistant *P. falciparum* parasites. It can be given by mouth or by intramuscular or intravenous injection. Side effects are mild: headache, dizziness, gastrointestinal dis-

***Riou B., Barriot P., Rimailho A., Baud F. J. (1988) Treatment of severe chloroquine poisoning. *New Eng J Med* 318: 1–6.**

orders and transient ECG abnormalities after oral administration.

Sulfones

The activity of diamino-diaphenyl sulfone (DDS or dapsone) against malaria parasites has been known since the 1940s, but the interest in this compound and sulfonamides has increased during the past two decades because of the appearance of resistance in *P. falciparum*. Early clinical trials confirmed the schizontocidal effect of dapsone, especially against *P. falciparum*, but the drug, which had a half-life of 25 hours, was much slower in action than chloroquine. Dapsone may produce side effects in susceptible subjects and this has limited its usefulness. It is now mainly used in combination with pyrimethamine as the chemoprophylactic drug 'Maloprim' or 'Deltaprim' (see below). This combination is often prescribed for travellers from Britain, is recommended by the Australian authorities for prophylaxis in Indonesia and Papua New Guinea and has been used for many years for mass malaria prophylaxis among plantation workers and others in Zimbabwe. More recently, it has been found to be safe and effective for prophylaxis in young Gambian children. The commonest side effect of Maloprim is probably methaemoglobinaemia in people with hereditary NADH methaemoglobin reductase deficiency. Affected individuals quickly develop dusky cyanosis, noticed first in the nailbeds, after taking a tablet. A nodular eosinophilic pneumonia attributed to the pyrimethamine component is rarely reported and, especially when the weekly dose is doubled to two tablets (each containing 100 mg dapsone, 12.5 mg pyrimethamine), there is an incidence of potentially fatal agranulocytosis of 1 in 2000.

Sulfonamides

Sulfalene (sulfamethoxypyrazine) has a plasma half-life of 65 hours. It is a good schizontocide and suppressive in chloroquine-resistant malaria, but some strains of *P. falciparum* respond less quickly. At a single dose of 1–1.5 g together with an antifolate compound, this is an acceptable therapeutic antimalarial combination in areas of drug-resistant malaria. The combination of sulfamethoxypyrazine with pyrimethamine is known as 'Metakelfin'.

Sulfadoxine (Fanasil) is rapidly absorbed from the gut and has a long half-life (120–200 hours) so that effective drug levels can be maintained by a single or weekly oral administration. This compound is less effective against *P. vivax* than against *P. falciparum*. Its real value lies in the synergistic combination with antifolate compounds such as pyrimethamine. This combination at a ratio of 20:1, known as 'Fansidar', was once valuable in the treatment of all chloroquine-resistant falciparum infections. A single adult dose of three tablets of Fansidar (total 1500 mg sulfadoxine, 75 mg pyrimethamine) has been found to be relatively safe and effective. However, resistance to Fansidar emerged in 1980 in South-east Asia, Indonesia and the Amazon area of South America (Plate 28).

Fansidar is also formulated for intramuscular injection. Since the combination acts only on the late trophozoite and schizont stages, theoretical concerns were raised about its efficacy and speed of action. However, in practice, it clears parasitaemia as quickly as chloroquine but, since it has no antipyretic effect, produces a less dramatic clinical cure. In patients who are hypersensitive to sulfonamide, these combinations may cause systemic vasculitis, Stevens–Johnson syndrome (Plate 26) or toxic epidermal necrolysis (Plate 27). In the USA in the mid 1980s the risk of fatal reactions was as high as 1 in 18 000 to 1 in 26 000 prophylactic courses. Aplastic anaemia and agranulocytosis can also occur. Pyrimethamine and sulfonamide cross the placenta and are excreted in milk. In the foetus and neonate, sulfonamides can displace bilirubin from plasma protein binding sites causing kernicterus. For these reasons, sulfonamide–pyrimethamine combinations are not recommended during pregnancy or lactation unless no alternative drug is available.

Co-trimoxazole (trimethoprim and sulfamethoxazole)

Co-trimoxazole is effective treatment for uncomplicated falciparum malaria in adults and children in malaria endemic regions of Africa. Since it is also recommended for acute lower respiratory tract infections in African children, it has been suggested as an effective single treatment for febrile illnesses in young children in areas where malaria is endemic, resources are few and diagnosis must rely on clinical findings alone.

Proguanil (chlorguanide)

The great advantage of this antifolate drug is safety, in which it excels against all other drugs. When given in proper doses it causes no ill-effects, although in recent years, since the daily dose for prophylaxis (usually in combination with chloroquine) has been increased to 200 mg, mouth ulceration, hair loss and mild gastrointestinal symptoms have been described. This drug has a slow schizontocidal action on the erythrocytic forms of malaria parasites but is highly effective against the primary exo-erythrocytic (hepatic) forms and has sporontocidal effects on *P. falciparum*. It is less active against *P. vivax*.

Proguanil was first used for treatment of malaria (300 mg twice a day for 10 days). Although it was successful in a proportion of cases, there were many failures and it is now not recommended for this purpose. However, recently, there has been renewed interest in its use for treatment in combination with dapsone. In Kenya the combination of chlorproguanil (1.25 mg/kg) and dapsone (4 or 8 mg/kg) proved effective in the treatment of uncomplicated falciparum malaria. Proguanil is rapidly absorbed after oral administration; peak plasma concentrations are reached in about 4 hours. Proguanil and chloproguanil are converted into the active triazine metabolites, cycloguanil and chlorcycloguanil. About 40% is excreted in urine and faeces. The elimination half-life of proguanil is from 11 to 20 hours and plasma concentrations fall to an undetectable level a week after dosage.

In Kenya there is evidence of two subpopulations with extensive or poor conversion of prodrug to the active metabolite by hepatic mixed functional oxidases. Because of its safety and relative efficacy in many malarious areas, proguanil (200 mg every day) in combination with chloroquine remains the standard prophylactic regimen recommended by authorities in the UK (see below).

Pyrimethamine

Resistance to this folate inhibitor is now widespread and it is used only in combination with chloroquine, sulfonamides or sulfones for treatment and prophylaxis.

Primaquine

This 8-aminoquinoline is currently the only drug available which kills the hypnozoites (latent liver stages) of the relapsing malarias *P. vivax* and *P. ovale*. It is essential for the radical cure of these infections. Primaquine is gametocytocidal for all species of malaria. Mass primaquine treatment of patients with *P. falciparum* infection could eliminate the sexual cycle in mosquitos. The principal drawback of primaquine is that it causes haemolysis in patients with congenital deficiencies of erythrocyte enzymes, notably glucose-6-phosphate dehydrogenase (G6PD). However, severe intravascular haemolysis is unusual even in G6PD-deficient patients, except in certain areas of the world such as Sardinia and Sri Lanka. Primaquine can cross the placenta and is excreted in breast milk and so it should not be used in pregnancy or lactation in areas where G6PD deficiency is prevalent. Primaquine, like sulfonamides and sulfones (e.g. dapsone, see above) can produce severe haemolysis and methaemoglobinaemia in patients with congenital NADH methaemoglobin reductase deficiency.

A single adult dose of 30–45 mg base is adequate for eliminating gametocytes. For radical cure of *P. vivax* and *P. ovale* 15 mg base is given daily for 14 days, but patients with G6PD deficiency tolerate better a weekly dose of 30–45 mg base for 8 weeks. Throughout South-east Asia and Oceania (Solomon Islands, Indonesia, Thailand, Papua New Guinea etc.) the primaquine-resistant Chesson-type strain of *P. vivax* requires a total dose of 6.0 mg/kg (twice the usual dose) usually given as 15 mg base per day for 28 days.

WR238,605

This new 8-aminoquinoline has been developed by the Walter Reed Army Institute of Research in Washington. It appears to be more than ten times more active as a hypnozoitocidal drug than primaquine and also has some blood schizontocidal activity.

Tetracycline

Tetracycline has proved a useful addition to quinine in areas of emerging quinine resistance such as South-east Asia. Although it has some blood schizontocidal activity, its slow and uncertain action justifies its use only in an ancillary role at an adult dose of 1–2 g daily for 7 days.

Doxycycline is an effective chemoprophylactic

drug for multiresistant falciparum malaria and is indicated especially in areas where mefloquine resistance is now common, such as Thailand and Cambodia. The daily dose is 100 mg. Unusually severe sunburn is evidence of photosensitization. Doxycycline prophylaxis is also effective against scrub typhus, travellers' diarrhoea (enterotoxogenic *Escherichia coli*) and leptospirosis.

Tetracyclines should not be used in pregnant or lactating women and in children under the age of 8 years because of its damaging effects on developing bones and teeth. In patients with severe falciparum malaria, tetracycline treatment should not be started until renal function has returned to normal.

Clindamycin

This is a synthetic derivative of lincomycin which has proved effective in uncomplicated falciparum malaria in various parts of the world used in 3–7 day courses in dose of 20 mg/kg body weight per day. In South America, Africa and the Philippines, it was effective against multidrug resistant *P. falciparum* infection. In Brazil, a 3-day course combining quinine 15 mg/kg twice a day and clindamycin 10 mg/kg twice a day proved more effective than a 3-day course of quinine–Fansidar. No serious side effects and, in particular, no *Clostridium difficile*-associated diarrhoea has been reported when clindamycin is used for antimalarial chemotherapy. Although its action is rather slow, and it should never be used alone, especially in more severe infections, it may be a useful drug in combination with quinine and other antimalarial drugs.

Fluoroquinolones

Evidence of slight activity of these expensive antibacterial agents does not justify their use in the treatment of malaria.

Artemisinin (qinghaosu)

This is a very interesting and important antimalarial compound, a sesquiterpine lactone, extracted from the herb *Artemisia annua* (sweet wormwood) which has been used as a treatment for fevers in China for more than 1000 years. Its peroxide (trioxane) configuration is responsible for its antimalarial activity. Artemisinin derivatives are very rapidly effective against malaria parasites including multiresistant strains of *P. falciparum* but recrudescences are commonly reported suggesting that these drugs should not be used alone for the treatment of falciparum malaria. Treatment of many thousands of patients in China and a very much smaller but rapidly increasing number outside China, has failed to reveal any serious toxicity, but animal studies suggest some effect on bone marrow (erythroid series), cardiotoxicity and foetal toxicity. In China, the drug has been used in the following forms:

Artemisinin suppositories have proved effective even in cerebral and other severe falciparum infections.

Artemether is dissolved in peanut oil and given by intramuscular injection. An adult dose of 200 mg is given on the first day and 100 mg each day on the subsequent 4 days or 3.2 mg/kg on day 1 and 1.6 mg/kg on days 2–5.

Sodium artesunate is prepared by dissolving anhydrous artesunic acid powder in 5% sodium bicarbonate solution just before intravenous injection to minimize the hydrolysis of the unstable solution. Both artesunate and its active metabolite dihydroartemisinin are rapidly eliminated (average elimination half-times 23 and 45 minutes, respectively).

Artesunate is also formulated as tablets and has proved effective for the treatment of uncomplicated falciparum malaria in China.

In a recent trial in Thailand, artesunate tablets (100 mg immediately followed by 50 mg every 12 hours for 5 days – total dose 600 mg) combined with mefloquine (750 mg followed by a further 500 mg after 6 hours) proved effective in curing adults with uncomplicated falciparum malaria and was more effective than artesunate or mefloquine given alone.

The artemisinin derivatives may well become the most important drugs for treatment of multiresistant falciparum malaria in the 1990s. Well-designed trials are now underway comparing the efficacy of artemether and quinine in patients with severe falciparum malaria.

Hydroxynaphthoquinones (atovaquone, BW566C80)

The antimalarial activity of naphthoquinone was first demonstrated in the early 1940s. There was some earlier interest in lapinone (M-72350), menoctone (WR49808) and BW58C, but the most promising compound has been atovaquone which clears resistant *P. falciparum* parasitaemia in Aotus monkeys and humans. Unfortunately, there was a high incidence of recrudescences in the early human studies attributed to the very rapid development of resistance, but combination with tetracycline or proguanil may prevent this problem.

Drugs which reverse chloroquine resistance

The mechanism of chloroquine resistance in *P. falciparum* is an active process by which chloroquine is excreted from the parasite's food vacuole and so does not reach lethal concentrations in its cytoplasm. This resistance has been effectively reversed in *P. falciparum* strains *in vitro* and in some cases *in vivo* in Aotus monkeys, and against chloroquine-resistant strains of *P. berghei* in mice by calcium channel blockers (e.g. verapamil and nifedipine), the antidepressant tricyclic desiprimine and a number of antihistamines (e.g. cyproheptadine, ketotifen and pizotifen). Although the doses and plasma concentrations of these drugs required to synergize the activity of chloroquine were not high, there was obvious concern about toxicity and no clinical trials have yet taken place in humans. Conversely, calcium agonists such as phenytoin may produce a clinically significant increase in resistance to chloroquine. Calcium antagonists may be found to reverse resistance to other drugs such as mefloquine.

Iron chelators (desferrioxamine)

Desferrioxamine suppresses the growth of *P. falciparum in vitro* and in Aotus monkeys and of *P. vinckei* and *P. berghei* in rodents. This compound also inhibits the hepatic stage of *P. falciparum* and *P. yoelii in vitro* in cultures of hepatocytes. Preliminary human studies in asymptomatic and uncomplicated falciparum malaria have demonstrated elimination of parasitaemia and in a recent study of Zambian children with cerebral malaria addition of desferrioxamine resulted in significantly shorter times to recovery of consciousness and parasite clearance than in controls treated with antimalarials alone, but there was no effect on mortality.

Practical antimalarial chemotherapy

Prescribing quinoline antimalarial drugs

The various salts of quinoline compounds (cinchona alkaloids and related compounds such as mefloquine and halofantrine, 4-aminoquinolines and 8-aminoquinolines) contain greatly differing amounts of base (Table 9.1). If the prescription fails to specify salt or base, or which particular salt is intended, serious problems of over- or underdosing can arise. Whenever possible the dose of base should be prescribed. This is generally accepted for mefloquine, chloroquine, amodiaquine and primaquine, but, in the case of quinine, quinidine and halofantrine doses of salts are usually quoted.

Table 9.1 Salt/anhydrous base equivalents of common quinoline antimalarial drugs

Antimalarial drug	Salt (mg)	Base (mg)
Amodiaquine sulfate	130	100
Chloroquine sulfate	136	100
Chloroquine phosphate	161	100
Chloroquine hydrochloride	123	100
Halofantrine hydrochloride	107	100
Mefloquine hydrochloride	110	100
Primaquine phosphate	18	10
Quinine sulfate	103	100
Quinine bisulfate	145	100
Quinine/quinidine dihydrochloride	122	100
Quinine/quinidine sulfate	121	100
Quinidine gluconate	161	100

Antimalarial chemotherapy: general considerations

Diagnosis

Ideally, the species of malaria parasite, the parasite density and the geographical origin of the infection should be known. In patients with features of severe malaria, a mixed infection including *P. falciparum* should be assumed even if parasites of one of the benign malarias alone are identified in the blood smear. A therapeutic trial is justified in patients who were exposed to infection and develop severe symptoms even if the blood smear is consistently negative.

Details of the patient

Choice of treatment will depend on the age and genetic origin of the patient, their presumed immune status and, in the case of women, whether they are pregnant or lactating or not. Dose must be calculated from the patient's weight whenever possible.

Clinical condition

A patient's clinical condition is of great importance. Patients with severe falciparum malaria and those who are vomiting will require parenteral treatment at least during the initial phase of management.

Prior treatment

Some prior treatment is extremely common particularly in developing countries where drugs such as chloroquine are sold across the counter for the treatment of fevers and suspected malaria. Malaria which breaks through prophylaxis (for example, with chloroquine) or which recrudesces or relapses after a recent course of chemotherapy is probably caused by a parasite resistant to that drug. People who have taken an antimalarial drug within the previous 24–36 hours may develop toxic blood levels if the same drug is given again or there may be adverse drug interactions if a different drug is given.

Objectives of chemotherapy

These will differ between mild and severe infections and in different geographical situations. In the treatment of uncomplicated infections in endemic areas the main objective may be to produce symptomatic improvement; radical cure may be an unrealistic objective where early reinfection is almost certain. In severe malaria, which can kill the patient within a few days, parasiticidal plasma concentrations of the antimalarial drug must be achieved as quickly and safely as possible and sustained for long enough to ensure rapid clearance of parasitaemia. Single dose regimens to ensure compliance, the prevention of recrudescences and the killing of gametocytes which may be important considerations in the treatment of uncomplicated malaria in endemic regions are of little importance in the treatment of severe disease. Symptoms which are troublesome to the fully conscious patient with uncomplicated malaria, such as cinchonism or pruritus, are acceptable in the treatment of life threatening disease and should not limit dosage.

Risk–benefit analysis

The choice of drugs for therapy and prophylaxis should depend on a proper assessment of the balance between the therapeutic needs and urgency in a particular case and the risks of toxicity.

Cost

Most malarious countries are relatively poor and so the choice of treatment will usually be determined by cost. In the UK at present the costs of some antimalarial drugs compared to chloroquine (= 1) are as follows: quinine 7.5, mefloquine 36.3, halofantrine 23.3; and in the USA: mefloquine 19.2, halofantrine 53.1, 'Fansidar' 1.3. In some estimates made by the WHO using European prices, the cost of a course of treatment relative to that of chloroquine (= 1) were as follows: halofantrine 66.4, mefloquine 24.0, quinine 18.4, amodiaquine 1.75, 'Fansidar' 1.6. Prices will vary a great deal in different countries and brand name antimalarial drugs are considerably more expensive than their generic equivalents on the international market.

Dosages

Recommendations for dosages of the principal antimalarial drugs are given in Tables 9.2 and 9.3.

Treatment of uncomplicated malaria

Table 9.2 outlines the antimalarial treatment available for those patients able to accept drugs orally.

Chloroquine remains the treatment of choice for *P. vivax*, *P. ovale*, *P. malariae*, monkey malarias and uncomplicated falciparum malaria in those geographical areas where this drug can still achieve a satisfactory clinical response. Chloroquine-resistant *P. vivax* has so far been reported only from New Guinea. Chloroquine-resistant *P. falciparum* is very widespread but even in areas where high level resistance is long established, such as Vietnam,

Table 9.2 Antimalarial chemotherapy in patients who can swallow tablets

Chloroquine-sensitive *P. falciparum* or *P. vivax*, *P. ovale*, *P. malariae* or monkey malarias	Chloroquine-resistant *P. falciparum* or origin of species unknown
1. *Chloroquine* Adults: 600 mg base on the 1st and 2nd days; 300 mg on the 3rd day Children: approximately 10 mg/kg on the 1st and 2nd days; 5 mg/kg on the 3rd day	1. *Mefloquine* Adults: 15–25 mg of the base/kg† given as 2 doses 6–8 hours apart Children: 25 mg/kg given as 2 doses 6–8 hours apart
	OR
For radical cure of vivax/ovale malaria add:	
2. *Primaquine* Adults (except pregnant and lactating women and G6PD-deficient patients): 15 mg base/day on days 4–17 or 45 mg/week for 8 weeks* Children: 0.25 mg/kg/day on days 4–17 *or* 0.75 mg/kg/week for 8 weeks*	2. *Halofantrine* Adults and children >37 kg (except pregnant or lactating women): 500 mg of the salt every 6 hours × 3 doses preferably with food Children: approximately 8 mg/kg every 6 hours × 3 doses In presumed non-immunes repeat after 1 week
	OR
	3. *Quinine* Adults: 600 mg of the salt 3 times each day for 7 days‡ Children: approximately 10 mg of the salt/kg 3 times each day for 7 days
	OR
	4. *Sulfonamide–pyrimethamine*§ Sulfadoxine (500 mg per tablet) or sulfalene (500 mg) plus pyrimethamine (25 mg) Adults: 3 tablets as single dose Children: <5 years ½ tablet, <9 years 1 tablet, <15 years 2 tablets

For salt/base equivalents see Table 9.1.
*For Chesson-type strains (South-east Asia, West Pacific) use double dose or double duration up to a total dose of 6 mg/kg in daily doses of 15–22.5 mg in adults.
†Depending on geographical area and presumed immunity.
‡In areas of quinine resistance (e.g. Thailand), add tetracycline 250 mg 4 times each day or doxycycline 100 mg daily for 7 days except for children under 8 years and pregnant women.
§Sulfadoxine + pyrimethamine (Fansidar); sulfalene + pyrimethamine (Metakelfin). Contraindicated if patient has known sulfonamide hypersensitivity or is pregnant or lactating.

chloroquine is still the most widely used treatment for uncomplicated falciparum malaria and still produces a clinical response albeit with RI or RII resistance in a majority of patients. Chloroquine is cheap, safe and in the usual 3-day course well tolerated but, despite the clinical improvement following chloroquine treatment, its failure to eliminate parasitaemia and the subsequent recrudescences may eventually lead to the development of profound anaemia. Primary health workers should be instructed routinely to look for anaemia, particularly in children, and if it is present should replace chloroquine with 'Fansidar' as soon as anaemia is clinically detected. In many parts of the malaria endemic area a decision may soon have to be made to replace chloroquine as the first-line treatment for falciparum malaria with a more expensive, more toxic and less well tolerated, drug. The switch to pyrimethamine–sulfonamide combinations has been made in many countries and, unfortunately, resistance usually develops within a few years. Combinations such as 'Fansidar' and 'Me-

Table 9.3 Antimalarial chemotherapy in adults or children with severe malaria (Table 3.2, p. 38) or in those who cannot swallow tablets **(all doses are given as base)****

Chloroquine-sensitive *P. falciparum** or *P. vivax*, *P. ovale*, *P. malariae* or monkey malarias	Chloroquine-resistant *P. falciparum* or origin unknown
1. *Chloroquine*† 25 mg base/kg diluted in isotonic fluid by continuous i.v. infusion over 30 hours (or 5 mg/kg over 6 hours every 6 hours) OR 2. *Quinine* (see above right-hand column)	1. *Quinine* Adults: 16.7 mg base/kg (loading dose)‡ diluted in 10 ml/kg isotonic fluid by i.v. infusion over 4 hours, then 8.4 mg/kg over 4 hours, 8–12 hourly until patients can swallow. Children: 12.5 mg base/kg (loading dose)‡ diluted in 10 ml/kg isotonic fluid by i.v. infusion over 2 hours, then 8.4 mg/kg over 2 hours, 12 hourly until patients can swallow. The 7-day course should be completed with quinine tablets approximately 8.4 mg/kg 8 hourly.§¶ OR 2. *Quinine* (in intensive care unit) 5.8 mg/kg (loading dose)‡ i.v. by infusion pump over 30 minutes followed immediately by 8.4 mg/kg (maintenance dose) diluted in 10 ml/kg isotonic fluid by i.v. infusion over 4 hours, repeated 8–12 hourly until patient can swallow etc.§¶ OR 3. *Quinidine* (in intensive care unit) 6.2 mg base/kg (loading dose)‡ i.v. by infusion over 1–2 hours, followed by 0.012 mg/kg/min by infusion pump for 72 hours or until the patient can swallow, then quinine tablets to complete 7 days treatment.§¶
If it is not possible to give drugs by i.v. infusion	
1. *Chloroquine*‡ Total dose 25 mg/kg given either (a) i.m. or s.c. 2.5 mg/kg 4 hourly; (b) i.m. or s.c. 3.5 mg/kg 6 hourly OR 2. *Quinine* i.m. (see above right-hand column)	1. *Quinine* 16.7 mg/kg (loading dose)‡ i.m. (anterior thigh), then 8.4 mg/kg 8–12 hourly until patient can swallow etc§¶

For salt/base equivalents see Table 9.1.
*Currently restricted to Haiti, Dominican Republic, Central America, parts of the Middle East and West Africa.
†Parenteral chloroquine should be used with great caution in young children.
‡Loading dose must not be used if patient started quinine or mefloquine treatment within preceding 24 hours.
§In areas of quinine-resistance (e.g. Thailand) add tetracycline 250 mg 4 times each day or doxycycline 100 mg daily for 7 days except for children under 8 years and pregnant women.
¶In patients requiring more than 48 hours of parenteral therapy reduce the dose to 4.2–2.8 mg/kg 8–12 hourly.
**Quinine 16.7 mg base = 20 mg dihydrochloride salt.
Quinine 8.4 mg base = 10 mg dihydrochloride salt.
Quinine 5.8 mg base = 7 mg dihydrochloride salt.
Quinine 4.2 mg base = 5 mg dihydrochloride salt.
Quinine 2.8 mg base = 3.3 mg dihydrochloride salt.

takelfin' have the great advantage of being single-dose treatments which are usually well tolerated except in people with hypersensitivity to sulfonamide (Plates 26 and 27). Quinine is an effective replacement for chloroquine in most areas where multidrug-resistant strains of *P. falciparum* are prevalent. However, it has the disadvantage of producing unpleasant symptoms (cinchonism – see above). In some countries a short course (3–5 days) of quinine followed by a single dose of pyrimethamine–sulfonamide is still effective. Quinine has also been combined with antibiotics such as tetracycline and clindamycin. Mefloquine, given as a single dose, or in divided doses 6–8 hours apart to reduce the risk of vomiting, was initially highly effective against multiresistant strains of falciparum malaria throughout the world. However, in some areas, notably in the border regions of Thailand, mefloquine resistance has developed rapidly and the dose has had to be increased from 15 to 25 mg/kg body weight to achieve reasonable cure rates. A proportion of patients, varying from 5 to 50% in different studies, suffer unpleasant gastrointestinal symptoms (nausea, vomiting, colicky abdominal pain and diarrhoea) and dizziness after taking mefloquine and a few develop more severe symptoms (see above). Halofantrine, the most recently marketed antimalarial drug, is coming into use for the treatment of uncomplicated multiresistant falciparum malaria. Because of its unpredictable absorption it is best taken with food, preferably a fatty meal. Three doses are taken at 6-hourly intervals and, in patients who are likely to be non-immune to malaria, the course is repeated after 1 week.

Most antimalarial drugs taste very bitter and must be given with a generous drink of milk, fruit juice or other flavoured fluid. Feverish patients, ill with acute malaria, may vomit the tablets and there will then be concern about whether the dose should be repeated. The risk of vomiting can often be reduced by insisting that the patient lies down quietly for a while after taking an antipyretic such as paracetamol (Acetaminofen). They may then be able to tolerate the antimalarial tablets. The oral administration of antimalarial drugs to infants and children with malaria is particularly difficult. Some antimalarial drugs are available as syrups or flavoured suspensions, or tablets can be crushed and attempts made to disguise their bitter flavour with honey, jam or chocolate. It is surprising that more effort has not been put into the development of suppository formulations of antimalarial drugs. The Chinese have used artemisinin suppositories with great success even in patients with cerebral and other severe forms of falciparum malaria. Many infants and children who, initially, will not tolerate oral treatment, will eventually be able to swallow and retain a tablet if they are laid quietly in bed, cooled, encouraged to take oral rehydration fluid and left 30–60 minutes before a further attempt is made to give the antimalarial drug. However, patients who vomit persistently will require treatment by injection, nasogastric tube or (where available) suppository. If these patients have no other features of severe malaria, they may soon be able to continue their course of treatment by mouth.

Ancillary treatment of uncomplicated malaria

Rehydration is important especially in hot climates where febrile patients may rapidly become dehydrated, and children and pregnant women whose tolerance of fasting is limited, may become hypoglycaemic. Mothers should be encouraged, through community education programmes, to give their children oral rehydration solutions containing extra glucose as in the home treatment of gastroenteritis.

Fever should be reduced by traditional methods such as removing the clothes, tepid sponging a large area of skin and fanning. Paracetamol (Acetaminofen) is the safest antipyretic drug which can be given by mouth or suppository. Crushed tablets can be administered via a nasogastric tube. Aspirin is out of favour because of its association with Reye's syndrome in children and with gastric erosions causing bleeding. Injectable antipyretics such as metamizole sodium (Dipyrone) are very convenient and widely used in developing countries. However, the risk of their causing agranulocytosis makes them unacceptable treatment.

Patients with uncomplicated malaria are often found to be anaemic. The causes are often multiple and complicated including the effect of repeated attacks of malaria, intestinal helminthic infections especially hookworm, inheritable erythrocyte abnormalities, malnutrition and sometimes the haemolytic effect of antimalarial drugs themselves. Treatment may be required with haematinics such as iron and folic acid, anthelminthics and, if the risk of blood-borne infections can be justified, with blood transfusion.

Treatment of severe falciparum malaria

The basic rules for the chemotherapy of severe malaria are as follows:

1. Treatment should be started immediately the diagnosis is proved or suspected.
2. Dosage should, wherever possible, be calculated according to the patient's weight.
3. The parenteral route must be used whenever possible as absorption of drugs through the gastrointestinal tract cannot be relied upon in severely ill patients who are often vomiting, may be shocked and in whom blood flow to the gut may be reduced. A loading dose is appropriate in order to achieve therapeutic blood concentrations of the drug as soon as possible. For quinine and artemether, the loading dose is double the maintenance dose. However, in the case of quinine, an initial loading dose should not be used if the patient has received quinine, quinidine or mefloquine during the previous 24 hours.
4. The therapeutic response must be carefully monitored by repeated clinical assessment, measurement of temperature, pulse, blood pressure etc. and examination of blood films.
5. Patients should be switched to oral treatment as soon as they are able to swallow and retain tablets.
6. Patients must be watched carefully for signs of drug toxicity. In the case of quinine and quinidine the commonest toxicity during antimalarial treatment is the development of hypoglycaemia. The blood sugar should, therefore, be checked frequently.

In patients with proven or suspected severe falciparum malaria, an intravenous infusion of quinine (usually quinine dihydrochloride) must be set up immediately. Delay in starting treatment is highly significantly correlated with mortality in patients with severe falciparum malaria in Thailand, and delays in diagnosis and treatment and the use of inappropriate antimalarial drugs account for most of the deaths among patients with imported malaria in western countries. Recommended parenteral regimes are given in Table 9.3.

At present, quinine is the only widely available drug that is effective for this condition, and should be used unless the patient is known to be hypersensitive to this drug. Chloroquine is less toxic than quinine and possibly more rapidly effective if the infecting strain is sensitive. However, chloroquine resistance is now so prevalent that most physicians would prefer to use quinine irrespective of the supposed geographical origin of the infection. Since chloroquine is still the most widely used first-line treatment and prophylaxis for malaria in tropical countries, many patients admitted to hospital with acute malaria will have failed already to respond to initial treatment with chloroquine or will have broken through chloroquine prophylaxis. In the USA, parenteral quinidine gluconate is now regarded as the drug of choice for the treatment of complicated *P. falciparum* malaria. The Centers for Disease Control Drug Service stopped supplying parenteral quinine dihydrochloride in 1991. Quinidine gluconate injection is often stocked by hospitals in the USA and continental Europe (but rarely in Britain) for treatment of cardiac arrhythmias and it can be used if there were likely to be any delay in obtaining parenteral quinine.

Further details about the administration and side effects of the cinchona alkaloids are given above. Therapeutic plasma concentrations of quinine and quinidine can be achieved rapidly and safely by the use of an initial loading dose which can be used in pregnant women and in severely ill patients with renal and hepatic dysfunction. There is evidence that the loading dose may reduce the duration of fever, parasitaemia and coma. To prevent accumulation, the maintenance dose should be reduced to a third to one-half after 48 hours of treatment, unless the patient is fit enough by that stage to switch to oral treatment. If it is possible to monitor plasma quinine/quinidine concentrations, the maintenance dose should be reduced if, at any stage, plasma concentrations exceed 15 mg/l (45 μmol/l).

It is likely that, during the next few years, artemisinin derivatives will become accepted outside China as the treatment of choice for severe resistant falciparum malaria. Uncontrolled studies in many thousands of patients in China and small pilot studies, some of them including comparisons with other antimalarial drugs in Burma, Vietnam, Thailand, Nigeria and the Gambia, have proved these drugs to be safe and rapidly effective. Results of further toxicity studies in animals and of large, well-designed comparative trials in adults and children should soon be available.

The importance of intramuscular administration of antimalarial drugs in situations where intravenous infusion is impossible has been discussed above. The considerable experience with intramuscular quinine in the past has been reinforced by recent studies in adults and children in Thailand, Vietnam, Papua New Guinea and several African countries. The high incidence of serious local complications (ulceration, muscle necrosis, peripheral nerve lesions, poliomyelitis, tetanus etc.) reported earlier this century with other formulations, some containing urethane and other dangerous adjuvants, has not been confirmed but it is clear that meticulous sterile technique must be employed when quinine is given by intramuscular injection. Other drugs which have proved effective against severe resistant falciparum malaria when given by intramuscular injection include 'Fansidar', artemether and artesunate.

Preliminary pharmacokinetic studies of an intravenous formulation of halofantrine have been carried out in animals.

Ancillary treatment of severe falciparum malaria (Table 9.4)

Hyperpyrexia

Ideally, core (rectal) temperature should be monitored continuously and should not be allowed to rise above 39°C as such temperatures are associated with clinical deterioration, febrile convulsions in children and foetal distress in pregnant women. Methods of lowering the body temperature have been described above. In the intensive care unit, the temperature of inspired gases and haemofiltrate can be reduced to aid cooling.

Cerebral malaria

Patients with impaired consciousness should be nursed in the lateral position with a rigid oral airway or endotracheal tube in place. Vital signs, level of consciousness (Glasgow coma scale in Table 3.4, p. 39) and incidence of convulsions should be recorded frequently. Generalized convulsions occur in more than 50% of patients with cerebral malaria. They are potentially harmful, leading to sustained neurological deterioration or aspiration pneumonia. Seizures must be treated promptly with a benzodiazepine drug such as diazepam, chlormethiazole or lorazepam. Convulsions may be prevented by controlling fever (in children) and by the use of prophylactic anticonvulsants such as a single intramuscular injection of phenobarbitone sodium (10–15 mg/kg body weight) or, in the intensive care unit, by phenytoin in a loading dose 10–15 mg/kg followed by an adult maintenance dose of approximately 100 mg every 6 hours controlled by daily measurement of blood phenytoin levels. Stomach contents should be aspirated through a nasogastric tube to reduce the risk of aspiration pneumonia. Elective endotracheal intubation is indicated if coma deepens and the airway is jeopardized.

Deepening coma and signs of cerebral herniation are indications for computer tomographic (CT) or magnetic resonance image (MRI) scanning or a trial of treatment to the lower intracranial pressure

Table 9.4 Principles of management of severe falciparum malaria

1. Suspect and attempt to confirm diagnosis
2. Make rapid clinical assessment, take blood etc. for laboratory investigations, check blood sugar and weigh the patient
3. Start appropriate parenteral antimalarial chemotherapy
4. Transfer to highest available level of medical care
5. Prevent convulsions (cerebral malaria) with prophylactic phenobarbitone
6. Detect complications such as hyperpyrexia and hypoglycaemia by monitoring and treat them
7. Correct fluid electrolyte and acid–base imbalance
8. Nurse the patient appropriately (e.g. comatose patients on their side, clear airway, turn frequently)
9. Avoid harmful ancillary treatments such as corticosteroids, heparin etc.

such as intravenous infusion of mannitol (1.0–1.5 g/kg of 10–20% solution over 30 minutes) or mechanical hyperventilation to reduce the arterial pCO_2 below 4.0 kPa. Two double blind trials of dexamethasone (2 mg/kg and 11 mg/kg intravenously over 48 hours) in adults and children with severe cerebral malaria showed no reduction in mortality but prolongation of coma and an increased incidence of infection and gastrointestinal bleeding. Low molecular weight dextrans, osmotic agents, heparin, adrenaline, cyclosporin A and prostacyclin have also been advocated for the treatment of cerebral malaria without adequate evidence and in some cases despite severe toxicity.

Anaemia

Where blood, competently screened for human immunodeficiency viruses (HIV), hepatitis B and other important pathogens, is available, transfusion with packed cells (90% of plasma removed) or whole blood should be considered when the haematocrit falls towards 20%. Exchange transfusion is a safe way of correcting the anaemia without precipitating pulmonary oedema in those who are fluid overloaded or chronically and severely anaemic (e.g. pregnant women in West Africa). The volume of transfused blood must be included in the fluid balance chart. Diuretics such as furosamide can be given intravenously in a dose of 1–2 mg/kg of the patient's body weight to promote diuresis during the transfusion. Survival of even compatible donor blood may be greatly reduced in patients during the acute and convalescent phases of falciparum malaria. This is not caused by quinine-mediated haemolysis.

Where screening of transfused blood is inadequate and infections such as HIV and HTLV-1 are prevalent, criteria for blood transfusion have become much more strict. This applies particularly to children in many parts of Africa.

Under these conditions plasma expanders (colloids) and oxygen should be used and clinical features such as shock, cardiac failure, hypoxia and extreme lethargy, rather than an arbitrary haematocrit value should be used as an indication for transfusion. However, a haematocrit of 15% in a normally hydrated child or adult is probably an absolute indication for blood transfusion. High parasitaemia, active or predicted bleeding (e.g. in a woman about to give birth) and other severe complications are other powerful indications for transfusion.

Hypoglycaemia

Frequent monitoring of the blood glucose (e.g. using a stix test such as Reflotest – Hypoglycemie and a Reflomat reader) is necessary especially in patients with severe or deteriorating symptoms. A therapeutic trial of 50% dextrose (1 ml/kg by intravenous bolus injection) should be given if hypoglycaemia is proved or suspected. This should be followed by a continuous infusion of 10% dextrose. In Malawi a continuous infusion of 5% dextrose (80 ml/kg over 24 hours) prevented quinine-induced hypoglycaemia in children who were initially normoglycaemic. However, in adults in the South-east Asia region, hypoglycaemia may develop or recur despite continuous intravenous infusions of 5% or even 10% dextrose. When the use of repeated doses of hypertonic dextrose for the treatment of quinine–quinidine-induced hypersinulinaemic hypoglycaemia is contraindicated (e.g. in patients with electrolyte disturbances or incipient fluid overload), the synthetic somatostatin analogue, 'Sandostatin' (SMS201–995), can be used in a single subcutaneous dose of 50 μg or a continuous intravenous infusion of 50 μg/hour (adult dose). Glucose (1 mg subcutaneously adult dose) must be given as well since somatostatin blocks glucagon release. Hypoglycaemia is easily corrected in patients receiving peritoneal- or haemo-dialysis or haemofiltration.

Metabolic acidosis

Lactic acidosis is treated by correcting hypovolaemia and improving oxygenation. Sodium bicarbonate may be given if the arterial pH falls below 7.0, but the value of this treatment remains controversial. Dichloroacetate which stimulates pyruvate dehydrogenase especially in skeletal muscle can reduce lactic acidosis.

Disseminated intravascular coagulation

If there is evidence of coagulopathy [spontaneous bleeding, oozing venepuncture sites, incoagulable blood, prolonged prothrombin time or international normalized ratio (INR)], vitamin K in an adult dose of 10 mg should be given by slow intravenous injection. Fresh frozen plasma or preferably cryoprecipitates should be given and platelet transfusion considered if the platelet count is less than 25 000 or the bleeding time prolonged.

Disturbances of fluid and electrolyte balance

Especially in tropical climates, patients with severe malaria may be salt and water depleted as a result of fever, diarrhoea, vomiting, high insensible losses and poor intake. Others, particularly those in renal failure, may be fluid overloaded because of excessive intravenous replacement. Hypovolaemia will lead to hypotension, shock, acute tubular necrosis and lactic acidosis, while circulatory overload may precipitate fatal pulmonary oedema. Fluid therapy should be controlled by measurements of jugular or central venous pressure. Mild hyponatraemia (plasma sodium concentration 120–130 mmol/l) is common in severe malaria and is probably explained by salt depletion. More severe hyponatraemia may be caused by inappropriate ADH secretion. Hypoalbuminaemia is common and may result in low plasma calcium concentrations. Hypophosphataemia is a feature of severe malaria and may be exacerbated by intravenous glucose therapy.

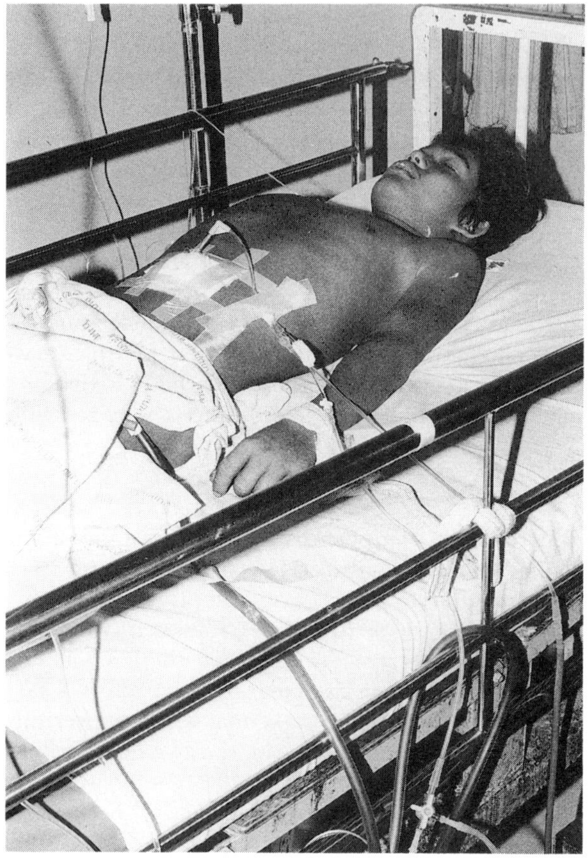

Fig. 9.6 Thai patient with severe falciparum malaria in acute renal failure receiving peritoneal dialysis. (Reproduced by courtesey of Dr R. E. Phillips.)

Renal failure

Renal dysfunction is seen in about one-third of adult patients with severe falciparum malaria but is uncommon in children. Most of these patients respond to cautious rehydration with an increase in urine output. In patients who have not been treated with diuretics, a urine specific gravity >1.015 or a urinary sodium concentration <20 mmol/l suggests dehydration. Indications for dialysis (Fig. 9.6) or haemofiltration include hyperkalaemia, uraemia, metabolic acidosis and pulmonary oedema.

Treatment of *massive intravascular haemolysis* (Blackwater fever etc.) involves correction of uraemia with dialysis and avoidance of fluid overload during blood transfusion which is invariably necessary to maintain life. Quinine should be given in usual doses as the risk of untreated falciparum malaria outweighs the risk of quinine-related haemolysis in malaria.

Pulmonary oedema

This results from increased pulmonary capillary permeability (resembling adult respiratory distress syndrome, ARDS) or, less commonly, from fluid overload. Where facilities allow, the use of positive pressure ventilation with positive end expiratory pressure/continuous positive airway pressure (PEEP/CPAP) to maintain adequate oxygenation, and haemofiltration to correct fluid overload, can be life-saving. Elsewhere, fluid overload must be prevented by maintaining the central venous pressure between 0 and +10–15 cm H_2O by nursing the patient propped up at 45° and by strict control of fluid intake. If pulmonary oedema develops, oxygen should be given by the most effective method available, a rapid-acting diuretic such as furosamide given by intravenous injection and, if all else fails, the patient should be venesected.

Septicaemic shock (algid malaria)

A secondary bacterial infection should always be suspected and blood, urine etc. sent for culture. Broad-spectrum antimicrobial treatment with an aminoglycoside such as gentamicin with ceftazidime or cefuroxime and metronidazole, should be started immediately. A less expensive combination would be gentamicin with benzyl penicillin or cephalothin. Other causes of shock syndrome in patients with malaria include hypovolaemia from dehydration or massive blood loss (e.g. ruptured spleen or gastrointestinal haemorrhage) and pulmonary oedema.

Treatment is the same as for septic shock: correction of hypovolaemia, the use of pressor drugs (e.g. noradrenaline) and inotropic agents (e.g. dobutamine).

Secondary bacterial pneumonia

Aspiration or hypostatic pneumonia is a common complication of severe falciparum malaria. Antimicrobial treatment consists of combinations of piperacillin or ceftazidime with gentamicin and metronidazole or, if this cannot be afforded, benzyl penicillin or cephalothin.

Hyperparasitaemia

In non-immune patients, mortality increases with parasitaemia, exceeding 50% with parasitaemias above 500 000/μl. It has been argued that exchange transfusion might reduce the parasitaemia more rapidly than chemotherapy alone and might also remove harmful metabolites, toxins, cytokines and other mediators and restore normal red cell mass, platelets, clotting factors, albumin and other depleted substances. These advantages must be balanced against the dangers of the procedure including electrolyte disturbances (e.g. hypocalcaemia), cardiovascular complications and infection. The use of exchange transfusion has been reported in approximately 70 patients. Some showed clinical improvement during or shortly after the procedure and most of the reported cases survived, although this may well reflect some selection. Manual exchange transfusion (alternating venesection and transfusion) or continuous cell separation (haemopheresis) have been used. There have been a few recent reports of ARDS developing during the procedure. Efficacy of exchange transfusion over optimal chemotherapy alone has not yet been proved. There is no consensus on the indications for this treatment and in most malarious parts of the world it is in any case out of the question because of the lack of adequate volumes of safe blood. Where facilities allow, this procedure should be considered in non-immune patients who are severely ill, who have deteriorated on conventional treatment and who have parasitaemias in excess of 10%.

Ruptured spleen

This potentially fatal complication of vivax and falciparum malaria must be suspected in patients who complain of abdominal pain (especially left upper quadrant), left shoulder tip pain and who become hypotensive with other signs of blood loss. Free blood in the peritoneal cavity and a torn splenic capsule can often be detected by ultrasound or CT and confirmed by needle aspiration of the peritoneal cavity, laparoscopy or laparotomy. A trial of conservative management is increasingly favoured so that the spleen with its important immunological functions can be preserved. This involves blood transfusion, close observation in an intensive care unit and rapid access to surgical help should there be any sudden deterioration.

Resistance to antimalarial drugs

About 40 years ago the detection of resistance of some strains of *P. falciparum* to proguanil and pyrimethamine signalled the ability of this organism to survive antimalarial chemotherapy through selection of resistant mutants. The development of resistance to pyrimethamine was blamed on its use for mass drug treatment and prophylaxis. It may have arisen in many geographical loci. Resistance to pyrimethamine may not persist if the drug is withdrawn from use for resistant parasites are at a biological disadvantage compared to sensitive ones.

An even more important event was the observation of resistance to 4-aminoquinolines (chloroquine and amodiaquine) in Thailand in 1957 and on the Colombian–Venezuelan border in 1959. In 1978 chloroquine resistance was reported in Africa, first in Kenya, later in the Comoro Islands, Madagascar, Tanzania, Uganda and Zambia. By the end of 1983 it had been detected in the Western Pacific, India and southern China. At April 1993 the only areas in which *P. falciparum* remains fully sensitive to chloroquine are: the Caribbean (Haiti and Dominican Republic), Central America northwest of the Panama Canal, parts of the Middle East (excluding Oman and the border area between Saudi Arabia and Yemen) and a few countries in West Africa such as Liberia, Senegal and Sierra Leone. Unlike pyrimethamine-resistant parasites, chloroquine-resistant strains are at a biological advantage over sensitive strains, having more robust metabolism and preferential 'tropism' for uptake by mosquitos. It seems inevitable that chloroquine resistance will eventually be found throughout the range of *P. falciparum*, although the epidemiology of the spread of resistance is not fully understood. Resistance to pyrimethamine–sulfonamide combinations (such as Fansidar) is now widespread in South-east Asia, parts of East, Central and Southern Africa and South America (such as the Amazonas area of Brazil). In Thailand there has been a progressive increase in the minimal inhibitory concentration (MIC) of quinine for the prevalent strains of *P. falciparum*, RI and RII resistance is increasingly common unless quinine is combined with tetracycline or some other accessory drug and there have been a few reports of suspected RIII resistance. Mefloquine resistance occurs in South-east Asia and in some African countries and in the border regions of Thailand there has been a dramatic reduction in the cure rate of *P. falciparum* infections by this drug even at the higher dose of 25 mg/kg. Halofantrine resistance is also reported.

Detection of resistance to antimalarial drugs

In vivo *tests*

In practice, drug resistance is suspected when acute cases of *P. falciparum* malaria do not fully and rapidly respond to standard regimens, or when recrudescence of symptoms and parasites in the blood is seen soon after their temporary disappearance after such treatment. Criteria for recognition of suspected resistance of malaria parasites to 4-aminoquinolines were adopted in 1974, and a standard procedure for determining the response of malaria parasites to chloroquine in the field has been recommended by the WHO (Fig. 9.7). *In vivo* tests involve the administration of standard treat-

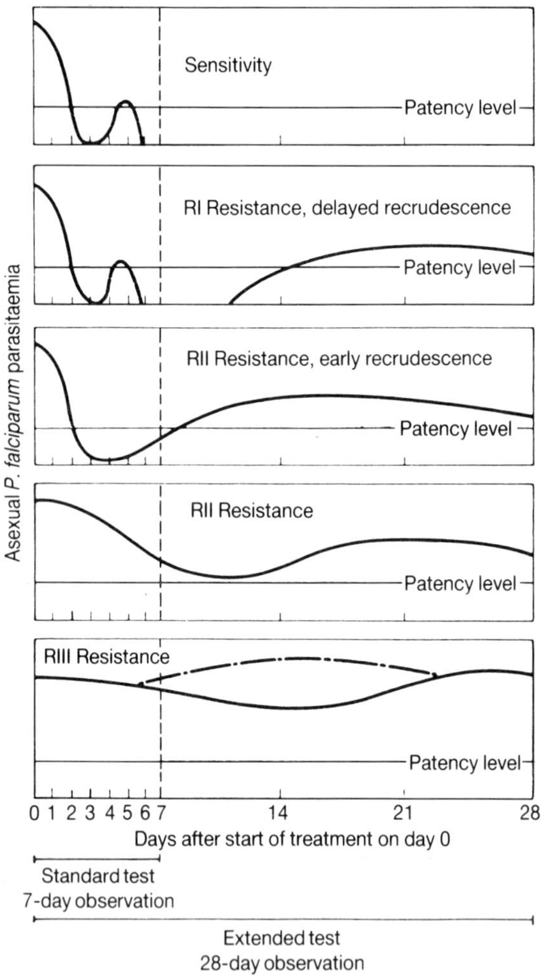

Fig. 9.7 A WHO field test for response of malaria parasites to chloroquine (and other antimalarial drugs). The diagram shows degrees of response ranging from sensitivity to high resistance. —— Patent parasitaemia may reappear by day 5; in sensitive (S) strains, however, it is absent on and after day 6. –·–·– There may be an increase in parasitaemia in RIII resistance. Note that it is not possible to distinguish between S and RI in the standard (7-day) test. (WHO, 1973.)

ment to a patient or group of patients followed by assessment during a period of 7 days (WHO standard field test) or during the next 28 days (WHO extended field test). The short test allows rapid detection of RII or RIII resistance while the longer test distinguishes sensitive strains from those with emergent RI resistance. It is of course essential to assess these responses parasitologically as well as clinically as patients may appear to be clinically cured (their fever and other symptoms disappear) with infection by parasites resistant at the RI or RII levels.

Interpretation of the WHO *in vivo* test may be vitiated by malabsorption of the drug (vomiting or transient gastrointestinal disturbance) or, in the case of RI resistance, by reinfection during the 28-day follow-up period.

To establish by clinical observations the geographical spread of resistance or an increase in the level of resistance it is important to confirm that a bona fide preparation of the drug in the correct dose was taken by the patient and was absorbed. Measurement of the concentrations of the drug in the patient's blood is the best way to achieve this. Antimalarial drugs sold in some developing countries may not be what they seem. For example, in the early 1980s a preparation of 'quinine' available in eastern Thailand turned out to consist entirely of chloroquine!

In vitro *tests*

Rieckmann's microtechnique is now the most widely employed. Standard test kits are distributed by the WHO (Manila). The same medium is used as in Trager's continuous culture. The test is carried out in 8 × 12 cm plastic culture plates, containing 12 drug dilutions (of chloroquine, quinine or mefloquine as needed) and controls. Blood can be taken from a finger puncture in a heparinized or EDTA-treated capillary tube and added to the growth medium. Aliquots of 50 μl of the suspension are added to the test wells. The plate is placed in a candle jar (according to Trager's method of culture) and the jar is put in an incubator. After incubation at 37.5°C for 24–26 hours, the plates are taken out, the supernatant is removed and thick films are prepared from the layers of erythrocytes. After staining, the count of the proportion of mature schizonts compared to controls gives the results of the test.

Mechanism of drug resistance in *Plasmodium falciparum*

Pyrimethamine and proguanil (cycloguanil) are dihydrofolate reductase (DHFR) inhibitors which act by binding to the parasites' enzyme. Point mutations in the active site of the DHFR enzyme, such as a change from serine to asparagine at position 108, reduces the binding of pyrimethamine. Other mutations are responsible for cycloguanil resistance. Wellems and his colleagues have used a polymerase chain reaction (PCR) method to screen *P. falciparum* isolates for the presence of this mutation. In the Brazilian Amazon they found that almost 90% of isolates contained the DHFR Asn-108 mutation, consistent with the high prevalence of Fansidar resistance in this region. However, proguanil has not been used in South America and another DHFR point mutation (Thr-108) associated with resistance to its active metabolite, cycloguanil, has not yet been found in that region.

Chloroquine, a dibasic compound, accumulates in a high concentration in the acid food vacuole of *P. falciparum* where it interferes with the functions of the vacuole and kills the parasite. The half-life of chloroquine in sensitive parasites is many hours but in resistant strains it is only a few minutes. The rapid leakage of chloroquine from the food vacuole of resistant parasites can be prevented by calcium channel blockers such as verapamil and other compounds (see above). The gene determining chloroquine resistance has been localized within a 200 kilobase segment of chromosome 7 of *P. falciparum*. The role of multiple drug resistance (MDR) genes is uncertain. The MDR phenotype shows over-expression of transporting P glycoprotein which increases the excretion of drugs four-fold, but this does not adequately explain the greatly increased release of chloroquine in resistant parasites.

Antimalaria prophylaxis

Infection by any of the human malaria species produces symptoms which, in non-immune subjects, are at least temporarily debilitating and, in the case of *P. falciparum* are potentially fatal. Malaria should therefore be prevented if possible.

Avoidance of infection

Non-immune people and other high-risk groups such as pregnant women, infants and young children, and people who are splenectomized or immunosuppressed should avoid entering the malarious zone. Infection via blood transfusion should be prevented by screening donors or transfused blood (by microscopy, DNA probes or PCR methods) or by treating donors, transfused blood or recipients with antimalarial drugs. Most but not all of the anopheline vectors of malaria bite in or near human dwellings during the hours of darkness (see Chapter 7). The risk of infective mosquito bites can therefore be reduced by insect-proofing sleeping quarters or by sleeping under mosquito nets, preferably those which have been impregnated with an insecticide such as permethrin (0.2 g/m^2 of material every 6 months). Bedrooms should be sprayed with a knock-down insecticide to kill any mosquitos that may have entered the room during the day. Mosquitos may also be killed or repelled by vaporizing synthetic pyrethroids on electrical heating devices (such as 'No Bite' and 'Buzz Off') (Bioallethrin 4.2% W/W) or by burning mosquito coils. N,N-diethyl-m-toluamide (DEET) is an effective repellant of mosquitos, flies, midges, ticks, leeches etc. when applied to skin and clothing. Very rarely, skin application results in allergy, dermatitis and neurotoxicity in children (behavioural changes, ataxia, encephalopathy, seizures or coma) and adults (confusion, irritability and insomnia). Light coloured protective clothing with long sleeves and trousers should be worn outside after sunset.

Indigenous communities in many parts of the tropics have been protected by impregnated bed nets, screens or curtains which can reduce the frequency of clinical attacks and density of parasitaemia and, among Gambian children, reduce malarial mortality.

Chemoprophylaxis

The widespread use of antimalarial drugs for prophylaxis with the inevitably poor compliance and resulting underdosing has provided the selection pressure for the emergence of resistance to dihydrofolate reductases, 4-aminoquinolines, pyrimethamine–sulfonamide/sulfone combinations and most recently to mefloquine. Over the last 40 years, the development of resistance to pyrimethamine, proguanil and chloroquine in particular has greatly complicated the choice of prophylactic drugs and the criteria for their use. These three drugs were remarkably safe, except for the cumulative retinal toxicity of chloroquine, whereas alternative compounds, forced into use as a result of the declining efficacy of the original chemoprophylactic agents, have proved toxic. Amodiaquine causes agranulocytosis and hepatitis, pyrimethamine–sulfonamide combinations cause Stevens–Johnson syndrome and toxic epidermal necrolysis, doxycycline causes photosensitization and mefloquine causes gastrointestinal symptoms and sometimes neurotoxicity.

People requiring prophylaxis

Those at most risk of contracting debilitating or life-threatening malaria are:

1. Indigenous populations in malarious areas before they have acquired protective immunity (i.e. infants and children up to the age of about 5 years), pregnant women, especially during their first pregnancy, people who have been away from the endemic area for several years and those with certain types of immunosuppression (but apparently not those with HIV infection).
2. Non-immune immigrant workers, military personnel, game wardens and other task forces working in malarious areas.
3. The increasing number of non-immune travellers visiting or residing in malarious areas.

Prophylactic drugs

(Fuller details of these drugs are given above.)

Causal prophylactic drugs prevent the infection from becoming established while most prophylactic drugs merely suppress the clinical symptoms of the disease. Recommended regimens of chemoprophylactic drugs and the choice of chemoprophylaxis and standby treatment for non-immune travellers in different geographical areas are given in Tables 9.5 and 9.6.

Biguanides

Biguanides such as proguanil are causal prophylactics for *P. falciparum*, *P. vivax* and *P. ovale* as they

Table 9.5 Recommended chemoprophylactic regimens for non-immune travellers

Regimen	Dose for adult	Dose for child (per kg body weight)
1. Chloroquine	300 mg base (2 tablets) once every week	5 mg base/kg
2. Proguanil	200 mg (2 tablets) once every day	3 mg/kg
3. Proguanil + chloroquine	(doses above)	
4. Maloprim	12.5 mg pyrimethamine + 100 mg dapsone (1 tablet) once every week	0.2 mg/kg* + 1.5 mg/kg
5. Maloprim + chloroquine	Weekly (doses above)	
6. Mefloquine	250 mg base§ (1 tablet) once every week	5 mg base/kg†
7. Doxycycline	100 mg (1 tablet/capsule) once every day	3 mg/kg‡

Not recommended for children: *<6 weeks; †<1 year; ‡<8 years; §228 mg base in USA.

Table 9.6 Choice of chemoprophylaxis and standby treatment for non-immune travellers

Geographical area	Prophylactic regimen*	Standby treatment†
A. Turkey (rural, Mar.–Nov.) and Side, Egypt (rural, June–Oct.), Iraq (rural, North, May–Nov.), United Arab Emirates (rural), Syria (rural, May–Oct.), Mauritius (rural)	1 or 2	C
B. Afghanistan, Iran, Oman, Saudi Arabia (rural SW Tihama), Yemen	3	F/M/H/Q
C. SubSaharan Africa including São Tomé, Principe, Madagascar and Comoro Islands (except D below)	3, 4 or 6	F/M/H/Q
D. Cameroon, Kenya, Malawi, Mozambique, Rwanda, Sudan, Tanzania, Uganda, Zaire, Zambia	6	M/H/Q
E. Mexico (rural), Central America, Haiti, Dominican Republic, Paraguay (rural, Oct.–May), Peru (below 1500 m), Argentina (few areas)	1	C
F. South America (except in E above and G and L below)	3	M/H/Q
G. Brazil (Amazonas)	6	M/H/Q
H. South-east Asia including some areas of rural China (except in I and L below)	6	M/H/Q
I. Thailand–Cambodia border region	7	H/Q
J. South Asia (Indian subcontinent, Nepal Terai, Bhutan, Indo-china, Indonesia etc.)	3	F/M/H/Q
K. West Pacific (Papua New Guinea, Irian Jaya and adjacent islands, Solomon Islands, Vanuatu)	5 or 6	M/H/Q
L. North Africa and Middle East (except in A and B above), Venezuala (coastal) tourist areas and cities of Peninsular (west) Malaysia, Bali, Thailand, China, Sarawak, Hong Kong, Macao, Philippines, Brunei, Singapore, Maldives	None	None

*Prophylactic regimen see Table 9.5
†Standby treatment: M = mefloquine; H = halofantrine; Q = quinine; F = Fansidar/Metakelfin; C = chloroquine.
Based on Bradley and Phillips-Howard, British Medical Journal (1989) **299**, 1087–89; and Bradley, British Medical Journal (1993), May.

kill the pre-erythrocytic tissue (liver) stages of these parasites. They are also slow-acting blood schizontocides. They do not kill hypnozoites of the relapsing malarias. They have been used for prophylaxis, either alone or more recently in combinations since the 1940s. Resistance developed rapidly in *P. falciparum* and has also been reported with *P. vivax*, but biguanides may remain active against the pre-erythrocytic stages of resistant parasites. Currently, proguanil is most often used in combination with chloroquine. The daily dose of proguanil has been increased from 100 to 200 mg daily based on observations made by Bruce-Chwatt in Nigeria many years ago. He found that increasing the dose from one to two tablets daily significantly reduced the breakthroughs of malaria among oil company employees. The increased recognition of side effects of proguanil in recent years (reversible hair loss, mouth ulcers, scaling of the palms and soles, indigestion and diarrhoea) may result partly from the higher dose now used and its combination with chloroquine. Warfarin is potentiated by proguanil and in patients with severe renal failure there may be accumulation of the drug causing megaloblastic anaemia and pancytopenia.

The proguanil–chloroquine combination is still an acceptably safe and partially effective prophylactic regime against *P. falciparum* (and other malarias) in most parts of the world, but increasing numbers of well-documented breakthroughs have been reported in South-east Asia, Papua New Guinea, East Africa, Amazonian Brazil and elsewhere. In Thai schoolchildren who possibly possessed some degree of immunity, encouraging results were obtained using a combination of 200 mg proguanil and 25 mg/kg sulfamethoxazole daily.

Pyrimethamine

Pyrimethamine is a causal prophylactic for *P. falciparum* and for some strains of *P. vivax* but resistance is now so widespread that it is used as a prophylactic only in combination with dapsone as Maloprim or Deltaprim or with chloroquine (as Daraclor).

Deltaprim is used widely in Zimbabwe for prophylaxis of plantation workers and their families. Over many years of use it has proved effective and no toxicity has been reported even in pregnant women and children. Maloprim proved safe and effective in young children in the Gambia, and in combination with chloroquine (to cover vivax malaria) it was effective in the West Pacific area.

Pyrimethamine has been blamed for cases of nodular eosinophilic pneumonia in patients taking Maloprim and Daraclor. Dapsone given every day in higher doses (50–100 mg) for the treatment of leprosy and other skin diseases has caused haemolysis, methaemoglobinaemia, Heinz body formation, leucopenia, agranulocytosis and pseudoleukaemia. When used in a single adult dose of 100 mg/week in combination with pyrimethamine 12.5 mg/week as Maloprim, serious toxicity is very uncommon, but mild haemolysis and methaemoglobinaemia is seen in children and in patients with erythrocyte enzyme defects (see above). The incidence of agranulocytosis is about 1 in 10 000 prescriptions at this dose but may be as high as 1 in 2000 if the dose is doubled. Haematological monitoring is recommended in people taking Maloprim prophylaxis.

Chloroquine

Chloroquine is an effective suppressive prophylactic against chloroquine-sensitive strains of *P. falciparum* and other malarias but does not prevent relapses of vivax or ovale malaria. For use on its own, chloroquine is now suitable only for areas where only vivax malaria occurs (e.g. Turkey) or for the few remaining areas where *P. falciparum* is sensitive to chloroquine. The use of chloroquine combined with proguanil has been described above. Chloroquine should be added to pyrimethamine–sulfone combinations in areas where vivax malaria is a problem.

Cumulative irreversible retinal toxicity from chloroquine is seen after a life-time dose of 50–100 g base (i.e. after 3 to 6 years of taking 300 mg base per week). Since chloroquine prophylaxis cannot prevent the establishment of hypnozoites in the liver and therefore relapses of vivax and ovale malaria, people who have been exposed to these infections for more than about 6 months should be given a course of primaquine for radical cure once they leave the endemic area.

Doxycycline

Doxycycline has proved effective for prophylaxis against resistant falciparum malaria in South-east Asia. Toxicity associated with prolonged use is uncertain but recognized problems include photosensitization, gastrointestinal symptoms (reduced by taking the capsules with a meal) and monilial vaginitis. There is a theoretical risk that widespread use of doxycycline prophylaxis might encourage the emergence of resistant strains of bacteria. Doxycycline and other tetracyclines should not be used in pregnant women or in children less than eight years of age.

Mefloquine

The WHO's original policy was to reserve mefloquine for treatment of multiresistant falciparum malaria. However, the increasing difficulties with prophylaxis in South-east Asia and, more recently, in East Africa and the Amazon region of Brazil, and other pressures have led to its use as a prophylactic drug. Early reports probably exaggerated the toxicity of mefloquine as comparative groups of subjects taking other antimalarial drugs were not included. There is also racial variation in the incidence of side effects. Mefloquine will probably produce dizziness or gastrointestinal symptoms in about 5–10% of people. The true incidence of neuropsychiatric complications is not yet known but at prophylactic doses it is likely to be less than 1%. It is now clear that other antimalarial drugs such as chloroquine can also cause psychosis and exacerbate epilepsy. Short-term prophylaxis with mefloquine proved effective and safe against multiresistant *P. falciparum* infection in pregnant Karen refugees in north-west Thailand, but reports of birth defects have caused concern. Mefloquine prophylaxis is not recommended in pregnancy, at least during the first trimester, until more information is available. Breakthroughs will occur unless the drug is taken every week in the recommended adult dose of 250 mg. The rapid increase in resistance to mefloquine resulting from its uncontrolled use as a prophylactic makes it unsuitable and ineffective now for prophylaxis in border areas of Thailand and Cambodia. Because of its neurological side effects, mefloquine prophylaxis was thought to be contraindicated in people such as airline pilots, drivers and soldiers, whose work requires fine coordination and spatial discrimination. Mefloquine is not recommended for prophylactic use in travellers known to be hypersensitive to the drug, for children less than 15 kg body weight, pregnant women, and those using beta-blockers and other drugs which may affect cardiac conduction. Since quinine, quinidine and mefloquine are pharmacologically similar, cumulative toxicity is a potential danger when they are used together, for example, if quinine or quinidine treatment were needed for a breakthrough of *P. falciparum* infection in someone taking mefloquine prophylaxis.

Non-recommended antimalarial drugs in chemoprophylaxis

The following antimalarial drugs are no longer recommended for chemoprophylaxis but are still used in some parts of the world: mepacrine, primaquine, quinine, pyrimethamine–sulfonamide combinations (Fansidar, Metakelfin) and amodiaquine. Halofantrine and artemisinin derivatives should not be used for prophylaxis: they should be reserved for treatment of multiresistant falciparum malaria.

Principles of chemoprophylaxis

Non-immune travellers

Before prescribing chemoprophylaxis a quick *risk–benefit analysis* should be carried out according to the algorithm in Fig. 9.8. This will ensure that the risk of malaria infection, as assessed by knowledge of the duration of foreign travel, itinerary and activities in the malarious area, balances the risk of toxicity of the prophylactic drug. The following points should always be borne in mind:

1. Although malaria may be widespread in a particular country, there may be a negligible risk of infection in the popular tourist sites. Thus, although Thailand is a malarious country, the most popular tourist sites – Bangkok, Pattaya, Phuket and Chiangmai – are malaria-free.
2. None of the chemoprophylactic drugs described above is now totally effective even when compliance is perfect, and all have some toxic effects. However, taking a chemoprophylactic drug reduces the risk of severe and fatal malaria even though it may not always prevent infection.
3. Following from 2 above, someone who has been to a malarious area should see a doctor and mention the possibility of malaria if they become febrile or ill within a few months of leaving the transmission zone.
4. Malaria may be acquired during stopovers or while the aircraft waits at an airport ('runway malaria') in the malarious country even though the traveller's country of final destination may be malaria-free. Rarely, people living near an international airport in a temperate country may be bitten by an infected imported mosquito ('airport malaria') and infection may result from routes other than mosquito bites, for example transfusion and syringe passage among drug addicts.

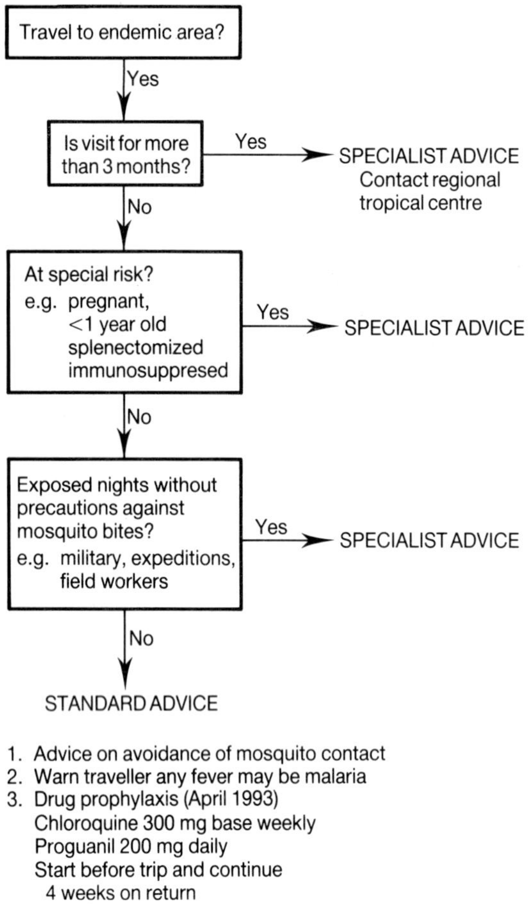

Fig. 9.8 A simple algorithm for malaria prophylaxis. (Adapted from Peto and Gilks, 1986.)

5. An alternative or supplement to chemoprophylaxis is 'standby treatment' (sometimes referred to as 'presumptive treatment') to be taken if the traveller becomes feverish and unwell more than 7 days after entering the malarious area in a place remote from medical care and diagnostic facilities. Rapid treatment with such 'standby drugs' or 'drugs in the pocket' may be preferable to chemoprophylaxis in those at increased risk of toxic reactions such as pregnant women, young children and people with drug allergies. Patients with acute intermittent and variegate porphyrias and hereditary coproporphyrinuria should never be given Maloprim, Fansidar, tetracycline, co-trimoxazole or other sulfonamides as this will precipitate attacks. It is uncertain whether chloroquine and pyrimethamine are porphyrinogenic, but quinine and primaquine are safe and can be used to treat attacks of malaria.
6. The cost of prophylaxis may be an important factor. Costs of prophylactic regimens relative to chloroquine (300 mg base/week adult dose) are as follows: chloroquine phosphate (= 1), Fansidar 4.1, Maloprim 1.5, proguanil (200 mg/day) 7.4, mefloquine (250 mg/week) 25.3, doxycycline (100 mg/day) 53.1.
7. When to start taking prophylactic drugs: most drugs need only be started on the day of entering the malarious area. However, reasons for starting earlier are:
   i. Because of its slow elimination from the body chloroquine is accumulated. Higher blood levels may afford better protection and so it makes sense pharmacologically to start weekly chloroquine 1 to 2 weeks before entering the malarious area or to start chloroquine prophylaxis with a loading dose of 5 mg base/kg/day on 2 consecutive days and to continue with a weekly dose of 5 mg/kg.
   ii. Relatively toxic drugs such as Maloprim and mefloquine could be started a week before departure so that side effects can declare themselves and another drug can be substituted. Haematological screening for haemolysis, methaemoglobinaemia and pancytopenia may be helpful. Suppressive schizontocidal prophylactic drugs should have reached effective blood concentrations by the time that merozoites first enter the bloodstream 6–14 days after first exposure to infection.
8. When to stop chemoprophylactic drugs: drugs must be continued for 4 weeks (mefloquine 2 weeks) after leaving the malarious area so that schizontocidal concentrations of the drug are present in the blood when merozoites emerge from the liver after a maximum pre-patent period. Most prophylactic drugs (with the exception of biguanides and perhaps pyrimethamine) have no effect on pre-erythrocytic (hepatic) forms.
9. The prophylactic drugs listed above cannot be relied upon to prevent development of hypno-

zoites of *P. vivax* and *P. ovale* in the liver. After substantial exposure to these infections (e.g. 6 months) it is therefore worthwhile to give a radical cure with primaquine.

Chemoprophylaxis for indigenous populations

There is reassuring evidence that in children under the age of 5 years who are growing up in malarious areas, continuous prophylaxis does not prevent the acquisition of immunity. Some degree of immunity will increase the efficacy of chemoprophylactic regimens. Chemoprophylaxis of the two groups most obviously at risk of severe malaria, young children and pregnant women, particularly primiparae, remains controversial because of the increasing difficulty in choosing acceptably safe chemoprophylactic drugs and because poor compliance further reduces their efficacy. Other strategies in these groups are to improve the speed of diagnosis and treatment in peripheral paediatric and antenatal clinics and to institute antimosquito measures such as the use of impregnated mosquito nets. However, it is clear from studies in the Gambia and elsewhere that many African children die of malaria without access to medical care and that even enthusiastic antenatal clinic surveillance without prophylaxis cannot prevent the damaging effects of acute malaria in pregnancy.

The strategy of giving antimalarial drugs to primiparae should be based on a knowledge of the parasitological and clinical findings in them; the general availability of antimalarial drugs, and the resistance status of the local *P. falciparum* strains, since these factors vary from one endemic setting to another.

We still adhere to the view that on present evidence, in most countries of Africa south of the Sahara, prophylactic chloroquine for primiparae is a reasonable antenatal strategy.

Chemoprophylaxis of long-term non-immune expatriate residents in the malarious area

Depending on the particular circumstances, long-term chemoprophylaxis with drugs of relatively low toxicity (and probably of only moderate efficacy) and/or early treatment of febrile illnesses with standby drugs, may be recommended. The cumulative toxicity of chloroquine must not be forgotten. Ophthalmological checks are recommended between 3 and 6 years of starting continuous chloroquine prophylaxis and, after 6 years, an alternative chemoprophylactic drug should be prescribed.

Recommended chemoprophylaxis

Recommendations are inevitably overtaken by developments in the emergence and geographical distribution of drug-resistant parasites, recognition of new toxic effects of drugs, by changes in drug supply and the global epidemiology of malaria. The recommendations given in Tables 9.5 and 9.6 are therefore tentative and based on information available at April 1993.

Chapter 10

Rationale and technique of malaria control

E. Onori*, P. F. Beales and H. M. Gilles

> Governments can trust no formulas devised in Geneva or elsewhere but must create the machinery necessary to define and resolve their own problems locality by locality.
>
> Hackett (1937)

Before considering in detail the concept and methods of malaria control, it may be useful to stress the great differences that exist between various epidemiological types of malaria. The epidemiological prototypes related to ecological and socio-economic conditions have been described in Chapter 8. The major eight prototypes are (1) African savannah, (2) desert fringe and highland fringe, (3) malaria associated with traditional agriculture in plains and river valleys outside Africa, (4) forest-related malaria, (5) malaria associated with extensive agricultural development, (6) urban malaria and malaria in planned human settlements, (7) coastland and marshland malaria and (8) malaria in war zones and areás with socio-political disturbances.

An understanding of the epidemiology of malaria based upon recognized ecotypes facilitates the understanding of malaria risks and also helps to identify the tools that are required to meet the local situation, which is dynamic rather than static.

Epidemiological types of malaria

The differences in the features of these types produce different pictures of the disease as it affects the whole community. Endemic malaria is constantly present in considerable degree and without great fluctuations in quantity; epidemic malaria shows great fluctuation in quantity and severity from time to time.

Apart from the endemic and epidemic types in some parts of the world a minor change in conditions may precipitate a great epidemic while in others the disease tends to be stable in its incidence and unexplained epidemics are rare. There is a high epidemic potential over very large parts of India, Sri Lanka, South-east Asia, North-west Africa and some countries in South America, and a low epidemic potential in much of equatorial Africa. In these areas of high epidemic potential disastrous outbreaks are easily precipitated, although control can be readily established. The explanation of this potential has been the subject of much study and controversy but can be rationally proved on the basis of the factors which influence the prevalence of the disease.

Endemic malaria of low epidemic potential

This type of malaria occurs over the greater part of equatorial Africa, in the hills and foothills of India, the plains of Assam and elsewhere. It is due to transmission by anophelines which preferentially bite humans and which commonly have a relatively long life, in places where the temperature and humidity are high for long periods. Malaria tends to be highly endemic, a fact often obscured by the

***Dr Erminio Onori died in January 1993, a few months before the publication of this book. This Chapter and Chapter 11 are dedicated to him.**

development of some degree of immunity by the local peoples, but made manifest in children and in immigrants who suffer severely. Epidemics in the indigenous population are almost unknown, except following a major increase in the numbers of mosquito breeding places. The disease can be maintained by relatively small numbers of mosquitos; entirely non-malarious parts are rare. Thus control measures which operate by reduction of mosquito numbers must be very nearly perfect to secure visible results, minor measures having little effect. Control by residual insecticides, which operates by reduction of expectation of life rather than by reduction of mosquito numbers, can be effective if it produces a sufficiently high *Anopheles* mortality, such as is attainable by the energetic use of the most effective insecticides, but which may not be reached when there is any degree of slackness in application.

Endemic malaria of high epidemic potential

This occurs over much of the plains of South America, India and Sri Lanka, and in South-east Asia. It is due to transmission by anophelines which tend to bite animals in preference to humans or which are normally relatively short lived. Its character is accentuated in areas where both these conditions apply. There are great variations in endemicity. In some places a high incidence is normal and the indigenous population may acquire some degree of immunity, with results comparable to those in the type previously described. Some non-malarious localities may be found, and all gradations between these extremes occur. Considerable fluctuations in the amount of malaria from year to year are common and there may be severe periodic epidemics in previously non-malarious parts.

The precipitating causes of these epidemics are difficult to explain as they may be quite minor in character; when they are major, epidemics such as those of 1934–35 or 1967–68 in Sri Lanka may occur. As a minor manifestation of this instability the disease may appear without apparent explanation in previously healthy places; it may disappear from them again with as little obvious cause.

The number of anophelines needed to maintain transmission is relatively high and control by reduction of breeding, though perhaps not easy, is at least readily feasible. Control by residual insecticides is effective provided a daily mosquito mortality of at least 25% is kept up. This is within the range of effect produced by the routine application of active insecticides.

Hill malaria

The greatest altitude at which malaria occurs differs very much from place to place in the tropics, from nearly 2500 m in Kenya to under 1000 m in Sri Lanka. Near the upper limit of its altitude range the disease is almost always unstable with a tendency to epidemic manifestations, which are likely to occur following unusually warm rainy weather. Control is relatively easy, when the method used is the application of effective residual insecticides.

Subtropical seasonal malaria

In those places where the temperature sinks below the minimum at which malaria is transmitted for most of the year, sharply defined summer epidemics occur. There may be three waves of the disease. In some places there is a spring epidemic occurring before transmission starts, due to relapses from the previous year and cases in which the incubation period has been prolonged to several months. The second wave consists of fresh cases, chiefly due to vivax malaria which may rapidly reach its peak. The third wave comes in the late summer of autumn and is characterized by the greater prevalence of falciparum malaria. These seasonal epidemic waves are annual; when the epidemic potential is high there may be great differences between the sizes of epidemic waves in consecutive years; when it is low a more or less uniform type is likely to occur. A high potential with great variations is to be seen in the subtropical parts of north-west India and Pakistan, the Punjab and Sind. To a lesser extent it can be seen in parts of the Middle East and in North Africa.

War and conflict malaria

War and other conflicts are notorious causes of an increased amount of malaria because of movements of large numbers of people, destruction of houses, damage to water distribution systems, loss of cattle and depletion of health services. During the colonial wars in the nineteenth century the losses due to malaria exceeded those resulting from weapons or other diseases. During the First World War (1914–1918) severe outbreaks of malaria occurred in England, France, Germany, Italy and other European countries; many of these outbreaks were caused by returning soldiers infected in south-eastern Europe; the post-revolutionary period in Russia was associated with a pandemic of malaria that affected millions of people for several years; the Spanish civil war spread the infection to many parts of the peninsula. During the Second World War (1939–1945) the impact of malaria on military operations in South-east Asia, Indonesia and the South-west Pacific was such that, without the most rigorous control measures it is doubtful if the American forces and their allies could have won a decisive victory. Another aspect of malaria related to movements of population are large numbers of refugees from tropical countries, who often bring the infection into Europe and North America. The same is true with regard to migrant labour forces and to some extent to the large numbers of tourists visiting the exotic parts of the world. Nomadism is common in the semi-desert belts of Africa and Asia; nomadic groups are exposed to the infection when on the move and may introduce the disease into new areas.

Urban malaria

Urban malaria was well known in India in the 1930s when serious outbreaks of the disease were described in some major cities such as Bangalore, Bombay, Calcutta, Lucknow and New Delhi. Most of the local transmission was related to methods of water storage in wells and large cisterns, where *A. stephensi* could breed in profusion. More recent instances of urban malaria were described in Karachi and also in West Africa, where the cities grow at a tremendous rate, so that at the periphery of the urban centre all the problems of water disposal and sanitation are permanent. The urbanization of the world continues at a fast pace and the overall population of large cities will increase from 16% in the 1960s to about 50% in the year 2000. It is certain that in the tropics urban malaria will become a serious problem. Control of urban malaria depends not only on technical measures but much more on administrative approach and on provision of proper sanitation.

Malaria of development workers

The assembly of a labour force in any part of the world always increases the epidemic potential of the locality, and for a number of reasons. Bringing people together, often from a considerable distance, always involves the introduction of some who have no tolerance to malaria as it is found locally. Not only do they suffer themselves but, by providing a focus from which infection spreads, they also increase the load on others and start epidemics amongst them. Their activities often include the clearing of land, exposure of streams and seepages, and other works which provide more facilities for mosquito breeding. In the early stages of development wild animals and birds tend to be driven away or may even be hunted for food. Also a labour force does not own cattle, so that mosquitos which might feed on cattle or wild animals are forced to feed exclusively on humans. Where the local vector prefers to feed on a person, as it does over most of equatorial Africa, this will make little difference; where it chooses cattle in preference, if it can find them, the result of the change may be marked.

Whatever the cause, epidemic malaria is extremely common in labour forces and particularly in those places where the epidemic potential amongst local inhabitants is high. Disastrous outbreaks have occurred on many occasions. Not only for the benefit of the workers but also for the success of the enterprise concerned, labour forces must have a degree of protection greater than the local population.

The building of dams for agricultural irrigation or hydroelectric projects is often responsible for serious health problems; in semi-arid parts of the world where malaria is usually seasonal, these perennial impoundments of water may greatly increase the amount of transmission. During the construction period, the mass movement of labour forces may be responsible for problems mentioned above.

Principles of malaria prevention and control

The control of malaria may be an individual matter, i.e. for the protection of one person or one house, or a community. It may have to be undertaken at short notice in the middle of an epidemic, or may be planned and arranged during the off-season; it may be necessary for a short period only, or for a long season throughout most of the year. In each of these cases different approaches are necessary (Table 10.1).

Generally speaking, the measures for prevention of malaria in individuals and for larger scale control of the disease can be divided according to the classification proposed by Russell (1952).

1. Measures designed to prevent mosquitos from feeding on humans.
2. Measures designed to prevent or reduce the breeding of mosquitos by eliminating the collections of water or by altering the environment.
3. Measures designed to destroy the larvae of mosquitos.
4. Measures designed to destroy adult mosquitos.
5. Measures designed to eliminate the malaria parasites in the human host.

Protecting people from bites of *Anopheles*, or curing the person from whom the mosquito gets its infection, is sound in theory, and as much as possible should be done to achieve this end in practice. However, experience has shown that, despite high hopes once rested in the latter method, it can never be relied upon to give complete control of the infection in a community. In the endemic types of malaria many people are free from symptoms and are not discovered or treated. Protection from mosquito bites should always be put into practice, and may be expected to yield valuable results, particularly in the presence of acute epidemic malaria, but which can rarely be relied upon exclusively.

Table 10.1 Principles of comprehensive malaria control

Type of control	Effect
*Individual protection**	
Mosquito repellents	
Impregnated mosquito nets	
Protective clothing	
House screening	Reduction of human–mosquito contact
House siting	
Pyrethrum house spraying	
Antimosquito fumigants	
*Vector control**	
Environmental modification and manipulation	Reduction of vector breeding habitats
Reduction of vector densities	
Chemical and biological larvicides	
Insecticide space spraying	
Residual insecticide spraying	Reduction of longevity of vector population
Antiplasmodial measures†	
Early diagnosis and treatment of acute cases of malaria	Elimination of malaria parasites and prevention of transmission
Chemoprophylaxis and suppression of malaria infection	
Radical treatment of relapses	
Mass treatment (epidemics)	
Social participation	
Health education	Motivation for personal and family protection

*Factors reducing the vectorial capacity.
†Factors reducing the parasite reservoir.

Protection against the bites of mosquitos

Nets

The use of mosquito nets as a protection from mosquito bites during the night has been practised from very early times. They still remain one of the most important of all measures of personal protection, not only from mosquitos but also from flies, beetles and other creatures. The size of the mesh is determined not only by the number of holes to the square unit of the material, but also by the thickness and the type of thread of which the netting is made. In woven cotton nets the mesh is stated in terms of the sum of the number of holes counted along a line of the warp and a line of the bobbin falling within an area of one square inch (6.45 cm^2), the hole at the corner of the square where the two lines meet being counted twice. A netting suitable for protection against most vector *Anopheles* is one of 25/26 mesh, woven of 30/s cotton. The number of holes to the square inch would be about 150. A band of cloth about 300 mm wide should form the lower part of the mosquito net at the mattress level to protect arms and legs from contact with the net during sleep, as the mosquito may easily bite through it.

Nowadays, mosquito nets are made of nylon or other synthetic material, which is lighter and easy to wash. The mean size of holes of nylon nets is 1.2–1.5 mm; there should be 6–8 holes to 10 mm.

The best pattern is the rectangular net with a reinforced lower end; there should be no tears and no openings in the side for the purpose of entering the net. When in use it should be tucked all round under the mattress or sleeping mat (Fig. 10.1). It should be let down before dark in the evening, and when going to bed a thorough search should be made for any mosquitos which may be inside it, preferably using an electric torch. A useful precaution is to spray the outside of the net with an aerosol dispenser or a hand-sprayer using an appropriate insecticide preparation. Attempts are now being made to produce cheap and effective mosquito nets for wider use of populations in developing countries.

During the last 10 years several field trials have demonstrated that the protective effect of mosquito nets can be greatly enhanced by treating them with a repellent or insecticide. The substances which are most commonly used for mosquito net impregnation are the pyrethroids, especially permethrin (0.2–0.5 g a.i./m^2), and to a lesser extent, deltamethrin (15–25 mg a.i./m^2). Good results have also been reported with the utilization of curtains on doors and windows and eave strips impregnated with permethrin (1.0 g a.i./m^2). Good reviews of this type of approach are given by Curtis *et al.* (1990), Rozendaal (1989) and WHO (1987, 1989).

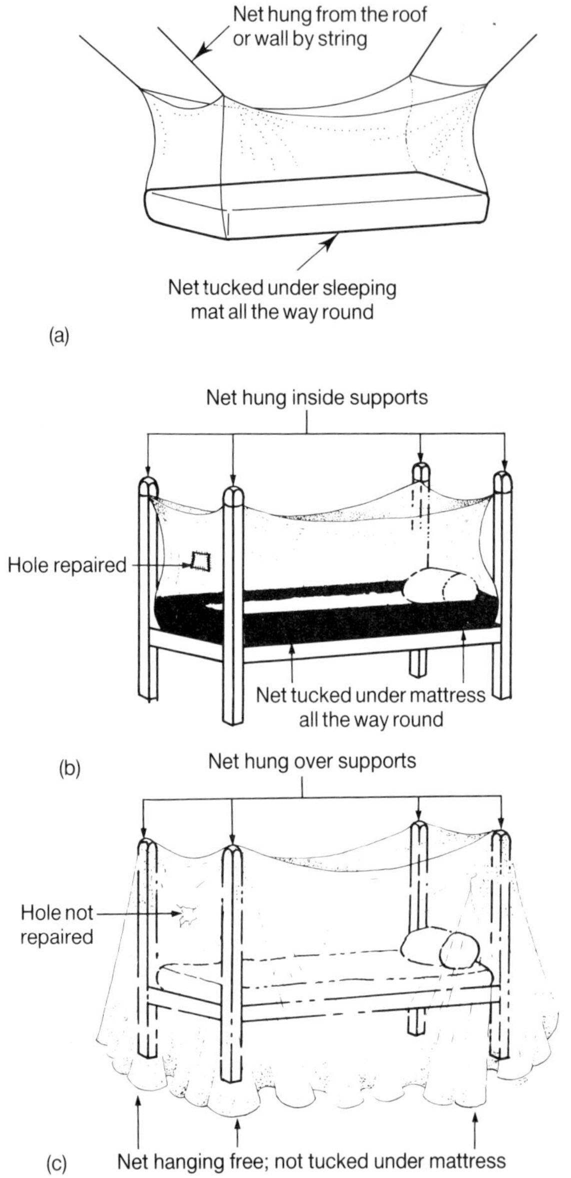

Fig. 10.1 A mosquito net hung the right way [(a) and (b)] and the wrong way (c).

Protective clothing

'Mosquito boots' made of soft leather or canvas are useful to protect the ankles in the evening. Alternatively, a pair of thick socks may be pulled up outside the bottoms of the trousers. Sleeves should be rolled down and trousers substituted for shorts or skirts after sunset. Mosquitos may pierce through clothing, which is in contact with the skin. Special hoods and gloves are sometimes used to protect persons on guard at night.

Repellents

These are substances applied to the skin, clothing or mosquito nets to repel mosquitos and prevent them from biting. In the past, citronella or eucalyptus oil were used on the skin but its effect is very short, not exceeding 15–20 minutes. Later a number of synthetic repellents were developed, with a duration of protection of 2–4 hours. The most useful of those developed are indalone, Rutgers 612, dimethyl phthalate (DMP), dibutyl phthalate (DBP) and a mixture known as 6-2-2. The most effective against *Anopheles* is DBP (average protection 4 hours) and DMP (average protection 3 hours). Several newer compounds are now available and among these N,N-diethyl-m-toluamide (DEET) appears to be the best repellent, active for at least 10 hours, and used in the form of a 50% solution in alcohol. A new group of mosquito repellents are dihydroacetone monoesters of carboxylic compounds. Their activity, while promising, does not exceed that of diethyltoluamide but the combination of the two prolongs their action.

Whatever preparation is used it should be applied liberally, especially about the neck, ankles and wrists. Eyelids and other sensitive skin surfaces or mucous membranes are irritated by these substances and should be avoided. Generally, repellents are applied at dusk or dawn when *Anopheles* are most active. Synthetic repellents are solvents of plastic materials and when spilled or carelessly spread they may damage plastic eyeglass, or watch lenses, stockings, fingernail polish, plastic pens, varnish and similar objects. For added protection, repellents may be applied to clothing (especially socks) or to mosquito nets; in the latter case, mosquito nets sprayed with pyrethrum solutions or diethyltoluamide will retain repellent action for a few days and may be particularly welcome for protection against midges which can pass through ordinary nets. Special wide-mesh netting impregnated with repellents for use as head nets etc. has been widely used in the former USSR. Mosquito-coils or joss sticks containing pyrethrum are useful as a type of repellent. Their value varies greatly, since it depends on the amount of the active substance that the smoke emits when the coil smoulders. A new type of the mosquito-coil principle has been recently developed and released commercially. It consists of a small semi-porous mat, similar to a miniature beer mat, impregnated with a synthetic pyrethroid compound, with the addition of perfume and a blue dye. When inserted in a small electrical heater, the mat slowly releases the insecticide and perfume by vaporization. The amount of insecticide released is sufficient for several hours to prevent mosquitos from entering the room and biting. Once spent the mat changes colour.

Screening

Mosquito-proofing of dwellings, especially where electricity is also available for light and fans, has made a great difference to the health and comfort in the tropics and its popularity is on the increase. There is no doubt that this type of protection is a practical and effective method of malaria control.

The building to be screened must be well constructed and in good repair. Door frames should be made of seasoned wood with metal brackets at the corners and should not sag on their hinges. They should open outwards and be made to fit against a batten all round; they should have a strong spring to ensure tight closing. It is an advantage to have double doors, with a porch at least 2 m in length between them. Every aperture in the building must be screened. Outside privies should also be made mosquito-proof.

The size of aperture in the screening material will vary with the diameter of the wire used. As there are several different gauges in use it is best to specify sizes of wire. It was found that 16–18 mesh [16–18 holes along the linear inch (2.5 cm)] and 28–30 Standard Wire Gauge or SWG (0.025–0.03 mm) is the optimum for general use; the aperture of such wire gauze is 1.2–1.3 mm, sufficient to protect from most mosquito species and leaving about 70% of free area for ventilation.

Many materials have been used for screening such as zinc-coated steel, brass, aluminium, monel-metal and plastic. A salt-laden atmosphere is very destructive to wire screening and under such conditions it is an economy in the end to install the most resistant screen available. Certain plastic screens are of good quality, fairly durable and not expensive. Frequent inspection is necessary for the detection of rents in the screen and defects in the wooden framework, the latter being especially likely to develop where there is extreme variation in humidity between the dry and wet seasons.

Site selection

Selection of a suitable site for new housing, temporary or permanent, may avoid much subsequent difficulty. The principles are simply to place the housing upwind from the nearest water source and that there is the minimum possible breeding of mosquitos within a half-mile (0.8 km) radius, and only a little within a mile (1.6 km); local specialist advice may enlarge on or modify these general points.

It may be less expensive to pump water some distance from the pond or river than to site the buildings near the water and then incur the heavy expense on some special methods of mosquito control. At one time such site selection was literally vital to the success of many projects, and it still considerably affects their prospects, although the availability of better methods of control nowadays makes it less important. Systematic malaria control measures should be practised in any village which may exist within 1 mile of the periphery of the new housing site or temporary camp.

Mosquito control

The control of mosquitos is undoubtedly the best method of protecting a community against the disease. Original attempts early in this century were by 'source reduction', namely, the prevention of breeding, the only means then available.

The spectacular achievements of sanitary measures employed during the building of the Panama canal were linked to large engineering projects; other equally successful projects were seen in Cuba, Brazil and the USA. Much pioneer work was carried out in Malaysia, where Malcolm Watson identified the characteristic breeding habits of the main vectors, the type of water in which they lay their eggs and the best methods to change their habitat in such a way that the vectors avoid these areas. This naturalistic approach, known as 'species sanitation', was not attempted as widely as it should have been. In many countries the majority of water types were dangerous; moreover, during the period 1955–75 the development of residual insecticides offered more promise. However, since then, environmental management for vector control has regained its popularity and is now widely advocated by the WHO.

Insecticides directed against the adult mosquitos (imagicides) were first used on a large scale about 1935. Pyrethrum was the first, and good results were achieved with it in southern Africa and in parts of India, but the new insecticides such as DDT, known as residual compounds, replaced it after the Second World War. They have had brilliant success, incomparably greater than many of the older methods which they soon almost entirely replaced throughout most of the world. Despite their general adoption, it would be wrong to conclude that prevention of breeding has now outlived its usefulness. Each of the two main methods of mosquito control has its place, according to epidemiological conditions of the area and other factors.

In places where malaria is of high endemicity, control by prevention of breeding cannot be effective unless it is very near perfect, the smallest observable density of adult anophelines being enough to keep the disease going on a substantial scale. Perfection, or near perfection, may be attainable where the breeding places are limited and of a distinct, easily recognizable type; it is not attainable where the breeding places are diffuse and various. High epidemic potential in areas of low endemicity offers conditions for easier control of malaria and the same perfection of technique is less important.

The pattern of amenability to control by residual insecticides is the same in principle but very different in degree. The object is not to kill all *Anopheles* at once, but to prevent a large proportion of them surviving for 12 or 14 days; even with the most potent vectors this can be achieved if the daily mortality inflicted on them is of the order of 40 or 50%. This is about the upper range of efficiency of insecticides applied using present techniques, but it can always be exceeded by a more thoughtful and generous application, which secures absolute control in most of the highly malarious places. In those places described as of low endemicity and high epidemic potential malaria is very sensitive to changes in the factors controlling it. A daily mosquito mortality of perhaps 20 to 25% will achieve the objective and this is well within the range of purely routine applications. Insecticides directed against the adult mosquito can therefore be prescribed to control the epidemic degrees of malaria, and routine applications by standard techniques will easily control the transmission of infection.

Another consideration is strictly economic. Prevention of breeding demands attention to a large area of ground around inhabited places, and varies little with the number of people in the area. It is therefore more costly per person in sparsely populated areas. On the other hand insecticides against the adult mosquitos are applied in the house, at a cost per house which varies only a little with the density of population. They are therefore very much preferable in rural areas but may lose some of their advantages in thickly populated places.

The techniques of larval control require real skill and discrimination on the part of the worker. Those involving insecticidal spraying against the adult mosquito require skill, but of another sort which can be acquired by routine drill and which does not demand the same degree of understanding or discrimination.

As a general principle the residual insecticides are faster in their effect than methods of prevention of breeding. There are, however, exceptions to their superiority, wherever the breeding places are few and easily accessible; in such places environmental management measures are preferable.

Antilarval measures of control are of particular value when employed in conjunction with other means such as environmental management. The use of larvicides should be governed by technical, operational and economic considerations.

Technical considerations include: (a) very brief seasonal activity of mosquito vectors, (b) behaviour characteristics (exophily) of the vector which makes residual spraying ineffective; (c) cultural or other objections to indoor house spraying.

Operational reasons refer to situations where the breeding areas of *Anopheles* vectors are limited and well known; obviously the advantages of antilarval measures are greater particularly in urban areas, unless permanent environmental measures are feasible.

Economic reasons are related to operational conditions. Generally, operational convenience is also more economical. Permanent measures while more expensive at first may be much more economical in the long run, especially when repetitive maintenance and supervision are not required.

Antilarval operations of any but the smallest sized projects should be based on technical requirements and on the assessment of the administrative and financial feasibility of the proposed method. Major items that should be considered are: personnel (permanent and temporary), equipment, chemical compounds, transport; supervision of field staff is of importance as is their training. Entomological evaluation of the effectiveness of the method used is indispensable. Among various ways of evaluating the results of antilarval control methods the use of *capture stations* is most advisable. These are selected shelters suitable as resting places for *Anopheles* mosquitos located in various quarters of the area to be protected. They are visited regularly and the mosquito collector sprays them with pyrethrum insecticide and picks up the killed mosquitos from a sheet previously placed on the floor. This is a valuable means of testing the efficacy of control measures; the presence of adult mosquitos is the most reliable test of antilarval work, and often leads to the detection of breeding places which would otherwise be overlooked.

Control of existing breeding places by any method must be carried out within the radius of flight of the local vector, commonly a mile (1.6 km), and throughout the entire transmission season which usually starts a month or so before the first clinical cases occur. It must be based on a knowledge of the local vector and particularly of its breeding habits, and depends on a detailed survey of the area showing all water surfaces of the potentially dangerous type within the radius prescribed. The collection of this information based on a preliminary survey demands knowledge, and the use of skilled labour; all of these may be available or possible in advanced communities or in highly organized industrial undertakings but they are not features of the general rural conditions in developing countries.

One cannot overemphasize the cardinal principle, true in both the urban and the rural areas, that one should avoid the creation of conditions in which the breeding of mosquitos does occur or can do so during the rainy season. Man-made malaria is a curse of the tropics, and much of it can be avoided. The breeding places may be created by digging large holes in the ground to obtain earth for road making; by faults in irrigation systems; by leaking taps in water pipes; by engineering works which interfere with the natural lines of land drainage. The correction of all these errors is usually much more difficult and costly than their prevention (Fig. 10.2).

The rising problem of resistance of mosquitos to insecticides used in public health programmes and in intensive agriculture, together with the growing concern for the environment exposed to repeated applications of potentially toxic compounds, has been responsible for the present interest in other less hazardous measures. Moreover, the high cost of new insecticidal compounds has increased the competitiveness of alternative techniques as components of integrated control strategies. Details of the use of chemical and other larvicidal methods are given in one of the following sections.

Environmental management for mosquito control

This section provides the basic information on environmental management for mosquito control. Those who are interested in the many engineering and technical details of environmental control of malaria vectors will find exhaustive information in the *Manual on Environmental Management for Mosquito Control* published by the WHO (1982).

As mentioned above the importance of measures against aquatic stages of malaria vectors has now been emphasized. The relatively new term of environmental management has been defined as 'planning, organization, implementation and evaluation of deliberate changes of environmental factors, with the view to preventing the propagation of vectors and reducing the human–vector pathogen contact'. Any long-lasting or permanent changes of land, water or vegetation aimed at the reduction of the habitat of the vector are often referred to as 'environmental modifications', while similar temporary or recurrent activity may be known as 'environmental manipulation'. The often used term 'source reduction' refers to any measure that will prevent or eliminate the breeding of mosquitos in their natural or man-made habitats.

Environmental modifications

Many engineering works greatly influence the amount of mosquito breeding; in the past and also at the present time highway and road construction, irrigation systems, agricultural drainage, flood control or impoundments have greatly increased the amount of malaria, wherever proper study of the presence and habits of the vector species have been neglected or adequate preventive measures have

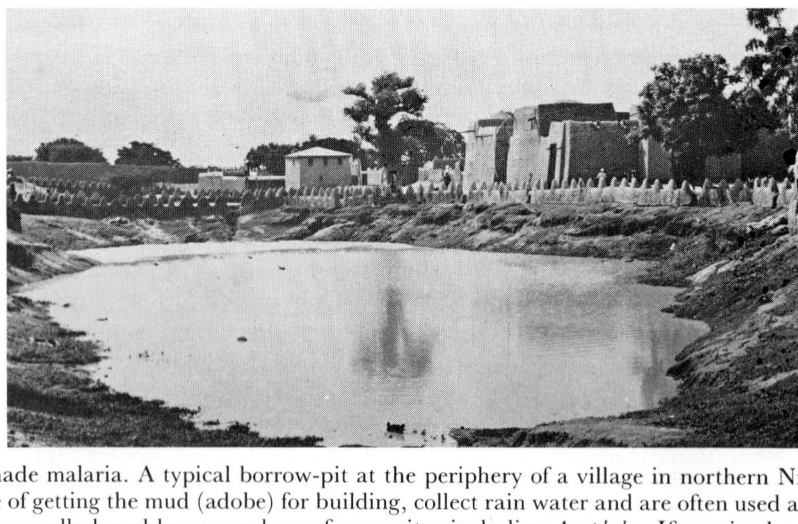

Fig. 10.2 Man-made malaria. A typical borrow-pit at the periphery of a village in northern Nigeria. These pits, dug for the purpose of getting the mud (adobe) for building, collect rain water and are often used as source of domestic water supply. They usually breed large numbers of mosquitos including *Anopheles*. If no piped water supply is available it is not easy to deal with such borrow-pits by filling in or oiling. Paris green or newer insecticides (such as temephos granules) will control the breeding of larvae, but the treatment must be regular in order to decrease the amount of local transmission. (Wellcome Museum of Medical Science.)

not been taken. Apart from health problems created by an increase of mosquito breeding, other water-related diseases may be a consequence of bad management of impounded water.

Impoundments are reservoirs for the storage of water behind dams, and its subsequent release for power generation, irrigation and other uses. The flooding of a large area following the construction of a dam may have a beneficial effect in controlling the mosquito population if, instead of innumerable scattered breeding foci, we have a large, well-defined water surface, more amenable to supervision and control. In the absence of floating vegetation, mosquitos do not breed in the deep water, far from the edges of the reservoirs. The usual habitats of mosquitos generally (and *Anopheles* in particular) is along the indentations of the shoreline, in shallow water covered with floating vegetation.

Thus, mosquito control related to impoundments should be based on the following considerations: (1) proper preparation of the reservoir site and particularly the clearance of trees and other vegetation at all levels between high and low water; (2) provision for fluctuating water levels of the reservoir; (3) appropriate marginal drainage to avoid pools along the margins of the reservoir; (4) maintenance of shoreline, vegetation control and drift removal.

This method of water management has been carried to perfection by the Tennessee Valley Authority in the USA. After the preparation of a clear shoreline, and dyking of shallow areas, the water level of the main reservoirs were subjected to periodic fluctuations to strand the mosquito larvae and pupae.

In deltaic regions such as Lower Bengal, the annual flooding of the land by the rise of water level in the great rivers provides a striking example of the natural control of malaria. The silty flood waters are inimical to the breeding of the local vectors, the extent of breeding edge is reduced, and the raising of the water level above that of the aquatic vegetation exposes the larvae to the attacks of fish and other predators.

Filling is a permanent measure of mosquito control, resulting in complete elimination of water-logged areas, if the source of fill material can be obtained without creating undrained borrow pits. Filling of small holes, abandoned ditches, borrow pits, ponds and similar water pockets is a simple operation, that can be carried out by unskilled labour and with simple equipment consisting of shovels, picks, wheelbarrows, or animal-drawn carts. It can be greatly speeded up when a tractor or motorized earth-moving machinery is available; at times, road contractors, public works departments or industrial firms may be requested to provide this equipment (with the driver) for a few hours. It is evident that the potential breeding places of *Anopheles* mosquitos are more dangerous the nearer they are to human settlements. Moreover, some discrimination in their recognition is needed; thus an old overgrown, water-filled ditch may be more likely to breed malaria vectors than a stagnant pond containing heavily polluted water. When the depression is on the sloping land and filled with ground water, the filling should start at the upper slope, so that the water runs towards the natural outlet.

Sanitary land-fills using refuse disposal for depressions of the ground are acceptable as a method of mosquito control, provided that nuisance and fly-breeding are avoided by compaction and earth cover. Filling on a large scale makes use of the spoil from such operations as harbour dredging, demolition, mining etc. Access to such material is extremely valuable since whole swamps and vast mosquito breeding areas can be converted into dry land. A special type of filling is that of 'hydraulic fill', when a slurry of silt or sand mixed with water is pumped from estuaries, lagoons and creeks into the coastal swamp, which is gradually filled and converted into valuable land.

Drainage is the removal of unwanted water from the land surface or below it. The purpose of a drainage system is the opposite to that of irrigation, but otherwise the hydrological concepts and techniques of the two systems are the same. While a well-constructed drainage system greatly reduces or prevents mosquito breeding, a system that is inadequate in coping with the excess water or that is technically faulty may contribute to the proliferation of mosquitos. The straightening and deepening of channels of natural streams, and the maintenance of their margins free from pockets and vegetation, allow the current to exert its greatest effect and to ease the access of larvivorous fish and other natural enemies. This has a marked effect in reducing the breeding of mosquitos.

Surface drainage involves the shaping of the land surface, the improvement of natural water courses and the construction of open ditches. It is particularly effective on flat, gently rolling lands, overlaying less permeable clay or hard rock. The planning and construction of a major surface drainage system is a matter for the specialist. However, small drainage schemes may be attempted by less experienced people and carried out by unskilled personnel with simple equipment. An important condition is a good topographical survey of the area, so that lines of drainage will follow the natural discharge flows (Fig. 10.3).

Open earth drains are the oldest and simplest structures for surface drainage. The cross-section of an earth drain is usually trapezoidal, with the sides sloping at an angle which depends on the type of soil that will withstand the flow of water. The ratio of horizontal to vertical projection of the drain varies between 3:1 and 1:1 (Fig. 10.4). Earth drains rarely maintain their original shape, since the rapid flow damages the channel, while slow water movement deposits silt. If the flow of water is very swift, undermining of the banks may occur, or if there is some temporary obstruction excessive local scouring may ensue, removing soil from below the grade line of the bottom of the drain and causing a pot-hole. Subsequently, if the rest of the drain becomes dry, as in storm-water drains, pools will remain, which may become *Anopheles* breeding places. A small temporary channel should then be made to connect these pools and drain off the water.

As a general rule the drains should be narrow and deep rather than broad and shallow; their banks should be kept clear of vegetation and sloped to an angle of 45°–60°; tributaries should enter at wide angles and not at right angles, in order to lessen the deposit of silt and debris at the point of junction. The bottom of a narrow drain should be rounded and not V-shaped, but in broad drains a shallow V is preferable to a flat bottom. A few simple precepts concerning the uniform shape of drains and the disposal of spoil are indicated in Figs 10.5, 10.6 and 10.7.

In the case of foot-hill seepages, the best method is to construct a system of contour drains at right angles to the direction of flow, to intercept the seepage at the point at which it arises.

Drains should be as few and short as possible, and their gradient should be carefully considered before starting work. The excavation for drainage

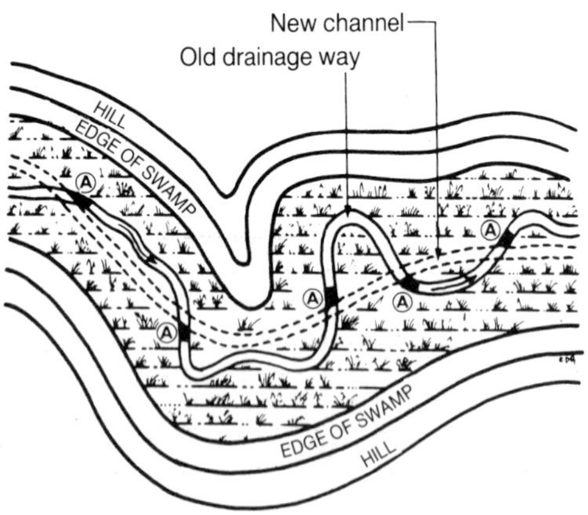

Fig. 10.3 Lay out drains as straight as possible, but the drain should follow the low land, so that deep drains will not be needed. When a new channel cuts across the old, winding watercourse, an earth dam should be built to prevent water from flowing into the old channel.

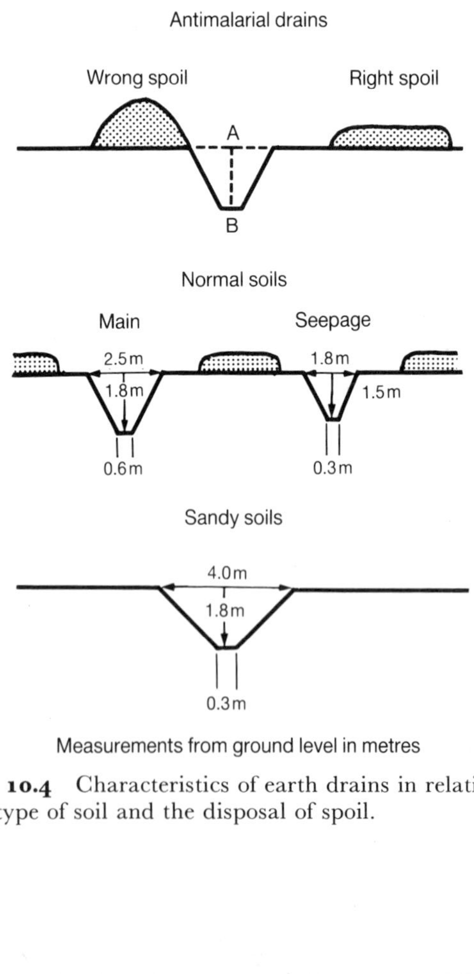

Fig. 10.4 Characteristics of earth drains in relation to the type of soil and the disposal of spoil.

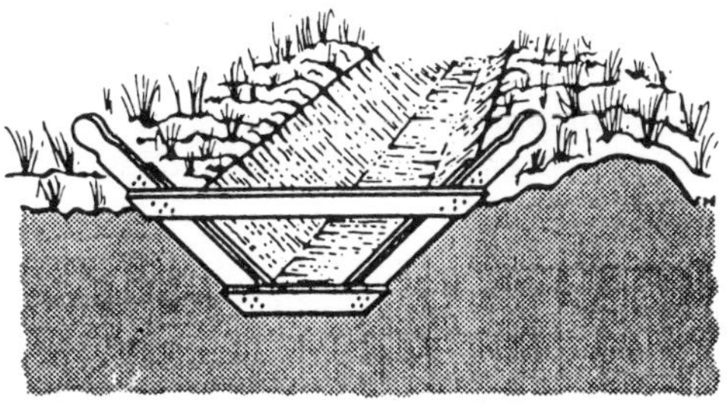

Fig. 10.5 The use of a wooden template facilitates the completion of a uniformly shaped slope of an earth drain.

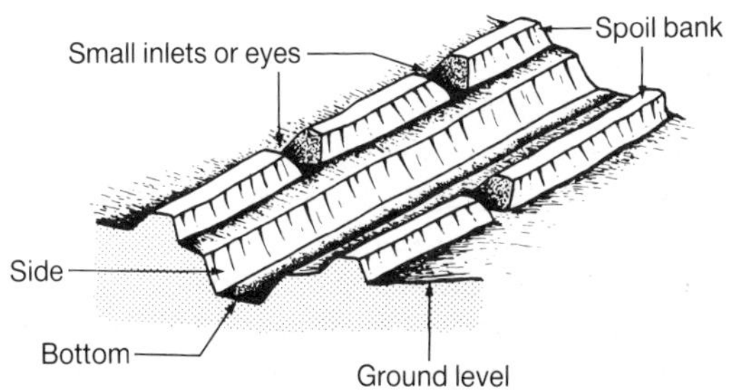

Fig. 10.6 When a drain is dug the removed 'spoil' is used to fill low spots near the drain or is spread or piled up evenly on each side at least 1–2 metres from the edge of the drain; such piles must be separated by small inlets to let the water run into the drain. If the drain crosses a sloping ground the spoil should be piled up on the low side.

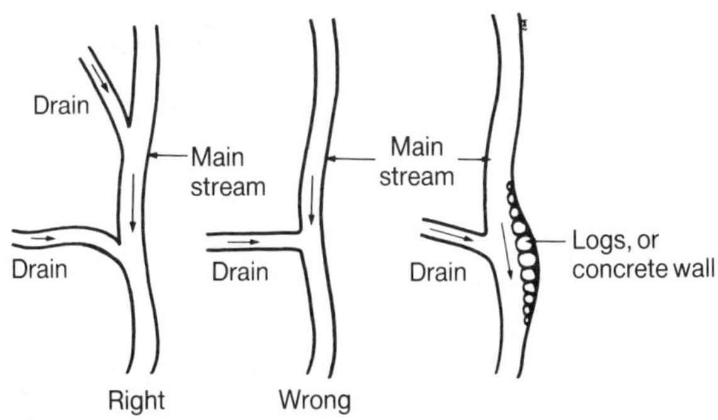

Fig. 10.7 Where two drains or a drain and a stream join, the smaller drain should enter the main stream at an angle of about 30° in the direction of the flow. When a drain must enter the main stream directly, the bank opposite the flow should be reinforced with stone, logs or concrete.

should start at the outfall end. Sharp bends should be avoided wherever possible. The main drain should be constructed first and the tributaries afterwards.

Field work should start by locating the centre line of the ditch by driving pegs at intervals of 25–50 m, and at some distance (2–3 m) from the actual ditch centre line. A guiding frame made up from two posts and a horizontal batten should be fixed at each point marked by a peg. A cord stretched from the centre of each batten to the next few will give a line above the ground parallel to a fixed height over the bottom of the ditch. Staffs (grade rods) marked to show the standard distance between the cord and the bottom of the ditch give the depth of the proposed excavation, which should be checked often (Fig. 10.8).

Manual ditching is generally used in tropical countries where labour costs are moderate. The width at ground level of trapezoidal earth drains, ranges between 1 m and 2.5 m. An average good worker can dig about 2 m^3 daily in not too compacted soils, at a depth of about 1 m; at depths greater than 1.5 m the output per worker drops rapidly because of the need to lift the spoil to the surface. However, ditching by machines is now becoming more common in developing countries in spite of high initial cost and the price of fuel.

While some mosquito breeding may be expected

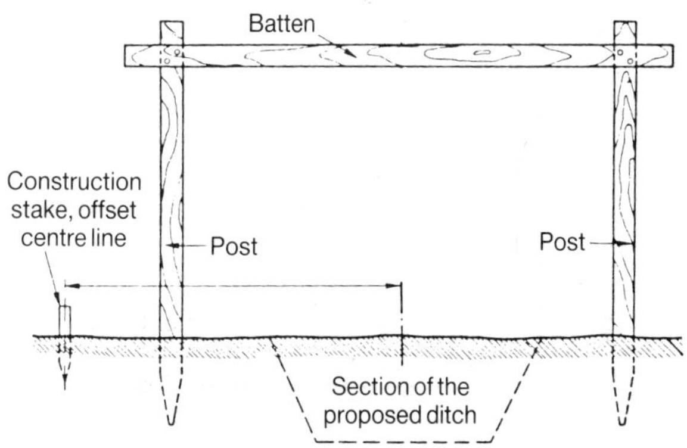

Fig. 10.8 Guiding frame for alignment and depth of earth drains. The height of the horizontal batten, when the frame is fixed over the centre line of the proposed drain gives the depth of the bottom of the drain when measured by grade rods. A cord stretched over a line of several guiding frames from the centre of the battens serves as a guide above the ground, parallel to the desired depth of the drain. The location of the centre line of the drain is given by its distance from the indicator pegs, driven into the ground every 30–50 metres. (Reproduced from *WHO Manual on Environmental Management for Mosquito Control*, 1982.)

in any part of the drainage system, the greatest amount occurs usually in the minor channels, where maintenance is neglected. If the water flow is sluggish, and the banks of drains eroded and covered by vegetation, mosquito breeding is at its most prolific (Fig. 10.9). Furthermore, drains with sharp bends are liable to erosion and silting, forming pockets of standing water. Erosion of the banks is accelerated by turbulence as it occurs downstream of culverts, bridges etc. Thus, wherever there is a change of water velocity the cross-section should be protected against the scouring action.

The 'Lido system', also known as filling and deepening, is useful if for any reason it is difficult to drain an extensive shallow water area covered with vegetation. In such circumstances the circumscribed shallow area may be widened and deepened below the depth of tolerance of emergent plants and the spoil used for an embankment. Providing that the side slopes are steep and stable, mosquito breeding rarely occurs and can be easily dealt with by the use of larvivorous fish. In this manner the shoreline can be greatly shortened and a public amenity may result. This technique is also applicable to fish ponds, or similar water reservoirs.

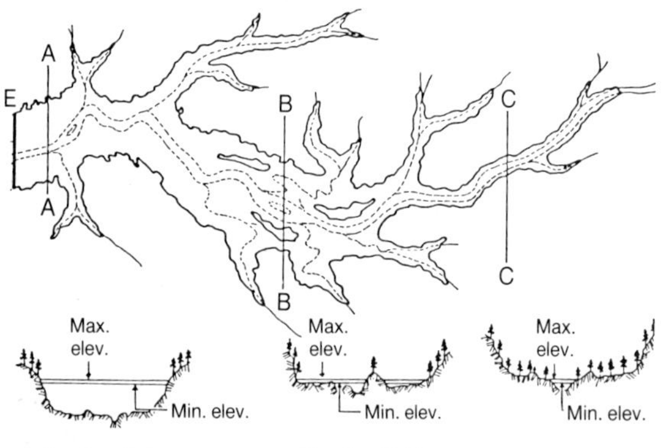

Fig. 10.9 Diagram of a water impoundment with different degrees of mosquito breeding potential. The section B-B is of the greatest importance, as the shallow water and extensive vegetation provide the best habitat for pond-breeding *Anopheles*. (Reproduced from *WHO Manual on Environmental Management for Mosquito Control*, 1982.)

Lining of earth drains is the best way of improving their performance and decreasing the cost of their maintenance. Open drains can be lined with cement concrete, asphalt concrete, stone or brick. When well-constructed and looked after, lined drains allow for faster flow of water, less silting and reduce the growth of weeds. Concrete lining can be made on-site but the use of connecting precast slabs is more common. The slabs for the bottom of the lined drain should have a central narrow invert (cunette) to give free water flow when its level is low. Stone lining may be used where this material is plentiful and cost of labour low. Recently, membrane lining made of asphalt-felt sheeting or of butyl rubber has been introduced. However, this type of lining is more affected by weather conditions and has a life expectancy of a few years only, as opposed to the much longer duration of cement concrete. A lined drain should never be constructed without first making an earth drain to determine the requisite depth of the drain, and to see whether the flow is satisfactory.

At the point of junction with a side channel, the opposite side of the drain should be strengthened and raised to prevent overflow. Weep-holes should be made in the sides of the lined drain so that the subsoil water may get into it; these should slope downwards towards the bottom of the drain. It is also an advantage to construct key-walls at right angles to the drain at intervals, especially where there is a curve in its course, to prevent water from outside from tearing away the earth supporting the side walls (Figs 10.6 and 10.7).

The necessity of repeated regrading, cleaning and oiling of open earth drains makes their upkeep expensive; however, lined drains which are more easily cleaned also require frequent inspection.

Subsoil drains (also known as 'subsurface drains') are widely used for irrigated areas; they prevent waterlogging, and improve aeration and leaching out of salts. There are many varieties of underground drains and the simplest of them, known as 'French drains', are made by half filling a deep trench with rocks, rubble, gravel etc. which present little resistance to water flow. The best way is to place three or four flat stones at the bottom of a deep trench to form a triangle or a square; this construction, when continued, will result in a stone-lined underground channel. This may be covered by coarse sand, palm leaves or straw to

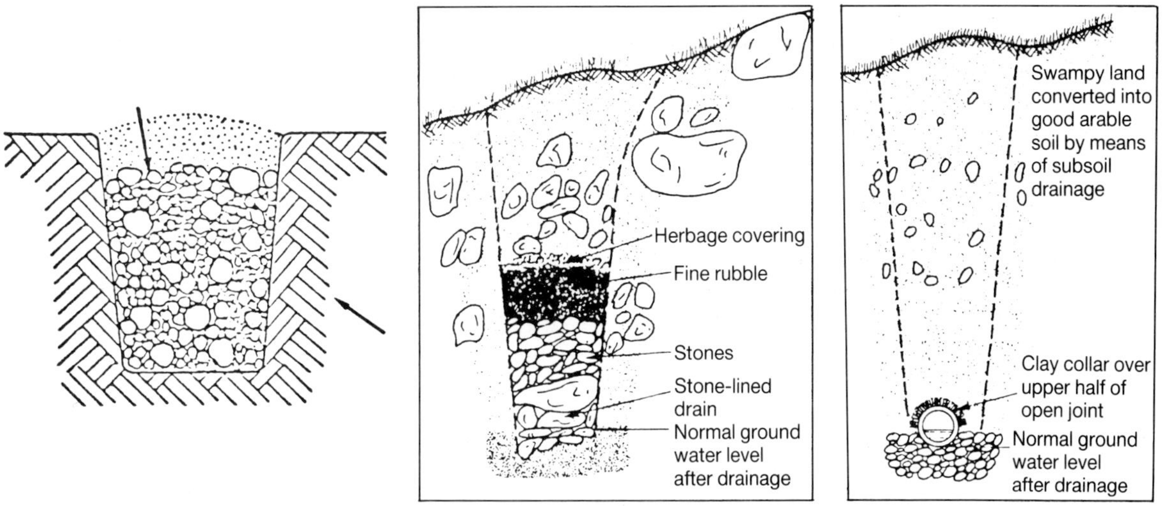

Fig. 10.10 Three types of subsoil drains. (Left) Common 'French' drain filled with rock, rubble or gravel and covered with layer of thatch, palm leaves or long grass. (Centre) Stones used for lining a drain provide a cheap and reasonably good subsoil system. (Right) Typical deep subsoil drains using fired clay-pipes. (Reproduced from *WHO Manual on Environmental Management for Mosquito Control*, 1982.)

prevent the silt and clay from clogging the pervious sections of the drain (Fig. 10.10).

A variant of primitive subsoil drains is that in which wooden poles, coconut husks, bamboo or faggots are used; the latter type refers to large twigs or tree branches being laid at the bottom of a trench, the water draining through the interstices when the ditch is filled in with layers of coarse grass.

A successful type of subsoil drainage evolved in Malaysia consists of using 'tile pipes'. The drain in this case is formed by a series of earthenware pipes laid end to end in trenches beneath the ground, the water entering from below at the joints between the pipes. If soft spots are found in the bottom of the trench (which must be properly graded), stones are rammed into place until a solid foundation is obtained. The laying of the pipes should commence at the outlet of the drain and continue upwards as the trench is made. Greasy water and house waste must not be allowed to discharge into any part of the system. Where pipes come near the surface, proper bridge crossings are necessary, to protect them from being crushed by wheeled vehicles. The pipes should be laid in an absolutely straight line, with as few changes in gradient as possible. Periodic inspections should be made to see that the outlets do not become clogged with silt or other deposits (Fig. 10.10).

It has been claimed that subsoil drainage is self-cleaning, permits a rapid inspection, needs little attention, and requires no oiling. But experience gained during the past 30 years has shown that it has many drawbacks; its main disadvantage is its high initial cost, added to the upkeep.

Design of drainage systems may be quite simple for a small area but its complexity increases with the size of the area and its topography; moreover, the climatic characteristics, type of soil, height of the water table and other factors must be considered. The layout of the drains is also determined by natural and artificial features such as lakes, roads, buildings etc. The most common layout in a flat land is that of a herring bone or grid iron pattern (Fig. 10.11).

The herring bone drainage system consists of a main drain with a series of parallel laterals set at an angle to the main drain. This system, while suitable for draining flat land, is often erroneously employed for swampy valleys. There, water running from the surrounding higher contours collects between the lateral drains and creates new breeding places for mosquitos. The alternative

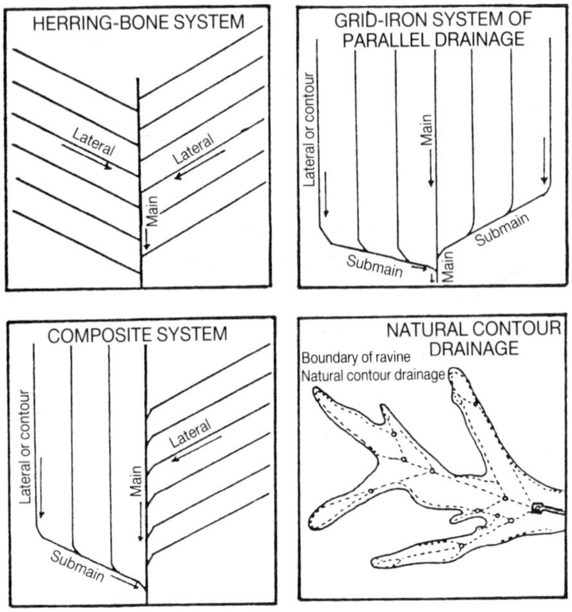

Fig. 10.11 Some typical layouts for surface drainage systems. The general principles are to assure efficient flow of water without exceeding water velocity that will erode the drains. This refers particularly to earth drains, but even concrete-lined drains may be subject to some erosion and silting. (Reproduced from *WHO Manual on Environmental Management for Mosquito Control*, 1982.)

system of grid iron design intercepts most of the water from the surface and underground. The use of the grid iron system avoids the multiplicity of junctions at which blockage may take place: moreover, its advantage lies in the possibility of using each drain at the outer end as a contour drain aiding in the removal of seepage water (Figs 10.9 and 10.11). Lateral drains are connected to a main disposal drain which discharges into a stream, river, lake etc. Interceptor ditches (contour drains) are needed to protect the sloping land from the flow produced by heavy rainfall. These drains run along the contour of the area with little gradient, or along the foot of hills where the land is flatter; they should also intercept seepages, which may cause heavy breeding of some species of *Anopheles*. Water collected by interceptor drains is carried away to the lateral and main drain.

Coastal swamp drainage presents special problems related to the topography of the shoreline, tidal levels, outflow of rivers, climate, coastal vegetation and many other factors. The silt carried by rivers tends to settle and forms deltas with lagoons that turn into swamps. Sand carried by tides and waves forms river bars, behind which brackish water is retained and where several species of important malaria vectors (e.g. *A. melas*, *A. sundaicus*) breed profusely. Some coastal swamps may be drained by constructing embankments (bunds) to prevent the inflow of seawater at high tides; fitting large pipes into the bunds with an automatic outflow gate allows for the removal of water from the lagoon into the sea (Fig. 10.12). In other conditions, large sluices (tide gates) operated manually or mechanically let out the water from the bunded area. When the land slope or low tides make it impossible to operate drainage by gravity, pumping may be necessary (Fig. 10.13).

Vertical drainage is sometimes used to drain

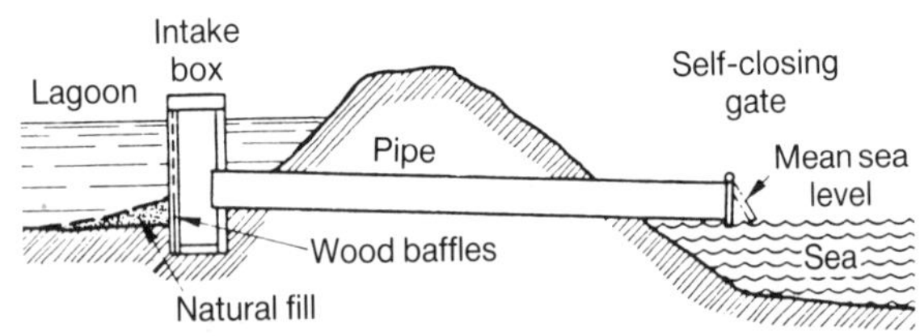

Fig. 10.12 Bund and gravity pipe-drain for a lagoon into the sea. The upper end of the pipe drain is at the level near the bed of the lagoon, and fitted with an intake box. Grooves at the open side of the box are provided to use wooden boards to adjust the sill height when the lagoon becomes filled with sand. The lower end of the pipe-drain is equipped with a self-closing gate, to stop the inflow of water at high tides. (Reproduced from *WHO Manual on Environmental Management for Mosquito Control*, 1982.)

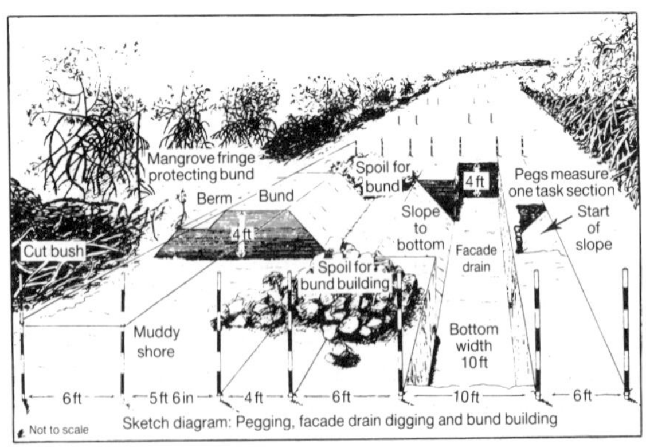

Fig. 10.13 Diagram of the method of coastal swamp drainage as carried out in Nigeria. (Gilroy, 1948.)

swamps or marshes. The bed of the marsh is probably of silt or clay, which retain the water, but beneath this there may be permeable or fissured rock which will afford drainage. A shaft is sunk down to the permeable rock, the exposed surface of which is blasted. A vertical pipe surrounded with stone or gravel is carried up to the level of the marsh bottom. A strainer is placed at the mouth of each sink-hole and a certain amount of grading is required in the marsh leading up to the holes.

Explosives have been successfully used in drainage and ditching operations with great saving of time and cost. Ditches varying from 1 to 10 m wide and from 0.75 to 3.5 m deep can be blasted using an appropriate amount of explosive and a precise method of placing the dynamite sticks.

Environmental manipulation

This recurrent activity aims at producing local conditions unfavourable for the breeding of mosquito vectors in their usual habitats. Many measures described below were classified as naturalistic methods of control; as they are usually directed against known species of local malaria vectors they were often referred to as 'species sanitation'. The success of such practices depends largely on the behaviour characteristics of local *Anopheles* and no general advice as to the use of this or that particular method can be given; thus, field trials are the best way of applying methods that were successful with regard to another vector of similar behaviour pattern.

Changing water levels has been mentioned before as one of the methods used in impounded reservoirs. A variant of this practice, known as 'intermittent drying', is of particular value for control of mosquitos in rice-growing areas, where the terraced or dyked fields are flooded during the planting and growing season. The basic practice is to drain the flooded plots periodically for a few days, to strand and kill the aquatic stages of mosquitos without any damage to the plants. The periodicity of such wet and dry cycles depends on the species of mosquitos present, on the type of irrigation, soil texture, variety of rice and other factors. Field trials of this method should be carried out in consultation with agricultural experts. Some mosquitos (*Psorophora*) may deposit masses of eggs on the dry soil, so that reflooding may be followed by an emergence of swarms of fiercely biting pests. Culicine mosquitos, including *Aedes aegypti*, breed in various water containers; enforcement of a 'dry pot day' when all exposed containers must be emptied and allowed to dry out is the usual method of control of peridomestic mosquito nuisance.

Stream sluicing or flushing methods are similar in principle to changing water levels. They were used extensively in tea gardens and rubber estates of South-east Asia, where *A. minimus* or *A. maculatus* prefer the edges of gently flowing streams. A periodical discharge into the stream of a large volume of water behind a dam after opening a hand-operated sluice or released from an automatic self-priming syphon or tipping bucket will carry the larvae and pupae from the edges of the stream and strand them on the banks. This method may also be used for the control of other stream-breeding malaria vectors such as *A. fluviatilis*, *A. maculatus*, *A. superpictus* and others (Fig. 10.14).

Changes of water salinity in coastal marshes or lagoons through increasing the flow of sea water, banked up by automatic tidegates or other devices, has been attempted with some success in several countries; in Albania *A. sacharovi* was eliminated

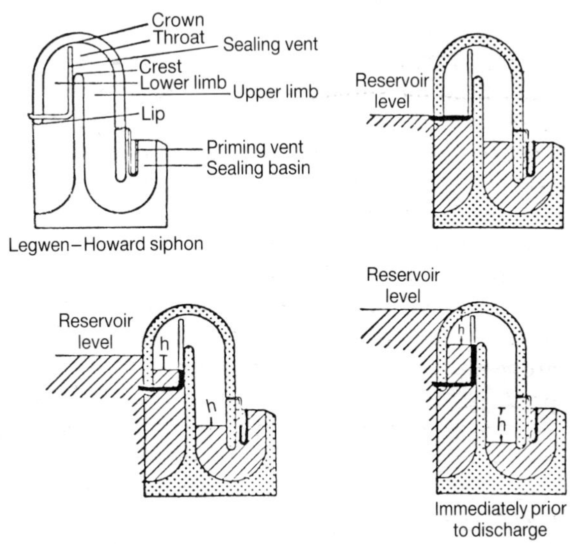

Fig. 10.14 Design of an automatic self-priming siphon for stream flushing as a method of mosquito control. The water level in the reservoir rises until it reaches the lip of the upper limb and seals the siphon, when the priming cycle begins. (Reproduced from *WHO Manual on Environmental Management for Mosquito Control*, 1982.)

by this method from a large coastal marsh. This measure may be of value if the major local vector cannot breed in sea water, especially if the salt content in the lagoon increases as a result of evaporation. However, in areas with heavy seasonal rainfall the measure is less likely to succeed, unless the area is properly drained. On the other hand, desalination of coastal swamps and irrigation with fresh water for growing wet crops may prove to be a risky procedure, if there is an alternative more dangerous vector. This was the case of the replacement of *A. aquasalis*, a secondary vector in Guyana, by *A. darlingi*. The same may be true in West Africa where the salt-water breeding *A. melas* would be replaced by the equally dangerous *A. gambiae*.

Shading of stream banks was used in Assam, India and elsewhere to deter *A. maculatus* and *A. minimus*, which prefer more open breeding spaces. Various shrubs, and especially the thorny Duranta, were planted to provide dense shade; this may be useful for partial control of other sun-loving species such as *A. gambiae*, *A. quadrimaculatus*, *A. fluviatilis* and *A. sundaicus*. A large number of other plants appear to have been used for this purpose with a variable degree of success. Under dense shade no vegetation can grow along the margins of a stream, so that the influence of the current extends right up to the bank and there are no longer any pockets of still water where mosquitos can deposit their eggs.

Clearing of vegetation in densely shaded areas has been used with success for the control of *A. balabacensis* in Sabah, and could be employed on a small-scale in other parts of South-east Asia where this elusive vector is important. Large-scale clearing of the forested areas may be dangerous, however, as it may favour the breeding of the sun-loving *A. minimus*. Generally speaking, clearing of scrub vegetation removes sheltering places of adult mosquitos; it promotes evaporation and therefore speeds up drying of water collections and discloses breeding places which otherwise may be overlooked. Indiscriminate clearing of jungle may, however, favour the breeding of various vector species which lay their eggs in water exposed to bright sunlight. Afforestation by planting eucalyptus and other trees has been introduced for partial drying up of waterlogged lands.

Some plants have a reputation for preventing mosquito breeding. Among these are muskgrass (*Chara*), floating leaf (*Brasenia*) and especially bladderwort (*Utricularia*); the latter is a carnivorous plant which may trap a few larvae in its specialized structures. All these plants grow preferentially where anopheline breeding is not heavy, in deeper waters. The duck-weed (*Lemna, Wolffia*) form occasionally dense mats where mosquito larvae may be less numerous. However, in practice, attempts to use plant growth for mosquito control are not to be recommended.

Deliberate water pollution has been used in India and Malaysia for control of *A. fluviatilis* and *A. maculatus*. *Anopheles* generally are clear-water breeders, but some species such as *A. gambiae* and *A. stephensi* may also breed in muddy waters, often containing organic waste. This is also the case for many Culicine mosquitos, and for this reason this method of control cannot be universally recommended. The technique consists simply of filling the large pool or pond with freshly cut grass, leaves, garden refuse etc. which, on decomposition by anaerobic bacteria, may deter some species of *Anopheles* from egg-laying and will kill larvae or pupae. Although this method may appear attractive, it does not offer any permanent solution and is often the source of pest mosquitos. The use of any industrial waste for deliberate pollution of water should be strongly condemned.

Biological methods

These methods of mosquito control are based on the introduction into the environment of various pathogens and predators of insect vectors of disease. Such agents range from viruses, bacteria, protozoa, fungi plants and nematodes to natural predators such as larvivorous fish.

The effective use of biological methods of control requires a good knowledge of bionomics of the vector species, as well as of local ecological conditions. The great potential of these methods lies in their use together with environmental manipulation, with agricultural practices and even with some pesticides. This is the essence of combined attack on multiple factors of disease transmission implied in the concept of 'integrated control'.

Several viruses (cytoplasmic polyhydrosis, baculovirus etc.) have been isolated and studied in mosquitos, but have shown little practical applicability. On the other hand, considerable attention has been given recently to two bacteria and their products. *Bacillus israelensis* (*B.t.i.*) also known as *B. thuringiensis* serotype H-14, forms spores and produces a toxin which can be isolated; it is a potent gut poison when ingested by mosquitos and other aquatic insects, but harmless to plants, animals and humans. The crystalline toxin, now produced industrially in large quantities as a wettable powder or an emulsion under various proprietary names (Baktimos, Teknar etc.), can be easily applied as a biological larvicide in waters for domestic supply or for irrigation of food crops. It is biodegradable and frequent periodic treatments are necessary. There is no evidence of any resistance of mosquitos to this product. Genes coding for the toxic component of the toxin have now been transferred to other bacteria and more potent compounds may be developed.

Bacillus sphaericus also produces a toxin in its spore envelope. This toxin, harmless to animals and humans, is also more potent and more specific to various mosquitos. Since *B. sphaericus* can multiply even in polluted waters, it has a longer action than *B. israelensis*; much field research on this method is now in progress. A good review of both these bactericides is given by de Barjac and Sutherland (1990).

Fungi of the genera *Coelomomyces*, *Culicinomyces*, *Lagenidium* etc. have been studied as a means of mosquito control. *Coelomomyces* have a complex life-cycle with an alternate crustacean host. Some species, such as some varieties of *C. iliensis*, are capable of causing massive mortalities in larvae of *Anopheles*. This parasite of mosquito larvae and adults has a high infectivity for *Anopheles* and decreases their ability to transmit malaria. However, field trials have not proved the economic practicability of microsporidia.

Nematodes of the family Mermithidae are now being studied as biological control agents. Three species of these parasites received some attention, but the most interesting of them is *Romanomermis culicivorax* which can greatly reduce larval populations and survives in a variety of habitats. Field trials showed certain limitations of the value of this type of mosquito control. Predatory mosquitos of the genus *Toxorhynchites*, the larvae of which feed voraciously on other mosquito larvae, have been investigated recently. They may be useful for destruction of container-breeding species but not for species breeding in ground water.

Of all biological mosquito control methods the use of *larvivorous fish* has been the most successful in many parts of the world. Larvivorous fish are natural enemies of mosquito larvae and have been utilized with advantage for malaria control in Spain, Italy, Greece and other countries in southern Europe and northern Africa, and also Georgia, India, Papua New Guinea, Malaysia, Madagascar and many other countries. Naturally, the use of larvivorous fish is limited to some special situations where the water and other conditions are suitable. Cisterns, shallow ponds, small streams, ornamental pools etc. are ideal places for mosquito control by fish.

The main indications for the selection of fish as a method of mosquito control are their preference for insect larvae over any alternative sources of food, their small size (less than 6 cm long), which makes for access to shallow waters, their rapid maturation and high fecundity, a degree of tolerance to salinity or pollution and harmlessness to other valuable species of the aquatic ecosystem. The most promising species belong to the family Cyprinodontidae of the genera *Aphanius*, *Valencia* (Mediterranean region and western Asia), *Aplocheilus*, *Oryzias* (southern Asia), *Epiplatys*, *Aphyosemion*, *Roloffia* (West Africa), *Nothobranchius*, *Pachypanchax* (East Africa), *Rivulus*, *Cynolebias*, and *Fundulus* (the Americas). In principle, indigenous fish should be selected in preference to imported species, if possible. The most important and best known is the top feeding minnow, *Gambusia affinis*, the guppy (*Poecillie reticulate*), and several others of the families Poecilidae, Cyprinidae and Cyprinodontidae. Of the latter, several species of 'annual fish' (e.g. *Nothobranchius* or *Cynolebias*) have been described and seem to hold some promise for control of mosquito larvae in certain situations. The special merit of these small fishes lies in their capacity to survive and multiply in non-permanent waters, where other species would perish. 'Annual fishes' occupy tropical habitats with a wide range of temperature, where surface water disappears during the dry season (Fig. 10.15). They survive until the next rainy season in the form of eggs buried in the soil. These eggs may be collected and transported in damp peat. Ripe eggs hatch within a few hours after being introduced into the water. The voracious young are hardy, mature rapidly and show high fertility. However, the most popular among

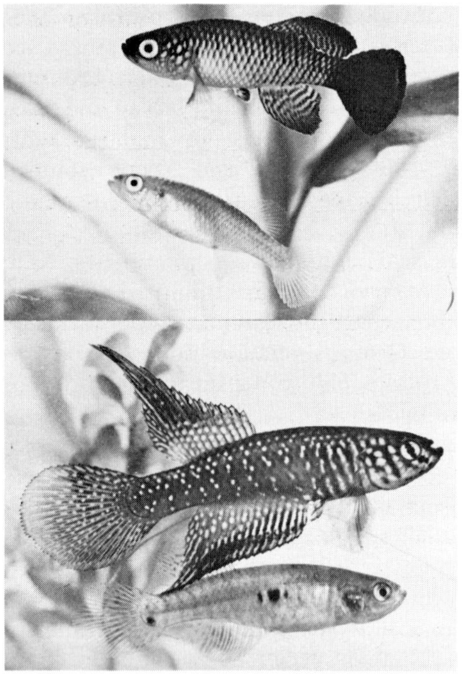

Fig. 10.15 Larvivorous fish used in some malaria control programmes. These are two species of 'annual fish' of the family Cyprinodontidae: *Nothobranchius guentheri* (above), male and female (× *c.* ⅓) and *Cynolebias whitei*, male and female (× *c.* ½). (Hildemann and Walford, 1963.)

larvivorous fish is still the *Gambusia affinis* of the family Poecilidae since it is small (30–65 mm), breeds rapidly (a single female may produce 200–300 offspring in a year) and its rearing and transport are easy. It adapts itself to a wide range of waters, warm and cold, fresh and brackish. Such adaptation is slow and it is advisable to transport the fish in water taken from an original source and gradually adjust it to the type of water in which the fish are expected to thrive for a considerable time. There is now a considerable amount of technical literature on the breeding and introduction of larvivorous fish.

Disadvantages of the use of fish as a mosquito control measure are that they are only effective if present in very large numbers; they are less effective for control of *Anopheles*, especially in the presence of weed and floating debris; constant inspection is necessary to see that the fish are flourishing and are in sufficient numbers and that the water is free from horizontal vegetation. Occasionally, *Gambusia* may become a predator of other ecologically useful aquatic animals.

For any mosquito control programme utilizing *Gambusia* the operational problems related to their rearing, transport and stocking must be solved. Rearing can be done in artificial tanks or natural bodies of water; the depth of water is a critical factor as the fish must be protected from the cold during winter months. For transportation of fish two methods were used. In Afghanistan, *Gambusia* were successfully carried for up to 12 hours in open containers holding 1500 fish, at temperatures between 13 and 18°C. In the Islamic Republic of Iran the fish were transported in double walled polyethylene bags of 30–40 litre capacity packed in wooden boxes, each bag half filled with water and inflated with oxygen (Fig. 10.16). Some 300 fish were transported in each bag for distances of over 2000 km. Plastic churns of 25 litre capacity or metal tanks equipped with an aerator have also been used. Releases of fish to the breeding place must be done so that the temperature of the water is balanced. It has been found that effective control requires 2–5 fish per square metre of water surface.

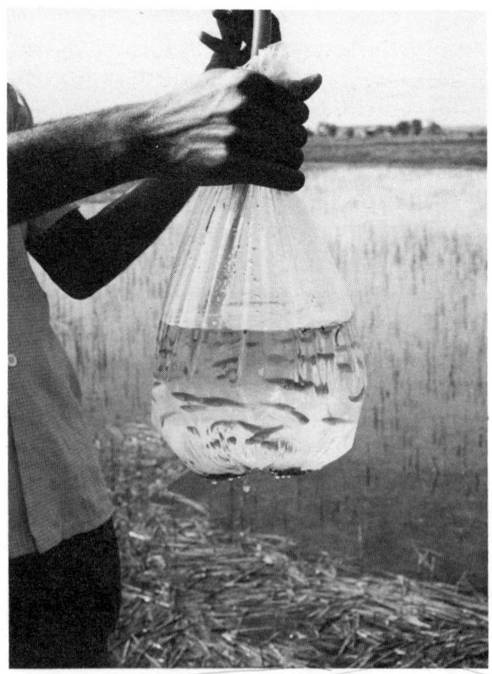

Fig. 10.16 Larvivorous fish (*Gambusia affinis*) widely used for mosquito control in many parts of the world. (WHO photograph by P. Almasy.)

Some species of fish have been found to have secondary uses for reducing the rooted aquatic vegetation and floating algae. These are the carp (*Cyprinus carpio*) and a species of *Tilapia*. Both species benefit larvicidal operations by ensuring a greater open water area in ponds and streams.

Genetic control is a special type of biological control; it has been defined as the use of any method that can reduce the reproductive potential of insects by altering the hereditary material of the vector species. Attempts at mass sterilization of insect pests have been the subject of much research since the early 1950s, when the eradication of the screw-worm in the southern states of the USA was largely successful.

Various methods of genetic control have been used, but the release of males sterilized by ionizing irradiation or chemical compounds has received most attention. The principle of this method is that the sterilized males seek out and mate with the wild females in the natural population, thus preventing the hatching of their eggs and lowering their reproductive potential.

Chemosterilant compounds fall into two main categories; the alkylating agents (e.g. apholate) and the antimetabolites (e.g. methotrexate), used for treatment of tumours in humans. A large number of the two groups have been tested during the past few years in order to find the lowest concentration which produces complete sterility in male mosquitos without causing excessive mortality, so that they should be able to compete with normal males. Various compounds have given promising results but the toxicological and mutagenic implications for mammalian species including humans present an additional difficulty. In a field trial in El Salvador some 4.3 million adults of *A. albimanus* were released after the sterilization of their pupae in a solution of an alkylating agent. In further releases, treatment of pupae by a juvenile hormone (methoprene) was also employed. Although the results seemed to be promising at first, the rapid influx of normal anophelines from the periphery of the area was a setback.

Another method of genetic control is based on crossing two sibling species of *Anopheles*. This leads to hybrid male sterility and when very large numbers of sterile males are released, their competition with fertile males is so great that eventually the size of the succeeding generation decreases below the threshold when transmission of malaria is possible.

The third method is that of incompatibility, in which the release of one sex of a certain species, infertile with the opposite sex of another population of the same species, achieves the same effect.

Introduction of mass hybrid sterility for control of the *A. gambiae* complex was tried in Burkina Faso of West Africa but little mating between sterile males and wild females occurred. The main and difficult requirement for success of all genetic methods of mosquito control is the production of very large numbers of healthy, competitive, though genetically different, mosquitos and their release in the right place and at the right time to mate successfully with wild insects.

Finally, a new concept of genetic control involves the mass release of mosquitos carrying genes that prevent the development of malaria parasites in female *Anopheles* or genes imparting greater susceptibility to some insecticides.

Zooprophylaxis

In describing the behaviour pattern of *Anopheles* and their feeding preferences (Chapter 6) it has been pointed out that several species of *Anopheles* are equally attracted to humans and animals and some species prefer feeding on the blood of domestic cattle, but will bite humans when they find no other source of blood. On the other hand, even such seemingly anthropophilic mosquitos as *A. gambiae* may be diverted to cattle and horses if these animals are easily accessible. Such diversion of vectors to animal hosts has been used deliberately in some parts of the world, including the former USSR, as an auxiliary method of malaria control. Indeed, it is likely that progressive deviation of the local *Anopheles* vectors was partly responsible for the decrease of malaria from northern Europe and much of North America. Many of the important vectors of malaria in India, Indonesia and Malaysia have zoophilic tendencies. While it may not be feasible to employ zoophrophylaxis as a practical antimalarial measure, the beneficial effects of deviation of some *Anopheles* species to cattle may have a bearing on agricultural practices in integrated vector control. The converse has occurred in recent years where cattle and buffalo have been redeployed in areas destined for new economic development (e.g. Vietnam). The depletion of animals from the areas from which the cattle and buffalo were taken resulted in a dramatic increase in malaria transmitted by not only *A. sundaicus* but also by *A. campestris*, which was previously feeding almost entirely on the animals.

Chemical methods

Chemical pesticides are still the mainstay of most vector control programmes, but the growing problem of resistance of many insects to insecticides and the present concern with the effect of some of these compounds on the environment has stimulated an intensive research programme coordinated by the WHO to develop a number of candidate insecticides and to test their activity and safety.*

The efficacy of chemical control measures depends on a number of factors: the species of vector involved; efficacy of the pesticide; type of its formulation; thoroughness of its application; nature of the surface treated and climatic conditions; acceptability to the inhabitants; and management of the control programme.

A detailed description of various chemical insecticides must be preceded by some knowledge of their classification.

Classification of insecticides

Insecticides can be classified as follows. (1) According to their chemical composition. (2) By the way of their entry into the body of the insect. (3) By the method of their application. (4) By the stage of the life cycle of the insect against which they are used.

1. *Classified by their chemical characteristics the most common insecticides applied in public health practice are*:
   - 1.1. Petroleum oils and their derivatives.
   - 1.2. Active constituents of flowers of pyrethrum (pyrethrins) or some newer synthetic compounds of this group (pyrethroids).
   - 1.3. Chlorinated hydrocarbons [dichloro-diphenyl-trichloroethane (DDT), hexachlorocyclohexane (HCH), dieldrin etc.].
   - 1.4. Organophosphorus insecticides (malathion, temephos etc.).
   - 1.5. Carbamates (propoxur, carbaryl etc.).
   - 1.6. Insect growth regulators (methoprene).
2. *Insecticides may be absorbed by the insect as follows*:
   - 2.1. By introduction into the plant or animal which is to be protected. These systemic insecticides are used mainly in agriculture and to some extent in veterinary medicine.
   - 2.2. By ingestion through the mouth (e.g. Paris green) of anopheline larvae. This is also the mode of action of various pesticides employed in agriculture (stomach poisons).
   - 2.3. By inhalation through the tracheae. All highly volatile insecticides (e.g. methyl bromide, dichlorvos) act in this way. Some contact insecticides (HCH) also have this type of 'fumigant' action.
   - 2.4. By contact with the cuticle and penetration into the body of the insect. Such contact insecticides are DDT, HCH, dieldrin; some of them may exert 'particulate' action through minute airborne particles without direct contact with the insect.
3. *According to the method of application insecticides may be*:
   - 3.1. Released into the surrounding air space (*space spraying*) in the form of vapour or aerosol such as fog, smoke etc. so that they are absorbed by inhalation or contact.
   - 3.2. Deposited on a solid surface, such as indoor walls and ceilings, for eventual contact with the insect. These long-acting or *residual insecticides* are generally used for control of malaria and other mosquito-borne infections and include a wide range of compounds from DDT to the newer organophosphates.
   - 3.3. Released on the surface of water or into it in the form of floating film, powder, granules, briquettes etc.
4. *Insecticides may also be classified according to the action on the life cycle of mosquitos into*: larvicides and imagicides. (The use of the term adulticides for the latter is not recommended.)

In selecting a suitable insecticide the following factors should be taken into consideration:

Specifications for Pesticides Used in Public Health*, **6th edn, World Health Organization, Geneva, 1985.

1. Its effective toxicity towards the target insect. (The problem of specific resistance to one or another compound must be considered.)
2. Duration of action on a surface to which it will be applied at a given dosage.
3. Ease of application in existing topographical and climatic conditions.
4. Toxicity towards humans, domestic or wild animals or fish.
5. Cost of insecticide and of transport and labour involved.

In the following section a simple classification by chemical composition will be used for convenience, although reference to the methods of application of these compounds is unavoidable. In addition reference is made to the WHO recommended classification of pesticides by hazard (WHO, 1992). In this regard the hazard referred to is the acute risk to health (that is, the risk of single or multiple exposures over a relatively short period of time) that might be encountered accidentally by any person handling the product in accordance with the directions for handling by the manufacturer or in accordance with the rules laid down for storage and transportation by competent international bodies. The classification is based primarily on the acute oral and dermal toxicity to the rat since these determinations are standard procedures in toxicology. Toxicity is expressed in LD_{50}, which is a statistical estimate of the number of mg of toxicant per kg of body weight required to kill 50% of a large population of test animals (Table 10.2).

Table 10.2 Toxicity and degree of hazard related to chemicals used as pesticides in agriculture and public health practice

Common name	Chemical type	Toxicity to rat LD_{50} (mg/kg)		Degree of hazard in use
		Oral	Dermal	
Larvicides				
Chlorpyriphos	OP	135	2000 (rabbit)	MH
Diflurobenzuron	IGR	4640	—	UH
Fenthion	OP	250	—	MH
Iodphenphos*	OP	2100	>1800	UH
Methoprene	IGR	34600	—	UH
Temephos (Abate)	OP	8600	>4000	UH
Imagicides				
Bendiocarb	C	55	—	MH
Chlorphoxim*	OP	500	—	SH
Cypermethrin	P	250	—	MH
DDT	Ocl	113	2510	MH
Dichlorvos	OP	100	>500	MH
Dieldrin	Ocl	37	60	MH
Deltamethrin	P	135	—	MH
Fenitrothion	OP	503	350	MH
γ-HCH	Ocl	88	900	MH
Lambda-cyhalothrin	P	56	—	MH
Landrin	C	119	>2500	MH
Malathion	OP	2100	>4000	SH
Parathion	OP	3	6.8	HH
Permethrin	P	4000	—	UH
Pirimiphos-methyl	OP	2018	—	MH
Propoxur	C	95	>2400	MH
Pyrethrum	P	200	>1800	UH

C, carbamates; IGR, insect growth regulators; Ocl, organochlorines; OP, organophosphates; P, pyrethroids; HH, highly hazardous; MH, moderately hazardous; SH, slightly hazardous; UH, unlikely to present hazard; HCH, hexachlorocyclohexane.

The list of imagicides contains those in common use and also some compounds* recommended for testing in the field by the WHO.

Petroleum oils

Petroleum oil fractions which include various paraffinic and other hydrocarbons, have played an important part in mosquito control by larvicides since the beginning of this century. These oils are applied on the water in such a way as to produce a continuous thin film on the surface. When larvae come up to the water surface to breathe, the oil penetrates into their tracheae and kills them either by suffocation or by poisoning. For larvicidal work the mineral oil selected should have high toxicity to larvae and pupae, should spread easily and evenly over the water surface to form a stable film, penetrate quickly into the tracheal system of larvae, have no offensive odour, and be harmless to fish, waterfowl and livestock.

There are many grades of oils on the market which may be used for mosquito destruction, ranging from the very light oils such as kerosene to the heavier forms known as crude or fuel oils. The choice of oil is largely determined by local conditions. Thus, with high temperature a thicker oil is required, while in the presence of vegetation a ligher oil with great spreading power is necessary. Again, in still water a heavy non-toxic oil applied in sufficient quantity to form a complete film will after some hours kill all the larvae; while in moving water a thin layer of rapidly spreading oil with a high toxicity is indicated. Full specifications for larvicidal oils are complex but the main points indicated in the *WHO Manual on Larval Control Operations* (1973) are: specific gravity at 15.6°C 0.82–0.85; viscosity at 37.8°C 33–45 cs; spreading pressure not less than 23 dynes/cm.

Larvicidal properties of mineral oils vary considerably in different consignments, according to the methods of refining. The addition of 1 to 2.5% of vegetable oil, such as castor or coconut oil, may increase the spreading power considerably. It is usually more satisfactory to use one of the proprietary oils (such as *Malariol*) which are specially designed for larvicidal work as it contains surface-active agents which increase its spreading property and toxic action.

Good mineral oils must be homogeneous, fairly stable, free-flowing and easily spreading over the water surface. The approximate amount of oils used in practice is between 200 and 600 ml for each 100 m^2 of water surface (20–60 litres per hectare). Addition of 1% of synthetic insecticides such as DDT greatly increases the toxicity of ordinary oils, but this contributes to the pollution of the environment.

Application of liquid larvicides can be carried out by simple oil cans, hand-operated continuous sprayers, compression sprayers or aerial spraying. Oils are usually applied from a knapsack sprayer, which must not be too heavy. The sprayer, fitted with a pump which has to be worked by hand, is preferable and less wasteful than a compression sprayer. All spraying requires supervision and regular (usually once a week) application.

Oil may also be applied from a garden watering can or garden syringe, by a used cotton waste soaked in oil and pegged into the ground for seepages and small pools, by means of a long stick with a bundle of old sacking attached, by balls of sacking tethered to the banks of streams or pools, by brushing over the surface with a sweeper's broom, by drip cans placed over streams and drains, by oil booms fixed across streams or irrigation channels, or it may be mixed with sawdust and thrown over breeding places after the manner of sowing grain.

The disadvantages of oiling are: it will not easily penetrate a barrier of grass and, to make it thoroughly effective, all vegetation and floating debris must be removed; wind will break up an oil film and carry it to one side of a sheet of water; it is cumbersome and costly for transportation; it may kill fish and render them unfit for human consumption; and it renders water unfit for drinking purposes. On the other hand, it kills the eggs and pupae of mosquitos; it is easy to see whether it has been properly applied.

Mineral oils are not cheap, especially at the present time when the cost of all petroleum products has sharply increased. However, the cost of oil is only a part of the total cost of the operation and good results can be obtained with oils used in moderate amounts by experienced teams.

As an alternative to mineral oils, synthetic monolayer films have been used with good results when the mosquito breeding activity is limited to a few large water surfaces. Aliphatic amines and polyoxyethylene stearyl alcohols have been employed for this purpose.

Paris green

Paris green (copper aceto-arsenite) was first applied as a mosquito larvicide in 1921. It is a microcrystalline green powder, practically insoluble in water. Its small particles will float on water and poison surface-feeding mosquito larvae. It should contain 50–55% arsenious oxide and be fine enough to pass through a 200–300 mesh sieve. It is dispersed in the field in the form of dust mixed with a cheap diluent such as powdered soap-stone, talc, slaked lime, road dust, powdered charcoal or some other locally available material. The dilution varies between 1 and 30% and depends on the equipment used. For hand-operated dusters or blowers a dilution of 10 to 20% is adequate. Various liquid suspensions of Paris green with water have been used in compression sprayers with satisfactory results; other formulations of Paris green have been developed, including granules and emulsion concentrates.

The application dosage of Paris green formulations ranges from 6 to 15 g of the active chemical per 100 m^2 of water surface. Larger doses are needed where the vegetation is dense. It is classified in class Ib 'highly dangerous' (LD_{50} 22 mg/kg).

Advantages of Paris green are its comparatively low cost, its high toxicity for *Anopheles* larvae, and its portability and ease of distribution by wind. There is no need to remove vegetation and no evidence of ill effects to domestic animals, fish or other natural enemies of larvae, or to crops. The water treated in the dosage recommended above is not rendered unfit for domestic purposes and it is equally effective in fresh or brackish waters. On the other hand, it has no effect on the eggs or pupae of mosquitos nor on any of the aquatic stages of culicines. It requires special apparatus for distribution, for screening the diluent and for mixing, and its use requires constant supervision. It is difficult to see whether it has been applied properly or not, except by dipping for larvae. With the development of highly effective and reasonably safe organophosphorus and other larvicidal compounds (synthetic pyrethroids or toxins of *B. israelensis*) the use of Paris green has markedly decreased.

Pyrethrum

This is the oldest effective insecticide known and its main advantage is its high immediate toxicity to insects while it is harmless to humans although classified in class II 'moderately hazardous' (LD_{50} 500–1000 mg/kg). It is obtained from the flowers of the plant *Chrysanthemum cinerariaefolium* grown commercially in many parts of the world, and cultivated on a large scale in Kenya, Zaire, Japan, India and South America.

Pyrethrum is used mainly in the form of a 10–25% extract of crushed dry flowers in kerosene or other organic solvents. This extract can be used when further diluted to 0.1–0.5% with kerosene. If a suitable emulsifier is added this extract can be diluted with water. Pyrethrum contains from 0.7 to 3.0% active principles. These are mainly esters of pyrethrins I and II which are rapidly oxidized and inactivated in sunlight with a loss of insecticidal activity.

Pyrethrins are nerve poisons, acting through the insect cuticle which is permeable to them. When sprayed, the droplets come into contact with the insect and their toxic action is fast. The addition of certain synergists increases the toxicity of pyrethrins to insects. Among these synergists, piperonyl butoxide is most commonly used.

Pyrethrins in crude form have been used for control of various insects for many years. Their rapid 'knock-down' effect is of particular importance, although this action is relatively short lived and frequent applications are necessary. There is no great evidence of mosquito resistance. Their use has greatly increased recently because of the popularity of aerosol dispensers for rapid insect control at home and for disinfestation of aircraft. Pyrethrum was also the first insecticide used for large-scale malaria control by attacking the adult *Anopheles*.

In malaria control programmes the common formulations of pyrethrum are: 0.2–0.4% dusts; 0.1–0.4% solutions in kerosene or petroleum distillate; as aerosol insect sprays (synergists are included in the formulations). The pattern of use of pyrethrum is very wide. It is applied as thermal fogs, mists for non-residual control by repetitive application in kitchens, food stores, factories etc. where toxic residual insecticides cannot be used. Thermal fogs of 0.05% pyrethrins with 0.4% piperonyl butoxide are used for fly control. Ultra-low volume (ULV) sprays are used against mosquitos, houseflies and tsetse flies. Pyrethrum is repellent to mosquitos; thus it is used in insect repellent creams and mosquito coils. Pyrethrins have a very low toxicity for warm blooded animals, but are toxic to fish; however, their persistence in water is brief.

Recently a number of synthetic compounds have been developed. They are as potent as pyrethrins and some of them present definite advantages over the natural products.

The first useful synthetic pyrethroid came from the USA in 1969; it was given the generic name of *allethrin*. Allethrin has eight possible isomers depending on the position of the hydrogen atoms on the one (cis) or other (trans) side of the cyclopropane ring.

The chemical names of the new compounds now available commercially are: allethrin, cismethrin, dimethrin, resmethrin, tetramethrin, deltamethrin, permethrin, lambda-cyhalothrin and others. The toxicity data for pyrethroids is highly variable according to Lisomer ratios, the vehicle used for oral administration and the husbandry of the test animals. The single LD_{50} value now chosen for classification purposes is based on administration to test animals in corn oil and is much lower than that in aqueous solution. These compounds are more stable when exposed to sunlight and are less volatile than the natural product; they are equally safe in use, since their acute toxicity to mammals is generally low.

The insecticidal activity (knockdown and kill) of synthetic pyrethroids is high, but each compound has a specific range of action, which is influenced by the formulation and the degree of synergism with other compounds. Synthetic pyrethroids are used as coarse space sprays, aerosols and smokes in mosquito coils. The exceptional toxicity of synthetic pyrethroids against mosquitos and other insects is important because they are expensive and must be used at dosage rates much lower than other insecticides. The new compounds are now available as usual formulations of solutions, emulsion concentrates and even as water-dispersible powders.

Deltamethrin, which has a fairly high mammalian toxicity (moderately hazardous; LD_{50} 135 mg/kg), was used at a dosage of 0.05 g/m^2 in a field trial in Africa and was safe and effective as a residual spray for at least 2 months. Permethrin, a safer pyrethroid (moderately hazardous; LD_{50} 500 mg/kg), when employed at a dosage of 0.5 g/m^2 was fairly effective as a residual spray for about 3 months. The latest synthetic pyrethroid, discovered in the early 1980s and developed as an insecticide for agricultural and public health applications is lambda-cyhalothrin. The formulations available for residual spraying are 2.5% and 5% emulsifiable concentrate and 10% wettable powder. Application rates are typically in the range of 10–25 mg per m^2, or for prolonged action (6 months) 25–30 mg per m^2 are suggested. It is classed as a 'moderately hazardous' pesticide with an LD_{50} of 56 mg/kg.

As already mentioned the pyrethroids are being used increasingly for the impregnation of mosquito nets and curtains. Comparative studies, which included deltamethrin, permethrin and lambda-cyhalothrin (Miller *et al.*, 1991), showed a 40% loss of permethrin after 12 weeks use compared with no loss and a 38% loss for deltamethrin and lambda-cyhalothrin, respectively. Each insecticide, especially lambda-cyhalothrin, caused significant mosquito mortality whilst permethrin-treated nets reduced the number of *A. gambiae* s.l. entering the experimental hut by 60%. Sleepers using the nets had no medical symptoms. Permethrin tends mainly to deter mosquitos from house entry at a high dose of 0.67 g/m^2, thus enhancing personal protection, whereas the other insecticides kill higher proportions of the endophilic mosquitos, which would give better community protection against malaria transmission.

Chlorinated hydrocarbons (organochlorines)

Insecticides of this group employed in public health practice are DDT, HCH and dieldrin; the latter two are collectively known as cyclodienes.

DDT

Dichloro-diphenyl-trichloroethane or DDT (known also under the name of dicophane or chlorophenothane) was originally synthesized in 1854, but its insecticidal properties were discovered in 1939 by Paul Muller of Switzerland. The first field trials of DDT took place during the Second World War. The abbreviated name DDT was given to this compound by the British Ministry of Supply.

DDT is still the most widely used insecticide in public health practice. The chemical structure of DDT and other organochlorine insecticides is shown in Fig. 10.17. The two chlorine atoms

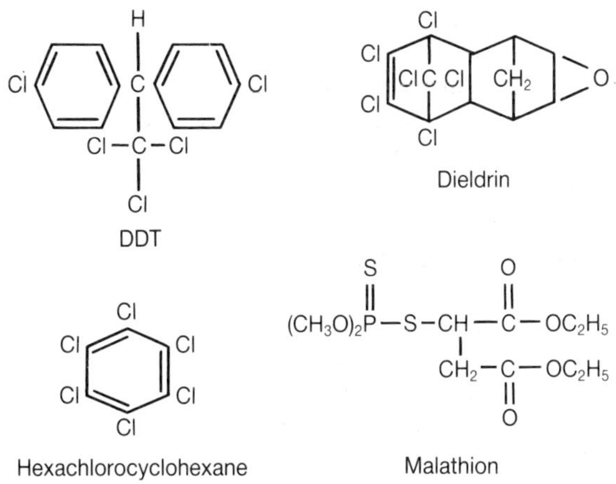

Fig. 10.17 Chemical structure of four common insecticides used for malaria control.

attached to the benzene rings may be linked with other carbon molecules giving different isomers of the compound, but the most effective of these is the para-para isomer of DDT. Technically DDT is a mixture of isomers, but it must contain at least 70% of para-para isomer to be acceptable. The content of the para-para isomer is usually stated on the container.

DDT is a white, amorphous, waxy powder with an aromatic smell. It is soluble in oils and organic solvents, but not in water. It is very stable and on suitable impervious surfaces it may remain active for as long as a year, but normally, if the DDT deposit is not rubbed off or covered up, it is applied twice a year. On sorptive surfaces like mud (adobe), DDT loses its insecticidal effect somewhat faster. It has a certain irritant effect on insects causing some of them to leave the treated surface soon after alighting on it, but its toxicity to most species of insects is high. Its toxicity to humans is very low and there is no evidence that the millions of people whose houses were treated with DDT are at any risk from exposure to it. It is classed as a moderately hazardous pesticide, with an LD_{50} of 113 mg/kg. On the other hand, it is true that DDT may adversely affect some animals including cats, chickens, predatory birds and fish. For this reason the use of DDT outdoors, when gross environmental contamination is likely, should be avoided. The amount of DDT for residual spraying of indoor surfaces is usually given in terms of technical DDT and the standard dosage is 2 g/m^2 of the treated surface every 6 months. DDT has also been used for its larvicidal properties, mainly as an additional compound to fortify the toxic action of oils; the required dosage is very small. Two methods were used: a 2–5% solution of DDT in 'high speed' oil employed at 0.3 to 0.6 litre to 1000 m^2 of water surface and an emulsion concentrate, to be diluted with water so that the final concentration of DDT is 0.1–0.15%, to be sprayed at a rate of 10–20 litres per 1000 m^2 (about 10–20 gallons per hectare) of water surface.

Like all chlorinated hydrocarbons, DDT has a short effect when used as a larvicide: the insecticide is diluted or washed away or absorbed by mud and vegetation. The use of all chlorinated hydrocarbons as larvicides today is frowned upon because of their adverse action on the environment.

The water-dispersible powder of DDT for residual spraying of houses contains 50–75% of active substance; the higher content of the insecticide is preferable for a number of reasons, mainly economic.

Hexachlorocyclohexane (HCH)

This compound, formerly called benzene hexachloride or BHC, was synthesized in 1825, apparently by Faraday. Its insecticidal action was discovered in the UK in 1942 when it was first known under the code name 666; it became widely used during the 1950s in agriculture, veterinary medicine and public health.

Its chemical constitution is remarkably simple ($C_6H_6Cl_6$), since it consists of a benzene ring with a chlorine atom attached to each carbon (Fig. 10.17).

The arrangement of the hydrogen and carbon atoms in space may vary, so that a number of optical isomers exist, the most active of which is the gamma isomer. This isomer when pure, or at least 99% pure, is called *lindane*. Technical HCH must contain at least 12% of the gamma isomer. It is soluble in organic solvents. Technical HCH is a whitish or light-brown, granular or flaky substance with a characteristic musty smell. It is relatively volatile and may kill insects fairly rapidly by fumigant action. However, because of this volatility, its residual action is generally half as long as that of DDT, although its toxic action is faster. It is classed as a moderately hazardous pesticide with an LD_{50} of 100 gm/kg based on the cumulative properties of the beta isomer. HCH may be used in the form of water-dispersible powder, containing 6.5% gamma isomer, as a residual insecticide for indoor spraying of walls; other formulations (solutions, emulsions) exist for use as larvicides or as insecticidal smoke. The usual dosage of HCH for residual spraying is 0.3 g/m^2 every 3 months or 0.5 g/m^2 every 4–6 months.

Dieldrin

This insecticide, together with aldrin, belongs to a small group of compounds obtained by the cyclodiene synthesis discovered by Diels and Alder, whose names were given to the first two products. The chemical structure of dieldrin is shown in Fig. 10.17.

The active principle is hexachloro-octahydro-epoxy-dimethano-naphthalene or HEOD which comprises some 80% of technical product soluble in organic solvents but not in water. Formulations of dieldrin may comprise powders, emulsions, granules or briquettes. Dieldrin is more toxic than DDT and HCH both to insects, other animals and to humans (highly hazardous; LD_{50} 37 mg/kg). Its residual activity at a dosage of 0.5 g/m^2 was expected to be of 6 months' duration, but it was found that it is shorter, being not more than 4 to 5 months. Dieldrin is less excito-repelling to mosquitos than DDT and its action is faster. However, it has two main disadvantages: fairly high toxicity to humans and other animals, and proneness rapidly to produce resistance to cyclodiene compounds and to HCH. Dieldrin has been responsible for poisoning spray operators, domestic animals and poultry. Because of this and other factors, its use in public health practice has now virtually ceased except for tsetse fly control in Africa.

Other chlorinated hydrocarbon insecticides comprise such compounds as chlordane, methoxychlor, heptachlor and many more. The increased trend of resistance to this group of chemicals has now led to a progressive search for and use of alternative compounds. However, the number of new potentially useful compounds has greatly decreased. The cost of research and the legal requirements concerning the toxicity of prospective insecticides are the main factors responsible for it.

Organophosphorus compounds

This group of insecticides, widely used in agriculture (e.g. parathion) is now commonly employed in public health practice, mainly because several insect vectors of disease have become resistant to chlorinated hydrocarbons. Most of the organophosphorus insecticides are esters or amides of organically bound phosphoric or pyrophosphoric acid. Their general mode of action is due to the inhibition of the enzyme cholinesterase in arthropods as well as in mammals. The normal mechanism of transmission of nerve impulses is through the liberation of acetylcholine, which acts on the effector cells of a muscle or a gland. Cholinesterase present in the nerves stops the effect of acetylcholine by hydrolysing it; organophosphorus compounds neutralize the enzyme and cause an accumulation of acetylcholine. This results in a blockage of the nervous system with consequent muscle paralysis, excessive gland secretion and finally death. Atropine is a specific antidote which counteracts these effects of organophosphorus poisoning. The suitability of organophosphates for use in public health programmes depends on their toxicity to the target insects and their danger to humans, but also on their properties of persistence, tendency to produce resistance in mosquitos, ease of formulation and cost. Generally speaking these insecticides are more volatile than chlorinated hydrocarbons and their activity is shorter. This also increases the cost of application of these compounds. The following organophosphorus compounds are in use for malaria control as imagicides or larvicides.

Malathion is now widely employed. It is an ester of dimethyl phosphorodithioate; the technical product is a brownish liquid with an unpleasant garlicky smell that can be masked by various additives. Its chemical structure is shown in Fig. 10.17.

Its formulation consists of emulsifiable 60–90% concentrates or of water-dispersible powders containing 50% of the active compound. Thus malathion can be used either for outdoor space spraying or for indoor residual applications. The duration of residual action of malathion depends on the substrate on which it is used but averages about 2–3 months, when the dosage of the active substance is at the standard 2 g/m^2 of sprayable surface.

Because of its higher cost and shorter residual action, the application of malathion is about three times as expensive as that of DDT at the same dosage.

While most of the organophosphates are very toxic to humans the toxicity of malathion is relatively low (slightly hazardous; LD_{50} 2100 mg/kg) and this compound has been widely used for indoor spraying of human dwellings and animal shelters. However, some formulations undergo rapid chemical degradation on storage in tropical conditions, and their toxicity can be much higher than expected. Thus, even with malathion, very strict safety precautions should be observed.

Fenthion (Baytex), another derivative of phosphorothioate, has a higher toxicity to insects and to mammals than malathion (highly hazardous; LD_{50} 330 mg/kg) and it was used with some success in Africa and Iran as water-dispersible powder at a target dosage of 1.5 g/m^2. However, because of its toxic hazards to sprayers, fenthion is not suitable for routine indoor spraying, although it is of some value as a larvicide for control of culicine mosquitos.

Fenitrothion is an ortho-dimethyl-nitro-tolyl-phosphorothioate known under the proprietary names of Sumithion or Folithion. It has been widely used in agriculture, but recent trials in Kisumu, Kenya showed that it can be of value for residual control of malaria vectors when used as a water-dispersible powder for house spraying. At a dosage of 2 g/m^2 this insecticide gave good results for about 3–4 months. This insecticide can be used for spraying houses provided that various precautionary measures are observed for protection of sprayers and domestic animals.

Dichlorvos (DDVP), a dichlorovinyl dimethyl phosphate, is a liquid product with a high volatility; the vapours thus produced are highly toxic to flying insect pests and of low toxicity to humans. The compound is now widely used when incorporated into various plastic resins (e.g. Vapona) for control of domestic flies. Despite many field trials carried out in Africa and elsewhere, dichlorvos has not found its place in the control of malaria vectors but has been employed for disinsectization of aircraft. In the Peoples Republic of China it has been used in houses for family protection on a communal basis. It is classed as highly hazardous, with an LD_{50} of 56 mg/kg.

Temephos (Abate) is a tetramethyl-thio-diphenylene phosphorothioate, highly active against aquatic larvae of mosquitos and other insects. It has been formulated as an emulsifiable concentrate or in the form of fine granules impregnated with 1–5% of the compound. The granules are applied on water surfaces at monthly intervals, in doses aiming at one part per million of the active product. This compound is highly effective against various species of mosquito larvae including those resistant to other insecticides. Its toxicity to fish, birds and mammals is very low (unlikely to present acute hazard: LD_{50} 8600 mg/kg). It is also used in liquid form as an emulsion at a rate of 37 to 100 ml per hectare and in granular form of 2% concentration at between 5 and 20 kg per hectare, depending on the type of water and the amounts of aquatic vegetation. This treatment can be repeated at 2–3 months' intervals, i.e. much less frequently than any other larvicide.

Chlorphoxim, at 2 g active ingredient per m^2, gave a satisfactory reduction of *A. gambiae* and *A. funestus* hut-resting populations for 3 months in Africa and of *A. aconitus* for 24 weeks in Indonesia, but a less satisfactory impact on indoor and outdoor human-biting rates. These conflicting results make it difficult to assess the potential effectiveness of chlorphoxim in malaria control. It is unlikely to present acute hazard in normal use, with an LD_{50} of less than 2500 mg/kg.

Pirimiphos-methyl is a broad spectrum, non-cumulative organophosphorus pesticide. It is a cholinesterase inhibitor with fast acting fumigant contact and stomach action. It is slightly hazardous to mammals (LD_{50} 2018 mg/kg). This insecticide has been used successfully for a number of years now. Studies conducted between 1979 and 1981 in Indonesia showed that the 50% emulsifiable concentrate was as effective as the 25% water dispersible powder at 2 g/m^2 and had the advantage of not leaving a brown deposit on the walls and did not cause rapid erosion of the nozzle tips. At a dosage of 2 g/m^2 it controlled DDT-resistant *A. aconitus* for about 12 weeks whilst at a dosage of 1 g/m^2 mosquito mortality in houses remained above 50% for 5 weeks by contact exposure and less than 2 weeks by airborne exposure. It was as effective or even better against *A. culicifacies* and *A. stephensi* in Pakistan, especially at 2 g/m^2 or sprayed twice with 1 g/m^2.

Carbamates

This fairly recent class of carbamic acid esters resembles in some ways the organophosphorus insecticides since they also affect the enzyme cholinesterase.

Carbaryl (Sevin) is an alpha naphthyl methylcarbamate and is in use as an agricultural pesticide. Field trials carried out in Haiti showed some promise at a dosage of 1–2 g/m^2 but the persistence of the compound was not as long as had been expected. It is classified as moderately hazardous, with an LD_{50} of 300 mg/kg.

Propoxur (Arprocarb) is an isopropoxy-phenyl methylcarbamate and underwent a number of field tests in various parts of the world. The results showed that at the dosage of 2 g/m^2 in the form of a water-dispersible powder, propoxur remains highly active against *Anopheles* for up to 3 months; it also has an airborne effect which extends to about 20 m from sprayed houses. It has moderate toxicity to humans (LD_{50} 95 mg/kg) and can be used with ordinary precautions in the field. However, its relatively high cost limits the application of propoxur.

Bendiocarb, although applied at low dosages (0.4 g of active ingredient per m^2) because of its high insecticidal activity, has a high mammalian toxicity. However, it is classed as a moderately hazardous pesticide with an LD_{50} of 55 mg/kg. This can be minimized by providing the 88 g/kg (80%) water-dispersible powder formulation in preweighed sachets: one sachet added to the water in the spray pump gives the required 10 g/l (1.0%) spray suspension. Because bendiocarb is virtually odourless and does not leave an unsightly deposit, it is acceptable to householders. In a recent study in Zimbabwe the insecticide remained active for up to 8 weeks (96% mortality) on thatch and in southern Mexico up to 3 months on most common indoor house surfaces.

Insect growth regulators

These are synthetic compounds which interfere with the larval growth and moulting of insects. These chemicals mimic the natural juvenile hormone, and prevent the formation of chitin during the pre-pupal stage. An isoprene compound (methoprene) and a chitin-inhibiting substituted urea (diflubenzuron) have shown much promise in early trials. It is likely that they will be more widely employed, although they are fairly rapidly decomposed in water. As granules or microcapsules they may show longer persistence.

Formulations of insecticides

Formulations of chemical compounds for mosquito control are numerous, ranging from fogs to fluid oils to solid briquettes.

Solutions are either in oil or kerosene, solvent naphtha or white spirit with concentrations of 10–15%; aromatic hydrocarbons such as benzene and cyclohexane permit higher concentrations, up to 25–40%, which can be diluted to the required spray concentration.

Insecticide solutions can be used either for larviciding or as imagicides for control of adult mosquitos by space- and residual spraying. The latter method has been used when spraying some types of houses in which the staining of walls by unsightly deposits of water-dispersible powder had to be avoided. For this reason the introduction of water emulsion concentrates found greater favour.

Emulsions are made up from two immiscible liquids, one of which is broken up into globules and scattered in the other liquid. To prevent the separation of the two, various emulsifying agents are added. Emulsions are prepared from various concentrates containing 10–35% of a chemical compound by dilution with water. Pastes are special types of emulsion concentrates.

Water-dispersible (or *wettable*) *powders* are composed of an active insecticides diluted with an inert carrier, to which various wetting, suspending and anticaking agents are added. Commercially available water-dispersible powders contain between 50 and 75% of the technical product. When mixed with water and stirred these powders form a suspension, i.e. a mixture of the liquid and of the insoluble small particles, which tend to settle more or less rapidly. This depends on various physical factors related to the composition of the water-dispersible powder, its amount, the type of water used and, naturally, the agitation of the suspended powder. Particle size and suspensibility are important factors in residual insecticide spraying. In standard formulations of water-dispersible powders the WHO specifications require that at least 50–70% of the insecticide content should have a particle size of less than 10–20 μm.

Solutions and emulsions are readily absorbed by porous surfaces of very rough walls in rural dwellings in the tropics; as a result the toxic effects on mosquitos may be decreased. Highly volatile compounds (HCH, propoxur, fenitrothion) still exert their action, especially at higher doses. Water-dispersible powders in suspension leave most of the active, crystalline particles of the insecticide on the surface; however, some particles penetrate beneath the surface and during the rainy season, when the humidity is high, an increase of the insecticidal effect takes place.

Solid formulations of insecticides are powders, microcapsules, granules, pellets or briquettes. All of these preparations used as larvicides are designed to disintegrate slowly in the water while releasing the toxic agent.

A new type of formulation is that of *granules*. These are produced from inorganic materials such as clays or organic polymers. The choice of carrier, solvent and binder provides some control over wetting and break-up, with subsequent release of the active ingredient. They are safe to handle, convenient and with little hazard of drifting away from the target. Another new procedure is that of microencapsulation. The tiny capsules containing the insecticide can be stored as suspension in water and diluted for spraying. Like the granules, microcapsules are designed to provide controlled release of the insecticide.

Space spraying formulations range from fumigants, through fogs, mists and other aerosols, to fine droplets.

Some insecticides (such as dichlorvos) have a low vapour pressure and volatilize spontaneously. This fumigant action has been proposed for aircraft disinsectization. However this insecticide is no longer recommended for this purpose. Instead aerosol applications of resmethrin, bioresmethrin, d-phenothrin or permethrin, each with 2% active ingredient in dichlorodifluoromethane (Freon 11) and trichlorofluoromethane (Freon 12), have been recommended either before take off (blocks away) or upon arrival. The use of chlorofluoromethanes as aerosol propellants is now questioned on environmental grounds. Recommendations have been made for the use of permethrin at a rate of 0.2 g a.i. m^2 on exposed surfaces of the aircraft cabin and cargo holds and at the rate of 0.5 g a.i./m^2 on the floor covering in the passenger cabin. The insecticide usually remains effective for up to 8 weeks and retreatment can be carried out to fit aircraft maintenance procedures.

Coarse sprays which consist of droplets over 400 μm volume median diameter (VMD) have a space spraying effect if the relevant liquid evaporates. *Fine sprays*, in which the droplets are between 100 and 400 μm VMD, also have this effect in addition to direct impact on flying mosquitos. When the droplets are between 50 and 100 μm VMD they are classified as *mists*. Finally, true aerosols or fogs have their particles less than 50 μm VMD; the latter type of aerosol remains suspended in the still air for about 1 hour.

Aerosols are produced from containers through the action of a compressed liquefied inert gas; for large-scale use, various thermal or rotary generators are available.

Larvicidal methods of mosquito control

The technique of application of larvicides to water surfaces depends on both the type of compound used and on the type of mosquito breeding place (Table 10.3). *Liquid larvicidal* compounds such as oils may be applied from a simple garden watering-pot or a hand sprayer on small pools or drains. Alternative simple methods such as using an ordinary sweeper's broom dipped into oil, drip cans improvised from tins with a hole in the bottom, sawdust mixed with oil and broadcast by hand etc. have been employed with reasonably good results provided the water surfaces are stationary and not too extensive. However, more commonly, *knapsack sprayers* are used, as by this means the oil can be distributed 5–10 m from the operator. Various designs of knapsack or shoulder-sling larvicide sprayers exist, but their general design is the same. It consists of a container with a 7–9 litre capacity, with a lever-operated plunger or diaphragm pump, connected by a rubber or plastic hose to a cut-off valve, lance and nozzle. The pressure developed by the hand-operated lever is low and the semi-continuous pumping can be maintained without much effort while the operator points the lance towards the target of the spray.

Various hand-operated or motor-driven modifications of these sprayers, mounted on wheels, on boats or now on small hovercraft, are available but their description exceeds the bounds of this book.

Larvicidal dusts such as Paris green may be broadcast by hand, small bellows-operated blowers,

Table 10.3 Selected insecticides suitable for larvicidal application in mosquito control

Insecticide	Dosage per hectare	Duration of effective action (weeks)	Remarks
Diesel oil (fuel oil) and other petroleum oils	142–190 litres in open ponds to cover water surface	1–2	With an addition of a spreading agent the amount can be reduced five times or more
Larvicidal oil	19–47 litres (with special spreading agents)	1–2	Various proprietary formulations
Paris green	*c.* 840–1000 g pure toxicant diluted at 1–5% in dust	2	Pellets containing 5% of Paris green may be applied at about 17 kg per hectare using ground machines or aircraft
Malathion	224–1000 g	1–2	As emulsion concentrate or granules. Avoid overdosing which may injure fish
Temephos (Abate)	56–112 g pure compound	2–4	As emulsion concentrate or granules. Higher dosages are used in polluted waters
Fenitrothion	100–1000 g	1–3	Not to be applied to waters containing fish or crustaceans (prawns, crabs). Caution in use
Fenthion	22–112 g	2–11	As above
Pirimipos-methyl	50–500 g	2–11	As emulsion concentrate
Chlorphoxim	100 g	2–7	As emulsion concentrate
Chlorpyriphos	11–25 g	3–17	As emulsion concentrate, granules or water dispersible powder
Permethrin	5–10 g	5–10	As emulsion concentrate. The lowest levels are recommended for fish-bearing waters
Deltamethrin	2.5–10 g	1–3	As above
Diflubenzuron	25–100 g	1–4	As granules or water dispersible powder
Iodofenphos	50–100 g	7–16	As emulsion concentrate or granules
Methoprene	100–1000 g	4–8	As slow release suspension
Phoxim	100 g	1–6	As emulsion concentrate
Bacillus thuringiensis	500–5000 g	1–2	Varies from liquid to granular formulation
Bacillus sphaericus	10000–20000 g	8	Against *culicinae* in pit latrines
Mononuclear film (oil)	3–5 litres	2–10 days	A very rapidly spreading oil greatly affected by wind movements

See also Table 3, page 21, in *Chemicals Methods for the Control of Arthropod Vectors and Pests of Public Health Importance*, WHO, 1984.

pump-type hand dusters, knapsack- or front-carried rotary blowers and power-operated, wheel-mounted dusting machines.

Gelatine capsules containing an emulsifiable concentrate of pyrethrins with piperonyl butoxide (Tossits), when tossed into the water, will disintegrate and release within minutes the contents, each capsule spreading over an unobstructed water surface of 5–9 m^2 (60–100 ft^2).

Briquettes containing 8% methoprene, an insect growth regulator (Altosid), have been devised to release an effective larvicide for 30 days on small bodies of water or for shorter periods in small streams.

For application of granulated compounds several modifications of standard equipment have now been developed and are increasingly used.

For large-scale application of larvicidal measures either in the form of large droplet sprays or as granulated insecticide formulations, fixed wing aircraft and helicopters are the best solution. In general, aerial spraying using rotary atomizers produces a broad spectrum of droplets, so that the resulting effect is due to direct action on larvae and adults of mosquitos as well as to some residual action on the vegetation.

Applications of larvicides must be repeated at intervals corresponding to the development cycle of the *Anopheles* species. Generally, the relevant period is between 7 and 14 days; longer periods are possible with some newer compounds.

Imagicidal measures aimed at control of adult mosquitos

Although individual protection from bites of adult mosquitos by smoke or various fumigant devices ('joss-sticks') was well known in the past, large-scale malaria control projects by indoor spraying with pyrethrum solutions proved to be unexpectedly successful some 40 years ago in southern Africa and India.

However, the introduction of DDT and other synthetic insecticides resulted in the revolutionary concept of malaria control by residual action of the new compounds. In contrast to the immediate knock-down effect of pyrethrum, which lasts only for a short time, the new synthetic insecticides retain their toxic action for a considerable period when applied to a surface with which adult *Anopheles* (and other mosquitos) may come into contact.

Residual insecticides are almost invariably applied in some liquid form which, on drying, leaves a crystalline deposit on the wall. Some wall surfaces absorb the original fluid which is put on, and if this is a solution or an emulsion, much of the active insecticide is drawn into the inner part of the wall where the insect cannot come into contact with it. This causes some loss of insecticidal power on mud and porous plaster walls. Surfaces such as wood may not absorb much of the insecticide which remains on the surface in an active form for many months.

These insecticides act slowly, and some of them irritate the mosquitos, leading to their flight towards the light out of the house. Their fate after that depends on whether or not they take away a small quantity of insecticide on their feet. Crystals formed after the evaporation of the solvents used in solutions and emulsions vary in size, but the range of insecticide particles in a wettable powder formulation is determined in the course of manufacture and is standardized to a specification that can be checked by suitable suspensibility tests to ensure optimum size for biological effectiveness. Volatility is important since a volatile product disappears in time whatever the quality of the wall, but exerts some fumigant effect which will kill insects not in actual contact.

The irritant effect, which occurs with DDT, nullifies the value of counts of mosquitos in treated houses as an index of efficacy since it always leads to the mosquito avoiding the house as a shelter, although it may still use it as a feeding place. The only reliable checking mechanism consists of trapping mosquitos leaving the house and noting the proportion of them dying in the next 12 or 24 hours. This demands the use of special traps and a rather elaborate technique which cannot be universally applied.

Obviously, large-scale application of residual insecticides will have a particularly marked effect on those species of mosquitos which feed preferentially on human beings inside their dwelling or which shelter in human houses or sheds for domestic animals.

A good residual insecticide should have the following characteristics: (1) high biological activity against the vector species, with a lethal effect for at least 3 months after application and without (or minimal) irritant reaction on the mosquito, to assure the full toxic action; (2) fairly rapid kill, after a brief contact with the toxic surface; (3) low acute or chronic toxicity to humans and domestic animals; (4) good stability on storage, easy formulations and application; (5) economy in use, and low cost.

The duration of residual activity of insecticidal compounds and their formulations depends not only on the intrinsic persistency of the chemical but also on its effectiveness, i.e. the biological action on the target insect. The latter varies considerably in relation to the type and composition of the sprayed surface. Thus, on porous walls made of unbaked clay or mud (adobe) the phenomenon of sorption interferes with the effectiveness of some insecticides incorporated into water-dispersible powders. This is the case for DDT which lasts much longer on non-porous surfaces (e.g. wood) than on mud; on the other hand, HCH may be effective even after sorption through its fumigant action. Organophosphorus insecticides formulated as water-dispersible powders may be less effective on sorptive walls after a few weeks.

All houses within the area to be protected should receive the appropriate dose of the insecticide before the start of the transmission season and at agreed intervals. The usual doses of insecticides (e.g. DDT at 2 g/m^2 every 6 months), although widely applicable, may vary somewhat depending on local conditions. The insecticide must be applied to the indoor walls and ceiling surfaces of all inhabited rooms and also animal shelters. Heavy furniture in the rooms must also be sprayed, particularly the back of it, close to the walls. Where wall surfaces and furniture are of good quality, emulsions or solutions of insecticides should be used rather than suspensions of water-dispersible powders which leave a whitish deposit (Table 10.4).

Space spraying

In spite of the tremendous success of the technique of residual insecticide spraying the method of space dispersion of fast acting compounds is still of value. A degree of local control of mosquitos (and other flying insects) may be achieved by 'space spraying', i.e. by releasing the insecticides into the air as smoke, or as fine droplets. Naturally, such measures of protection must be frequently repeated to result in any significant effect. However, in epidemics of insect-borne diseases the 'space spraying' technique can rapidly reduce the numbers of mosquitos not only in dwellings but also temporarily in outside breeding grounds.

Table 10.4 Insecticides suitable as residual spray applications for control of *Anopheles* vectors of malaria

Insecticide	Dosage (g/m^2)	Average duration of effectiveness (months)	Chemical type	Remarks
DDT	2.0	6 or more	OC	In some conditions 1.0 g/m^2 may be used
γ-HCH	0.2–0.5	3 or more	OC	Some sorption by mud. Used in some areas to control DDT-resistance in the absence of dieldrin resistance
Malathion	1–2	2–3	OP	Widely used although sorption by mud
Fenitrothion	1.0–2.0	3 or more	OP	Reasonably safe when usual precautions are observed, but expensive. Airborne toxicity
Chlorphoxim	2.0	1–3	OP	Rarely used in malaria control
Pirimiphos–methyl	1–2	2–3 or more	OP	Long-lasting airborne toxicity
Propoxur	1–2	2–3	C	Rather expensive. Sorption by mud
Bendiocarb	0.4	2–3	C	High mammalian toxicity
Permethrin	0.5	2–3	Py	Low mammalian toxicity.
Deltamethrin	0.05	2–3	Py	High costs which are partially neutralized by low dosage
Cypermethrin	0.5	4	Py	There may be cross-resistance with DDT
Lambda-cyhalothrin	0.03	6	Py	Limited experience to date
Fenthion	1–2	2–3	OP	Contact effect

OC, organochlorine compounds; OP, organophosphorous compounds; C, carbamate; Py, synthetic pyrethroids; HCH, hexachlorocyclohexane.

Equipment for vector control operations*

Equipment for control of mosquitos can be classified in many different ways. The following classification is convenient and relevant to the malaria control strategy. It was followed by the WHO Expert Committee on Vector Biology and Control (WHO, 1990).

Pesticide application equipment
- Hand compression sprayer
- Motorized knapsack mistblowers
- Thermal foggers
- Aerosol generators
- Dusting equipment
- Household equipment
- Aircraft

Equipment for biological control
- Equipment for application of insect pathogens
- Equipment for rearing, transporting and distributing larvivorous fish

Equipment for environmental management
- Light machinery
- Heavy machinery
- Domestic equipment
- Water management devices

The choice of equipment depends on the size of the control operation and knowledge of the vector involved, and it must be consistent with the recommended method of control. Moreover, one has to bear in mind: (1) the frequency and duration of control measures; (2) the extent and accessibility of the target area; (3) the ease of use of the equipment by the operator; (4) the amount of maintenance; and (5) initial and recurring costs. Only the briefest description of conventional equipment can be given here.

Pesticide application equipment

Evaluation according to standard specifications is necessary for appropriate selection and purchase of pesticide application equipment for use in programmes for the control of disease vectors, disease reservoirs, and pests. Evaluation is also needed to ensure that equipment is suitable for a specific application, and that it is durable, reliable and easily maintained. To achieve this WHO established the WHO Pesticide Application Equipment Evaluation Scheme (WHO, 1977).

Selection of properly designed equipment for the recommended method of control is an important part of any vector control programme (WHO, 1990). Routine maintenance is essential and personnel need to be properly trained to do this.

Most vector control programmes continue to give preference to properly designed hand-operated equipment, with the compression sprayer being the most commonly used for various control operations such as residual treatment, and the application of larvicides and insect pathogens.

The operation and maintenance of motorized equipment need additional skills, and problems will occur unless specially trained personnel are placed in charge.

Aerosols are used to apply insecticides for temporary control of adult mosquitos and other flying insects, especially during epidemics of mosquito-borne diseases such as malaria, yellow fever, dengue, or dengue haemorrhagic fever.

Hand compression sprayer

Most of the residual insecticidal spraying for control of *Anopheles* is carried out now by means of hand-compression sprayers. However, in some parts of the world the much simpler and cheaper *stirrup pumps* or bucket sprayers have been extensively used in the past and may still be of value. These pumps consist of a bucket containing the liquid to be sprayed and a pump with a double-acting piston operated manually. A hose attached to the pump leads to the spraying lance ending with a nozzle (Fig. 10.18). Obviously this equipment must be operated by two persons: one working the pump and the other directing the spray lance. Moreover, the pressures are erratic and do not make for even application. Nevertheless, stirrup pumps are adequate for use in malaria control if no other sprayers are available.

In 1979 Coffee (1979) announced a revolutionary new concept of electrodynamic spraying. As the name suggests this sprayer operates on electrodynamic energy, capable of atomizing liquid pesticide

***See:**
WHO (1990). ***Equipment for Vector Control*****, 3rd edn, Geneva.**
WHO (1977). ***Engineering Aspects of Vector Control Operations.*** **Technical Reports Series No. 603. Geneva.**

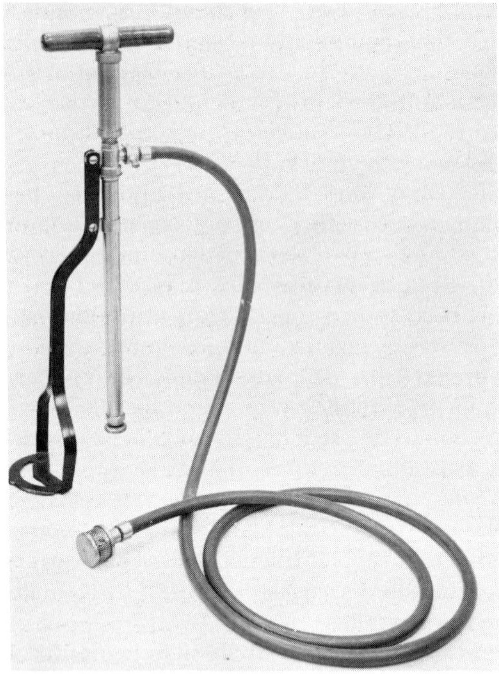

Fig. 10.18 Stirrup pump, a simple and robust type of sprayer used for residual indoor spraying of insecticides. (Wellcome Museum of Medical Science.)

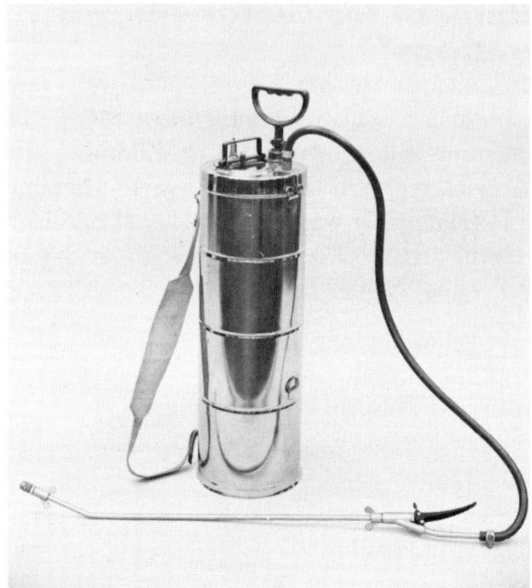

Fig. 10.19 Compression sprayer, a standard type of equipment for residual insecticide spraying in malaria control and eradication programmes. (Wellcome Museum of Medical Science.)

into evenly sized droplets which are attracted by the surface being sprayed. The sprayer runs on four torch batteries (60 hours' operation) generating an electric charge of 25 000 volts at the sprayer nozzle, thus atomizing the pesticide packed in a special disposable container. The resulting spray cloud, because it is electrically charged, is attracted by the surface, giving perfect coverage. Electrical attraction, in addition to increasing the spray efficiency, prevents pesticide wastage and losses. This sprayer was designed for use in agriculture, and especially for cotton. Its use for malaria control has yet to be evaluated, especially from the point of view of cost efficiency. It is very safe, light and easy to use.

The *hand compression sprayer* is universally regarded as standard equipment for residual insecticide spraying (Fig. 10.19). This type of sprayer (e.g. Hudson Expert) consists of a cylindrical tank made of stainless steel about 9–13 litres (2–3 gallons) capacity in which the liquid insecticide formulation (usually a suspension of water-dispersible powder) is contained. The internal pressure in the tank is raised by a hand-operated pump incorporated in the sprayer; the cover is of the 'inner seal' type which tightens when the pressure is high. It is fitted with a hose, a cut-off valve, a lance and a nozzle. Some types of sprayers also have a constant pressure valve and a pressure gauge. One or more straps are attached for carrying the sprayer. This equipment is designed to produce a uniform insecticide dosage on sprayed surfaces and to be simple, robust and durable so that it can be used by sprayers with elementary technical knowledge. The important requirement is a controllable and uniform nozzle discharge rate. Nozzle spray patterns of different forms have been tried, the flat-fan shape being favoured because it facilitates the application of parallel, vertical spraying swaths on interior surfaces.

In practice, the rate of application of an insecticide is regulated by three controlling factors: its concentration in the liquid carrier, the nozzle discharge rate and the speed of spraying.

The generally recommended operating pressure in the delivery lance and nozzle to give the most efficient application is 2.8 kg/cm^2 (40 lb/in^2). To maintain this pressure until the sprayer is empty, after a single filling and pumping, involves a constant pressure in the tank and a pressure control valve in the lance. The required cylinder pressure may be achieved by a given number of strokes of the pump or more accurately read from a pressure gauge (Fig. 10.20).

The ideal nozzle to ensure uniformity of application is the Tee-Jet Nozzle 8002, delivering a fan-type spray, with a spray angle of 80° and an output of 0.76 litre (0.18 gallons) per minute at the standard pressure. Held at a distance of 45 cm (18 inches) from the surface to be sprayed, such a nozzle will deposit a swath of spray 75 cm (30 inches) wide, of which the middle half is effective. In practice, therefore, the marginal 18–20 cm of one swath should be overlapped by the margin of the next swath to produce a uniform deposit.

Irregularities in spraying and uneven dosage are due in part to faults of the operator, and in part to faults of apparatus. The first can be overcome by thorough training in which the operator is taught how to apply a standard dose, usually 4.5 litres to 100 m^2 (1 gallon to 1000 ft^2), with complete regularity. The training having been given, supervision must continue to ensure its maintenance. The principal faults in maintenance are wear in the nozzle, and fall of pressure as the quantity of fluid in the tank decreases. The ordinary brass nozzle may wear very quickly, particularly when wettable powders are used, because their composition may be abrasive. The nozzle should be made of very hard material, for which various metal alloys and ceramic materials are used.

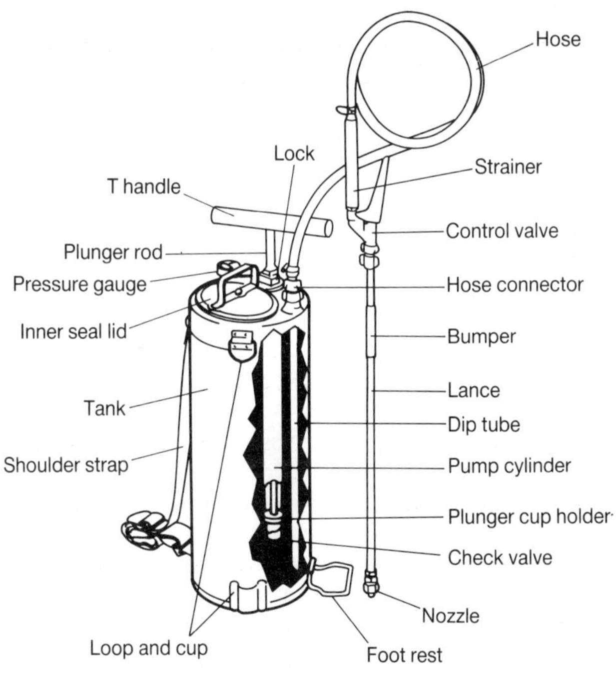

Fig. 10.20 Cutaway diagram of a compression sprayer.

Important from the standpoint of spraying efficiency is frequent and regular maintenance of sprayers, in particular the replacement of worn washers, pressure hose, nozzles and hose clips.

An essential requirement of spraying equipment is that it should be of a standard type, constructed of durable materials, with a standard lance and a cut-off valve which does not leak, thus ensuring uniform application of insecticide with minimal risks of toxicity to sprayers. (Specifications of hand-operated compressing sprayers will be found in *Application and Dispersal of Pesticides*, WHO Technical Report Series no. 465, 1971; for revised specifications see *Engineering Aspects of Vector Control Operations*, WHO Technical Reports Series no. 603, 1977). It is also important to make provision ahead for sufficient supplies of equipment and for ample spare parts and replacements to be available at all field depots. At least one person in each spraying team should be trained in the maintenance of equipment.

Motorized knapsack mistblowers

Motorized knapsack mistblowers, powered by a small two-stroke (two-cycle) internal combustion engine, produce a high velocity airstream (0.5 m^3 air/minute) to a hand directed vertical nozzle. An air flow sucks the spray from a 1 litre plastic container to the nozzle via a metering restrictor. The volume of liquid insecticide applied can be up to 350 ml/min. They are widely used in mosquito and tsetse fly control as they are the only portable equipment that can project spray into the eaves of houses or thickets around villages where exophilic vectors can occur. They are useful for areas which are difficult to access by road.

The vast majority of these machines have a recoil starter; however, some new machines are equipped with an electrical starter, which makes the engine easier to start. The main difficulties in starting occur because fuel mixture (oil and petrol) left in the engine after use evaporates, leaving an oily residue over the ignition plug, which prevents ignition. Also, the use of an incorrect fuel mixture can rapidly cause wear, especially when the engine is left idling. When sprayers are used without full air output, poor atomization of the spray liquid occurs. With poor atomization droplets are generally far too large to be effective for vector operations, and there is increased fall-out of spray, contaminating the ground.

Constant output is dependent upon positive pressure in the tank, but this will not be achieved if, as often happens, the lid gasket has been affected by the pesticide formulation and no longer fits properly. Other components can also be adversely affected by some insecticide formulations, especially those used in ultra low volume (ULV) applications.

The spray operator walks along the street directing the lance of the mistblower through the doors or windows. Persons working with these generators for long periods must wear ear protectors because of the high level of noise. There is a risk of burns from unguarded exhausts with some types of these machines and proper precautions should be observed.

Thermal foggers

These machines (Fig. 10.21) are preferred in many vector control programmes, despite the extra cost, because the highly visible fog is psychologically more acceptable to the user and to those who wish to see that control operations are being carried out. Where thermal foggers are used consideration should be given to increasing the concentration of insecticide and decreasing proportionally the flow rate, in order to reduce formulation costs. A reduction in flow rate will decrease fuel consumption in the combustion chamber as less heat is required to atomize the lower volume. Manufacturers of thermal foggers should be consulted on appropriate insecticide flow rates and combustion chamber temperature settings.

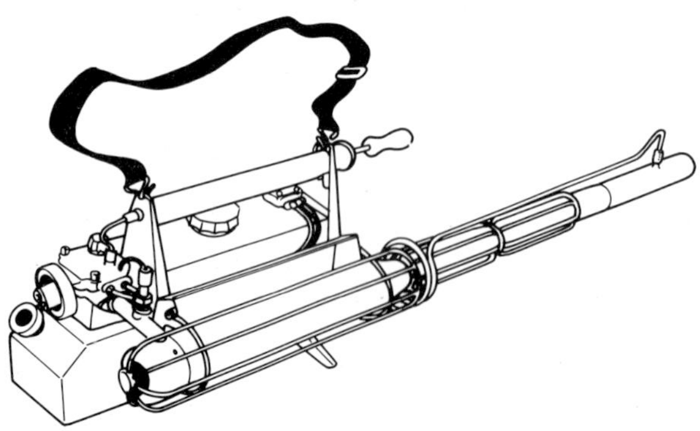

Fig. 10.21 Hand-carried thermal fog generator.

There is a potential fire hazard when thermal foggers are used, especially when the pulse-jet type foggers are carried indoors. It is important that they are operated only by well trained personnel using appropriate insecticide formulations and with access to a fire extinguisher. When manufacturers' instructions are followed carefully the fire risk with equipment that meets WHO specifications is minimal, since safety devices on the machines are designed to stop the flow of insecticide if the engine stops. The main advantage of the pulse-jet type fogger is its simplicity of design and construction, as there are no rotating parts and no lubrication is required, but its loud noise can be objectionable and harmful to hearing unless suitable ear protection is used. Large pulse-jet type foggers may be vehicle-mounted, but it is usual, when treating extensive areas with fog, to use equipment with a rotary blower to move more hot gas through the nozzle and thus vaporize higher volumes of insecticide diluted in kerosene or a similar refined oil.

Aerosol generators

Insecticidal aerosols are used both for indoor and outdoor space treatments for the control of adult vectors. The optimum droplet size range is 8–18 μm volume median diameter (VMD). Some residual effectiveness may be achieved with high doses of persistent insecticides applied indoors because the small droplets eventually deposit on surfaces. Ground applications of aerosols alone may provide satisfactory vector control on a temporary basis for interruption of disease transmission, but they are used principally as a supplement to other vector control methods.

Aerosol generators used to disperse insecticides are designed for the control of flying insect pests and vectors with ULV applications. One type uses a high volume of air at low pressure in a vortex nozzle to atomize concentrated or technical formulations of insecticide whilst other aerosol generators use high-pressure, low-volume air flow to atomize the insecticide, or a rotary nozzle driven by an electric motor.

ULV applications, in which the minimum volume of liquid insecticide formulation is applied per unit area, provide maximum effectiveness against target vectors. Most organophosphorus insecticides can be applied as technical formulations, but other insecticides, such as carbamates and pyrethroids, must be formulated with compatible solvents for ULV application. These non-volatile formulations permit improved control of droplet size. (In contrast, thermal foggers may present a fire hazard and can contribute to environmental pollution through production of exhaust gases. They also require costly oil diluents and increased insecticide storage capacity, and entail higher formulation costs.)

Vehicle mounted aerosol generators (Leco, Micro-Gen) are particularly useful in reducing the numbers of adult mosquitos in urban and suburban areas with adequate access roads. Where roads are inadequate, hand-carried or knapsack-type aerosol generators are available. For adequate coverage inside open houses and other buildings the vehicle mounted equipment should be capable of discharging an aerosol cloud on either side of the vehicle; this discharge should extend more than 8 m from the vehicle. For outdoor space treatment a swath at a 100 m interval should be achieved by wind dispersal of the cloud.

Although portable ULV aerosol generators are used primarily indoors or for small-scale applications outdoors, large-scale treatments can be carried out when several machines and operators are used in a team. In some circumstances portable ULV aerosol generators are more efficient since the aerosol can be placed precisely into a dwelling, whereas virtually none of the aerosol cloud from vehicle-mounted equipment may penetrate the interior of dwellings.

The smaller hand-carried and shoulder-slung machines are usually powered by a two-cycle internal combustion engine, as on the knapsack mistblowers. These require more care in operation and maintenance than four-cycle engines, which are more reliable and convenient to use. The larger machines have a solvent-flushing system and remote control in the vehicle cab; thus the operator has less direct contact with the insecticide.

Factors that need to be considered when choosing a method for ground application of aerosols include: cost, efficiency, convenience and safety of operation; environmental impact; reliability, ease of maintenance, durability and availability of the equipment; insecticide formulations; fuel oil diluents; and the availability of trained staff.

The ULV technique of applying insecticides proved to be a particularly useful and economical method of temporary control of adult mosquitos. This method is based on the production by special machines (Buffalo Turbine and others) of insecticide droplets of 10–20 μm diameter for ground aerosols and 20–50 μm diameter for aerial sprays.

The great advantage of the ULV technique is that the total amount of insecticide distributed per unit area is the same as or slightly less than used in thermal fogging, while the total volume of the carrier is very much less. Thus, about 0.5–1.0 litre of the liquid carrier per hectare are sufficient and this results in great savings in materials and labour involved.

Both thermal fogging and ULV spraying should be undertaken preferably at dawn or in the late evening because of thermal currents that build up during the day. The area to be treated should be divided into sections related to the desired frequency of spraying. Ultra low volume methods can cover a much greater area in a given time than any fogging units.

For indoor fogging the usual formulation consists of 0.5% pyrethrins, 1% piperonyl butoxide in high-grade deodorized kerosene; the dosage is 25–30 ml per 100 m^3 of space. For outdoor application 6% malathion or 1% DDVP in no. 2 fuel oil are commonly used.

Some liquid proprietary concentrations (e.g. Cythion) used for ULV sprays in populated areas may permanently damage paint on houses, boats, motorcars etc.; to avoid this the droplet size produced by the machines must be accurately determined and not exceed the VMD range of 50 μm.

It must not be concluded that ULV methods briefly described in this section represent the best techniques for mosquito control, although they have been used in some projects in India, Indonesia, Venezuela and more widely in the USA.

Difficulties encountered are: lack of uniformity of dosage of the insecticide and of coverage, high initial and recurrent costs, shortage of trained staff for maintenance and repair, and contamination of non-target areas.

Dusting equipment

Although dusts contain only a small proportion of active ingredient, the main concern in the field is the risk of inhalation of pesticide particles smaller than 10 μm in diameter. This problem is accentuated if the equipment is carried in front of the operator, or if the operator walks into a cloud of dust. Nevertheless, in some situations application of dusts is considered to be important, particularly in emergencies such as epidemics.

The trend has been away from the use of heavy, well constructed metal dusters to those made of plastic components. So far there has been no feedback on the reliability of these machines in vector control.

With all the dusters that use a rotary blower, there are problems of metering the dust accurately.

One of the oldest types of dust and granule applicator is the 'horn seeder', originally used for sowing seeds. Early commercial versions used a metal horn fitted to a bag container, but new plastic versions have recently been marketed. Simple equipment of this type is useful for spreading larvicides on water surfaces, especially to control mosquito larvae.

Household equipment

The simplest hand-operated atomizers (e.g. Flit guns), used for space spraying of pyrethrum solutions of bedrooms in the evening, need no elaborate description. They are composed of a pump, container and nozzle; they are often crudely made and easily damaged. The spray they produce is usually coarse and much of the insecticidal solution is wasted. Some better sprayers have a continuous, instead of an intermittent, action which produces finer droplets, and are more effective. In using the simple sprayers it is important to keep the nozzle upward during the operation and to start with the corners of the room, finishing in the centre. If there is a mosquito net over the bed of the treated room, the net should be fitted over the bed before spraying; a few strokes should also be directed over the sides of the mosquito net. Moreover one should be certain that the solution of insecticide (usually about 0.05–0.1% of pyrethrum extract in kerosene with various synergists) is of good quality. The number of strokes required depends on the size of the room and the type of insecticide solution but on average about 10 ml per 30 m^3 (about 1000 cubic feet) of space are generally adequate. To obtain the best effect of space spraying the room should be closed during application and for 10–15 minutes after.

Pressurized aerosol dispensers and smokes

At the present time the hand-operated pumps have been largely replaced by aerosol dispensers which contain liquid insecticides under pressure of a liquefied gas. The amount of pressure and the size of the orifice of the container determine the rate of discharge of the liquid and its droplet size. The time required to produce an effective dosage of the insecticidal solution for a given volume of space is indicated by the manufacturers, although it averages 3–5 seconds per 30 m^3. The aerosol dispensers must always be operated in an upright position and kept away from excessive heat. There is increasing concern about the effect of the propellant gas on the ozone layer and aerosols are being replaced increasingly by pump-action sprayers.

Smokes are special types of aerosols produced by a chemical mixed with an insecticide compound. Mosquito coils containing pyrethrum are produced in large numbers in eastern Asia. Each coil consists of a flat spiral of material which will smoulder slowly when lit; it releases smoke which deters mosquitos from entering the room and prevents them from biting. These coils are made of a vegetable filler, a starch binding agent, and contain 0.1–0.4% of natural or synthetic pyrethrins. More recently, electrically heated fumigation mats have become available which last from 6 to 8 hours.

Other smoke generators such as 'HCH bombs' for outdoor use are of limited value since a proportion of the insecticide is decomposed by the heat.

Nets and screens

In addition to household applications of pesticides by use of mosquito coils, fumigation mats and hand sprayers, and the use of nets and screens, there has been a recent trend towards treatment of household materials such as wallpaper, plaster, mosquito nets and curtains. Pyrethroids have been widely tested in recent years for impregnating mosquito nets.

Treatment of mosquito nets is particularly suitable for community action within an integrated strategy for malaria control. Chemical treatment of netting is simple and can be conducted seasonally under the supervision of community health workers. There is potential for large-scale local manufacture of treated nets in areas where malaria is a major public health problem, particularly when nets can be made from local fibre. The use of treated mosquito nets should be integrated with other available methods, on the basis of comparisons of the cost-effectiveness of each method in the particular epidemiological situation.

Aircraft

Aerial space sprays are commonly used in agricultural practice and also occasionally in malaria control. There are a number of aircraft especially suited for this purpose. Two different principles are employed. The solution of insecticide may be pumped or gravity-fed into a boom with nozzles along it. The spray so produced is further broken up by the slipstream of the aircraft or by a rotary atomizer. An alternative system, in which the insecticide is introduced into the exhaust of the aircraft's engine to produce a thermal aerosol, is less favoured because of some decomposition of the active compound. At the present time the use of ULV atomizers has been generally adopted. Helicopters are increasingly used because of the downdraught of this aircraft and better distribution of the spray. As mentioned before, aerosol generating machines and aircraft are of particular value when rapid elimination of mosquitos from a relatively small area is needed, as in the case of epidemic outbreaks of a vector-borne disease.

Several types of atomizers are used for aerial ULV spraying. The most widely employed consist of a metal gauze cylinder rotating around a fixed spindle which is attached to a bracket on the aircraft wing or to a boom designed for helicopter operation. The rotating power comes from the slipstream through a fan clamped in a hub that carries the bearing assembly. The pitch of the fan blades is adjustable and this controls the particle size of the insecticide solution, introduced through the hollow spindle under pressure and dispersed by a diffuser tube over the rotating gauze of the cylinder. Normally four to six such units are mounted on the aircraft. Another type of ULV atomizer uses an electrically driven rotating multidisc. In this type the particle size is independent of the speed of the aircraft; such atomizers are particularly suited for low speed helicopter operations.

Aircraft have been used for aerial application of pesticides for the past 50 years but only recently on a larger scale. The early aircraft used occasionally for antimosquito spraying were standard military (such as the USA Air Force C-123 cargo) or commercial planes, equipped with a range of D2–13 nozzles on a boom at a 45° downward angle. This produced 170 m swath at the flight altitude of 50–60 m. In some antimosquito spraying programmes Twin Beech aircraft equipped with a boom carrying four Tee-jet 8004 nozzles, spraying at a pressure of 100 psi, and producing a 100 m swath at a height of 50–60 m were used. More commonly in the USA the Stearman (PT-17), in the UK and Canada the DHC-2 (Beaver), and in the former USSR the Antonov (AN-2M) were employed. Except in an absolutely flat country, four-engined piston-driven aircraft have to fly much higher than twin-engined planes. Spraying at high altitudes produces a wide but uneven dispersion of insecticides and a relatively small aircraft designed specifically for pesticide spraying is greatly superior. The Piper Pawnee (PA-25) is now the most popular, but further developments in this field are in progress. The present technique of aerial spraying tends to decrease the size of the spray drops while maintaining the concentration in order to get the spray to drift across wide swaths (ULV drift spraying). For large spraying programmes such as for tsetse and locust control the Avro Anson was widely used, but now Piper Aztec, Beechcraft Baron, Cessna 310 and Britten-Norman Islander are increasingly popular. For vector control, aircraft need higher operating speeds than for agricultural work and thus must have special navigational instruments, flow meters and a 'black box' to record all the information on airspeed and height. The spraying equipment should be an integral part of the aircraft.

Helicopters have been used in some field projects

but they require special equipment such as a rotary nozzle which must be mounted behind and below the boom to minimize the effect of air turbulence.

Generally speaking, fixed-wing aircraft are to be preferred when high payload and speed are more important for the planned task; they are also less expensive to operate than helicopters; the latter have the advantage of good manoeuvrability, better delimitation of the coverage in population areas and safety of unprepared landing in any emergency.

Large-scale and emergency vector control programmes often benefit from the use of aircraft to apply chemicals. Aircraft are especially well suited for rapid treatment of large areas or areas where wet soil, water, rough terrain, or dense woody vegetation prohibit or render impractical the use of ground or hand-carried equipment. The use of aircraft over or near populated areas, especially during daylight hours when adult insects are most vulnerable to chemical control, may create concern about safety and requires coordination with governmental agencies responsible for aviation safety.

Accurate placement of sprayed chemicals is usually more difficult from aircraft than with ground or hand-carried sprayers since many interacting factors affect the trajectory of the spray particles after they are released. Therefore, the decision to use aerial sprays, as opposed to alternative methods, should be carefully considered, including safety, timeliness, cost, meteorological conditions, vector habitat and biological effectiveness, as well as the availability of suitable equipment, operational sites and trained crews.

Both fixed-wing aircraft and helicopters have been used successfully to apply larvicides rapidly to large and remote breeding areas. Such applications require precise targeting of the chemical, either in granular or liquid form, to ensure thorough coverage of the treated area and a high level of effectiveness. The remote location and inaccessibility of many of the breeding areas often makes the use of ground personnel for flagging aircraft swaths impossible or impractical. There is a need for affordable electronic swath guidance systems for use on small fixed-wing aircraft and helicopters to increase the precision of application. Since breeding sites are often covered by dense canopies of vegetation, penetration by either liquid or dry particles to the breeding sites is often critical to the success of the application.

Equipment for biological control

The biological agents considered over the years for malaria control are:

1. Fish e.g. *Gambusia affinis*, *Poecilia reticulata* and *Tilapia* spp.
2. Bacteria e.g. *Bacillus thuringiensis* serotype H-14 (*B.t.* H-14), *Bacillus sphaericus*.
3. Nematodes e.g. *Romanomermis culicivorax*, *R. jingdeensis*, *R. iyengari*, *Octomyomermis muspratti*.
4. Predatory mosquitos e.g., *Toxorhynchites* spp.

The most promising have been bacteria and fish. Nematodes have a potential use in specific situations but their use requires mass rearing facilities and mass handling of live parasites. The use of predatory mosquitos has not been particularly useful since the breeding habits of the predators rarely coincide with that of anopheline vectors.

Equipment for the application of insect pathogens

The use of formulations of *Bacillus thuringiensis* in operational programmes is limited due to its short residual effect. However, improved formulations with longer residual effect are being developed. *Bacillus sphaericus* on the other hand can multiply in polluted habitats rich in organic matter giving extended periods of mosquito control, but its value for *Anopheles* has not been well demonstrated. All the bacteria for vector control form spores and potent, stable toxins and can be stored for long periods. They can be formulated as suspensions, wettable powders and dusts for easy application with conventional equipment.

The equipment required for application of *B.t.* H-14 and *B. sphaericus* will vary according to the formulation used. Compression sprayers or other sprayers used for chemical control can be used to apply particulate suspensions. Granular formulations, including those using corn cob as a base, are usually applied by hand, although the horn seeder and knapsack dusters can be used. Briquettes can be applied by hand, but where there is running water, especially in rice fields, the larvicide may be introduced using a constant-flow dripping device. Such a device can be connected directly to the formulation container and the rate of application adjusted either by a stopcock or a flow control with different sized holes. Aerial application of *B.t.* H-14 to large bodies of water has been carried out in the USA for mosquito control. For this operation light planes were fitted with a hydraulic spray system and cone nozzles (D6 and D12 type).

In the Onchocerciasis Control Programme in West Africa special formulations have been developed for aerial application of *B.t.* H-14 to large rivers for the control of blackflies. The latest formulations are applied by helicopter (cross-river) or by fixed-wing planes, with a discharge of up to 200 m^3/second, during the dry season in rivers by dropping predetermined quantities of the formulation upstream of the target area. The river's current disperses the formulation to the breeding sites.

Equipment for rearing, transporting and distributing larvivorous fish

Larvivorous fish have been used extensively. Indigenous species should be selected wherever feasible as they are adapted to local conditions and are less likely to have an adverse ecological impact. Laboratory evaluations of indigenous larvivorous fish have shown that they can be highly effective in mosquito control. Fish can also be employed at low cost and can be used at the village level, with community participation.

Gambusia affinis, *Tilapia* spp, and *Poecilia reticulata* are most often used for larval control, mainly against *Anopheles* and to some extent against *Culex* and *Aedes* spp.

The advantage of biological vector control is that the predators that are used can be produced and reared within the local community. The equipment needed for production and rearing, i.e. tanks, aerators, nets, is simple and can be manufactured or bought locally.

Wherever possible suitable local fish species should be utilized for larvicidal programmes. Since transport distances and times will then be relatively short the need for sophisticated equipment is reduced.

Fish should preferably be reared in their natural habitats or, if this is not practicable, in specially prepared breeding ponds, which can be simply constructed according to accepted fish farming practices. Where the soil is pervious a plastic sheet or cement lining may be necessary.

Fish can be collected using conventional netting techniques, involving a 'butterfly' net of 60–90 cm in diameter, a sweep net stretched between two sticks, or other traditional methods. Care must be exercised to avoid injury to the fish.

The fish can be transported in any convenient carrying device, e.g. buckets, with provision to avoid spillage, or plastic bags about half full with water. Containers should be protected from heat and bright sunlight. No other special measures are necessary for journeys lasting for less than about 4 hours. Beyond this time the container should be insulated, the water may be chilled by addition of ice and provision must be made for aeration or oxygenation. Naturally occurring water should be used for transport and topping up. The fish can be dispersed manually.

Equipment for environmental management

Environmental management, using appropriate equipment, is a principal measure in integrated disease control. The major modifications and manipulations are land filling, land clearance, drainage, waterway construction and maintenance, land forming, weed control, pumping, reservoir operation and salt-marsh management. Such activities should not preclude community planning and collaboration with government or private agencies.

The advantages of environmental management are that they are long-lasting and not damaging to the environment, and that they minimize the need for application of pesticides. Environmental management measures in vector control vary from regular maintenance of small-scale, existing schemes to large-scale or emergency activities. The equipment required may range from simple, easily available, hand-held, lightweight tools to heavy, sophisticated machinery.

Selection of the appropriate equipment must be based on the needs and resources of the programme. Local leaders, professionals and community representatives should participate in establishing the selection criteria.

The main criteria to be considered when specific

equipment for environmental management for vector control is being selected include (but are not necessarily limited to): durability of equipment; reliability; operation and maintenance costs; the capability of local technicians or residents to operate and maintain the equipment; environmental compatibility; effectiveness; safety; and cost-effectiveness.

Light machinery

Members of local communities can contribute a wide range of skills and equipment of great potential value in environmental management. Skills in carpentry, ironwork and farming will usually be available. Equipment will include a range of agricultural tools and machines which, depending on the local farming system, may be operated by hand, by animals or by tractor. The use of available equipment and skills will encourage local understanding and participation in environmental management, and will also bring economic benefits to the community. The infrastructure to support continuing use of the equipment will already exist in large measure. Through the use of local skills, equipment and services, the community will realize that it is able to execute and maintain environmental management works from its own resources. This process is an important advantage of community based methods, and is the basis for the pride of community ownership and understanding which make such programmes long-lasting.

The equipment available will mostly be light agricultural machinery, ranging from hand tools to equipment drawn by tractors of up to about 50 kW (65 horsepower). In many rural communities the hoe is the most widely available tool and is used in a wide range of operations such as land clearance, soil preparation, formation and maintenance of ditches and bunds etc. Other widely available hand tools include the machete, spade, sickle and various forms of rakes or levelling boards. A hand-operated winch, which may have to be purchased, is able to clear large trees at lower cost than heavy tractor-driven land-clearing machines and with less environmental disturbance.

There is a wide range of activities to which animal-drawn equipment might be able to contribute. Equipment that can be used with tractors of low to medium power, much of which may already be in use locally, includes the bulldozer blade, heavy-duty cultivator (which may be used as a light ripper), land leveller, scraper, bund former, trailer, and various types of cultivation equipment such as the plough or rotary hoe. Other tractor-drawn equipment of a more specialized nature, which may not be in local use but is readily obtainable through commercial channels, includes ditch formers, ditch cleaners and trenchers used for laying underground drainage pipes.

The applications for which this equipment would need to be used include land clearance, drainage, soil preparation, soil movement, land forming, waterway construction, waterway maintenance and vegetation control.

Heavy machinery

Community environmental management programmes should use to the fullest extent the equipment and manpower available locally. However, when local resources are not sufficient, there may be a need to look beyond the community.

Major construction and maintenance work requiring the use of large machines should be considered only after careful planning and design of the project and in the light of a complete understanding of the vector ecology. Some large machines that have been used successfully are backhoes, draglines, excavators, bulldozers, rotary ditchers and mowers.

Domestic equipment

Several simple measures for improvement of housing, such as plastering of walls, screening of houses, installation of roof and wastewater drains, collection of solid waste and proper disposal of refuse should be included in the basic community approach to vector control.

Many mosquitos, particularly some *Aedes* species which are vectors of arboviral diseases, breed in a wide variety of water storage tanks and vessels, discarded containers and other scrap materials. Screens and other materials have been used successfully to cover water storage containers to prevent mosquitos breeding in them. In both urban and rural communities only an efficient refuse collection and disposal service can reduce the tremendous number of discarded containers which provide sources of mosquito production. Refuse can be disposed of by burial, incineration or composting, using hand tools such as shovels, picks and wheelbarrows. Community vehicles such as donkey carts can be used for collection and disposal of refuse.

Water management devices

Technical devices that have been successfully used in water management as part of vector control programmes are diesel and electric pumps, pipes and culverts, gates, gate valves and weirs, siphons, artesian wells and porous drains.

Technique of residual spraying

In view of the importance of correct technique for application of residual insecticides some details of the relevant practice may be of value. Knowledge of the number, location and accessibility of the houses and field shelters is of great importance and this is the real aim of *geographical reconnaissance*, which should be carried out during the preparatory phase of the programme and kept up to date as much as possible.

The main data to be provided by geographical reconnaissance are as follows. (1) The extent of the area must be clearly known – maps showing the location of villages, roads and other features must be available, if not they should be prepared by a properly trained team. (2) The number, type and size of dwellings and other sprayable structures must be identified and recorded. (3) The mean sprayable surface per dwelling must be calculated, in order to know the amount of insecticide needed for one spray round. This is done by measuring the walls and ceilings of a sample of dwellings. (4) The maps are useful for preparing itineraries and for plotting the location of villages, houses and roads for the squad leaders to follow. Each dwelling should receive a reference number, painted on the wall or on the door, to enable the spraying squad leaders to check the work done. (5) Information on the population in each locality is important, for epidemiological evaluation of the prevalence of malaria and any subsequent changes. (6) The timing of spraying operations is important; in areas with a short transmission period the spraying should be planned so that it is completed before the onset of the high activity of the vector. Certain customs and cultural patterns of the local population must be taken into consideration. Replastering of indoor walls, whitewashing, smoke deposits, rethatching etc. may greatly decrease or nullify the insecticidal effect and require changes of spraying routine or additional spraying. (7) Population movements related to seasonal migration, planting, harvesting and cattle grazing may result in locked houses or building of temporary shelters away from the locality; this would often require special insecticide applications.

The spraying is done at stated intervals. The operation of spraying in one locality is known as the *spraying round*, while the spraying of all houses in a given area, repeated at regular intervals, is known as the *spraying cycle*. Focal spraying is limited to a group of houses forming a distinct focus of transmission. The progress of spraying operations is measured by comparing the number of houses sprayed and localities with the totals included in the programmes. Special measures are put into action to ensure the complete spraying of all houses, localities and the area involved.

The dosage is the amount of insecticide applied to a unit of indoor surface of the inhabited or other premise; it is expressed in terms of grammes of active compound per square metre of surface (g/m^2). Dosages and cycles must be determined according to local conditions and depend on the results of an entomological study of the habits of the vector species. Each type of residual insecticide requires an optimum dosage depending on the toxicity of the compound to the mosquito, the type of surface to which it is applied (wood, adobe, thatch), climatic conditions, and the transmission season; if the latter is of short duration (3–4 months) one spraying cycle per year may be sufficient. Dried mud (adobe) surfaces usually decrease the duration of insecticidal effect, while wood increases it markedly.

The total amount of the insecticide formulation required for each spraying round depends on the dosage. For example, if a group of villages had 10 000 houses, each averaging 200 m^2 of sprayable surface, requiring a dosage of DDT at 2 g/m^2, the total amount of the active compound needed would be 4000 kg; however, if the formulation consists of 75% water-dispersible powder, then 6000 kg of the formulation will be required. Usually, about 10%

of the product is added to cover possible waste or spillage; thus the total amount to be supplied would be 6600 kg per spray round (Table 10.5).

The personnel required for a spraying operation depends on the size of the proposed activity and on the intended degree of supervision and evaluation. Normally, the whole area is divided into sectors, with a sector chief in charge. The sector chief's responsibilities include the preparation of work schedules, maintenance of personnel rosters, checking on performance, filling in spraying reports, ordering of supplies, coordination of transport, public relations etc. The squad leaders should be responsible to the sector chief.

The basic field unit for carrying out a spraying operation is a *spraying squad* which consists of two to six spraymen and a squad leader. The predetermined area of work and itinerary must be established in advance. The task of the spraymen consists of proper application of the insecticide formulation to all sprayable surfaces of all the dwelling units and other premises in the locality. This must often include animal sheds and temporary field shelters, away from the centre of the village.

The number of spraying personnel required depends on the number of houses that one sprayman can deal with in a day, but also on many other factors, such as accessibility, number of rooms, distances between villages etc. As an average, it can be stated that one sprayman can treat 8–10 houses, with a 200 m^2 surface, in a day; thus in a month of 22 working days, some 500–600 houses can be sprayed by a squad of three spraymen with one squad leader. In addition to the squad leader a squad often has a mixer to prepare the spray, to fill the sprayers, to help with moving the furniture, stored water and food out of the house, to clean up at the end of the day etc. A tentative calculation for spraying 10 000 houses every 4 months would require 5–6 squads each with a squad leader and one sector chief, making a total of 25–30 men, not counting drivers of vehicles.

Although residual insecticides may be applied by a variety of spraying equipment, the hand-operated compression sprayer continues to be the most effective and commonly used method. The five factors governing the application of a uniform dosage rate are:

1. The insecticide concentration in the liquid.
2. The air pressure in the sprayer.
3. The nozzle aperture.
4. The distance from the nozzle tip to the sprayed surface.
5. The speed of application to the surface.

The need for *total coverage* was of particular importance in malaria eradication campaigns where it was rigidly observed. However, in malaria control projects a more flexible approach can be adopted, adjusting the type of coverage by residual insecticides to epidemiological conditions and entomological assessment of results. The following modifications may be considered. *Selective spraying* of ceilings, parts of the walls and other parts of the house where *Anopheles* mosquitos rest may be effective, with a consequent saving of insecticide. *Focal coverage* of villages, groups of buildings or parts of the area, closest to the main breeding places of vectors, will give a measure of control while at the same time reducing the workload of available staff. *Barrier spraying* of groups of houses or of a concentric zone of dwellings at the perimeter of the protected area may intercept the influx of vector mosquitos from the non-controlled outer area. It may be preferable to spray the inner area, if there is evidence of a marked influx from outside. *Partial coverage* may exclude from spraying those buildings which are not inhabited such as grain stores, shops, schools, etc.

Cooperation of the population is essential; the people in an area to be treated should be given adequate warning of the day and time of spraying, being asked to arrange that houses are open, foodstuffs removed or covered, and furniture pulled out into the middle of the rooms (Fig. 10.22). Spraymen must be accompanied by a responsible local resident whose main function is to secure cooperation and vouch for the safety of persons and property in the houses treated, as without their support future work may be hampered by misunderstandings. After spraying, a printed form should be left on the indoor wall of the house, with the date of spraying and the date of next visit, which gives needed information to inspectors checking the work and to the householder about provision for the next spraying.

The public response may be that of suspicion in the early stages, but this soon gives way to active

Table 10.5 Quantities of formulations for standard spraying*

Insecticide	Formulation	Active insecticide content (%)	Dilution required for field use†	Remarks
DDT	Water-dispersible powder	50	90 g/litre (14 oz/ gallons)	Imperial gallons (4.5 litres) throughout
DDT	Water-dispersible powder	75	60 g/litre (9.5 oz/ gallon)	
DDT	Liquid concentrate	20	1 part to 3½ parts of kerosene or water	Kerosene for solutions, water for emulsion concentrates
Hexachlorocyclohexane (HCH)	Water-dispersible powder	25	40 g/litre (6 oz/ gallon)	
Hexachlorocyclohexane (HCH)	Water-dispersible powder	50	20 g/litre (3 oz/ gallon)	
Hexachlorocyclohexane (HCH)	Liquid concentrate	20	1 part to 22 parts of kerosene or water	Kerosene for solutions, water for emulsion concentrates
Dieldrin	Water-dispersible powder	50	26 g/litre (4.2 oz/ gallon)	Now rarely used
Malathion	Water-dispersible powder	50	90 g/litre (14 oz/ gallon of water)	}
Malathion	Water-dispersible powder	25	180 g/litre (28 oz/ gallon of water)	} For dosage of 1 g/m² add twice the amount of water
Malathion	Emulsion concentrate	20	1 part to 4 parts of water	}
Lambda-cyhalothrin (ICON)	Water-dispersible powder	10	7.5 g/litre	
Lambda-cyhalothrin (ICON)	Emulsion concentrate	2.5	1 part to 50 parts water	
Bendiocarb	Water-dispersible powder	80	10 g/litre	1 preweighed sachet added to water in the standard spray-pump gives the required dosage as a spray suspension
Pyrimiphos–methyl	Emulsion concentrate	50	1 part to 10 parts water	For dosages of 1 g/m² add twice the amount of water
Fenitrothion	Water-dispersible powder	40	112 g/litre	
Fenitrothion	Emulsion concentrate	20	1 part to 4 parts water	
Permethrin	Water-dispersible powder	25	45 g/litre	
Permethrin	Emulsion concentrate	25	1 part to 20 parts water	
Deltamethrin	Water-dispersible powder	6	22 g/litre	

*This table indicates the quantity of different formulations required to prepare one gallon (4.5 litres) of diluted spray for application using a sprayer with an average spraying rate of one gallon per 1000 ft² of surface (4.5–5.0 litres/100 m²) to obtain the usual application rates of DDT 2 g/m², dieldrin 0.5 g/m² and malathion 2 g/m².

†The generally used standard type of sprayer operating at the recommended pressure and with the usual nozzle aperture allows the sprayman to cover 1000 ft² or close to 100 m² of treated surface in the time required to deliver 1 gallon (4.5 litres) of diluted spray.

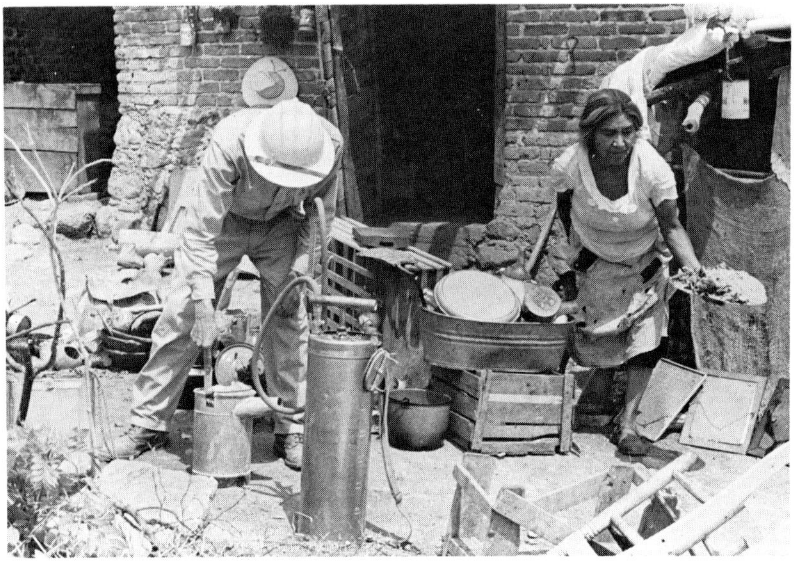

Fig. 10.22 Temporary removal of part of the furniture and food supplies from dwellings before residual spraying begins. The assistance of local inhabitants in this procedure is an important factor of cooperation with the spraying squad. (WHO photograph by E. Schwab.)

cooperation when the benefits of treatment become apparent, and for the most part such schemes run smoothly.

Transport facilities for moving equipment, materials and personnel play an important part in most vector control programmes. In developing countries, vehicles must generally be imported and delays in receiving them can seriously impede the planned operations which are timed to coincide with an appropriate season of the year. Several months may occur between placing the orders and the arrival of the vehicles, but even then, the delivery may be delayed by various customs formalities. Similar delays may occur in the delivery of spare parts. It is essential that all vehicle service centres have an experienced mechanic and are provided with workshop manuals and proper tools. Drivers should receive adequate training and perform simple maintenance tasks. The type of transport facilities required in developing countries may range from bicycles to four-wheel vehicles and boats. Detailed assessment of the type of transport and quantities needed must be made at an early stage of planning so that specific needs of the programme are taken into account (Fig. 10.23).

As the residual spraying aims specifically at the adult anopheline vectors of malaria it is evident that the role of entomological methods, in measuring the impact on the target insect, is of primary importance. The choice and interpretation of the results of sampling of the vector population is the responsibility of an experienced professional entomologist, with the aid of auxiliary personnel. Baseline data collected before the start of control will have provided information on the vector species

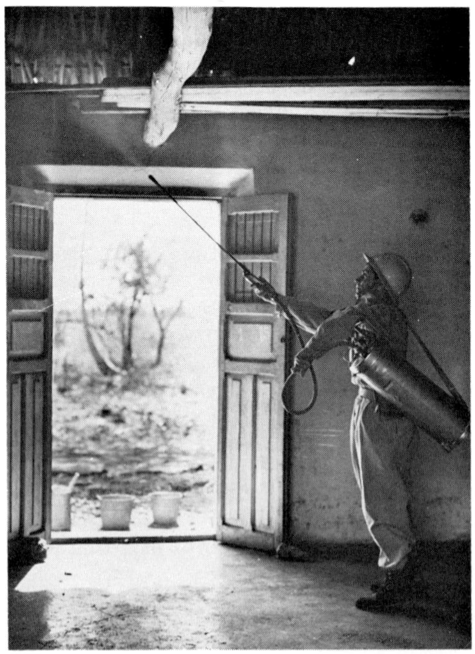

Fig. 10.23 Residual house spraying as carried out in the state of Yucatán in Mexico. (WHO photograph by P. Almasy.)

concerned, its distribution, behaviour, susceptibility to the insecticide etc.

After the first and subsequent spray rounds, entomology provides information on:

1. The impact of the spraying on the vector population.
2. The duration of insecticidal effect.
3. The need for alteration in the spray cycles and rounds.
4. The need to change the insecticide dosage.
5. The need to change insecticides because of incipient resistance or other problems.
6. Changes in mosquito behaviour induced by insecticidal exposure.
7. Incidental effects on domestic animals and insects such as bedbugs, cockroaches, fleas and flies.
8. Harmful effects on beneficial insects (honey bees, silkworms).

Many sampling methods for *Anopheles* have been used, and only the briefest mention of them can be given here. They vary from the measuring of indoor resting densities (by the spray sheet method), through outdoor resting densities (collections in natural or artificial resting places), to the use of window-exit traps, outdoor biting collections on human or animal bait, bioassay tests (exposing samples of 20–25 mosquitos in a plastic conical chamber held against the treated wall), to testing vector susceptibility in contact with a known dosage of insecticide. (See *WHO Manual on Practical Entomology in Malaria*, parts I and II, 1975.)

Resistance of mosquitos to insecticides

General considerations

Resistance to insecticides has been defined as the 'ability of a population of insects to tolerate doses of an insecticide which would prove lethal to the majority of individuals in a normal population of the same species'. It is understood that this biological phenomenon develops as a result of selection pressure by the relevant insecticidal compound or its analogue.

The above definition refers to what is known as *physiological resistance* affecting the direct mortality of a proportion of a population of insects exposed to the toxic compound. Another, different, aspect of this phenomenon is the change of behaviour pattern of a population of insects, so that they acquire the ability to avoid contact with the insecticide. This phenomenon is known under the term '*behaviouristic resistance*' or '*insecticide avoidance*'.

Both types of resistance may interfere with the results of malaria control measures, especially when the main method comprises residual insecticide spraying. Although 'physiological resistance' is by far the most important of the two and more easily measurable, insecticide avoidance can become an obstacle to malaria control.

The efficacy of indoor residual spraying depends, among other things, on the feeding and resting habits of the vector. Obviously any changes in the house-entry pattern, a shift to outdoor biting to avoid insecticide treated surfaces, and exophilic and exophagic tendencies will affect the result of the control programme. This has been observed in some species of the *A. gambiae* complex in Africa, in *A. nuneztovari* in Venezuela, in *A. punctulatus* in New Guinea, in *A. farauti* in the Solomon Islands, *A. dirus* and *A. minimus* in Thailand, *A. balabacensis* in Bangladesh and *A. philippinensis* in India. It is not certain that this change of behaviour is due to a specific selection pressure of the insecticide.

Changes in the environment have also been shown to alter the ecology of various vector species. For example, urbanization development activities and insecticide use have led to a decline in the density of *A. culicifacies* in India; other studies have shown that *A. stephensi* has assumed importance in areas where water is stored in tanks and wells and, although essentially endophilic, this species was found to rest outdoors in southern Iran and southern India.

In Afghanistan, agricultural development led to the replacement of *A. pulcherrimus*, an established vector, by *A. hyrcanus*, which was found to be resistant to DDT and also exophilic and exophagic. Observations in Kisumu, Kenya, revealed that before spraying with the insecticide fenitrothion, *A. gambiae* was the dominant species and was more endophilic than *A. arabiensis*, although the two species did not differ in infectivity and host preferences. After spraying, the density of both species was reduced, but there were increases in the degree of exophily and the relative proportion of

A. arabiensis. In Ethiopia, *A. gambiae* s.l. and *A. funestus* have been shown to be partly exophilic while *A. pharoensis* and *A. nili* were strongly exophilic. *Anopheles aconitus* in Central Java or Indonesia was found mostly resting outdoors and the endophilic fraction rested only on the lower parts of walls so that effective control could be achieved by selective spraying of the lower portion of the walls only.

Although the physiological resistance of *Anopheles* to DDT was recognized as a potentially serious problem already 45 years ago, the impact of this phenomenon on malaria control and eradication has become fully obvious during the past two decades.

The extension of resistance from DDT to other chlorinated hydrocarbons (HCH and dieldrin) led to giving up these compounds in many parts of the world. The alternative use of organophosphorus and carbamate insecticides proved to be expensive and few developing tropical countries are able to afford it without external help. Moreover, mosquito vectors have developed a degree of resistance to several newer insecticides, and particularly those widely used in agriculture. Research on and development of new insecticidal compounds is expensive and increasingly difficult, so that the possibility of having in the immediate future a vast array of valuable compounds is not very likely. Nevertheless, even in the present, less than satisfactory, situation, the available insecticides, if properly used, can still play a major role in the decrease of malaria transmission.

Nature and cause of resistance

Much research in the laboratory and in the field has been devoted to our understanding of the nature and mechanism of the development of resistance. Only the briefest review of this complex problem can be given here.

The multiple factors that influence the development of resistance to insecticides in a population of mosquitos can be classified into genetic (e.g. presence of specific genes and their frequency), operational (e.g. type of insecticide and its method of application) and biological (e.g. size and characteristics of the insect population).

Resistance to insecticides arises not through a process of gradual adaptation of mosquitos to a toxic compound. It is a speeded up process of Darwinian selection which can occur when in the original population of mosquitos there was a small proportion of mutant individuals genetically endowed with the capacity to withstand, at least partly, the toxic action of the insecticidal compound (Table 10.6).

Such a protective mechanism may depend on a single genetic factor, which is recessive, partially dominant or dominant in the process of inheritance. Resistant individuals are rare when they first appear in the heterozygous state in a mosquito population. Heterozygotes that survive the contact with the insecticide (which gradually eliminates the susceptible mosquitos) mate with other heterozygotes and produce a proportion of homozygotes, with a higher degree of resistance. If the resistance gene is dominant it will spread rapidly through the whole population.

Some types of resistance are due to one single gene while other types are related to several genes. Studies which revealed that certain types of resistance can be assigned to specific loci on chromosomes of relevant mosquitos allowed us to distinguish between different biochemical mechanisms of resistance. While some such mechanisms involve detoxification by enzymatic processes of the chemical compound, other mechanisms are due to the change of the site of the toxic action or reduced penetration of the toxicant. These largely unknown protective mechanisms may be specific for a particular compound or active against several compounds. They probably depend on the reduced penetration and increased detoxification of the given chemical poison.

When resistance due to the selection of one or more genes by a certain insecticide extends to other chemical compounds, we are dealing with the phenomenon of *cross-resistance*. The spectrum of cross-resistance may be narrow as in the case of the cyclodiene group (HCH, dieldrin) or it may be wide, also covering other groups (e.g. organophosphate compounds).

It has been known for some time that resistance to DDT caused by the action of the *kdr* gene also imparts cross-resistance to pyrethroid insecticides. It was subsequently demonstrated that selection of mosquitos by pyrethroids confers or enhances resistance to DDT.

Resistance to carbamates and organophosphorus compounds in *A. albimanus* in Central America is primarily caused by the selection of acetylcholinesterase that is less sensitive to the action of these chemicals. The mechanism was later also found in *A. sacharovi*, *A. atroparvus* and *A. nigerrimus*. In most instances this mechanism has produced a broad spectrum of resistance to many organophosphorus and carbamate insecticides. The low level of resistance to fenthion of *A. albimanus* and of *A. sacharovi* to malathion are notable exceptions.

A distinction between monogenic resistance and the more complex polygenic type is important, as the former is more amenable to countermeasures such as the addition of synergists or change to a different insecticide.

The insecticide selection pressure depends also on the relative toxicity of the compound, the degree of coverage of the area, the developmental stage and density of the mosquito population, the number of generations exposed, the behaviour characteristics of the respective species of mosquitos, and many genetic factors.

Resistance to dieldrin (and HCH) is more common and develops more rapidly than does DDT resistance because the former is of a higher degree and since the gene for dieldrin resistance is fully or partially dominant. On the other hand, the DDT resistance is of a lower degree and recessive in its genetic expression; even if DDT resistance in *Anopheles* is confirmed, its development may be slow and the continued use of DDT may still have a sufficient impact on the mosquito population to achieve a fair degree of control.

Insecticide resistance often develops within a small part of the population of one species of *Anopheles* and assumes different patterns depending on the type of selection pressure. Thus, *A. funestus* populations in a few parts of Africa show only dieldrin–HCH resistance without any other chemical group being involved.

A multiple resistance pattern covering organochlorines, organophosphates and carbamates is rare but has been described in some populations of *A. albimanus*, *A. atroparvus* and *A. sacharovi*. This is generally due to the widespread use of various insecticides for control of agricultural pests in neighbouring areas and severe contamination of anopheline breeding places. The knowledge of genetic factors involved in insecticide resistance allows for making some predictions of the speed of its selection and the ways to avoid it, if possible.

Determination of resistance

The standardized WHO method entails a comparison of mortality of a number of female *Anopheles* of a known species exposed in special tubes to filter papers impregnated with various concentrations of a given insecticide dissolved in mineral oil (Fig. 10.24).

Some comments on the criteria and interpretation

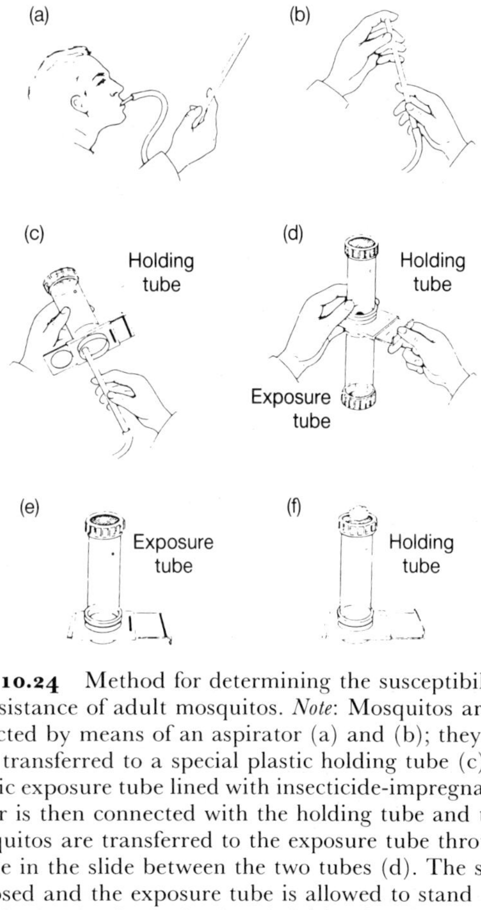

Fig. 10.24 Method for determining the susceptibility or resistance of adult mosquitos. *Note*: Mosquitos are collected by means of an aspirator (a) and (b); they are then transferred to a special plastic holding tube (c); a plastic exposure tube lined with insecticide-impregnated paper is then connected with the holding tube and the mosquitos are transferred to the exposure tube through a hole in the slide between the two tubes (d). The slide is closed and the exposure tube is allowed to stand upright for the determined period (e); after the exposure period the mosquitos are transferred back to the holding tube, which should stand upright for 24 hours, with a piece of moist cotton wool on the gauze end (f). Counts of dead mosquitos killed by the contact with the insecticide are made at the end of this recovery period. (WHO 1970 Technical Report Series, No. 443.)

Table 10.6 Insecticide resistance in 34 *Anopheles* which play an important role in malaria transmission, as reported by the World Health Organization

Species	DDT	Organophosphate compounds	Other compounds
A. aconitus	Bangladesh, India, Indonesia, Nepal, Thailand	—	—
A. albimanus	Belize, Colombia, Costa Rica, Cuba, Dominican Republic, Ecuador, Guatemala, El Salvador, Haiti, Honduras, Mexico, Nicaragua, Panama	Costa Rica, El Salvador, Guatemala, Honduras, Mexico, Nicaragua	Costa Rica, El Salvador, Ecuador, Guatemala, Haiti, Honduras, Panama
A. albitarsis	Brazil, Colombia	—	—
A. annularis	Bangladesh, India, Myanmar, Nepal, Pakistan, Thailand	Sri Lanka	—
A. arabiensis	Ethiopia, Mauritius, Saudi Arabia, Senegal, Sudan, Swaziland, United Republic of Tanzania (Zanzibar)	Sudan	Sudan
A. atroparvus	Portugal, Roumania, Spain, United Kingdom, former USSR	Portugal, Spain	Portugal, Roumania, Spain
A. barbirostris	Myanmar, India, Indonesia, Sri Lanka	Sri Lanka	—
A. coustani	Egypt, La Reunion, Saudi Arabia	Egypt	—
A. culicifacies complex	Afghanistan, Bhutan, India, Islamic Republic of Iran, Myanmar, Nepal, Oman, Pakistan, Sri Lanka, Thailand	India, Oman, Pakistan, Sri Lanka, United Arab Emirates	India, Oman, Sri Lanka, United Arab Emirates
A. darlingi	Colombia, Venezuela	—	—
A. d'thali	Islamic Republic of Iran	Egypt, Jordan	Egypt
A. farauti	Solomon Islands	—	—
A. fluviatilis	Afghanistan, India, Nepal, Pakistan	—	Nepal
A. funastus	Sudan	—	—
A. gambiae sensu stricto	Benin, Burkina Faso, Cameroon, Central African Republic, Congo, Ghana, Liberia, Mali, Niger, Nigeria, South Africa, United Republic of Tanzania (Zanzibar), Togo, Zaire	—	Nigeria (only in the laboratory)
A. hyrcanus	Afghanistan, Myanmar, Pakistan, Turkey, former USSR	Turkey	Turkey
A. labranchiae	Algeria, Morocco, Tunisia	Italy	—
A. maculatus	Bhutan, India, Myanmar, Nepal, Pakistan, Thailand	—	—

Table 10.6 *cont.*

Species	DDT	Organophosphate compounds	Other compounds
A. maculipennis	Bulgaria, Greece, Islamic Republic of Iran, Roumania, Turkey, former USSR	Turkey, Greece, Roumania	Bulgaria, Greece, Roumania, Turkey
A. minimus	Thailand	—	—
A. nigerrimus	India, Indonesia, Myanmar, Pakistan, Sri Lanka, Thailand	India, Sri Lanka	Sri Lanka
A. pharoensis	Angola, Egypt, Ethiopia, Sudan	Egypt	Egypt
A. philippinenesis	Myanmar, Thailand	—	—
A. pseudopunctipennis	Bolivia, Guatemala, Honduras, Mexico, Panama, Peru	Guatemala, Honduras	Guatemala, Honduras
A. pulcherrimus	Afghanistan, Iraq, Pakistan, Saudi Arabia, former USSR	—	—
A. punctimacula	Colombia, Ecuador	—	—
A. quadrimaculatus	Mexico, USA	USA	USA
A. sacharovi	Bulgaria, Greece, Islamic Republic of Iran, Lebanon, Syrian Arab Republic, Turkey, former USSR	Bulgaria, Greece, Lebanon, Syrian Arab Republic	Bulgaria, Lebanon, Syrian Arab Republic
A. sergentii	Egypt	Egypt, Jordan	—
A. sinensis	China, Japan, Nepal, Vietnam	China, Hong Kong, Japan, Republic of Korea	—
A. stephensi	Afghanistan, India, Oman, Iraq, Pakistan, Islamic Republic of Iran, Yemen, United Arab Emirates	India, Iraq, Islamic Republic of Iran, Pakistan	Dubai, India, Pakistan
A. subpictus	Afghanistan, Bangladesh, India, Indonesia, Myanmar, Nepal, Pakistan, Sri Lanka, Vietnam	India, Sri Lanka	Sri Lanka (only larvae)
A. sundaicus	Indonesia, Malaysia, Thailand, Vietnam	—	—
A. superpictus	Afghanistan, former USSR	—	—
A. vagus	Bangladesh, India, Indonesia, Malaya, Myanmar, Nepal, Sri Lanka, Thailand, Vietnam	Sri Lanka	Sri Lanka

Note: This list, based on data provided by the World Health Organization in the Technical Report Series Nos 737 and 818, refers only to the most important vectors of malaria. It should be remembered that in each of the species quoted the phenomenon of resistance and its degree do not cover the whole geographical area of distribution of the species concerned. Information on the latter point will be found in the reports quoted above.

of tests for vector resistance to insecticides will be of practical value. The detection and measurement of this phenomenon is based on the comparison with a strain of the *Anopheles* species of normal susceptibility, tested under similar conditions. Preferably the response of the susceptible strain should be known before the control campaign, but it may be possible to compare the results of tests in treated and untreated areas. The more elaborate test consists of exposing samples of female *Anopheles* for a standard time (usually 1 hour) to a forced contact with a range of three concentrations of a given insecticide on impregnated filter papers. The mortality after 24 hours recovery of exposed mosquitos, when plotted on logarithmic probability graph, gives a dosage/mortality regression line (Fig. 10.25). If the regression line flattens out at high concentrations of the insecticide-impregnated papers this indicates a resistance in the mosquito population. If the regression line remains parallel to the line seen in susceptible strains then the sample exhibits only a higher tolerance, due to physiological conditions of mosquitos (gravid) or to microclimatic factors of the test. A simpler test has been widely used. It consists of exposing samples of *Anopheles* to one single diagnostic concentration of a given insecticide on impregnated papers prepared by the WHO. These diagnostic concentrations which kill all susceptible *Anopheles* are: DDT 4%, dieldrin 0.4%, malathion 5%, propoxur 0.1% and fenitrothion 1%. They require the exposure of mosquitos in special plastic tubes for 1 hour, with the exception of fenitrothion which needs 2 hours' exposure. The proportion of surviving mosquitos after the 24-hour period of recovery indicates the development of resistance and its degree in the vector population. Another method is applicable to anopheline larvae. Appropriate test kits for determination of resistance are issued by the WHO, which also periodically circulates the latest reports on findings in the field (Fig. 10.26).

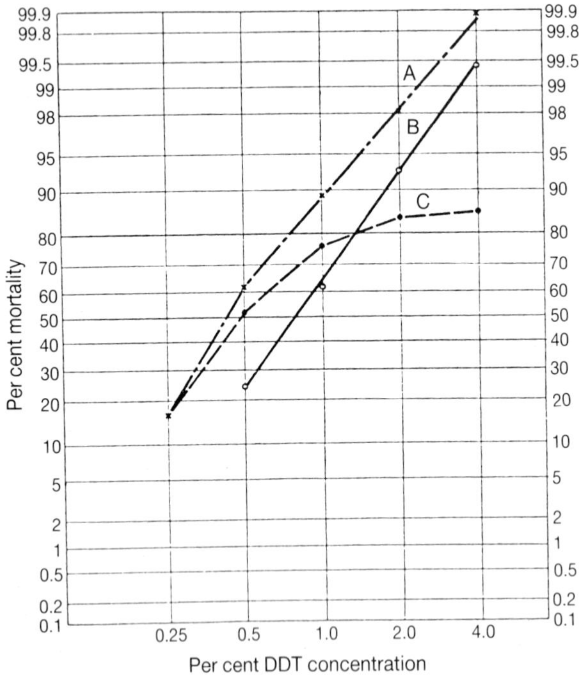

Fig. 10.25 Dosage/mortality regression lines for DDT indicating susceptibility of a sample of vectors: (A) to the insecticide; (B) seasonal fluctuation or tolerance; (C) presence of resistance in the vector population. (Reproduced from WHO 1976 Technical Report Series. No. 585.)

In any malaria control programme based on a wide use of residual insecticides one should attempt an early detection of resistance. Once the presence of resistance has been established its progress should be monitored; this means the assessment of its operational importance and planning of countermeasures. The chances of an early detection of resistance are greater if the surveillance operations concentrate on areas where agricultural pesticides have been widely used. A suitable policy for detection of resistance in vector control programmes should provide for investigation of 5–10% of villages or groups of houses over the entire control area. When the presence of resistance is confirmed the operational significance of it requires studies of vector density as well as epidemiological appraisal of the origin of human infections. If it is established that a low degree of insecticide resistance is the cause of increased transmission then insecticide spraying at shorter intervals or at higher dosage of the active compound, combined with better detection of cases and their treatment may be a temporary solution. However, when the degree of resistance is high and transmission continues, a change of insecticide becomes imperative, together with other attack measures to decrease the amount of transmission. Detailed discussion of these prob-

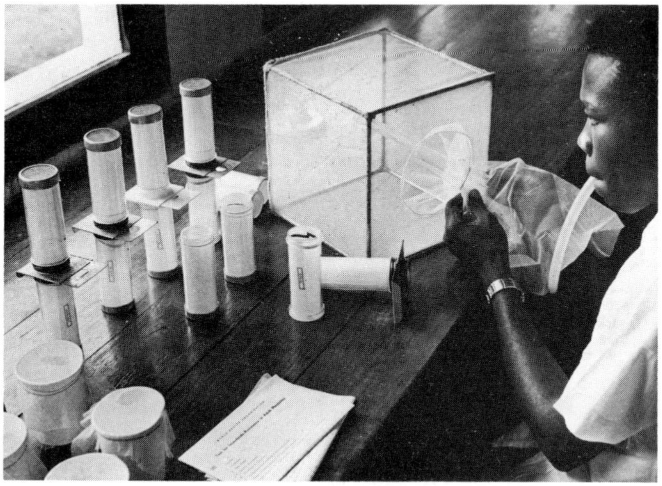

Fig. 10.26 Testing *Anopheles* mosquitos collected in the field for insecticide resistance in West Africa. (WHO photograph by P. Almasy.)

lems will be found in the WHO Technical Report Series no. 585 (1976) and no. 655 (1980).

More recently, new biochemical and immunological resistance assays have been developed. These methods detect resistance mechanisms in single insects in the field and are both cheap and simple to use.

Resistance can be detected at very low frequency, allowing efficient monitoring of vector populations.

As biochemical insecticide susceptibility assays are more widely used as diagnostic procedures there is a need for standardization. Criteria should be set for good practice in applying methods, allowing their consistent use anywhere, and encouraging a more careful use of the new techniques in the field.

Present state of resistance to insecticides in malaria vectors

In 1946, only two species of *Anopheles* were resistant to DDT, but by 1991 a total of 55 species showed resistance to one or more insecticides. Of the 55 species, 53 show resistance to DDT, 27 to organophosphorus compounds, 17 to carbamates and 10 to pyrethroids; 16 species show resistance to three or four chemical compounds.

Twenty-one of the 55 resistant species are very important vectors of malaria, namely: *A. aconitus*, *A. albimanus*, *A. albitarsis*, *A. annularis*, *A. arabiensis*, *A. culicifacies*, *A. darlingi*, *A. fluviatilis*, *A. gambiae*, *A. labranchiae*, *A. maculatus*, *A. pharoensis*, *A. pseudopunctipennis*, *A. pulcherrimus*, *A. sacharovi*, *A. sergentii*, *A. sinensis*, *A. stephensi*, *A. subpictus*, *A. sundaicus* and *A. superpictus*. They are listed in Table 10.6 which has been taken from a table reported by WHO in 1986 which showed the insecticide resistance of 51 anopheline species in countries or areas, and adjusted following later information contained in two subsequent reports in 1991 and 1992.

The following findings of resistance in malaria vectors are of particular significance: *A. aconitus* is resistant to DDT in central and western Kalimantan, Bangladesh, India, Nepal and Thailand. *Anopheles albimanus* is resistant to organophosphorus compounds and carbamates in most of Central America and in some parts of Mexico. *Anopheles annularis* is resistant to DDT in Bangladesh, Myanmar, India, Pakistan and Thailand, to DDT and cyclodienes in Nepal, and to DDT and organophosphates in Sri Lanka.

It seems that nearly all members of the *A. gambiae* complex are resistant in various degrees to DDT and other organochlorine insecticides over most of tropical Africa, but *A. arabiensis* (formerly *A. gambiae* B) in the Sudan has become resistant also to malathion. *Anopheles culicifacies* is resistant to DDT and HCH in several countries of the Middle East and in the Indian sub-continent; it has developed resistance also to malathion especially in the Gujarat and Maharastra states of India and in Oman, Sri Lanka and the United Arab Emirates. *Anopheles minimus* has shown a decrease of susceptibility to DDT in Thailand. *A. sacharovi* is now resistant to DDT, organophosphates and carbamates in certain areas of Bulgaria, Greece, Turkey and the former USSR and to fenithrotion in parts of Lebanon and the Syrian Arab Republic. *Anopheles sinensis* has been found to be resistant to DDT, cyclodienes and malathion in southern China and partly in Vietnam.

Anopheles stephensi is resistant to malathion in Afghanistan, India, Iraq, the Islamic Republic of Iran, Oman, Pakistan, Saudi Arabia and the United Arab Emirates, and has shown resistance to permethrin in India and the Islamic Republic of Iran.

The method formerly followed to meet the problem of insecticide resistance to a specific compound was to use an alternative insecticide. However, this is now less and less feasible. A WHO Programme for the Evaluation of Insecticides has been in operation since 1957 and by 1982 over 1800 compounds were screened for their activity and safety; only a small number of some 20 compounds passed the stringent tests and a few of them were tentatively tried in the field.

In 1982 the Programme was revised to cover a wider range of vectors and formulations, and was renamed the WHO Pesticide Evaluation Scheme. It now comprises four progressive phases: laboratory examinations, small-scale and large-scale field trials and, if all other phases have successfully passed, specifications for purchase.

The aim of the revised Programme is the same as that of the original, namely, the assessment of new candidate insecticides and formulations in order to provide suitable alternatives for pesticides used for all types of vector control to which resistance has appeared or is likely to appear.

In recent years, however, there has been a decline in the number of compounds submitted by industry, primarily because of the high cost of insecticide development, and particularly the cost of mounting large-scale field trials.

DDT still remains the cheapest and probably the most widely employed insecticide for malaria control. Its use is expected to continue with a preference for emulsifiable instead of water-dispersible powder formulations. The demand for malathion is also expected to remain high as it is still effective against many malaria vectors. Fenithrotion may be used instead of malathion in some countries however its cost is higher than that of malathion and resistance to it is most likely to include resistance to malathion, whereas the converse is not the case. This implies that malathion should be used before fenitrothion for malaria vector control. Permethrin, deltamethrin, pirimiphos–methyl and propoxur may be used in special circumstances, especially in view of the increasing resistance of vectors to organochlorine and organophosphorus compounds.

Operational approaches of malaria control to counteract insecticide resistance

As mentioned before, the development of insecticide resistance is related to two main factors: (1) the biological characteristics of the species and of the local population of the respective vector, and (2) the type and degree of the selection pressure of the insecticide. Research carried out in the past has improved our capacity to judge the relative speed with which a specific resistance pattern may appear under certain circumstances; however, it is still impossible to predict the time when the resistance gene will attain a certain frequency and present operational problems. It is now clear, that the selection pressure is related to the degree and time of action of the toxic compounds on the heterozygote individuals within the insect population and on the house haunting habits of *Anopheles*. Thus, the appearance of resistance might be slower with less persistent residual deposits and, if the susceptible mosquitos enter the target area from the outside, cross-breeding with the resistant ones would lower the frequency of heterozygotes. In practice, it would mean that in an area where new houses have been built after the last spraying cycle, it may be preferable to leave the new houses unsprayed and to respray only the houses that were sprayed before. However, these considerations may not be acceptable in practice when prolonged residual activity is required for an acceptable degree of control.

In order to prolong the useful life of the insecticides currently available for public health use, methods need to be devised to minimize or counteract the selection pressure exerted on vector populations by insecticide applications. This would involve both close coordination in insecticide use by health and agricultural authorities and the introduction of a new practical rationale of pesticide application based on vector population genetics.

In view of the fact that contamination of mosquito breeding sites by extensive use of agricultural pesticides often leads to marked resistance of *Anopheles* vectors, the coordination of antimalaria activities with other schemes, based on the outdoor use of pesticides, is imperative.

The results of susceptibility tests alone may be misleading if the sample size is small; these tests should be supplemented by studies of vector density, survival rates from window traps and malaria prevalence. All these indices provide a more precise picture of the extent of the problem. Collaboration between entomologists and malariologists will make it possible to continue adequate monitoring and provide early warning of any deterioration of the situation.

Monitoring vector resistance is essential in assessing its operational importance. This monitoring can be limited to its simplest form, namely, continuation of entomological vigilance without any change of the diagnostic concentration of tests of resistance to determine the distribution and proportion of susceptible vectors. In its more complex form it may involve the longitudinal determination of the phenotypic composition of the vector population with a periodic assessment of cross-resistance characteristics and detailed epidemiological studies to correlate resistance levels with possible failures of control operations. However, the substitute compound may not remain useful for very long especially in areas where various insecticides are widely applied in agriculture. This has happened already in cotton growing areas of Central America and in other parts of the world.

Other solutions have been proposed, although not often used on a realistic scale. One of them is to use sequentially or in rotation two or three unrelated insecticides, thus maintaining an overall insecticide coverage of the whole operational area. The other is to use combinations of various compounds, on the assumption that the genes of resistance to each chemical compound exist in such low frequency that they are not likely to occur within a given population of the vector. These methods have a number of logistic or economic constraints in residual insecticidal programmes, but present some advantages in larvicidal control.

When the presence and degree of resistance of malaria vectors in the area have been confirmed, often the only solution is to change to a different insecticide, taking into account the operational and financial consequences of this decision. Should resistance to both groups of chlorinated hydrocarbons occur it may be necessary to change either to one of the organophosphate compounds or to a carbamate. Although there are some cases of cross-resistance between these two groups this is uncommon and usually one may employ one or the other of these compounds as an alternative solution, although operational and financial consequences may be serious. This is particularly important in areas of socio-economic importance, where residual house spraying needs to be maintained, using either DDT or a suitable alternative insecticide wherever DDT is no longer effective. Where insecticidal attack is not feasible, large stocks of antimalaria drugs should be made available for the protection of at least the most vulnerable group of the human population and for the prevention of morbidity and mortality in general. It is understood that any insecticidal attack should be considered as a temporary measure until more permanent environmental control measures become feasible.

Integrated vector control

The development of resistance to insecticides as well as the growing concern about environmental contamination, human safety and increased costs of alternative chemical compounds led to the present emphasis on the value of integrated vector control. This has been defined as the utilization of all appropriate technological and management techniques to bring about an effective degree of vector suppression, in a cost-effective manner. In fact, this is the nineteenth century concept, revived and improved through the use of appropriate new chemical and biological compounds. The essential requirement for integrated vector control is the ability to use one method that favours (or at least does not interfere) with another method. Thus, in several countries such as Italy, Hawaii and Japan larvicidal treatment of ponds with an insecticide is combined sequentially with various source reduction methods and the use of larvivorous fish. An adequate knowledge of the biology, ecology and behaviour characteristics of the vector, of some agricultural practices and of aquatic animal life is necessary to avoid costly mistakes; naturally, human safety must also be taken into account. The trend of integrated vector control is in the direction of community involvement through well planned sustained measures, related to socio-economic conditions. Generally speaking, personal protection, better sanitation, skilful agriculture and water management, source reduction, waste disposal and acceptable pesticides will remain the major components of integrated mosquito control schemes.

Safe use of insecticides

General principles

All pesticides are in some degree harmful to animals and to humans, but there is a major difference between the *toxicity* of a given compound and the *hazard* that it presents. Highly toxic compounds are excluded from use in vector control because of the difficulty of reducing human exposure to them. A measure of potential toxicity of a given pesticide to humans or other mammals is the oral or dermal LD_{50} value, i.e. the estimate of the amount of toxicant per kilogram body weight required to kill 50% of experimental animals (usually rats) used for testing (Table 10.2). According to this table parathion (an agricultural pesticide) is the most toxic and temephos the least toxic organophosphorus compound if taken by mouth. The apparently low toxicity of malathion may be misleading since some formulations may become toxic in tropical conditions. Such an unexpected change in an insecticide with a previous good safety record was seen in 1976 in Pakistan where about 2500 cases of illness occurred among spraymen, five of whom died. An investigation showed that the major toxic component was isomalathion formed in malathion-dispersible powder during prolonged storage in tropical conditions. This unfortunate episode, while revealing a new problem, indicated ways for improvement of pesticide formulations.

During the past few years there have been few changes in the use of pesticides for public health, except for the introduction of pyrethroids and insect growth regulators. A number of operational field trials provided information on the safety precautions concerning malathion, fenitrothion, chlorfoxim, pirimiphos–methyl, landrin, some pyrethroids and insect growth regulators. It appears that, although acute mammalian toxicity of permethrin and decamethrin is quite high, no serious problems have been encountered in the field.

The degree of hazard is estimated by the dangers involved when the insecticide is used under the particular conditions of usage. Thus the factors relevant to hazard depend not only on the intrinsic toxicity of the compound but also on the type of formulation used, concentration of the pesticide, method of use, accidental exposure of food and drink, poor storage conditions, bad labelling of containers or improper use of contaminated barrels and tins. Illiteracy and lack of training are also important factors. The type of exposure is also of importance: people are generally aware of the danger of the ingestion or inhalation of pesticides but many field workers are not aware that some compounds may be absorbed through the skin, particularly in hot climates.

Precautionary measures

The safe use of insecticides depends on the availability of up-to-date information on the compounds and formulations selected for use, on their storage conditions and on the way they are going to be used. Naturally, both the compounds and the formulations must conform to the WHO specifications. Detailed instructions on the safe application of any pesticide have been prepared by the WHO. Only the main points of these instructions can be given here.

In the first instance any vector control campaign must include provision for the safe transport and secure storage of pesticide concentrates. These should not be stored in rooms in which people live or in which food is kept. Protection against theft, misuse and accessibility to children must be provided. Safe disposal of empty insecticide containers must be taken care of. All pesticide containers should be adequately labelled in a form or language understood by the local operators. All equipment used for distribution of pesticides should conform to the WHO recommendations with regard to design and manufacture. There should be regular systematic inspection of all equipment to ensure that it is adequate.

With careful handling there is little real risk to the occupants of treated houses, but as a safety measure all foodstuffs should be removed or carefully covered before a house is sprayed. There is some risk to domestic animals, especially with dieldrin; casualties have occurred amongst cats which lick their contaminated fur, and chickens which have pecked along the floor near the sprayed walls.

Pre-packing of pesticides into small labelled plastic bags, containing enough material for a single tank charge, eliminates the need to measure the amount of the formulated compound in the field and this lowers the risk of contamination and ensures the correct application dose. This also reduces the spillage and wastage and minimizes the accidental poisoning of children.

Spraymen, mixers and baggers should report any symptoms of illness promptly to the supervisor. A medical examination is advisable, including the determination of blood cholinesterase, of those applying organophosphorus compounds, and regular medical surveillance of spray operators should be enforced. (These instructions, and also field kits for monitoring the degree of exposure to organophosphorus insecticides by measuring blood cholinesterase activity in the workers are available on demand from the World Health Organization, 1211, Geneva 27, Switzerland.)

Training in the safe use of pesticides should be provided for the supervisory medical and other personnel so that they are able to recognize the signs and symptoms of accidental poisoning and to give immediate treatment in an emergency. Equally important is the training of the foreman and other responsible field operators in the technique of proper spraying, safety precautions and maintenance of protective equipment.

Any extensive spraying should be carried out under adequate supervision. Spraymen should wash, using soap or detergent, at the end of each working day and whenever the insecticide is spilled in quantity on the skin or clothes. Spraymen should not smoke or eat while on duty, or after duty unless they first wash their hands. Insecticide should be scooped out with proper implements and not by hand.

Protective equipment

There are various items of protective equipment that should be used by field staff directly involved in insecticide spraying. The most important of these are the following:

Hats – these should be of impermeable material with a broad brim to protect face and neck.

Veils – a plastic mesh net loosely attached to the hat will give protection from large drops of spray and permit sufficient visibility.

Overalls – should be of light, durable cotton fabric; they should be washed regularly with soap or detergent.

Aprons – of rubber or plastic will protect from liquid concentrates.

Impervious gloves, capes, respirators and rubber boots are often advised but they are seldom acceptable in tropical countries (Fig. 10.27).

Greater risk occurs when handling oil solutions, such as concentrates or emulsions, which should be poured through threaded taps, or by pumps arranged to prevent contact of the solution with the skin.

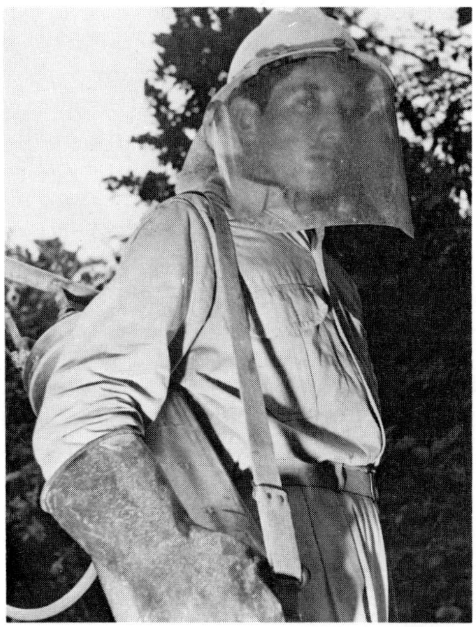

Fig. 10.27 Sprayman employed by the Malaria Eradication Programme in Mexico wearing full protective clothing. (WHO photograph by E. Schwab.)

Emergency treatment of poisoning by insecticides

As with all other types of poisoning the emergency treatment of accidental ingestion or other contact with a toxic compound comprises: (1) action to deal with life-threatening symptoms; (2) removal of the toxicant; and (3) administration of antidotes and alleviation of other symptoms.

Immediate action in case of life-threatening effects

When vomiting and difficulty of respiration occurs lie the patient flat on the stomach with the head to one side, the lower jaw extended and tongue pulled forward; clear the mouth and pharynx of vomit manually or by endotracheal intubation if necessary; give oxygen and apply artificial respiration if needed but do not attempt mouth-to-mouth respiration to avoid further accidental poisoning. If the poisoning occurred by ingestion then gastric lavage is needed except in the case of paraquat, Diquat and zinc phosphide. Some toxic material may be present on the skin and clothing, from which absorption may continue. Clothing should be removed and the skin washed with soap and water. Contamination of the eyes must be dealt with by washing them with water. If several people show symptoms of poisoning, without any evidence of previous exposure, then the most likely cause is contamination of food or water by the pesticide.

The symptoms of acute poisoning by *chlorinated hydrocarbons* such as DDT, HCH, dieldrin, include convulsions followed by an adverse effect on the liver tissue. Acute poisoning due to ingestion (except paraquat, Diquat and zinc phosphide) should be met, if the person is unconscious, by inducing vomiting by tickling the back of the throat with the tip of the finger. Consult doctor as soon as possible. Chronic poisoning due to the continued intake of smaller quantities is heralded by nervous symptoms which include hyperexcitability, anxiety and tremors. In addition, there is a very marked loss of appetite which quickly leads to loss of weight. Convulsions should be controlled by doses of injectable phenobarbitones, diazepam or paraldehyde. Blood samples for organochlorine levels may be necessary for confirmation of the cause of poisoning but this is a complex analytical procedure. Treatment must not be delayed pending the results of laboratory tests.

Any person who has suffered toxic effects due to handling chlorinated hydrocarbon insecticides should be removed from risk of contact with the insecticide.

Symptoms of poisoning by *organophosphate insecticides* are similar in many respects to those of chlorinated hydrocarbon poisoning, but also include giddiness, nausea, vomiting and diarrhoea; excessive sweating and salivation may be present. In severe cases cyanosis, respiratory difficulties, convulsions and loss of consciousness may follow. In such cases artificial respiration by mechanical means may be necessary before the administration of atropine sulfate intravenously or intramuscularly (if intravenous route not possible) at 0.4–2.0 mg for adults and 0.05 mg/kg body weight for children under 12 years. Repeat injections every 15–30 minutes until signs of atropinization occur (dry mouth, flushing, mydriasis, tachycardia). Do not limit dosage, signs of atropine toxicity need not be unduly alarming. A total of 25–50 mg or more may be necessary during the first day. Diazepam may be helpful in controlling intractable convulsions not controlled by antidotes. Atropine prophylaxis is not recommended. In addition, in severe poisoning one might administer 1–3 g of a soluble salt of pralidoxime by slow intravenous injection for adults or 50 mg/kg body weight for children. Morphine and tranquillizers *must not* be given to persons poisoned by anticholinesterase compounds. Organophosphorus insecticides inhibit cholinesterase (one of the vital body enzymes) and blood samples should be taken for cholinesterase determinations before and after the treatment of a case of poisoning. Supplies of atropine should be available in first-aid kits when organophosphorus or carbamate insecticides are being applied and the spraying supervisor should be trained to administer atropine in emergencies. Medical help should be sought immediately if poisoning is suspected. It is advised that people habitually handling these insecticides should have their blood cholinesterase levels checked periodically. Operators should be withdrawn from exposure if this level decreases by 25% or more from a well-established pre-exposure value.

The insecticidal *carbamates* give rise to a more rapidly reversible cholinesterase–inhibition complex. This makes it impossible to use estimates of cholinesterase activity as an accurate index of the levels of this enzyme in the tissues. In cases of poisoning by carbamates all the methods used for treating poisoning by organic phosphorus compounds are useful, with one exception: pralidoxime and other oximes are not recommended for routine use. Recovery from carbamate poisoning is usually quite rapid.

Generally, insecticides that are more toxic than DDT undergo faster degradation in the environment and are more acceptable to the ecologist. However, the hazard that they present to the operators is very much higher. Prevention and treatment of accidental poisoning should be given high priority in all spraying programmes.

Pesticides and the environment

The application of residual insecticides and especially of DDT has been the main factor responsible for eradication of malaria from large parts of the world and remains an important method for control of this disease in the tropics. However, anxiety about the pollution of the environment by pesticides has increased during the past few years to such an extent that all the virtues of these compounds tend to be forgotten, while their disadvantages receive much sensational publicity.

It has been estimated that during the period 1978 to 1982 the annual amount of DDT used for public health programmes all over the world was of the order of 30 000 tonnes, without any major adverse effect on the human population living in areas where this compound was employed. Studies carried out under the auspices of the WHO have shown that even high degrees of continued exposure to DDT of workers in industries that produce it, have not led to any health problems when proper precautions are observed. The continued availability of DDT and other insecticides is imperative, until better methods of vector control are devised. There is no doubt that indiscriminate use of organochlorines and organophosphates affects various species of wild fauna, especially birds. However, one should stress that the commonest method of malaria control by residual spraying of houses has practically no effect on the environment, since the insecticidal compounds are confined within the house.

DDT and other more toxic pesticides (like parathion) have been used in very large amounts, mainly for protection of agricultural crops; it is the aerial spraying of fields that has been responsible for contamination of mosquito breeding sites by run-off. This led to the phenomenon of multiresistance to a number of organochlorine and organophosphate compounds. The most complete study, carried out under the joint sponsorship of the United Nations Environment Programme and the World Health Organization, reported that the only demonstrated effects of DDT on the general population are the storage of this compound in the tissues and its excretion in urine and milk. No confirmed ill-effects of DDT have been reported in babies, even in the communities with the highest concentrations of the compound in human milk. There is no evidence that DDT is carcinogenic in humans; nor is there any indication that DDT affects human reproduction. DDT appears to have some depressant effect on the immune system, but the evidence of this is not conclusive.

Calls for limitation of pesticides used in agriculture have not been very successful in many tropical countries, where food and cash crops are of great economic importance. Information on the adverse impact of such agricultural practices is often difficult to collect and to interpret. This was demonstrated in a much publicized controversy, in which the introduction into India of high yield rice (which needs more irrigation and protection from pests) was alleged to be responsible for the spread of insecticide resistance and increase of malaria. A further complication arises from the widespread anxiety about harmful effects of chemical compounds and very expensive screening of potentially valuable new candidate insecticides, so that many manufacturers are unwilling to invest in costly research and development.

Thus, in the final account, it seems that for the immediate future insecticides will continue to play a major role in agriculture and in the control of vector-borne diseases of humans and animals. Environmental contamination, accidental toxicity to humans, resistance and rising costs of pesticides are all serious problems. But a solution may be found in devising, and applying for each area concerned, appropriate methods of integrated control which will not preclude the use of chemical compounds, if they are effective and safe, and applied at the right place and at the right time. All other methods, such as source reduction, water management, biological control, treatment and prevention of infection, will have to be used increasingly by well informed and well trained health service personnel. Although integrated control of malaria is still more of a concept than a practical reality, this is the present major trend.

Planning malaria control

Malaria control methods vary from the simplest to the most elaborate, but the success of the former and the failure of the latter are equally likely if they are applied with what Paul Russell, the great American malariologist called 'prejudice of experience' due to the blind belief in cherished fetishes.

This view expressed nearly 40 years ago is of even greater significance today, when as a result of disappointments with some overambitious goals of malaria eradication the need for a less rigid approach to malaria control has become urgent.

The revised strategy of malaria eradication and control approved by the WHO in 1979 stressed the need for flexibility of antimalaria programmes, namely, the adaptation of any and all available methods to realistic aims, set by national health authorities and feasible within the limitations of their human and material resources. Thus, a malaria control programme has been redefined as an organized effort to institute, carry out and evaluate activities that are appropriate in prevailing epidemiological and socio-economic conditions and are likely to achieve the greatest possible improvement of the health situation in the country concerned (WHO, 1979).

A realistic formulation of the control programme requires an answer to the question whether the expenditure on it will be covered wholly from the central government budget, or if some proportion of it will come from other sources. It is also important to know the degree of commitment of the authorities to any long-term programme. Evidently, the cost of malaria control within an area will vary inversely to the density of its population. Preference should be given to permanent measures of control rather than to those of a temporary character, unless the environmental conditions favour the latter methods. Permanent measures often require high capital expenditure but the cost of their maintenance is low; moreover, their results may be of considerable indirect benefits if the land becomes suitable for agriculture or housing. Evidently, the objectives of any malaria control programme depend on the prevailing epidemiology of malaria, on the effectiveness of available methods and on the national commitments, as well as on the financial possibilities of the relevant health authorities, and on the degree of support of the community.

Article VIII of the World Declaration on the Control of Malaria (WHO, 1992) made at the WHO Ministerial Conference on Malaria held in Amsterdam on 26 and 27 October 1992 states: 'We commit ourselves and our countries to control malaria and will plan for malaria control as an essential component of health development and will incorporate health development as an essential component of national development'. This collective statement of political will may well prove to be a historic landmark in our quest to conquer this disease. Planning for malaria control is clearly an intersectoral matter, which should be carried out carefully by an intersectoral team of responsible persons. It is a dynamic process and follows a cycle of planning, implementation, evaluation and replanning.

Today countries are faced with the difficult task of controlling malaria as a disease problem (not as a parasitic infection) in the face of parasite resistance to antimalaria drugs and vector resistance to insecticides.

Control programmes need to be developed which:

- have no time limit;
- use available national resources or resources that can be mobilized;
- are designed to ensure that the gains can be sustained;
- take into account the local epidemiological conditions.

Malaria is naturally an acute disease, not chronic; however it may be a chronic parasitic infection. Its clinical manifestations may be modified by the inappropriate use of antimalaria drugs and by parasite resistance to them. Malaria disease control therefore means undoubtedly a continuing presence of infection in the community, maintained by mosquito transmission. Malaria transmission control implies keeping malaria transmission to a minimum by the effective use of the available resources and technology. It does not necessarily mean complete interruption of transmission as in an eradication campaign.

Malaria control requires careful, pragmatic planning and replanning and necessitates frequent evaluation. Malaria control is inherently difficult in the sense that there are no general prescriptions that can be equally effective everywhere. Approaches have to be constantly modified to take account of local variability. This demands a greater epidemiological capability at the periphery than is necessary for the control of most other diseases and certainly more than was necessary for the malaria eradication campaign of the 1950s and 1960s.

In an attempt to facilitate malaria control a sequence of objectives and relevant action were classified into four 'tactical variants' (WHO, 1979). These were Tactical Variant No. 1: reduction and prevention of mortality due to malaria; No. 2: reduction and prevention of morbidity and mortality; No. 3: decrease in the prevalence of malaria; and No. 4: countrywide malaria control with the ultimate objective of eradication. The intention was that any one of these or their combination may be used within the same country or area. However, it was stressed that no single approach should exclude elements drawn from other approaches, since these four tactical variants should not be considered as the only possibilities. This was however a first attempt to standardize and simplify the approach to malaria control.

The experience of countries in applying the four tactical variants was reviewed in 1985 and revealed a number of problems. The tendency was to view the variants as mutually exclusive compartments to be selected and implemented according to the resources available instead of planning antimalaria action based upon epidemiological stratification. Thus the variants, while serving to highlight the need to view malaria more as a disease problem than as a parasitic infection, had not inspired countries to develop flexible approaches suitable to their individual needs through a process of planning (WHO, 1986).

Antimalaria objectives need to be developed as part of the planning process relevant to each identified epidemiological stratum. However, it is possible to recognize that methods of attacking the problem can be graded according to their complexity and that these methods require a range of different resources and development activities to ensure the long-term maintenance of any results obtained. One possibility is to begin malaria control with a sophisticated attack on malaria transmission, as attempted by eradication programmes, but this proved to be successful and sustainable in only a few areas. Thus a hierarchy of objectives and activities can be envisaged as a broad spectrum of possibilities. This implies that a more complex plan of malaria control should not be adopted unless there is assurance that earlier objectives would be reached. Two substantially different approaches, aimed at attaining the objectives at the two extreme ends of the spectrum, can be identified:

> Improvement in the general health services to ensure adequate diagnosis, accessibility to health care, treatment for malaria cases, provision of adequate protection for the population at risk and the promotion of personal and community protection. This incorporates the tactical variants 1 and 2 and is aimed at obtaining objectives such as the reduction of morbidity and mortality and of the duration of sickness.
>
> Establishment of the capability for the long-term control of malaria transmission. This will require the planning of specific antimalaria actions designed to change the epidemiological equilibrium. This includes the objectives of preventing epidemics, reducing the foci of *P. falciparum* malaria and transmission control in selected areas or in the entire country. This incorporates tactical variants 3 and 4.

At one end of the spectrum, as an absolute minimum, all countries would need to provide diagnosis and appropriate treatment for the sick, curative treatment and prophylaxis throughout pregnancy, and improved education to the population concerning the better use of health services, the non-tolerance of illness and the use of personal protective measures. At the other end of the spectrum planned interference in malaria transmission on a large scale should only be considered if this will effectively change the epidemiological equilibrium and if this change can be sustained.

Intermediate approaches between these two extremes would be the progressive strengthening of the referral system and the development of a meaningful information system, as well as epidemiological surveillance with appropriate recognition of abnormal situations, delimitation of problem areas and the provision of an adequate response capability. This will progress from the control of epidemics to their prevention, and to the control of the most serious foci. It will include monitoring problems such as drug resistance and the evaluation of the response to control measures.

The art of planning is to identify which approaches should be implemented, where and when, to achieve and sustain desired objectives within the resources available, or that can be made available, based upon a sound scientific knowledge of the local epidemiological, sociological and environmental circumstances.

The planning process

Planning involves identifying and analysing problems, examining solutions, setting priorities, making choices and decisions, setting objectives, developing approaches to achieve these objectives, allocating resources and organizing them into programmes for effective and efficient delivery and measuring progress towards those objectives. In an environment of scarcity, such as is found in many developing countries, planning takes on all the more importance in order to get as much accomplished with what little there is in the way of staff, supplies, equipment, drugs, transport, funds and so on.

Planning is a systematic and continuous process for allocating resources to achieve objectives. It is a way to define why, how, when, where and by whom these objectives can be achieved. In health planning we are concerned with extending coverage and improving the effectiveness and efficacy of health care services. An integral part of this approach is intersectoral collaboration for programmes that will impact the total health environment of which malaria control is one component.

The aim of disease control is to reduce the impact of the disease on the health of the population to the lowest possible level that can be achieved within the available financial and manpower resources, in the context of other health priorities and according to existing technology and feasibility.

The intensity of the required disease control effort will depend upon the magnitude of the disease problem and the objectives being pursued and may vary from one situation to another. The required action will take the form of a coordinated set of activities with targets and dates for their achievement designed to achieve well defined objectives. These objectives should be regarded as intermediate steps towards the achievement of the ultimate goal. The objectives and the approaches decided upon will determine the form and the content of the national antimalaria action, which implies the expenditure of valuable resources.

It is difficult to establish meaningful objectives because of the complexity and uncertainty surrounding many of the factors that must be taken into account.

Defining the objectives, formulating approaches and setting operational targets are closely interrelated and are best considered in a practical sequence. Setting the goal, priorities, and deciding upon and supporting control approaches is primarily a political decision (political will). The planning process enables a logical approach to be taken to determine the appropriate combination of measures to use for control purposes, and where and when to use them, based upon an assessment of the local situation and the technical, operational and economic feasibility. It is suggested that the planning process should consist of an analysis of the malaria situation, stratification of the problem, formulation of objectives and approaches to achieve these objectives, the selection and definition of evaluation methods, establishment of the operational outputs and targets, programme budgeting, and finally preparation of an implementation plan.

The planning environment

There are certain characteristics of the planning environment in developing countries which should be recognized and taken into consideration. Health planners must work in an environment of scarcity, or at best inadequacy. Resources of all kinds may be in short supply: staff, staff accommodation, materials and supplies, facilities and equipment, drugs and vaccines, petrol, transport and communications, etc.

Another aspect of the planning/management environment is the problem of organizing and managing health data. There is no lack of data, but rather the problem is in its collection and organization into a usable form. Also much data is collected which is not used at all. Some of it could be eliminated; and other data should be used closer to the source of collection for monitoring, evaluation and control at lower levels in the health system (e.g. at health centres, medical field units, mobile clinics, etc.).

This calls for intuition and creativity in approaching problems. The health planner manager must use judgement and educated guesses of their experience and understanding of conditions that can contribute to the decision making process. Furthermore, simple techniques should be used for sample surveys and field observation to set baseline data; and easily measured indicators should be applied to monitor, evaluate and control health programmes.

The health planner should be a good observer; they should know what to look for and how to evaluate information reaching their senses as they conduct field inspections, visit clinics and walk through the market place and villages.

Analysis of the malaria situation

Analysis of the malaria situation is the essential basis for planning antimalaria action based upon the epidemiological characteristics. A complete analysis would include a description of the distribution of malaria (infection) and its consequences (morbidity, mortality, economic losses) and an explanation of that distribution in terms of its causal factors (geophysical, environmental, biological, social, political and economic). It is clear that a really complete analysis is practically impossible and malaria control therefore will often have to be planned using imperfect knowledge. However, an important component of any plan should be to collect the additional, valid information necessary for replanning purposes, thereby improving the programme as it progresses.

The analysis of the malaria situation has six major components:

1. The current malaria problem can be analysed by considering the impact of malaria on the health of the community, the economic and social effect of malaria, the economic and social effect on malaria, the infection in man and clinical manifestations, parasitological factors, the vector mosquito and other aspects of the environment.
2. The current malaria control activities and their effects on the malaria problem. This would include a critical review of individual current control activities, overall evaluation of the malaria control activities and current field research.
3. The health services resources that are available and that could be used for malaria control.
4. Community involvement, which would include community structures and groups, the extent to which the community is involved in health matters and the potential for community involvement in antimalaria activities.
5. Intersectoral cooperation. The sectors will need to be identified which are associated with malaria transmission and/or its control. The analysis would also include the extent of intersectoral cooperation to date for malaria control and the mechanisms available at different levels.
6. The history of the problem, which would include past infection and especially history of epidemics, major changes occurring over time in the epidemiology of the disease and identification of socio-economic changes over time, and the resulting amount of malaria.

Based upon the analysis of the malaria situation certain key decisions need to be made. These include the relative importance of malaria in the politico-socio-economic context warranting action; opportunistic resources for antimalaria action; the magnitude of the planning process necessary for malaria control (which parts of the country are more involved than others, what other agencies/organizations should be involved, how can resources be mobilized); the budgetary resources and limitations; and the extent of investment in infrastructure development.

Stratification of the malaria problem

Very often, the same degree of reduction cannot be achieved simultaneously all over the national territory due to administrative, operational, financial and technical constraints. Hence the necessity to proceed to a stratification of the country, with the definition of different objectives and consequently the selection of appropriate control measures in the different strata which have been defined.

Stratification is a process intended to reduce and simplify a complex problem, to facilitate its understanding and to formulate solutions. Many factors contribute to the epidemiology of malaria, such as the distribution and relative prevalence of different *Plasmodium* species and their response to drugs, the distribution of vector species and their susceptibility to insecticides, the intensity of transmission etc. In addition, the ecological and geographical characteristics of different areas, socio-economic conditions of the populations, climatic and meteorological factors, which are not usually uniformly similar throughout a national territory, also play a major role.

In order to simplify this heterogeneity it may be possible to identify common factors and to use this knowledge to delimit new areas, populations or situations which exhibit a relative similarity through specific characteristics which distinguish them from other areas dissimilar by the same characteristics.

An epidemiological stratification is essential and it should be considered as the preliminary step prior to arriving at an operational stratification of the country. Once the degree and distribution of the malaria problem have been assessed, and the interplaying climatic, geographical, logistical and socio-economic factors involved in the epidemiology of the disease have been analysed, then homogeneous zones with similar epidemiological, socio-economic and ecological characteristics can be delineated. For each defined stratum, specific objectives and targets can then be formulated and the intervention methods selected for the objectives to be met.

Strategy for malaria control

A strategy for malaria control has recently been formulated by the WHO to address the serious worldwide malaria situation. It was presented to the Ministerial Conference on Malaria in Amsterdam in 1992. It is generally accepted that, *with few exceptions*, malaria eradication is not a realistic goal where it has not already been achieved. Reduction of malaria morbidity and mortality with their consequences on human performance and socio-economic development is a more modest and realistic goal. This will require an improvement in the capacity of existing health services to provide diagnosis and early treatment within the umbrella of primary health care, a reorientation of existing malaria control programmes to take into consideration epidemiological, ecological, environmental and social factors; as well as the primary goal of the new strategy.

The variability of malaria has already been pointed out and hence no uniform strategy applicable to all areas can be formulated. Nonetheless, four fundamental elements can be identified.

1. Early diagnosis and treatment.
2. Selective application of vector control including human–mosquito barriers.
3. Development of epidemiological information systems.
4. Early detection or forecasting of epidemics and rapid application of control measures.

Early diagnosis and treatment

Malaria is a curable disease and timely diagnosis and treatment is a basic human right of all populations in endemic areas whatever their social or economic circumstances.

Since complications of *P. falciparum*, in children in particular, develop rapidly, children should ideally receive treatment within 24 hours after the onset of symptoms; in adults the antecedent history before severe manifestations occur is usually longer (4–5 days).

In many of the highly endemic countries, the diagnosis of malaria is made on clinical grounds, since microscopy is unavailable at the peripheral health posts; moreover, in these areas a positive blood film does not necessarily mean a definitive diagnosis, although the density of infection can be a valuable index. Clinical diagnostic criteria should be defined according to the local epidemiology, bearing in mind in particular the transmission season, and the age and sex of the patient. Thus, any febrile illness in a child or other risk group, for example, primigravidae women, should be regarded as malaria, while in partially immune adults, only fevers without symptoms suggesting another disease should be considered as malaria. This approach will reduce the wastage which is inevitable in these circumstances.

The choice of drugs will depend on a variety of factors, such as pattern of resistance, cost, side effects and compliance. At the first referral level, health personnel should be trained to have enough clinical competence to diagnose and treat malaria and to recognize severe anaemia especially in children. An unusually large number of children with anaemia may indicate that RII resistance to chloroquine is occurring and an alternative drug, for example, sulfadoxine–pyrimethamine may be indicated. National guidelines will determine which antimalarial drugs should be used as first and second line treatments, the quantities required and their distribution. Patients with severe disease could be given parenteral treatment or a suppository preparation (if available) and referred to the next level of health care with greater facilities for diagnosis, monitoring and treating the patient.

Self-medication is increasingly common, almost universal, yet knowledge among those who provide or sell antimalarial drugs is abysmally low resulting in inappropriate or incomplete treatment. Persons like shopkeepers, teachers, priests, traditional birth attendants, traditional healers and mothers could be taught the importance of early treatment and the proper use of antimalarial drugs in different age groups at different times of the transmission season; using up-to-date and culturally acceptable means of communication.

Evidence from several countries indicates that self-medication accounts for as much as half of all consumption of antimalarial drugs in rural areas.

Except under special circumstances such as epidemics, non-immune migrant labourers, soldiers and others living temporarily in endemic areas; special risk groups, such as pregnant women (especially primiparae); children with homozygous haemoglobinopathies; and immunosuppressed persons, mass prophylaxis is no longer recommended.

Although early diagnosis and drug treatment is the first element of the new strategy, it must be realized that neither the distribution nor the use of antimalarial drugs have hitherto followed a clear and tidy pattern, as is often assumed. An objective review of the situation is given by Foster (see Selected References).

Selective application of vector control including human–mosquito barriers

The aim is the progressive reduction of malaria transmission where this is sustainable and cost effective. Decisions on whether to apply vector control and which methods to choose must depend on an assessment of the relevant epidemiological, ecological, social and operational determinants including the local identification of epidemiological types. The various methods available have been described earlier and are aimed at (a) a reduction of mosquito breeding, (b) a reduction in the longevity and/or density of adult mosquitoes, and (c) reduction in human–mosquito contact.

Residual spraying is now recommended for special situations, for example, epidemic control or protecting particularly vulnerable populations. Impregnated mosquito nets or curtains are justifiably receiving considerable attention. However, their value in areas of intense perennial transmission remains to be proven.

Development of epidemiological information systems

The collection and handling of malaria data should be part of the general health service information system and is an essential prerequisite for the early detection and forecasting of epidemics. They are a means of monitoring the potential rapid changes in malaria transmission and disease. As much as possible, data should be analysed and appraised as peripherally as possible – at regional or event district level.

Early detection or forecasting of epidemics

The aim here is the forecasting or early detection of epidemics in order to ensure rapid and effective control. Monitoring meteorological data and population movements might be useful since unusually heavy rains and/or increased temperatures are possible causes of malaria epidemics as are man-made ecological changes often associated with the influx of many non-immune persons. A relatively high rate of slide positivity among fever patients, or an increased demand for antimalaria drugs, could suggest an outbreak of malaria, while follow-up of therapeutic results could indicate that an alternative second line medication may be required. Remote sensing may prove useful in the future for the early detection of epidemic malaria. Once an epidemic occurs the rapid use of appropriate drugs, mass drug administration and residual spraying are appropriate measures.

Prevention and control of outbreaks of introduced malaria

Factors related to the origin of epidemics of malaria were discussed before (see Chapter 8). There is no doubt that the most important practical method for monitoring the malaria situation is a continued and regular surveillance of fever cases by examination of blood films from all or a reasonable proportion of such patients. An additional approach for determining the warning threshold of a possible malaria epidemic is the knowledge of the malariogenic potential, which is the product of receptivity and vulnerability of the area concerned. From the purely practical point of view one may distinguish two different circumstances of an epidemic outbreak: (1) in a non-endemic area, and (2) in an endemic area. In both situations one may take into account the ratio between indigenous and immigrant populations. Where the area is non-endemic, an outbreak would develop only when a large parasite reservoir has been imported. On the other hand, when there is an influx of a large number of non-immune people into an endemic area, an outbreak of malaria may occur rapidly, unless the new population is protected. Naturally, all the factors of the environment, as well as those related to the vector and the species of the parasite will have to be considered. As mentioned before, *P. vivax* malaria is much faster in multiplying than *P. falciparum* and an outbreak due to the latter species reaches its epidemic peak when some 50% of the population are infected. There is in both cases a stage of slow growth before a sudden rise. When secondary, locally transmitted cases occur, the emergency insecticidal and chemotherapeutic measures cannot act as rapidly as they would if earlier action had been taken.

Two needs arise when dealing with a malaria epidemic: one is to recognize it at its earliest stage; and the other is to stop it by all the methods available. In planning control measures against a potential malaria epidemic two degrees of prevention have been advocated; (1) first-degree prevention, in which measures are taken against the importation of vectors or suspected sources of infection, and (2) second-degree prevention, in which measures are taken against the re-establishment of transmission.

If the infected vectors arrive from outside the area there are no fully reliable defences, although protection of the border zone by residual spraying may be of some value. Protection against the influx of infected persons comes under the vigilance mechanism, which should detect all cases of imported malaria and provide some information on the possibility of the introduction of drug-resistant strains of *Plasmodia*. The activities required for second-degree prevention comprise the following: study of patterns of population movements, provision of diagnostic facilities, maintenance of case detection posts, epidemiological investigation of active foci of malaria, radical cure of patients with malaria, and re-introduction of residual spraying in the area involved. However, any such measures must be preceded by the wide use of antimalarial drugs, and especially those that can combine treatment of acute malaria with good preventive properties. For most circumstances 4-aminoquinolines are still the most appropriate, except when highly resistant strains of *Plasmodia* have been identified. In such cases other appropriate drugs will have to be used, together with the wide use of primaquine for a radical cure of relapsing cases.

All necessary imagicidal measures of vector control should be instituted, including space spraying and aerial spraying if feasible. However, these measures have no immediate impact and additional action is necessary.

A force of auxiliary health workers should be maintained to search for malaria cases and apply the required remedial measures. It is important to follow up the foci from which malaria has been eliminated. It is doubtful whether any basic health service, unless it is of exceptional competence, can take appropriate and rapid action in cases of extensive or even localized epidemics, but the local health units are of great help in detecting and reporting the incidence of malaria and administering the necessary drugs. It is only during a malaria epidemic that the value of a centrally directed service, specializing in the control of malaria and other vector-borne diseases, is fully appreciated. The tendency to integrate prematurely the malaria control units into the general health services, in countries where the menace of epidemics exists, may have serious adverse effects.

Malaria control in development projects

Development projects and industrial undertakings in the tropics are often a rife ground for outbreaks of malaria due to the fact that many among a large labour force, including newcomers to the area, are either non-immune to the local strains of *Plasmodia* or introduce strains to which the local population is particularly susceptible. Moreover, the living conditions of the labour force may often be less than adequate and the construction activity contributes to environmental pollution. For detailed guidance on malaria control related to immigration into development areas see *WHO Manual on Personal and Community Protection* (1974).

A point made in Chapter 8 concerning 'man-made malaria' deserves some amplification. It refers to the creation of breeding places of malaria vectors and other mosquitos as a result of human activities. The list of such potential breeding places, which are usually close to human habitations, is very long. It comprises barrels, badly designed or blocked soakaway pits, garden pools, cisterns, disused wells, borrow-pits left by building projects, obstructed drains, etc. Much malaria has been due to bad handling of water in irrigation channels, poorly sited ditches, culverts, leaking sluice gates, seepages and fallow rice-fields. No major operations involving water supply should be undertaken without considering their possible impact on malaria and other water-related diseases and requesting appropriate advice on the malaria situation of the area involved and on methods of prevention and control of the disease.

Three principles should be adhered to in all engineering projects in the tropics: the *first* is not to make additional breeding places of mosquitos, the *second* is to know how to correct the errors once made and the *third* is to involve the health authorities from the very beginning of the project.

The duty of the resident medical adviser is to foresee the potential dangers, to protect the health of the working force as well as their families and to be ready to act in an emergency.

Selection of a suitable site for new housing, temporary or permanent, may avoid much subsequent difficulty. The principles of this have been described in the earlier section. Such site selection may be vital to the success of many projects, though better methods of control, if available, should be fully used.

Existing breeding places may be dealt with by the use of larvicides, drainage, or modification of the water to make it unsuitable as a breeding place. It must be carried out within the radius of flight of the local vector, commonly a mile (1.6 km) but more in some places, and throughout the entire transmission season. It must be based on a knowledge of the local vector and particularly of its breeding habits, and on a detailed survey of the area showing all water sites of the potentially dangerous type within the radius prescribed.

The prevention of malaria among the non-immune labour force entails the provision of personal protection measures and regular chemoprophylaxis with an appropriate antimalarial drug.

If malaria is already prevalent on any scale among the labour force the right policy is to eliminate the infection and thus reduce its transmission.

The most practical way of doing this is to muster the work force and each adult be given and seen to swallow four tablets of chloroquine (600 mg base) on each of 2 days and two tablets (300 mg base) on day 3. In areas with high chloroquine resistance other curative regimens will have to be considered (see Chapter 9).

This initial curative treatment should be followed by appropriate and regular chemoprophylaxis. 'Breakthroughs' should be promptly treated.

Space spraying of insecticides is of limited practical value and the expense of this method is considerable. However, at times noisy and clearly visible applications of thermal or other aerosols has some value, in addition to having a psychological effect which may inspire confidence in the health authorities and increase the cooperation of the population and of administrative echelons.

The regular use of commercial low pressure aerosol containers for disinsectization of premises of the technical and managerial staff (usually at their own expense) should be encouraged.

For more permanent malaria control, residual insecticides should be used. This does not make great demands on personnel; several small schemes could be amalgamated into one. The most economical working unit is a population of between 10 000 and 20 000. Where amalgamation into units of such size is possible, one skilled assistant can be employed full time on organization and management. In smaller schemes supervision must be part time, but should not be, for that reason, of minor importance. For the initial rounds of spraying the choice will in most cases be DDT at a dose of 2 g/ m^2. This application should be repeated every 6 months or more often in case of interference with the insecticide deposit on the walls.

Workers should be carefully trained in the use of sprayers and in the regular and even application of given quantities of fluid, using water only for this training. An even dosage of the spray can be attained by practice, provided that the supervisor has personally taken the trouble to become competent at it. All houses and animal sheds in the area should be sprayed unless reliable experience shows that discrimination between different dwellings is possible.

After establishing full control by such means, a revision programme can be considered. The chief intention will be to prolong the interval between insecticide applications, but before this is contemplated the frequency with which walls are replastered should be carefully examined. If they are often whitewashed or replastered, frequent re-sprayings are essential. In this case the insecticide of choice is DDT at a standard dose or half of it, according to local conditions, to be applied at intervals never exceeding 3–4 months during the malaria transmission season.

After the initial treatment has been operative, transmission of malaria within the treated area should decrease. The size of the treated area and the extent to which people move out of it at night will clearly affect the resulting incidence of malaria, but in a labour group of 10 000 or more people, the amount of malaria should be reduced to negligible proportions.

Managerial and senior staff should also be protected by residual insecticide spraying. As they normally occupy houses in which the discoloration caused by wettable powders would be objectionable, solutions or emulsions of insecticides should be used. Such houses may well be screened or provided with some screened rooms, and for this purpose it is best to use plastic screen cloth. The use of mosquito nets, preferably impregnated, for labour forces and staff, even in screened houses, should be encouraged and the importance of regular drug prophylaxis emphasized.

Summary of main control measures for the major malaria prototypes

1. *African savannah malaria*
   a. Provision of early diagnosis and treatment
   b. Impregnated mosquito nets or curtains may be useful
2. *Desert highland fringe malaria*
   a. Provision of early diagnosis and treatment
   b. Monitoring climatic and ecological changes
   c. Early detection and control of epidemics
3. *Malaria in plains and valleys outside Africa*
   a. Provision of early diagnosis and treatment
   b. Sustainable vector control methods
   c. Early response to situations of increased risk
4. *Forest related malaria*
   a. Provision of early diagnosis and treatment
   b. Personal protection measures (repellents/impregnated mosquito nets)
   c. Chemoprophylaxis
5. *Agricultural development malaria*
   a. Provision of early diagnosis and treatment
   b. Personal protection measures (as above)
6. *Urban malaria*
   a. Provision of early diagnosis and treatment
   b. Environmental sanitation
   c. Personal protection measures (as above)
7. *Coastal and marshland malaria*
   a. Provision of early diagnosis and treatment
   b. Engineering methods
   c. Personal protection measures (as above)
8. *War and sociopolitical malaria*
   a. Provision of early diagnosis and treatment
   b. Temporary chemoprophylaxis
   c. Spraying of shelters
   d. Personal protection measures (as above)

A classification of malaria control measures is given in Table 10.7 and a summary of main control measures for the major malaria prototypes are given in Appendix IV.

Table 10.7 Classification of malaria control measures

Type of measures	Individual and family protection	Community protection
Prevention of human–vector contact	Repellents, protective clothing, impregnated mosquito nets, screening of houses	Site selection, screening of houses
Destruction of adult *Anopheles* vectors	Use of domestic space sprays including aerosols	Space spraying, ultra low volume sprays, residual insecticide spraying
Destruction of mosquito larvae	Peridomestic sanitation, intermittent drying of water containers	Larviciding of water surfaces, intermittent drying, sluicing, biological methods
Source reduction of mosquitos	Filling, small-scale drainage and other forms of water management	Prevention of man-made malaria, environmental sanitation, water management, drainage schemes, naturalistic methods of control
Measures against the malaria parasites	Diagnosis and early treatment, chemoprophylaxis	Diagnosis and early treatment, chemoprophylaxis to primigravidae, mass drug administration (in epidemics)
Social participation	Motivation for personal and family protection	Community involvement, health education, expansion of rural health services. Training of staff

Cost of malaria control

The cost of malaria control varies considerably in relation to a number of factors such as the type of insecticide, the method involved, the degree of surveillance, the cost of labour, transport, administration etc. Thus, it is difficult if not impossible to give any idea of an average cost of a programme, unless full information on it is available. Nevertheless, it should be possible to plan malaria control measures, that are within the budgetary limitations of the programme and could be extended as economic development proceeds. Effective malaria control depends on the regular application of appropriate procedures. This can be assured only if a regular budget is provided and maintained over the whole duration of the programme, which should also be so planned that its eventual extension may be beneficial for the future development of the country.

The estimated cost, in 1991, of malaria control in an endemic area inhabited by a population of 1 million based on one round of spraying or single-dose treatment is shown in Table 10.8.

Generally speaking, the average expenditure in extensive programmes involving the protection of a million people is not comparable with the estimation of costs of antimalaria activities aimed at protection of a few thousand people over a limited period (e.g. construction phase of a development project). In the latter case the overall costs may be lower if the degree of performance is adjusted to the temporary needs of the project over a relatively short time. However, such savings may be illusory if the degree of exposure to malaria is considerable. Normally, any measures of malaria control can be easily incorporated into the general medical and community health budgeting of an important development project. The application of vector control methods based on motorized equipment or various technically advanced machinery may be less expensive where local salaries are high. However, it is always preferable to involve the local population as much as possible in participating in all environmental methods of malaria control and to extend the benefits of it to the peripheral localities and villages.

Personal protection measures and provision of mosquito-proof houses is important. Communal places such as cafeterias should also be protected by screened windows and doors. It goes without saying that the proper organization of antimalaria

Table 10.8 Estimated costs, in 1991, of malaria control in an endemic area inhabited by a population of 1 million, based on one round of spraying or single dose treatment (WHO Supply Service, Geneva: prices at May 1991)

Type of spraying	Requirements for one round or single dose	Price per unit	Total cost of insecticide or drug	Cost of insecticide or drug per person
Residual spraying with DDT 75% water-dispersible powder	147 tonnes	US$3150 per tonne	US$463 000	US$0.46
Residual spraying with malathion 50% water-dispersible powder	220 tonnes	US$4160 per tonne	US$915 000	US$0.9
Single dose treatment using chloroquine (10 mg base/kg)	4.5 million tablets at 100 mg base	US$6.05 per 1000 tablets	US$27 225	US$0.03

Note: The annual number of spraying rounds depends on the endemicity of malaria and on the degree of control to be achieved. In order to obtain a good control in holoendemic areas, two rounds of DDT or 3–4 rounds of malathion would be required. The above figures do not include the cost of application of vector control measures or the distribution of drugs, that is to say that costs of transport, storage and cost of salaries and travel of personnel have not been considered.

activities for a development project demands the availability of competent technical supervisory and executive personnel. Unreasonable budgetary restrictions on trained and experienced staff are a false economy as they jeopardize the very aim of some development projects.

Cost-effectiveness and choice of interventions

A critical review of the economics of malaria control was recently published by Anne Mills (see Selected References).

Clearly, the nature of the different epidemiological prototypes will have an impact on the choice and cost of intervention. Since chemotherapy is common to all the situations, it must be borne in mind that the cost of this intervention should take into account both the costs of the treatment itself as well as the costs of getting the patient to seek treatment which will vary from area to area. At 1987 prices the costs for one adult course of drug treatment were as follows: chloroquine $0.23; sulfadoxine–pyrimethamine $0.50; mefloquine $1.20; quinine and tetracycline $3.00. The cost of impregnated mosquito nets will be different if locally manufactured or subsidized.

In evaluating the economics of malaria control Mills concentrates on the following five areas of concern: (1) the determinants of malaria transmission; (2) the resource costs of malaria; (3) the demand for malaria treatment and prevention; (4) the characteristics of the supply of malaria control; and (5) economic evaluation which includes cost analysis, cost-effectiveness analysis, cost–utility analysis and cost–benefit analysis.

Our knowledge on whether and how individuals adapt their behaviour to influence their malaria risks is rudimentary.

The resource costs are two-fold – the costs of prevention and treatment, and the indirect costs expressed in terms of production. The latter have often been exaggerated and have not taken into consideration factors such as parasite species and immune status; frequency of proven attacks of malaria; efficacy and rapidity of treatment; time of year of alleged attacks and substitution by non-salaried members of the family; low value of labour at certain times of the year; and variation in productivity by age and sex.

Few studies on factors influencing demand for drug treatment and mosquito nets have been carried out while the supply role of the private sector has until recently been ignored. Waste in health centre prescribing practices often observed has only occasionally been documented.

Chapter 11

From malaria eradication to malaria control: the past, the present and the future

E. Onori, P. F. Beales and H. M. Gilles

I myself have been infected with malaria only once in spite of nineteen years' service in India and thirteen subsequent 'malaria expeditions' to warm climates; and I attribute this good fortune to my scrupulous use of the bed net.

Ronald Ross, *Studies on Malaria* (1928)

Stimulate the Phagocytes. Drugs are a Delusion.

G. B. Shaw, *The Doctor's Dilemma* (1906)

Principles of malaria eradication

Soon after the Second World War the World Health Organization recognized that malaria not only killed more people than any other disease but also interfered with the development of agriculture and industry, especially in the new independent countries. The intensive control methods carried out in some western countries and in certain tropical territories gave satisfactory results but could not be applied in many rural tropical areas. The advent of DDT presented the world with a new method of interrupting the transmission of malaria infection by attacking the adult *Anopheles* vector during its epidemiologically most important stage, when it feeds on humans in their dwellings or when it shelters indoors in the nearest house or animal shelter.

The epidemiological concept of the interruption of malaria transmission by residual insecticide spraying is simple. After taking her blood meal the female *Anopheles* usually rests on a nearby indoor surface such as a wall, ceiling etc. for several hours while the blood meal is digested and the batch of eggs matures. Spraying of all inside surfaces of dwellings with a long-lasting insecticide creates conditions in which a substantial proportion of *Anopheles* would be killed before they could transmit the disease (see Chapter 8).

This concept proved to be correct as shown in several examples of early campaigns in Italy, Cyprus, Greece, Guyana and Venezuela. It appeared that the widespread use of DDT and other residual insecticides was the most reliable, feasible and economical methods for the interruption of transmission. Any remaining foci of malaria could be detected by proper surveillance and eliminated by distribution of antimalarial drugs and local application of insecticides.

This simplified description of the principle of malaria eradication gives only a perfunctory idea of the operational complexity of a large-scale programme (Pampana, 1969).

The malaria eradication programme has been defined as an operation aimed at cessation of transmission of malaria and elimination of the reservoir of infected cases in a campaign limited in time and carried to such a degree of perfection that, when it comes to an end, there is no resumption of transmission.

Three main epidemiological principles of malaria eradication can be tersely summarized as follows:

1. Female *Anopheles* of vector species feed prefer-

Table 11.1 Differences between malaria control and eradication

	Control	Eradication
Objective	Reduction of incidence until no longer a major public health problem	Cessation of transmission and elimination of the human reservoir of infection
Duration	Indefinite	Limited in time
Area of operation	Only where transmission is intense	All areas where transmission occurs
Total coverage (by spraying and surveillance)	Not necessary	Indispensable
Operational standards	Good	Perfect
Cost	Recurring	Capital investment; after completion no recurring annual cost except for surveillance
Assessment of results	Sampling of population for parasite rates and spleen rates (malariometric surveys)	Case detection (active and passive) in advanced stages. Surveillance procedure
Imported cases	Not relevant	Of concern in advanced stages of the programme

ably on humans, who are the only host of human malaria parasites. Frequency of feeding is related to the gonotrophic cycles of mosquito (usually every 2–3 days). After feeding, the female mosquito rests on a surface inside the house to digest the blood.

2. Duration of cycle of development of malaria parasites in the mosquito depends on the temperature. For *P. falciparum* at 26°C, it takes about 12 days. During that period there are 4–6 mosquito feeds on a human being and this increases the chance of mortality of female mosquitos alighting on indoor surfaces covered by an insecticide deposit.
3. Residual insecticides maintain their toxicity for several months and, as a result of this, the local population of *Anopheles* decreases its mean longevity to a point when maintenance of transmission becomes impossible and the malaria infection of the community is gradually eliminated. Any remaining foci of infection are dealt with by case detection and treatment.

The substantial differences between malaria control and malaria eradication are given in Table 11.1.

Because of the size and cost of the undertaking, a malaria eradication programme is usually organized on a national scale. The planning of a full-scale programme presupposes that its practical feasibility has been assured. If there is doubt that the proposed attack measures will stop transmission it must be first tested in a pilot project on a limited scale.

The programme is usually carried out over 8 or more years, in four phases (Fig. 11.1). The phases of the programme are described below.

1. *A preparatory phase* of 1 or 2 years' duration is devoted to geographical reconnaissance of the area, training of field staff, identification and numbering of sprayable houses, collection of equipment and vehicles etc.

2. *The attack phase*, during which residual house

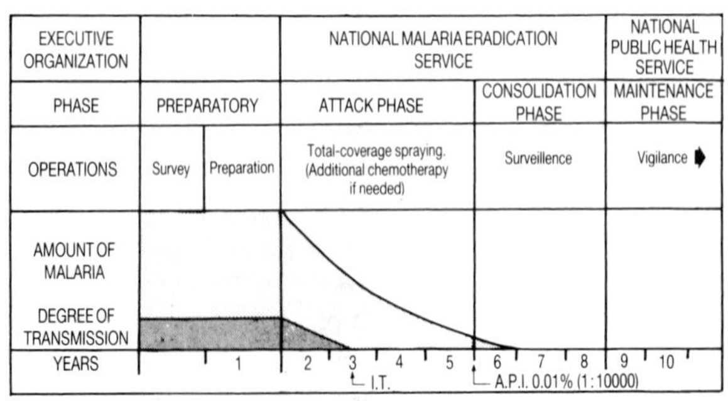

Fig. 11.1 Diagram of theoretical sequence of phases in malaria eradication programmes.

spraying and other measures aimed at the vector population are instituted, so that the principle of 'total coverage' of all premises and areas is observed. The dosage and frequency of spraying depend on local epidemiological conditions. This may be supplemented by chemotherapy. The duration of the attack phase is 4 years or longer.

The decrease of transmission is followed by taking blood slides from samples of the population to determine the parasite rate according to age groups. When the parasite rates reach a level of 5% the evaluation methods must be changed to measure the amount of malaria not in samples of the population but in all possibly infected individuals.

This basic process of surveillance is *case detection*, in which the presence or recent occurrence of fever is used as a screening device, to be confirmed by blood examination. Active case detection is carried out by house-to-house visits at fortnightly intervals; passive case detection is based on reporting from static medical units such as dispensaries and hospitals. The number of blood slides examined from fever cases in any given area should be not less than 1% of the population for each month of transmission. As the parasite reservoir falls full surveillance is instituted; this comprises, besides case-finding, epidemiological investigation and remedial measures. If the transmission is interrupted then the parasite rate of infants born after the start of the attack phase should be zero, while the successive parasite rates in population age groups over 3 years should decline annually to the value of less than 22% of the previous annual figure. The remedial function of surveillance is the treatment of cases by administration of a 'presumptive' (single) dose of an antimalarial drug, at the time of blood examination, followed (in confirmed cases) by full (radical) treatment (Fig. 11.2).

3. *The consolidation phase* of malaria eradication begins when the surveillance activity shows that the annual parasite incidence (API), which is the proportion of positive slides per 1000 population, is below 0.1 per 1000. Cessation of complete coverage by residual spraying is allowed when there is no more transmission of malaria throughout the area. Experience of successful programmes showed that surveillance operations alone should be effective to mop up the remaining foci of infection. However, the receptivity and vulnerability of the area to introduced infections must be considered.

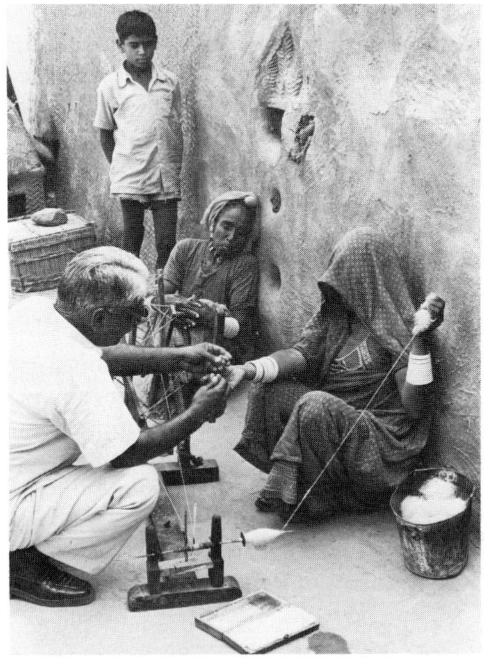

Fig. 11.2 Surveillance of malaria eradication programme in Rajastan, India. (WHO photograph by A. S. Kochar.)

Receptivity is the degree of probability of resumption of transmission, largely dependent on the presence and abundance of local vectors of malaria and climatic or other conditions favouring the infectivity. *Vulnerability* is the probability of importation of the sources of infection, either from abroad or from nearby malarious areas, through immigrants or through infected mosquitos.

4. *The maintenance phase* begins at the end of the consolidation phase and the entry into it demands that, during three consecutive years, there is no evidence of transmission of malaria, after the cessation of anopheline control by residual spraying. The preventive activities during the maintenance phase are known as *vigilance*, which consist of watchfulness for any occurrence of any imported or indigenous cases of malaria, and the application of appropriate measures. Thus, normally the maintenance of malaria eradication is the responsibility of general health services.

Certification of malaria eradication by the WHO can

be, and has been, requested by several countries. The inspection and review of the accomplishments of the programme are vested in a special certification team acting on behalf of the WHO and subject to confirmation of its findings by the WHO Expert Committee on Malaria.

In the light of present experience and accepting the fact that malaria eradication cannot be achieved in a number of countries for technical or other reasons, the alternative course of action is *malaria control* defined as follows (WHO, 1979):

> A malaria control programme is an organized effort to institute, carry out and evaluate such antimalaria measures as are appropriate for achieving the greatest possible improvement of the health situation of a population living in given epidemiological and socio-economic conditions and subjected to the burden of this disease or exposed to the risk of its resurgence.

As the resurgence of malaria in many parts of the world gives cause for anxiety, a number of countries intensified their efforts by adapting their health policies to the epidemiological situation and mustering their resources. The WHO aims at merging the antimalaria activities at the peripheral level with the work of expanding health services. Promotion of international and bilateral assistance for application of environmental methods of malaria control and stimulation of training courses for all cadres of medical and health personnel are long-term programmes which are closely related to the pace of socio-economic advance of developing tropical countries where malaria will remain a serious health problem for many years.

Trends in the world malaria situation

The worldwide programme of malaria eradication was formally endorsed by the Eighth World Health Assembly in 1955, and in 1957 the WHO took over the coordinating activities and the provision of technical assistance.

The concept of malaria eradication was accepted by all the member governments of the WHO. Previous control programmes were converted to eradication programmes and these were initiated in all malarious countries in the Americas and Europe, and in the majority of countries in Asia and Oceania. But only pilot projects were attempted in Africa.

Within 15 years of the start of this remarkable international endeavour malaria had been eliminated from the whole of Europe, the Asian part of the former USSR, several countries of the Middle East, most of North America including the whole of the USA, most of the Caribbean, large areas of the northern and southern portions of South America, Australia, Japan, Singapore, Korea, and Taiwan (Table 11.2). Some examples of country-wide malaria eradication programmes are illustrated in Figs 11.3, 11.4 and 11.5.

By 1970, the eradication programmes had freed 727 million people from the risk of malaria; this number then represented 53% of the population of the originally malarious areas. This progress had saved a great number of lives, and had contributed to economic development of many areas, particularly in Asia, South and South-east Europe, and the Americas. In addition to promoting a general improvement in health, malaria eradication measures in certain countries had reduced the prevalence of other vector-borne diseases, such as leishmaniasis and plague. They had also stimulated the recruitment and training of thousands of health workers, who later formed the backbone of general health services.

During the years which followed the conversion of malaria eradication programmes into malaria

Table 11.2 Progress of malaria eradication and control in 1961 and 1976, in terms of millions of population according to WHO

Description of area	Population in millions (approx.)	
	1961	1976
Areas freed from endemic malaria (under vigilance)	317	436
Areas under surveillance	75	809
Areas under mosquito control or protected by drugs	576	451
Areas without specific antimalaria measures	452	352
Grand total of the population in originally malarious areas	1420	2048

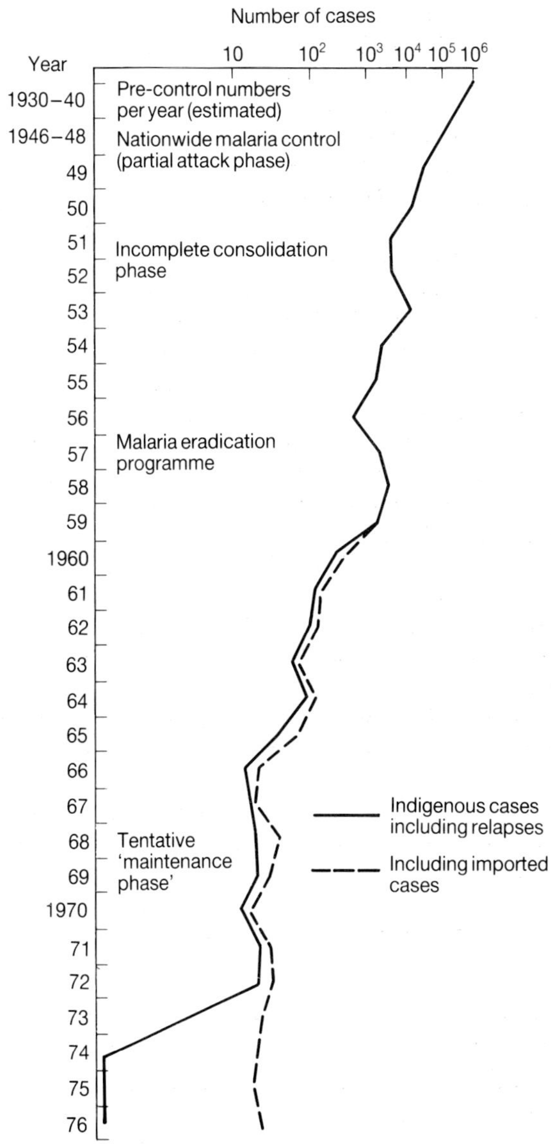

Fig. 11.3 Progress and achievements of malaria eradication in Greece. (Reproduced from Bruce-Chwatt and de Zulueta, 1980.)

control (1969), the malaria situation greatly deteriorated. The resurgence of the disease affected several countries in southern Asia and Latin America as well as the south-eastern part of Turkey. The number of reported cases of malaria throughout the world had more than doubled in 1977 in comparison with 1974 (Table 11.3).

This was due to the reduction of malaria control activities in many countries, because of a sudden withdrawal of external resources which was then aggravated by the energy crisis and subsequent economic strains; other factors were the rising costs of insecticides and development of resistance to DDT and other organochlorines.

Moreover, resistance of *P. falciparum* to some drugs was responsible for an increase of malaria incidence in South-east Asia and parts of South America. Although the achievement of malaria eradication in the whole of Europe and most of North America was maintained, a number of countries in the temperate regions saw a marked increase of cases of malaria imported from the tropics.

The figures in Table 11.3 would indicate that the situation remained stagnant between 1984 and 1988: however, they represent much less than the true situation, as case detection activities in many countries have been greatly reduced because of the high cost of maintaining full surveillance systems. Moreover, in tropical Africa, most countries report only cases of malaria that attend health institutions, which cover not more than 10–20% of the whole population. Only a small proportion of these cases is confirmed by blood examination and for this reason the figures from Africa have not been added to the totals in Table 11.3.

An evaluation of the global epidemiological situation by the WHO (1991) indicates that at the end of 1989, out of a world population of about 5160 million people, 1400 million (27%) lived in areas where malaria never existed or disappeared without specific malaria interventions; 1650 million (32%) lived in areas where endemic malaria disappeared after the implementation of a specific control campaign and the malaria-free situation has been maintained; 1620 million (31%) lived in areas where endemic malaria had been considerably reduced after control measures had been introduced, but transmission was reinstated and the situation is unstable or deteriorating; 490 million (10%) lived in areas, mainly in tropical Africa, where endemic malaria remained basically unchanged and no national antimalaria programme was ever implemented. Broadly speaking, it can be stated that the resurgence of transmission in the mid-1970s was reduced during the years 1977–82, but this reduction did not reach the low levels seen during the first decade of the 1960s. In recent years the

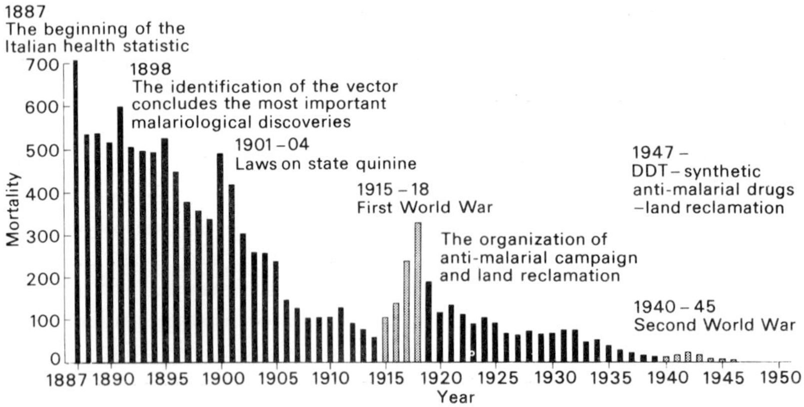

Fig. 11.4 Progress and achievements of malaria control in Italy between 1900 and 1950. (Reproduced from Bruce-Chwatt and de Zulueta, 1980.)

overall situation has remained stagnant, but the trends in individual countries of the different regions vary and a continuous upward trend has been observed in the number of malaria cases reported in the American region and some Asian countries.

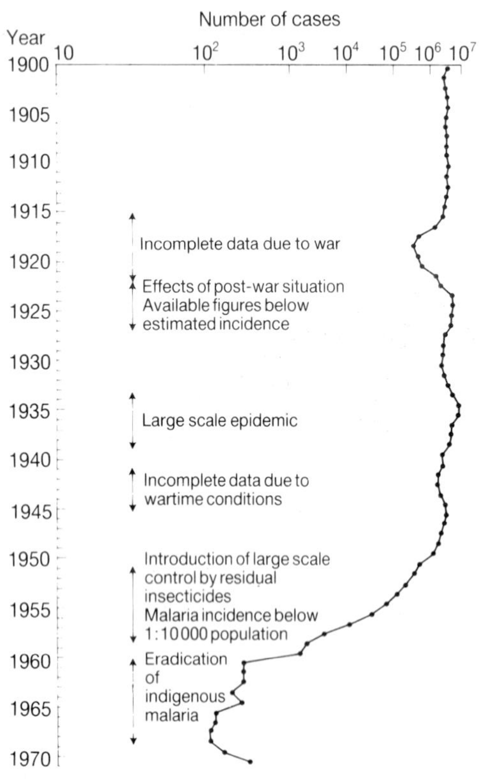

Fig. 11.5 Progress and achievements of malaria eradication in USSR. (From Bruce-Chwatt and de Zulueta, 1980.)

Summary of the world malaria situation in 1990

The last available summary review of the world malaria situation can be found in the *WHO Weekly Epidemiological Record*, 1992, No. 22, pp. 161–7, and No. 23, pp. 169–74 (Figs 11.6–11.8; Plate 28).

Africa north of the Sahara

In Africa north of the Sahara malaria transmission is very low and confined to rural areas. The total number of cases reported has fluctuated around 1100 during recent years.

Africa south of the Sahara (Tropical Africa)

In Africa south of the Sahara, between 12 and 22 million cases per year were reported during 1985–1989 but it can be estimated that about 100 million clinical malaria cases occur every year, and that prevalence of infection may be of the order of 275 million parasite carriers, of which some 85–90% are caused by *P. falciparum*. In this area endemicity reaches the highest levels in the world, but varies greatly from place to place. Based on available epidemiological data Onori defined four broad epidemiological strata:

1. *Very high endemicity* is found in areas where malaria transmission is intense and perennial with essentially minor seasonal variations, due to extremely favourable meteorological conditions, such as rainfall and relative humidity, for most if not all the year round.

Table 11.3 Numbers of malaria cases (in thousands) reported during the period 1974–1990 by WHO region (WHO, 1992)*

Region	1974	1975	1976	1977	1978	1979	1980	1981	1982	1983	1984	1985	1986	1987	1988	1989	1990‡
Africa†‡	5120	4136	5212	4477	6682	5720	7146	6754	6042	2726	4523	11634	17442	19463	21957	13835	–
Americas	269	357	379	399	469	515	603	638	718	831	932	911	951	1018	1120	1114	1057
South-east Asia	4162	6059	7304	5540	4800	3666	3706	3566	2964	2731	3004	2503	2689	2823	2789	2957	2614
Europe§	7	13	41	119	93	34	38	60	66	73	62	57	47	28	24	21	12
Eastern Mediterranean	480	424	349	227	162	125	137	207	308	305	335	391	611	566	602	532	566
Western Pacific¶	179	188	211	4457	3422	2706	3654	3464	2487	1839	1410	1178	1012	893	774	829	761
Total (excluding Africa)	5097	7041	8284	10742	8946	7046	8138	7935	6543	5779	5743	5040	5310	5328	5309	5453	5010

*The information provided does not cover the total population at risk in some instances.
†Mainly clinically diagnosed cases, and not included in total figures. Actual numbers of unreported malaria cases are very much higher.
‡Incomplete figures.
§In 1976–1980 there was an epidemic of vivax malaria in Asian Turkey.
¶Data from China became available in 1977. The totals for 1974–1976 do not include figures from China.

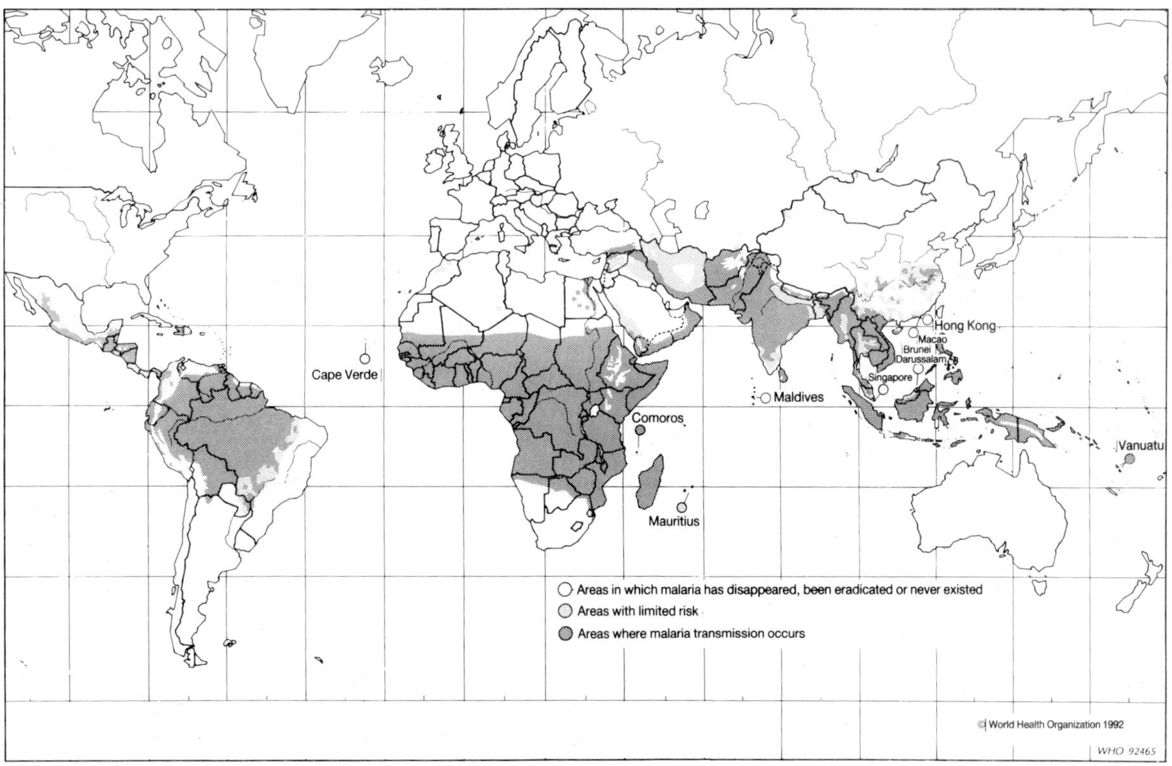

Fig. 11.6 Epidemiological assessment of status of malaria. (Reproduced, by permission of WHO, from *Weekly Epidemiological Record*, 1992, **22**: 162.)

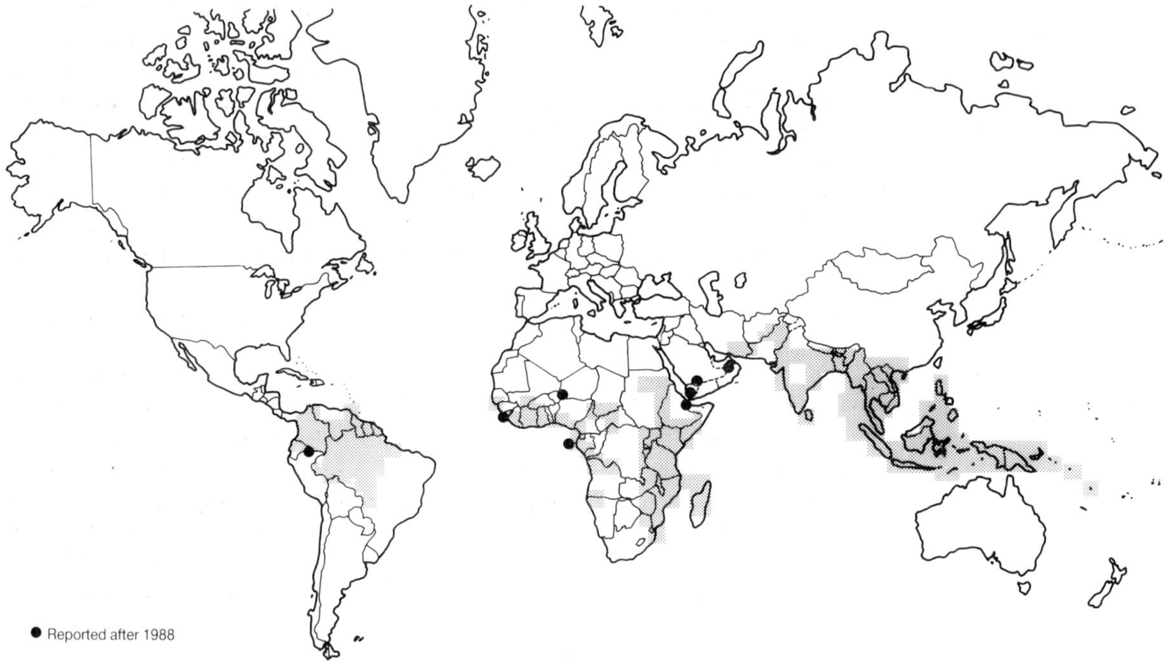

Fig. 11.7 Areas where chloroquine-resistant *P. falciparum* has been reported. (Reproduced, by permission of WHO, from *Weekly Epidemiological Record*, 1991, **22**: 162.)

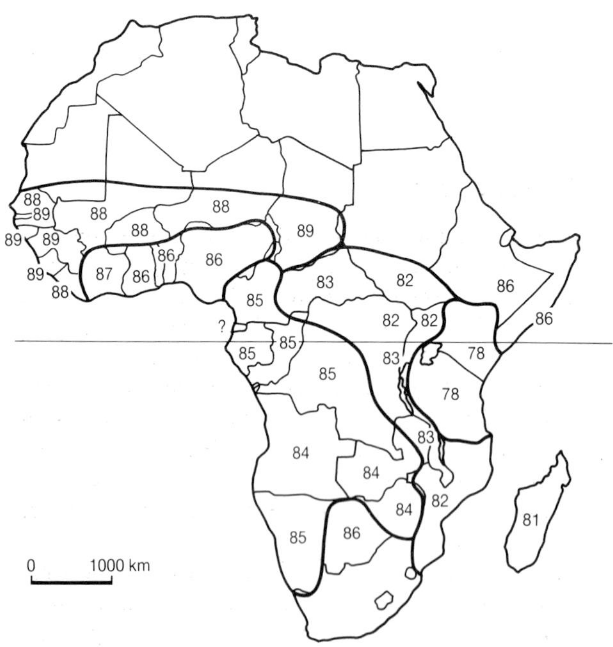

Fig. 11.8 Spread of chloroquine resistance in Africa. Numbers refer to year of detection. (After Charmot *et al.*, 1991.)

The immunity of the population builds up quickly so that by the age of 5 years local residents are almost free from clinical attacks.

The majority of deaths occur in infants and children under the age of 5 years. Mortality rates are of the order of 6 per 1000 in infants and 11 per 1000 in children aged 1–4 years, representing 10% and 25% of all deaths in these age groups, respectively. Cerebral malaria constitutes less than 1% of all cases of hospitalization in paediatric clinics but death due to cerebral malaria is relatively high (up to 25%). A number of children undoubtedly die before reaching any health post; while deaths from malarial anaemia are significantly under recorded.

The area affected by this highly endemic and stable malaria corresponds to the degraded forests of Central Africa.

2. In *high endemicity areas*, transmission is heavy but essentially seasonal, reaching its peak during the rainy season and then disappearing or remaining at a very low level during the dry season. This is reflected in important seasonal variations in parasite prevalence. Malaria morbidity affects mainly children of the pre-school age. Immunity

develops relatively quickly, depending on the local epidemiological situation, and reaches a steady level during adolescence.

This type of malaria can be found in the savannah zones of West, East and Central Africa.

3. *Mesoendemic malaria* is usually found in areas where transmission of the disease is of short duration, usually 2 months, corresponding to the rainy season, with an almost complete interruption in the remaining 10 months. Malariometric indices show great seasonal variations and may vary from year to year depending on the prevailing meteorological conditions. Development of immunity is delayed so that not only children, but also adolescents and even adults can have clinical manifestations.

In the areas belonging to this epidemiological stratum which are actually at the extreme limits of malaria distribution in Africa, seasonal epidemics may occur following exceptional meteorological phenomena, i.e. heavy rainfall after several years of drought.

The areas involved correspond to the saharian zones with semi-desert or arid climate in the north, and to the plateaux of Madagascar, the highlands of Zimbabwe, limited areas of Lesotho, some low altitude areas of northern and eastern Transvaal and some of the coastal areas of Natal in South Africa in the south.

4. *Low malaria endemicity* is usually found in areas where malaria transmission is absent but in which it may occur following exceptionally favourable meteorological changes. The immunity of the population in these areas is practically non-existent and when transmission starts it may rapidly reach epidemic proportions with high mortality among all the different age groups of the population. These conditions exist in the valleys of high mountains in Central Africa, Kenya and Ethiopia.

There are also areas where malaria never existed or has been eradicated: they include nearly all Cape Verde and Lesotho, Réunion, Saint Helena, the Seychelles and most of South Africa. *Plasmodium vivax* transmission in Mauritius, re-established in the early 1980s after the disease had been eradicated from the island, has been gradually and constantly reduced.

Although there are few studies on malaria mortality in Africa, it is obvious that in highly endemic areas it is concentrated in the younger age groups. In 1969, it was estimated that malaria might be responsible for the death of 1 million infants and children per year in tropical Africa. From data collected in 1970–75, it was concluded that in Kenya (Kisumu) and Nigeria (Garki) malaria was responsible for about 20–30% of infant mortality. A study in The Gambia in 1987 indicated that about 25% of the childhood (1–4 years) mortality may be attributable to malaria.

The lack or shortage of trained personnel for the planning, organization, monitoring and evaluation of programmes remains one of the major constraints. The WHO Regional Committee for Africa adopted a policy to encourage the development of malaria control within the framework of primary health care at district level. The aim is to prevent and reduce malaria mortality by providing prompt diagnosis or recognition and adequate treatment of malaria cases through the basic health services and primary health care. This implies the creation of efficient referral systems for the management of severe and complicated cases as well as for treatment failures.

Chloroquine resistance has been extensively reported – most recently in West Africa, and in East and Central Africa the level has increased, hampering its effectiveness as first line treatment in certain areas.

Resistance to sulfadoxine–pyrimethamine has been sporadically reported from several African countries.

The Americas

In 1990 the number of malaria cases notified was 1057 000 compared to 1 114 000 in 1989. More than half of the cases were found in Brazil (53%); 25% originated from the Andean countries; and 14% from Central America including Mexico.

Vivax malaria continued to predominate (67% of all infections) but *P. falciparum* is still highly prevalent in Brazil, the Dominican Republic, French Guyana, Guyana, Haiti and Surinam. Of all falciparum infections registered in the Americas, 73% originated from Brazil.

In Central America including Mexico in 1990 more than 90% (75 104) of all cases originated from Guatemala, Honduras, Mexico and Nicaragua; the highest incidence (16.1 per 1000) occurred in Belize.

In the *Andean sub-region* of South America, which

includes Bolivia, Colombia, Ecuador, Peru and Venezuela, 267 000 cases were reported in 1990, with nearly half of the cases occurring in Colombia (99 489).

In *Brazil* 99% of cases were recorded in the Amazon region, mainly from Rondonia (33% of the total cases).

In the southern cone of South America *P. vivax* is the predominant parasite. Malaria is endemic only in Paraguay and in a small area in northern Argentina.

Europe (including Turkey and the former USSR)

In Europe endemic malaria (*P. vivax* only) occurred in the south-eastern part of Turkey and in some small foci in Azerbaijan and Tajikistan.

Asia

In Asia the situation is very variable and for some countries, e.g. Afghanistan, Iran and Yemen, incomplete recording makes an assessment futile.

Many countries have remained malaria-free – Bahrain, Israel, Jordan, Kuwait, Lebanon, Qatar, the United Arab Emirates. In others – Oman, Syria, the Arab Republic, Saudi Arabia – the number of cases is small.

In Pakistan the number of reported cases decreased in 1990, with more than 54% of them due to *P. falciparum*.

In Bangladesh *P. falciparum* prevalence remained about the same (63.2% in 1990), nearly all cases originating from Chittagong Division. An increase in the number of cases from 11 000 in 1988 to 19 000 in 1989 was observed.

In India, malaria cases decreased from 2.02 million in 1989 to 1.78 million in 1990. This represents 35% of the cases reported outside Africa. Of the total of 746 000 falciparum infections in 1989 30% were from Orissa, 27% from Gujarat and 14% from Madhya Pradesh. Meanwhile in Sri Lanka in 1990 the number of reported cases of malaria was 287 384.

Eastern Asia and Oceania

Australia, Brunei Darussalam, the Democratic People's Republic of Korea, Hong Kong, Japan, Macao, Mongolia, the Republic of Korea, Singapore, large areas of China and most of Oceania continued to remain free from indigenous malaria.

In China *P. falciparum* is confined to five areas – Hainan, Yunnan, Guizhou, Guangxi and Anhui.

About nine-tenths of the population of peninsular *Malaysia* live in malarious-free areas. Malaria has increased over the last 4 years in relation to newly opened land development schemes. The majority of cases (55% are *P. falciparum*) were recorded in the rural areas of Pahang, Kelatan and Perak States. In Sabah malaria remains a significant problem.

In the Lao People's Democratic Republic, Myanmar, Papua New Guinea, Solomon Islands and Vanuatu, the malaria situation has not changed significantly in recent years.

In Thailand, incidence has increased in the border provinces with Cambodia (Trat) and Myanmar (Tak). In certain areas multidrug resistance including to mefloquine has occurred.

The future of malaria eradication and control

The reasons for the reverses of the global malaria eradication programme are complex. Technical obstacles such as the exophilic habits of some anopheline species, resistance of malaria vectors to insecticides, resistance of *Plasmodia* to antimalarial drugs, inaccessibility of outlying groups of houses, and the primitive structure of dwellings, are of undoubted importance. It has also been realized in recent years that failures to achieve or maintain control depends not only on the previous intensity of transmission but also on new trends in agricultural exploitation and the distribution of rural populations. Extensive agricultural development projects attract large numbers of temporary workers who are often concentrated in labour camps where inappropriate sitings and quality of shelters, the shabbiness of the environment and the overcrowding create optimal conditions for malaria transmission.

Other serious difficulties that have stopped the former advance of global malaria eradication are administrative, socio-economic, financial and political which affect the improvement of health conditions in developing countries with inadequate basic health services and a shortage of trained personnel.

The importance of the latter point will be fully understood when it is remembered that in the attack phase, but especially in the consolidation phase, there is great need for a reliable surveillance system capable of monitoring the interruption of transmission. In this phase, adequately developed public health services should carry out much of their task of case detection of malaria. This also explains why the proper organization and country-wide coverage of public health services are necessary for the transition from the consolidation phase to the maintenance phase of malaria eradication.

A re-examination of the global strategy of malaria eradication was carried out during the 1960s and the results were presented at the 22nd World Health Assembly in 1969.

The main conclusions of this report stressed that malaria eradication should remain the final aim: it is a long-term investment because of its overall impact on health, and its socio-economic benefits. Wherever malaria eradication programmes have good prospects they should be pursued with vigour towards their defined goal. In countries where eradication does not appear to be feasible because of the inadequacy of financial resources, personnel requirements, or shortcomings of basic health services, malaria control operations should form a transitional stage toward the future launching of an eradication programme. In 1979 the WHO Expert Committee reviewed the status of antimalaria programmes in the world. Out of 143 countries or areas where malaria was originally endemic (in part or all of the territory), 37 countries or areas had been freed from malaria, the malaria risk was minimal in 16 others, and in large areas of the remaining 90 the risk ranged from moderate to high.

Further study of the malaria situation, especially in developing countries, confirmed the existence of many constraints to malaria control. Among these were some social factors (e.g. nomadics, refusal to spray dwellings or extreme simplicity of their construction, replastering of sprayed walls), financial stringency (increased cost of materials, equipment, transport), shortage of trained personnel, rudimentary health infrastructure, uncontrolled development of irrigation, deforestation etc.

As a result of this report the 31st World Health Assembly adopted in 1979 a resolution on the new strategy of malaria control stressing its five principles: (1) the national will to control the disease should be expressed through a government decision to support antimalaria activities on a long-term basis; (2) malaria control should be an integral part of the country health programme; (3) the feasibility and practicability of reducing malaria to a low level should be demonstrated; (4) the participation of the community should be obtained since the success of various methods of control will greatly depend on this; (5) wherever applicable, permanent measures for the control of malaria should be made an integral part of the relevant development programmes.

This resolution was in line with the general requirements for health development stressed at the International Conference on Primary Health Care held in Alma-Ata in 1978. Many national strategies for malaria control are now based in conformity with these principles but the role of primary health care in relation to antimalaria activities requires some elucidation (WHO, 1982).

The concept of primary health care, adopted by the World Health Assembly, on the basis of recommendations of the International Conference on Primary Health Care, held in Alma-Ata in 1978, includes as one of the priorities 'the prevention and control of endemic diseases, with the full participation of the relevant communities, at a cost that the community can afford and in the spirit of self-reliance and self-determination'. The report of the Alma-Ata conference stresses that primary health care should be based on 'practical, socially acceptable methods and technology, made universally accessible to individuals and families within the community'. According to this concept, one of the paramount responsibilities of the system of primary health care is the control of malaria. The effective coordination of antimalaria activities with other responsibilities at various levels of the health system has often been interpreted as 'integration'. While administratively all antimalaria programmes are part of the health services, there remain some ill-defined areas concerning the level of specific technical competence required, the lines of command, the areas of responsibility and the degree of supervision to be exerted. Different patterns of 'integration' have been proposed or applied, depending on the epidemiological, socio-economic, cultural and other variants in the health care systems and malaria services. Planning of primary health care cannot be carried out as a separate programme, nor can it dismantle the existing health services; but from the very beginning all the resources of the health sector and of the related departments (e.g. agriculture) should be co-ordinated. Some unrealistic planning during the early stages of the process of 'integration' had produced an overburdening of the peripheral health workers, who had no knowledge of the level of their responsibility or the authorities for issuing instructions, receiving reports and supervising the work. The various phases of a process of integration need to be introduced gradually. The concept of primary health care, which provides the malaria control programme with a structure at the village level that is essential for securing community involvement, epidemiological information and application of control measures, is sound in theory. In practice, however, insufficient definition of the lines of competence, supervision and responsibility for an integrated programme is bound to affect the control of malaria. Thus in planning it in a country that adopted the system of primary health care, there still remains the need for expertise and responsibility at the central level of health authority. This is particularly evident when one must be flexible in adapting various control approaches to local epidemiological conditions in relation to all social, economic and political factors. When malaria is recognized as a major health problem and when its importance has been assessed in relation to other aspects of national health the first responsibility of the relevant authorities is to provide access for the population to diagnosis and treatment of the disease, as well as to its prevention. The primary health care approach requires the selection of feasible activities; and, as Russell stressed 50 years ago, striving for continuity of a modest effort should be preferred to some spectacular attempts which are only of short-term value. The creation of a network of treatment units at the village level, with an appropriate referral system to more advanced health centres, may become a channel for further preventive activities. The main aim of primary health care is the projection of its possibilities to the community through the training and activities of health workers whether volunteers or those in salaried employment. As the primary health system develops and the participation of the community is stimulated it may be possible to embark on specific vector control programmes.

One of the most important functions of those responsible for providing primary health care at the village level is the provision of health education aimed at encouraging community involvement in planning, acceptance and implementation of antimalaria activities. Such community participation is part of the national culture in some countries, but in others it must be stimulated in order to produce the desired effect.

It would be wrong to assume that the involvement of primary health care in malaria control in developing countries is an easy way of solving the present difficulties related to administrative, social or economic obstacles. While some countries were undoubtedly successful, a number of others were unable to achieve a proper degree of cooperation between different levels of their health care system and, consequently, the malaria situation deteriorated. Present experience indicates that many problems of malaria control within the system of primary health care can be rapidly solved if, as a result of good planning of field activities, staff members and personnel of every grade have full knowledge of the tasks involved, of the expected degree of their competence, provision of supplies and equipment, system of supervision, and other administrative and technical details, including the support of the community.

All these and many other aspects of malaria control through integration with primary health care have been outlined in the *Seventeenth, Eighteenth and Nineteenth Reports of the WHO Expert Committee on Malaria* (WHO, 1979, 1986, 1992). Certain specific aspects of existing programmes were described at the *Seventh Asian Malaria Conference on Malaria Control and National Health Goals* (WHO, 1982), in the USA also in the AID *Manual on Malaria Control and Primary Health Care in Africa* (1982) and recently in *Malaria – Obstacles and Opportunities* (1991).

Socio-economic considerations

The important role of human behavioural, social and economic factors in the epidemiology of malaria have long been recognized, yet we remain relatively ignorant of the social and economic effect of malaria in those countries where it is most prevalent. Several studies have been undertaken in recent years to improve our knowledge.

The consequences of ignoring *human behaviour* can be illustrated by two recent examples. Sociological studies in Malawi revealed that the bitter taste of chloroquine was associated with traditional herbs which cause abortion, and pregnant women were advised to avoid all bitter medicine during pregnancy. When enteric coated tablets were substituted compliance significantly increased. Similarly in New Guinea, it was found that maternal chemoprophylaxis was affected by the local knowledge that a large dose of chloroquine would produce abortion. This created an impression that the drug was dangerous in pregnancy.

The *economic* impact would clearly vary with the different epidemiological prototypes – whether children are predominantly affected or all age groups; how much self-treatment is undertaken; costs involved in reaching the local clinic; costs to governments supplying the antimalarials and other protection against the disease; indirect effects of mortality; the cumulative effect on health by malaria superimposed on other infections that are commonly found in the same community; the knowledge, attitude and practices of the community.

Days of disability per case of malaria have ranged from 3.5 to 20; in some studies no difference in working capacity has been found between parasitized and non-parasitized adult workers. The detrimental effect of malaria on the education of children, whether due to absenteeism or reduced ability to assimilate, has never been satisfactorily analysed. In many countries the burden of malaria is borne disproportionally by the poor or by migrant labourers.

Clearly the analysis of the socio-economic impact of malaria is multifactorial and requires a multidisciplinary approach.

Malaria research

From the very beginning of malariology as a well-defined discipline, aiming at our understanding of all aspects of this disease and at forging better tools for fighting against it, research has been the foundation on which the gradual successes were built. In the 1950s the general trends were mainly related to the concept and practice of eradication. Development of new antimalarial drugs and insecticides, together with the formulation of epidemiological basis of surveillance activities were then the main themes of scientific interest. Most of the applied research during that period was carried out by various national institutes, industrial laboratories and independent scientists.

Although the sum total of this activity produced very important results the increasing technical and operational problems encountered during the 1960s indicated that the difficulties, due to the advent of resistance of *Plasmodia* to the available drugs and the resistance of *Anopheles* vectors to our best insecticides, present a major challenge that must be met by a better coordination and a greater stimulation of international research of both a basic and applied character. In 1975 the Special Programme for Research and Training in Tropical Diseases was established jointly by the United Nations, the World Bank and the World Health Organization. This programme covers the six main tropical diseases including malaria. Its objectives are not only the development of new methods for control of these infections but also strengthening of research capabilities in developing parts of the world. Such research has now assumed a multidisciplinary approach.

Although basic research into all aspects of malaria and its transmission form the backbone of the coordinated scientific activity of the Special Programme, research is also undertaken in order to try out and improve the application of available technical tools in given epidemiological conditions.

The latest tenth report of the Special Programme on Research and Training in Tropical Diseases covers the years of 1989–90 (UNDP/World Bank/WHO, 1991) and the results related to studies on malaria are now summarized.

Drug developments

Work continues on new drugs, on the optimization of available drugs, for example, new drug combinations; on defining the factors that impair utility of current drugs such as drug resistance and adverse drug reactions and on basic research.

The programme supported the first identification, cloning and sequencing of the genes for multidrug resistance. Wellems located the gene for *chloroquine* resistance on a 200 kb region of chromosome 7. In collaboration with Knoll Chemische Fabriken AG, advanced preclinical studies of a candidate resistance reverser are in progress.

A study of *mefloquine* prophylaxis in the second and third trimesters of pregnancy has shown the drug to be highly effective and without significant maternal or foetal toxicity. Research to study the mechanism of resistance to mefloquine is in progress.

Clinical studies of efficacy, bioavailability and pharmacokinetics of *halofantrine* have been supported in Thailand, Africa and Colombia.

Efficacy and pharmacokinetic trials comparing intravenous and intramuscular *quinine* have been undertaken. Clearly if intramuscular quinine could be used at the periphery of the health system, treatment of severe cases could be given earlier.

Clinical trials of the artemisinin derivatives, arteether and artemether, both given intramuscularly and artesunate intravenously are in progress. The Tropical Diseases Research Programme (TDR) is also assisting China by providing consultants in pharmaceutical manufacturing and good manufacturing practices to the Kunming Pharmaceutical Factory.

A toxicity and dose-finding trial to test an anti-tumour necrosis factor monoclonal antibody in human cerebral malaria has taken place in the Gambia.

Simple *in vitro* microtest kits for assessment at the field level of drug resistance against chloroquine, amodiaquine, quinine, mefloquine and the sulfadoxine–pyrimethamine combination have been developed and evaluated.

TDR has advanced knowledge on several unique aspects of the biochemistry of the parasite at the molecular level.

Vaccine developments (see also Chapter 5)

Vaccine research continues on the development of three types of vaccine: antisporozoite, asexual blood stage and transmission blocking. The most useful future vaccine may combine two or more of these components.

With regard to the *pre-erythrocytic* (antisporozoite) vaccine, the important role of γ-interferon (INF) and CD8+ cytotoxic T cells in antisporozoite immunity in a mouse model has been demonstrated. In human malaria, a *P. falciparum* liver stage specific antigen (LSA-I) and an antigen shared by *P. falciparum* sporozoites and liver stages (SALSA) have been cloned. The circumsporozoite protein of *P. vivax* has proved to be polymorphic.

From the many antigens identified in the blood stages of *P. falciparum* interest focussed on the precursor to the major merozoite surface antigen protein (PMMSA). A single fragment of the PMMSA has been shown to remain on the merozoite surface during red cell invasion and antibody to this fragment inhibits merozoite invasion *in vitro*.

Ring-infected erythrocyte surface antigen (Pf 155/RESA) is another *P. falciparum* vaccine candidate found in the membrane of newly infected erythrocytes.

As a potential antigen for a *transmission-blocking vaccine*, Pfs 25, an oökinete surface molecule of *P. falciparum*, has been cloned and sequenced. Three other leading candidate antigens have been identified: Pfs 230 and the doublet Pfs 48/45.

Diagnosis

The development of systems based on DNA probes and monoclonal antibodies for epidemiological diagnostic studies are being developed. Substantial progress has been made on developing kits for the immunological detection of sporozoites in infected mosquitos using monoclonal antibodies, and test kits are now available for the detection of antisporozoite antibodies in human serum. Micro-assays for lymphocyte activation, as an indication of immunity system activity, have been adapted for use with finger-prick samples.

Other activities

Multicentre trials have begun in African countries to determine the impact of impregnated mosquito nets on general mortality. The genetic engineering of an uninfectable mosquito is being pursued. A case control study is in progress of host, parasite and environmental factors determining the severity of clinical malaria in Kenya.

The *social and economic* processes that may influence the epidemiology of malaria and facilitate or hamper the effectiveness of potential control measures are being given increased and justified prominence.

Outside the TDR programme, a great deal of

research on malaria is taking place which is quite impossible to summarize here. Clinical trials in human volunteers in South America using the Patarroyo asexual blood stage vaccine have taken place, the results of which are awaited with interest.

There is much hope that these and all future achievements of research in experimental pharmacology, industrial chemistry, mosquito genetics and ecology, biochemistry, immunology and especially molecular biology, will eventually produce new weapons against malaria.

However, the conquest of this disease, rooted in the physical environment and closely linked with the socio-economic conditions of vast populations of tropical developing countries, cannot be achieved by the new technical tools alone. Each of these tools will be needed, but their proper use will depend on the other factors, and especially on the national ability of the countries of the Third World to relieve the poverty of their large rural areas and on generous and sustained international aid.

The last thoughts of Professor Leonard Jan Bruce-Chwatt

In the modern history of man's fight against malaria three dates are of special significance: that of 1957 when the global eradication of this ancient disease was considered to be feasible and was planned with an excessive optimism, appropriate to that decade. The second historical date is that of 1969 when a more realistic appraisal of technical and socio-economic obstacles to global eradication led to the acceptance of an alternative goal of malaria control in developing countries. Such a drastic change of strategy had a profound psychological impact. It confronted the WHO, all the other international bodies and the countries concerned with the need to replace the rigid rules and tactics of eradication by the much more flexible, not time-limited and often untried aspects of malaria control. Consequently, a number of important points became obvious. In the first instance, the malaria control programmes in many countries had to be re-orientated to the reduction of malaria incidence to a 'tolerable level' but this level could not be easily determined, whether in terms of morbidity or mortality. Secondly, concentration of control operations on one specific part of the country created difficulty in delimiting such priority areas. Thirdly, malaria control, in contradistinction to malaria eradication, held no promise of rapid and permanent effects but had to be planned as a long-term, continuous and unspectacular commitment, demanding great devotion to a distant goal. The fourth point is the frequent tendency of *ad hoc* transfer of the responsibility for malaria control from specialized units to general health services; this may give a broader basis for cooperation, but often delays the implementation of a necessary action. The fifth factor is the depletion of technically competent national and international staff, capable of advising the complex malaria control programmes.

> The present trend of expert opinion is fully in favour of a malaria component of a comprehensive primary health service; but few countries understand that integration of malaria control into the general health system does not mean the abdication of expertise and responsibility for technical planning at the central level.
>
> Bruce-Chwatt (1987)

The third important date is that of 1975 when the Special Programme for Research and Training in Tropical Diseases came into being. Its latest achievements in the field of malaria have been outlined in the preceding pages and this justifies the hopes that various new means and methods for control of malaria will become available in the near future. Its increasing emphasis on training at all levels of scientific institutions and national health services is of special significance.

Much fundamental and applied research continues unabated, and the most promising aspect of it is the involvement of national scientists and medical staff of developing countries.

In several resolutions passed at recent World Health Assemblies the member states of the WHO have stressed the need to improve the number and qualifications of antimalaria personnel. In the past, various excellent centres for such training were available. However, many of these centres have closed down and the staff already trained went to other fields of activity. There is now the opportunity of reviving or extending training activities specifically orientated towards malaria control. The many aspects of malariology should not be taught in isolation but in the context of varying priorities of national public health programmes and in relation to the needs of the community. Modern teaching methods should be introduced and the participants must be directly involved in the training process. Learning by doing practical field work must be emphasized.

The subject of malaria in its epidemiological, parasitological, clinical and public health aspects should be reflected in the undergraduate and post-graduate curricula of medical schools in developing countries. Extensive reorientation is required for the existing malaria personnel, at both national and international levels. The concept of the community orientated health team should be in the centre of training activities. Ways and means must be found to train a large number of primary health workers and medical auxiliaries with sufficient knowledge and skills with regard to treatment of malaria and its prevention.

Every health project in a developing country, which is supported by an advanced country or by an international agency, should contain a training component. Moreover, every such project should be co-ordinated with the relevant country's overall health programme.

The general consensus is that training facilities for the diagnosis of malaria, its treatment and its control should be provided for medical, professional and auxiliary personnel involved in clinical and public health aspects of communicable disease in developing and developed countries. The old generation of 'blood, mud and sweat' malariologists has nearly disappeared and much of their experience has been largely forgotten. The author of the present book hopes that he has contributed to forging a link between the not so distant past and the new generation of primary health workers and specialists in tropical community health.

Selected bibliography

The bibliography on malaria is immense and the following section concentrates on publications of the past 10 years, although they comprise some important titles of the previous period. The most extensive list of references on various aspects of malaria up to about 1946 will be found in M. F. Boyd's *Malariology*, two volumes (1949). An even more extensive list of references up to 1987 is to be found in W. H. Wernsdorfer and Sir I. McGregor's *Malaria, Principles and Practice of Malariology*, two volumes (1988), Churchill Livingstone. For those interested in parasitology of malaria, P. C. C. Garnham's *Malaria Parasites and other Haemosporidia* (1966), and G. R. Coatney *et al.* (1971) *The Primate Malarias* provide a rich source of references. Many basic references on various aspects of malaria up to 1962 are quoted at the end of each chapter of the substantial (and still valuable) *Practical Malariology* by P. F. Russell, L. S. West, R. D. Manwell, and G. Macdonald, (1963).

For chemotherapy of malaria the following books are a mine of bibliographical data: G. M. Findlay, *Recent Advances in Chemotherapy* Vol. II (third edition), (1950–51); W. Peters, *Chemotherapy and Drug Resistance in Malaria*, two volumes, 2nd edition (1987); P. E. Thompson and L. M. Werbel, *Antimalarial Agents* (1972). A complete and up-to-date monograph on all relevant aspects is *Practical chemotherapy of malaria* (1990), the report of a WHO Scientific Working Group, Technical Report Series No. 805.

For most aspects of malaria eradication the text and references contained in E. J. Pampana's *A Textbook of Malaria Eradication*, 2nd edition (1969), are still of great value, while for a revised approach to malaria control in Africa *Malaria and Planning for its Control in Tropical Africa* (1989) WHO/UNDP emphasizes the reorientation that will be required within the context of the implementation of the Global Strategy for Health for All by the Year 2000.

The various indepth facets of forest-related malaria, including numerous pertinent references, are available in *Forest Malaria in South East Asia* (1991) (Sharma V. P., Kondrashin A. V., eds) WHO/MRC Meeting, New Delhi.

Malaria – Waiting for the Vaccine (Targett G. A. T., ed.) indicates what one can do now and in the near future to control malaria, utilizing the resources available.

Malaria – Obstacles and Opportunities (1991) (Oaks S. C., Mitchell V. S., Pearson G. W., Carpenter C. C. J., eds) Institute of Medicine, National Academy Press, Washington DC, is a wide ranging review of the problems and possibilities relating to the global control of malaria.

Finally a recent French text on malaria *'Paludisme'*, (1992) edited by Danis M. and Mouchet J., Ellipses, Paris, gives the most comprehensive Francophone viewpoint on the subject.

For keeping abreast of the large volume of publications on all subjects directly or indirectly related to research on and control of malaria the *Tropical Diseases Bulletin*, issued monthly by the Bureau of Tropical Diseases in London, is invaluable.

In the present book, particular attention has been given to the sources of authoritative and abundant information on problems of malaria and its control, provided over the past decade by the World Health Organization. Catalogues of WHO publications are produced by the Organization's headquarters in Geneva and by the regional offices. The complete catalogue of the World Health Organization's publications for 1948–89 is available.

The *Bulletin of the World Health Organization* is its main regular scientific journal.

WHO *Technical Reports Series* present the findings of international groups of experts, who provide the latest scientific advice on specific medical and public health problems. Summaries of these reports are often included in the *WHO Chronicle* which regularly reviews all activities of the Organization.

WHO *Weekly Epidemiological Record* brings important news of significance for the control of communicable diseases. Many issues of *WER* contain valuable reviews such as: (1) synopsis of the world malaria situation (with periodic information on areas where resistance of *P. falciparum* to present drugs has been recorded); (2) information on malaria risk for international travellers; (3) advice on chemoprophylaxis of malaria; (4) reports on malaria surveillance in certain countries and areas.

Among other publications, sponsored or otherwise, linked with the World Health Organization a number of excellent manuals on the practice of malaria control are highly recommended. Important series of documents on malaria are released by the UNDP/World Bank/WHO Special Programme for Research and Training in Tropical Diseases. These publications comprise comprehensive progress reports, proceedings of research meetings and also quarterly bibliographies of major tropical diseases.

Finally, two series of cyclostyled documents dealing with various aspects of research on and control of malaria are distributed by the World Health Organization to institutes and individual scientists or public health workers. Special issues containing abstracts in English of Chinese publications on malaria are available. These documents known as WHO/Mal, WHO/CTD or WHO/VBC reports can be forwarded on request to interested professional persons by writing to the World Health Organization, Documents Distribution Section, 1211, Geneva, Switzerland.

In view of the many new bibliographical facilities now available for most of the topics dealt with in this book, a simplified presentation of references has been adopted. The following pages indicate predominantly recent publications, except for some older titles important or relevant to the origin of illustrations. They are presented in alphabetical order.

Selected references*

Abel L., Cot M., Lambertus M., Carnevale P., Feingold V. (1992) Segregation analysis detects a major gene controlling blood infection levels in human malaria. *American Journal of Human Genetics* **50**: 1308–17.

Agency for International Development (1982) *Manual of Malaria Control in Primary Health Care in Africa.* Washington DC: AID Bureau for Africa.

Agency for International Development (1983) *AID Malaria Strategy Workshop.* Baltimore: Insect Control and Research.

Aikawa M., Miller L. H., Johnson J., Rabbege J. (1978) Erythrocyte entry by malaria parasites: A moving junction between erythrocyte and parasite. *Journal of Cell Biology* **77**: 72–82.

Aikawa M., Miller L. H., Rabbege J. R., Epstein N. (1981) Freeze fracture study on the erythrocyte membrane during malaria parasite invasion. *Journal of Cell Biology* **91**: 55–62.

Aikawa M. (1988) Human cerebral malaria. *American Journal of Tropical Medicine and Hygiene* **39**: 3–10.

Aikawa M., Atkinson C. T. (1990) Immunoelectron microscopy of parasites. *Advances in Parasitology* **29**: 151–214.

Aikawa M., Iseki M., Barnwell J. W., Taylor D., Oo M. M., Howard R. J. (1990) The pathology of human cerebral malaria. *American Journal of Tropical Medicine and Hygiene* **42**: 30–7.

Aikawa M., Miller L. H. (1983) Structural alterations of the erythrocyte membrane during malaria parasite invasion and development. In *Malaria and the Red Cell* (Evered D., Whelan J., eds), pp. 45–59. London: Ciba Foundation.

Aikawa M., Suzuki M., Gutierrez Y. (1980) Pathology of malaria. In *Malaria*, Vol. 2 (Kreier J. P., ed.) pp. 47–102. New York and London: Academic Press.

Allison A. C., Eugui E. M. (1982) A radical interpretation of immunity to malaria parasites. *Lancet* **ii**: 1431–3.

Alonso P. L., Hill A. G., David P. H., Fegan G., Armstrong J. R. H., Andreas F., Cham K., Greenwood B. H. (1992) The impact of treated bed-nets on childhood mortality in the Gambia. *The World Bank Policy Research Working Papers. WPS* 383.

Ambroise-Thomas P. (1980) La vaccination contre le paludisme. *Cahiers ORSTOM* **18**: 132–48.

American Journal of Tropical Medicine and Hygiene (1990) Symposium on cytoadherence and cerebral malaria. **43**: Supplement 1–42.

Anderson W. K. (1927) *Malaria Psychoses and Neuroses. Their Medical, Sociological and Legal Aspects.* London: Oxford University Press.

Banguero H. (1984) Socio-economic factors associated with malaria in Colombia. *Social Science and Medicine* **19**: 1099–104.

Bannister L. H., Sinden R. E. (1982) New knowledge of parasite morphology. *British Medical Bulletin* **38**: 141–6.

Barker R. H. (1990) DNA probe diagnosis of parasitic infections. *Experimental Parasitology* **70**: 494–9.

Bateman D. N., Dyson E. H. (1986) Quinine toxicity. *Advances in Drug Reactions and Poisons Review* **4**: 215–33.

Baudon D., Roux J., Carnevale P., Guigembde T. A. (1983) La chimiotherapie systematique des accés febriles dans la lutte contre le paludisme en milieu rural. *Médecine Tropicale* **43**: 341–6:

Beale G. H. (1979) *Genetics of Drug Resistance of Malaria Parasites.* WHO/Mal 79.911. Geneva: World Health Organization.

Beales P. F., Orlov V. S., Kovzaetsov R. L. (1989) *Malaria and Planning for its Control in Tropical Africa.* Moscow: WHO/UNDP.

Beier J. C., Asiago C. M., Onyango F. K., Koros J. K. (1988) ELISA absorbence cut-off method affects malaria sporozoite rate determination in wild Afrotropical *Anopheles. Medical and Veterinary Entomology* **2**: 259–64.

Belkin Y. N. (1962) *The Mosquitoes of the South Pacific (Dip-*

***Some of the older references included in the 2nd edition have been omitted.**

tera, Culicidae), Vols I and II. Los Angeles: University of California Press.

Bennish M. L., Azad A. K., Rahman O., Phillips R. E. (1990) Hypoglycemia during diarrhea in childhood. Prevalence, pathophysiology and outcome. *New England Journal of Medicine* **322**: 1357–63.

Berendt A. R., Simmons D. L., Tansey J., Newbold C. I., Marsh K. (1989) Intercellular adhesion molecule-1 is an endothelial cell adhesion receptor for *Plasmodium falciparum*. *Nature* **341**: 57–9.

Black R. H., (1968) *Manual of Epidemiological Services in Malaria Programmes*. Geneva: World Health Organization.

Black R. H. (1982) *Malaria in Australia* (Tropical Medical Technical Papers). Canberra: Australian Government Publishing Services.

Blocker W. W., Kastle A. J., Daroof R. B. (1968) The psychiatric manifestations of cerebral malaria. *American Journal of Psychiatry* **125**: 192–6.

Boland M. E., Brennand Roper S. M., Henry J. A. (1985) Complications of quinine poisoning. *Lancet* **i**: 384–5.

Borrelly R. (1974) *L'Economie du Paludisme*. Grenoble: Institut de Recherche Economique et de Planification.

Bown D. N., Rodriguez M. H., Arrendondo-Jimenez J. I., Loyola E. G., Rodriguez M. C. (1991) Age structure and abundance levels in the entomological evaluation of an insecticide used in the control of *Anopheles albimanus* in southern Mexico. *Journal of the American Mosquito Control Association* **7**: 180–7.

Boyd M. F., ed. (1949) *Malariology*, Vols I and II. Philadelphia: W. B. Saunders Co.

Brabin B. (1990) An analysis of malaria parasite rates in infants: 40 years after Macdonald. *Tropical Diseases Bulletin* **87**: R1–R27.

Brabin B. J. (1991) The risks and severity of malaria in pregnant women. *UNDP/World Bank/WHO. Applied Field Research in Malaria Reports No. 1*. Geneva: WHO.

Bradley D. J. (1993) Prophylaxis against malaria for travellers from the United Kingdom. Report of a meeting convened by the Malaria Reference Laboratory and the Ross Institute. *British Medical Journal* (in press, May).

Bradley D. J., Newbold C. I., Warrell D. A. (1987) Malaria. In *Oxford Textbook of Medicine*, 2nd edition (Weatherall D. J., Ledingham J. G. G., Warrell D. A., eds) pp. 5.474–5.502. Oxford: Oxford University Press.

Bray R. S., Garnham P. C. C. (1982) Life-cycle of primate malaria parasites. *British Medical Bulletin* **38**: 117–22.

Brewster D. R., Greenwood B. M. (1993) Seasonality of paediatric diseases in the Gambia, West Africa. *Annals of Tropical Paediatrics* **2**: 139–52.

Brewster D. R., Kwiatkowski D., White N. J. (1990) Neurological sequelae of cerebral malaria in children. *Lancet* **336**: 1039–43.

Brooks M. H., Kiel F. W., Sheehy T. W., Barry K. G. (1968) Acute pulmonary edema in falciparum malaria. *New England Journal of Medicine* **279**: 732–7.

Brown A. W. A. (1986) Insecticide resistance in mosquitos: a pragmatic review. *Journal of the American Mosquito Control Association* **2**: 123–40.

Brown A. W. A., Haworth J., Zahar A. A. (1976) Malaria eradication and control from a global standpoint. *Journal of Medical Entomology* **13**: 1–25.

Brown K. N. (1980) Host resistance in malaria. In *Critical Reviews in Tropical Medicine* (Chandra R. K., ed.) pp. 6–182. London: Plenum Press.

Bruce-Chwatt L. J. (1979) Man against malaria. Conquest or defeat? *Transactions of the Royal Society of Tropical Medicine and Hygiene* **73**: 605–17.

Bruce-Chwatt L. J. (1982) Chemoprophylaxis in Africa: the spent magic bullet. *British Medical Journal* **285**: 674–6.

Bruce-Chwatt L. J. (1982) Imported malaria: an uninvited guest. *British Medical Bulletin* **38**: 179–86.

Bruce-Chwatt L. J. (1982) Transfusion malaria revisited. *Tropical Diseases Bulletin* **79**: 827–40.

Bruce-Chwatt L. J. (1983) Malaria control and primary health care: or the art of squaring the circle. *Bulletin de la Société de Pathologie Exotique* **76**: 477–85.

Bruce-Chwatt L. J. (1987) Quinine and the mystery of blackwater fever. *Acta Leidensia* **55**: 181–96.

Bruce-Chwatt L. J. (1987) Malaria and its control. Present situation and future prospects. *Annual Review of Public Health* **8**: 75–110.

Bruce-Chwatt L. J., de Zulueta J. (1980) *The Rise and Fall of Malaria in Europe*. Oxford: Oxford University Press.

Burkot T. R. (1988) Non-random host selection by anopheline mosquitos. *Parasitology Today* **4**: 156–62.

Burkot T. R., Dye C., Graves P. M. (1989) An analysis of some factors determining the sporozoite rates, human blood indexes, and biting rates of members of the *Anopheles punctulatus* complex in Papua New Guinea. *American Journal of Tropical Medicine and Hygiene* **40**: 229–34.

Busvine J. A. (1978) The future of insecticidal control of medically important insects. In *Medical Entomology Centenary Symposium*, pp. 106–11. London: Royal Society of Tropical Medicine and Hygiene.

Cairncross S., Feachem R. G. (1983) *Environmental Health Engineering in the Tropics*. Chichester, New York: John Wiley.

Campbell C. C., Collins W. E., Nguyen-Dinh P., Barber A., Broderson J. R. (1982) *Plasmodium falciparum* gametocytes from culture *in vitro* develop to sporozoites that are infectious to primates. *Science* **217**: 1048–50.

Canfield C. J. (1980) Antimalarial aminoalcohol alternatives to mefloquine. *Acta Tropica (Basel)* **37**: 232–7.

Canfield C. J., Rozman A. S. (1974) Clinical testing of new antimalarial compounds. *Bulletin of the World Health Organization* **50**: 203–12.

Carlson J., Helmby H., Hill A. V. S., Brester D., Greenwood B. M., Wahlgren M. (1990) Human cerebral malaria: association with erythrocyte rosetting and lack of anti-rosetting antibodies. *Lancet* **336**: 1457–60.

Carnevale P., Mouchet J. (1980) Le paludisme en zone de transmission continue en région afrotropicale. *Cahiers ORSTOM* **18**: 162–70.

Centres for Disease Control (1992) *Health Information for International Travel 1992*. HHS Publication No. (CDC) 92–8280. Atlanta.

Centers for Disease Control (1992) Recommendations for the prevention of malaria among travellers. *Morbidity and Mortality Weekly Report.*

Chanthavanich P., Looareesuwan S., White N. J., Warrell D. A., Warrell M. J., Digiovanni J. H., von Bredow J. (1985) Intragastric mefloquine is absorbed rapidly in patients with cerebral malaria. *American Journal of Tropical Medicine and Hygiene* **34**: 1028–36.

Chapman H. C., ed. (1985) *Biological Control of Mosquitoes*. Fresno: American Mosquito Control Association.

Charmot G. (1980) Facteurs congenitaux et facteurs génetiques dans la résistance au paludisme en Afrique tropicale. *Médecine Tropicale* **40**: 657–66.

Charmot G., Amat-Roze J. M., Rhodun F. *et al.* (1991) Abord géographique de l'epidemiologie de la chloroquino-résistance de *Plasmodium falciparum* en Afrique tropicale. *Annals de la Société Belge de Médecine Tropicale* **71**: 187–97.

Charoenpan P., Indraprasit S., Kiatboonsri S., Suvachittanont O., Tanomsup S. (1990) Pulmonary edema in severe falciparum malaria. Hemodynamic study and clinicopathophysiologic correlation. *Chest* **97**: 1190–7.

Chinese Society of Protozoologists (1982) *Malaria and Other Protozoal Diseases*. Zhongshan (Sun Yatsen) University, Guangzhou, China.

Chow C-Y. (1991) Malaria vectors in China. *Chinese Journal of Entomology Special Publication* **6**.

Christophers S. R., Sinton J. A., Covell G. (revised by Jaswant Singh and Puri I. M.) (1959) *How to do a Malaria Survey*. Delhi: Government of India Press.

Cisgriff T. M., Boudreau E. F., Pamplin C. L., Doberstyn E. B., Desjardins R. E., Canfield C. J. (1983) Evaluation of antimalarial activity of the phenanthrene methanol, halofantrine. *American Journal of Tropical Medicine and Hygiene* **31**: 1075–9.

Clark H. C., Tomlinson W. J. (1949) That pathologic anatomy of malaria. In *Malariology*, Vol. 2 (Boyd M. F., ed.) pp. 874–903. Philadelphia: W. B. Saunders.

Clark I. A., Cowden W. B., Butcher G. A. (1983) Free oxygen radical generators as antimalaria drugs. *Lancet* **i**: 234.

Clark I. A., Rockett K. A.,Cowden W. B. (1992). Possible central role of nitric oxide in conditions clinically similar to cerebral malaria. *Lancet* **340** 894–6.

Clyde D. F. (1967) *Malaria in Tanzania*. London, New York, Toronto: Oxford University Press.

Clyde D. F., McCarthy V. C., Miller R. M., Woodward W. E. (1975) Immunization of man against falciparum and vivax malaria by use of attenuated sporozoites. *American Journal of Tropical Medicine and Hygiene* **24**: 397–401.

Coatney G. A., Collins W. E., Warren McW., Contacos P. G. (1971) *The Primate Malarias*. US Department of Health, Education and Welfare, National Institutes of Health, Bethesda, Maryland.

Cochrane A. H., Aikawa M., Jeng M., Nussenzweig R. S. (1976) Antibody induced ultrastructural changes of malarial sporozoites. *Journal of Immunology* **116**: 859–67.

Cockburn A., ed. (1967) *Infectious Diseases: Their Evolution and Eradication*. Springfield, Illinois: Charles Thomas.

Coffee R. A. (1979) Electrodynamic energy – a new approach to pesticide application. *Proceedings 1979 Crop Protection Conference – Pests and Diseases*, **22**: 777–89.

Cogswell F. B. (1992) The hypnozoite and relapse in primate malaria. *Chemical Microbiology Reviews* **5**: 26–35.

Cohen S. (1979) Immunity to malaria. *Proceedings of the Royal Society* **203**: 323–45.

Cohen S. (1982) Progress in malaria vaccine development. *British Medical Bulletin* **38**: 161–5.

Cohen S., ed. (1982) Malaria. *British Medical Bulletin* **38**: 115–218.

Collins F. H., Finnerty V., Petrarca V. (1988) Ribosomal DNA probes differentiate five cryptic species in the *Anopheles gambiae* complex. *Parassitologia* **30**: 231–40.

Collins F. H., Petrarca V., Mpofu S., Brandling-Bennett A. D., Were J. B. O., Rasmussen M. O., Finnerty V. (1988) Comparison of DNA probe and cytogenetic methods for identifying field collected *Anopheles gambiae* complex mosquitos. *American Journal of Tropical Medicine and Hygiene* **39**: 545–50.

Collins R. T., Dash B. K., Agarwala B. S., Dahl K. B. (1983) *An Adaptation of the Gel Diffusion Technique for Identifying the Source of Mosquito Blood Meals*. WHO/Mal./83.992. Geneva: World Health Organization.

Coluzzi M., Petrarca V., Di Deco M. (1985) Chromosomal inversion intergradation and incipient speciation in *Anopheles gambiae*. *Bolletino di Zoologia* **52**: 45–63.

Coluzzi M., Sabatini A., Petrarca V., Di Deco M. A. (1979) Chromosomal differentiation and adaptation to human environment in the *A. gambiae* complex. *Transactions of the Royal Society of Tropical Medicine and Hygiene* **73**: 483–97.

Conly G. N. (1975) *The Impact of Malaria on Economic Development: A Case Study*. Washington DC: Pan-American Health Organization Publication No. 297.

Cova-Garcia P. (1961) *Notas Sobre los anofelinos de Venezuela y su Identification*, 2nd edition. Caracas: Editoria Grafas.

Covell G. (1950) Congenital malaria. *Tropical Diseases Bulletin* **47**: 1147–67.

Curtis C. F. *et al.* (1990) Impregnated bed nets and curtains against malaria mosquitos. In *Appropriate Technology in Vector Control* (Curtis C. F., ed.) pp. 5–46. Boca Raton: CRC Press.

Curtis C. F., ed. (1990) *Appropriate Technology in Vector Control*. Boca Raton: CRC Press.

Daškova N. G., Rasnicyn S. P. (1982) Review of data on susceptibility of mosquitos in the USSR to imported strains of malaria parasites. *Bulletin of the World Health Organization* **60**: 893–7.

David P. H., Hommel M., Miller L. H., Udeinya I. J., Oligino L. D. (1983) Parasite sequestration in *Plasmodium falciparum* malaria: spleen and antibody modulation of cytoadherence of infected erythrocytes. *Proceedings of the National Academy of Sciences* **80**: 5075–9.

Davidson G. (1964) *Anopheles gambiae*, a complex of species. *Bulletin of the World Health Organization* **31**: 625–34.

Davidson G. (1980) Overview of genetic mechanisms as an alternative to chemical control. *Miscellaneous Publications of the Entomological Society of America* **11**: 12–27.

Davidson G. (1982) Application of genetics in studying vector control and evolution. In *Recent Developments in the Genetics of Insect Disease Vectors* (Steiner W. W. *et al.*, eds). Champaign: Stipes Publishing Co.

Davis T. M. E., Supanaranond W., Pukrittayakamee S., Karbwang J., Molunto P., Mekthon S., White N. J. (1990) A safe and effective consecutive-infusion regimen for rapid quinine loading in severe falciparum malaria. *Journal of Infectious Diseases* **161**: 1305–8.

de Barjac H., Sutherland D. J. (1990) Bacterial control of mosquitos and black flies. *Biochemistry, Genetics and Applications of Bacillus thurgiensis israelensis and Bacillus sphoericies*. London: Unwin Hyman.

Delforme D. R., Wirtz R. A., Loong K. P., Lewis G. E. (1989) Identification of sporozoites in *Anopheles maculatus* from Malaysia by enzyme-linked immunosorbent assays. *Tropical Biomedicine* **6**: 21–6.

Department of Health, Republic of China (1992) Mosquito-borne diseases in mainland China. *Epidemiology Bulletin* **8**: 184–5.

Deroff P., Reuger M., Simitzis A. M., Boudon A., Saleun J. P. (1982) Depistage des donneurs de sang susceptibles de transmettre *P. falciparum*. *Revue Française de Transfusion et d'Immunohématologie* **25**: 3–11.

Desowitz R. S., Miller L. H. (1980) A perspective on malaria vaccines. *Bulletin of the World Health Organization* **58**: 897–908.

Detinova T. S. (1962) *Age-grouping Methods in Diptera of Medical Importance: With Special Reference to Some Vectors of Malaria*. Monograph Series No. 47. Geneva: World Health Organization.

Dietz K. (1988) Mathematical models for transmission and control of malaria. In *Malaria – Principles and Practice of Malariology*, Vol. 2 (Wernsdorfer W. H., McGregor Sir I., eds) pp. 1091–113. Edinburgh: Churchill Livingstone.

Diggs C. L. (1980) Prospects for development of vaccines against *P. falciparum* infection. In *Malaria*, Vol. 3 (Kreier J. P., ed.) pp. 299–316. New York and London: Academic Press.

Doberstyn E. B., Phintuyothin P., Noeypatimanondh S., Teerakiartkamjorn C. (1979) Single-dose therapy of falciparum malaria with mefloquine pyrimethamine–sulfadoxine. *Bulletin of the World Health Organization* **57**: 275–9.

Draper C. C., Sirr S. S. (1980) Serological investigations in retrospective diagnosis of malaria. *British Medical Journal* **284**: 1575–6.

Duarte M. I. S., Corbett C. E. P., Boulos M., Amato Neto V. (1985) Ultrastructure of the lung in falciparum malaria. *American Journal of Tropical Medicine and Hygiene* **34**: 31–5.

Dye C. (1992) The analysis of parasite transmission by blood-sucking insects. *Annual Review of Entomology* **37**: 1–19.

Edington G., Gilles H. M. (1982) *Pathology in the Tropics*, 2nd edition. London: Edward Arnold.

Edington G. M. (1967) Pathology of malaria in West Africa. *British Medical Journal* **i**: 715–18.

Editorial (1983) Pyrimethamine combinations in pregnancy. *Lancet* **ii**: 1005–7.

Editorial (1984) Human malaria gene cloned. *Science* **225**: 607–8.

Evered D., Whelan J., eds (1983) *Malaria and the Red Cell*. Ciba Foundation symposium 94. London: Pitman Books.

Field J. W., Sandosham A. A., Fong Y. L. (1963) *The Microscopical Diagnosis of Human Malaria*, Parts I and II. Kuala Lumpur: Institute for Medical Research Federation of Malaysia.

Findlay G. M. (1950–51) *Recent Advances in Chemotherapy*, 3rd edition, 2 vols. London: J. & A. Churchill Ltd.

Fitz-Hugh T., Pepper D. S., Hopkins H. U. (1944) The cerebral form of malaria. *Bulletin of the US Army Medical Department* **83**: 39–48.

Fogarty International Center (1982) Can infectious diseases be eradicated? *Report of the International Conference* (Stuart Morris C., Western K. A., Chamberlayne E. C., eds). *Review of Infectious Diseases* **4**: 913–84.

Fontaine R. E., Pull J. H., Payne D. Pradhan G. D., Joshi G. P., Pearson J. A., Thymakis M. K., Ramos Camacho M. E. (1978) Evaluation of fenitrothion for the control of malaria. *Bulletin of the World Health Organization* **56**: 445–52.

Foster S. D. F. (1991) The distribution and use of antimalarial drugs – not a pretty picture. In *Malaria*

Waiting for the Vaccine (Targett G. A. T., ed.) pp. 123–40. Chichester: John Wiley.

Friedman K. Y. (1978) Erythrocytic mechanism of sickle cell resistance to malaria. *Proceedings of the National Academy of Sciences* **75**: 1994–7.

Friedman M., Trager W. (1981) The biochemistry of resistance to malaria. *Scientific American* **225**: 113–19.

Gabaldon A. (1969) Global eradication of malaria: Changes of strategy and future outlook. *American Journal of Tropical Medicine and Hygiene* **18**: 641–56.

Gaffigan T. V., Ward R. A. (1985) Index to the second supplement of 'A catalog of the mosquitos of the world', with corrections and additions. *Mosquito Systematics* **17**: 52–63.

Gale K. R., Crampton J. M. (1988) Use of a male-specific DNA probe to distinguish female mosquitos of the *Anopheles gambiae* species complex. *Medical and Veterinary Entomology* **2**: 77–9.

Garnham P. C. C. (1966) *Malaria Parasites and Other Haemosporidia*. Oxford: Blackwell Scientific Publications.

Garnham P. C. C. (1977) The continuing mystery of relapses in malarias. *Protozoological Abstracts* **1**: 1–12.

Garnham P. C. C. (1980) Malaria in its various vertebrate hosts. In *Malaria*, Vol. 1 (Kreier J. P., ed.) pp. 96–144. New York and London: Academic Press.

Garnham P. C. C. (1988) Swellengrebel lecture. Hypnozoites and 'relapses' in *Plasmodium vivax* and in vivax-like malaria. *Tropical and Geographical Medicine* **40**: 187–95.

Garnham P. C. C., Krotoski W. A., Bray R. S., Killick-Kendrick R., Cogwell F. (1983) Relapse in primary malaria: A reply. *Transactions of the Royal Society of Tropical Medicine and Hygiene* **77**: 736–7.

Garnham P. C. C., Pierce A. E., Roitt I., eds (1963) *Immunity to Protozoa*. Oxford: Blackwell Scientific Publications.

Gentilini M. (1993) Paludisme. *Santé Cahiers d'Etudes et de Recherches Francophones* 3, No. 2.

Gerberich J. B. (1985) Update of annotated bibliography of papers relating to the control of mosquitos by the use of fish for the years 1965–1981. Mimeographed document. WHO/VBC/85.917. Geneva: World Health Organization.

Gilles H. M. (1991)— Malaria. In *Current Medicine*. Edinburgh: Churchill Livingstone.

Gilles H. M. (1991) Management of severe and complicated malaria. *A Practical Handbook*. Geneva: World Health Organization.

Gilles H. M., Lawson J. B. Sibelas M., Voller A., Allan N. (1969) Malaria, anaemia and pregnancy. *Annals of Tropical Medicine and Parasitology* **62**: 245–63.

Gillet J. D. (1985) The behaviour of homosapiens, the forgotten factor in the transmission of tropical disease. *Transactions of the Royal Society of Tropical Medicine and Hygiene* **79**: 12–20.

Gillies M. T. (1977) Confidence and doubt in the history of anopheline control. *Patrick Manson Centenary Symposium Proceedings*, pp. 26–9. London: Royal Society of Tropical Medicine and Hygiene.

Gillies M. T., Coetzee M. (1987) *A Supplement to the Anophelinae of Africa South of the Sahara (Afrotropical Region)*. Johannesburg: South African Institute of Medical Research.

Gillies M. T., De Meillon B. (1968) *The Anophelinae of Africa South of the Sahara*. Johannesburg: South African Institute for Medical Research.

Gilroy A. B. (1948) *Malaria Control by Coastal Swamp Drainage in West Africa*. London: Ross Institute of Tropical Medicine.

Glik D. C. *et al.* (1989) Malaria treatment practices among mothers in Guinea. *Journal of Health and Social Behaviour* **30**: 421–35.

Gopinanthan V. P., Subramanian A. R. (1982) Pernicious syndromes in plasmodial infections. *Medical Journal of Australia* **11**: 568–72.

Gorduek V., Thuma P., Brittenham G. *et al.* (1992) Effect of iron chelation therapy on recovery from deep coma in children with cerebral malaria. *New England Journal of Medicine* **327**: 1473–4.

Gorduek V., Thuma P. E., Brittenham G. M. *et al.* (1992) Iron chelation with desferrioxamine B in adults with asymptomatic *Plasmodium falciparum* parasitemia. *Blood* **79**: 308–12.

Goreham J. R., Stojanovich C. J. (1973) Clave ilustrada para los mosquitos anofelinos de sudamerica occidental. Illustrated keys to the anopheline mosquitos of western South America. *Mosquito Systematics* **5**: 97–156.

Gozal A., Hengg C., Fadat G. (1991) Prolong malaria prophylaxis with chloroquine and proguanil (chloroguamicide) in a non-immune resident population of an endemic area with a high prevalence of chloroquine resistance. *Antimicrobial Agents and Chemotherapy* **35**: 373–6.

Gramiccia C., Hempel Y. (1972) Mortality and morbidity from malaria in countries where malaria eradication is not making satisfactory progress. *Journal of Tropical Medicine and Hygiene* **75**, 187–92.

Gratz N. G. (1977) The importance of chemicals in the control of tropical diseases. In *Chemie der Pflanzenschutz – und Schadlings Bekampfungsmittel*, Vol. III (Wegler R., ed.) pp. 86–180. Berlin, Heidelberg, New York: Springer-Verlag.

Grau G. E., Taylor T. E., Molyneux M. E., Wirima J. J., Vassalli P., Hommel M., Lambert P. H. (1989) Tumor necrosis factor and disease severity in children with falciparum malaria. *New England Journal of Medicine* **320**: 1586–91.

Greenwood B. (1991) An analysis of malaria parasite rates in infants: 40 years after Macdonald. A response. *Tropical Diseases Bulletin* **88**: R1–R3.

Greenwood B. M., Bradley A. H., Greenwood A. M. *et al.* (1987) Mortality and morbidity from malaria among children in a rural area of the Gambia, West Africa. *Transactions of the Royal Society of Tropical Medicine and Hygiene* **81**: 478–86.

Greenwood B. M., Greenwood A. M., Bradley A. H. *et al.* (1987) Deaths in infancy and early childhood in a well-vaccinated rural West African population. *Annals of Tropical Paediatrics* **7**: 91–9.

Greenwood B. M., Greenwood A. M., Bradley A. H. *et al.* (1988) Comparison of two different strategies for control of malaria within a primary health care programme in the Gambia. *Lancet* **i**: 1121–7.

Greenwood B. M., Marsh K., Snow R. (1991) Why do some African children develop severe malaria? *Parasitology Today* **7**: 277–81.

Guan W. B., Huang W. J., Zhou Y. C., Gong J. Z. (1982) Effect *in vitro* of artemisinine and its derivatives on *Plasmodium falciparum*. *Acta Pharmacologica Sinica* **3**: 139–41.

Gutteridge W. W., Coombs G. H. (1977) *Biochemistry of Parasitic Protozoa*. London: Macmillan Press.

Guyer R., Candy D. (1979) Injectable antimalarial therapy in tropical Africa: iatrogenic disease and wasted medical resources. *Transactions of the Royal Society of Tropical Medicine and Hygiene* **73**: 230–2.

Hackett L. W. (1937) *Malaria in Europe*. London: Oxford University Press

Hamilton D. R., Pikacha D. (1982) Ruptured spleen in a malarious area: with emphasis on conservative management in both adults and children. *Australia and New Zealand Journal of Surgery* **52**: 310–13.

Hamon J., Mouchet J., Brengues Y., Chauvet G. (1970) Vector ecology and behaviour before, during and after application of control measures. *Miscellaneous Publications of the Entomological Society of America* **7**: 28–41.

Handunnetti S. M., Gilladoga A. D., Van Schravendijk M.-R., Nakamura K.-I., Aikawa M., Howard R. J. (1992) Purification and *in vitro* selection of rosette-positive (R+) and rosette-negative (R−) phenotypes of knob-positive *Plasmodium falciparum* parasites. *American Journal of Tropical Medicine and Hygiene* **46**: 371–81.

Harinasuta T., Dixon K. E., Warrell D. A., Doberstyn E. B. (1982) Recent advances in malaria with special reference to Southeast Asia. *The Southeast Asian Journal of Tropical Medicine and Public Health* **13**: 1–35.

Harrison B. A. (1980) Medical Entomology Studies – XIII. The Myzomyia series of *Anopheles* (*Cellia*) in Thailand, with emphasis on intraspecific variations (*Diptera*: *Culicidae*). *Contributions of the American Entomological Society* **17**: 1–195.

Harrison B. A., Scanlon J. E. (1975) Medical entomological studies – II. The subgenus *Anopheles* in Thailand (*Diptera*: *Culicidae*). *Contributions of the American Entomological Society* **12**: 1–307.

Harrison G. (1978) *Mosquitoes, Malaria and Man*. London: John Murray.

Hatton C. S. R., Peto T. E. A., Bunch C., Pasvol G., Russell S. J., Singer C. R. J., Edwards G., Winstanley P. (1986) High incidence of severe neutropenia associated with amodiaquine prophylaxis for malaria. *Lancet* **i**: 411–14.

Haworth J. (1991) Malaria in man. Its epidemiology, clinical aspects and control. *Tropical Diseases Bulletin* **88**: R1–R80.

Heymann D. L. *et al.* (1990) Antenal chloroquine chemoprophylaxis in Malawi: chloroquine resistance, compliance, protective efficacy and cost. *Transactions of the Royal Society of Tropical Medicine and Hygiene* **84**: 496–8.

Hien T. T., White N. J. (1993) Qinghaosu. *Lancet* **341**: 603–8.

Higgins Hardin E., Nussenzweig R. S., Bryan J. H., McGregor I. A. (1981) Congenital transfer of antibodies against malaria sporozoites detected in Gambian infants. *American Journal of Tropical Medicine and Hygiene* **30**: 1159–61.

Hildemann W. H., Walford R. S. (1963) Annual fishes: Promising species as biological control agents. *Journal of Tropical Medicine and Hygiene* **66**: 163–6.

Hill A. V. S. *et al.* (1992) Common West African HLA antigens are associated with protection from severe malaria. *Nature* **352**: 595–600.

Hill A. V. S. *et al.* (1992) Molecular analysis of the association of HLA-B53 and resistance to severe malaria. *Nature* **360**: 434–9.

Ho M., White N. J., Looareesuwan S., Wattanagoon Y., Lee S. H., Walport M. J., Bunnag D., Harinasuta T. (1990) Splenic Fc-receptor function in host defence and anemia in acute falciparum malaria. *Journal of Infectious Diseases* **161**: 555–61.

Hoffman S. L., Rustama D., Punjabi N. H., Surampaet B., Sanjaya B., Dimpudus A. J., McKee K. T., Paleologo F. P., Campbell J. R., Marwoto H., Laughlin L. (1988) High-dose dexamethasone in quinine-treated patients with cerebral malaria: a double-blind placebo-controlled trial. *Journal of Infectious Diseases* **158**: 325–31.

Hongvivatana T., Leerapan P., Chaiteeranuwatsiri M. (1985) *Knowledge Perception and Behaviour of Malaria*. Bangkok: Monograph Series, Center for Health Policy Studies, Mahidol University.

Hongvivatana T., Leerapan P., Smithisampan M. (1982) An observational study of DDT house-spraying in a rural area of Thailand. *Journal of Tropical Medicine and Hygiene* **85**: 245–50.

Howard R. J., Gilladoga A. D. (1989) Molecular studies related to the pathogenesis of cerebral malaria. *Blood* **74**: 2603–18.

Institut de Médecine Tropicale du Service de Santé des Armées (1982) Le Paludisme. *Médecine Tropicale* **42**: 363–462.

Jeffery G. M. (1975) Malaria control in the twentieth century. *American Journal of Tropical Medicine and Hygiene* **25**: 361–70.

Jennett B., Plum F. (1972) Persistent vegetative state after brain damage. A syndrome in search of a name. *Lancet* **i**: 734–7.

Jing-Bo Jiang, Xing-Bo Guo, Guo-Aiao Li, Yun Cheung Kong, Arnold K. (1982) Antimalarial activity of mefloquine and qinghaosu. *Lancet* **2**: 285–8.

Jing-Bo Jiang *et al.* (1982) Long incubation of *Plasmodium vivax multinucleatum* as demonstrated in three experimental human cases. *Transactions of the Royal Society of Tropical Medicine and Hygiene* **76**: 845–7.

Kaewsonthi S., Harding A. G. (1984) Cost and performance of malaria surveillance in Thailand. *Social Science and Medicine* **19**: 1081–97.

Karbwang J., Harinasuta T. (1992) *Chemotherapy of Malaria in South East Asia*, pp. 147. Bangkok: Ruamtesena Co. Ltd.

Kaul D. K., Roth E. F., Nagel R. L., Howard R. J., Handunnetti S. M. (1991) Rosetting of *Plasmodium falciparum*-infected red blood cells with uninfected red blood cells enhances microvascular obstruction under flow conditions. *Blood* **78**: 812–19.

Kelton J. G., Keystone J., Moore J., Denomme G., Tozman E., Glynn M., Neame P. B., Gouldie J., Jensen J. (1983) Immune-mediated thrombocytopenia of malaria. *Journal of Clinical Investigation* **71**: 832–6.

Kemp D. J., Cowman A. F., Walliker D. (1990) Genetic diversity in *Plasmodium falciparum. Advances in Parasitology* **29**: 75–149.

Keusch G. T., ed. (1982) The biology of parasitic infections. *Reviews of Infectious Diseases* **4**: 735–905.

Killick-Kendrick R., Peters W. (1978) *Rodent Malaria.* London and New York: Academic Press.

Kitzmiller J. B. (1982) *Anopheline Names: Their Derivations and Histories.* Washington: Thomas Say Foundation.

Knight K. L. (1978) *Supplement to a Catalog of the Mosquitoes of the World (Diptera: Culicidae).* 6 Supplement. Washington: Thomas Say Foundation. Maryland: Entomological Society of America.

Knight K. L., Stone A. (1977) *A Catalog of the Mosquitoes of the World.* Washington: Thomas Say Foundation.

Knüttgen H. J. (1987) The bone marrow of non-immune Europeans in acute malaria infection: a topical review. *Annals of Tropical Medicine and Parasitology* **81**: 567–76.

Kofi-Ekue J. M., Ulrich A. M., Rhabwogo-Atenyi J., Sheth U. K. (1983) A double-blind comparative clinical trial of mefloquine and chloroquine in symptomatic falciparum malaria. *Bulletin of the World Health Organization* **61**: 713–18.

Kortmann H. F. (1972) *Malaria and Pregnancy*, Thesis. Elinkwijk, Utrecht: University of Utrecht.

Kramer S. G., Campbell C. C., Moncrieff R. E. (1983) Fulminant *P. falciparum* infection treated with exchange blood transfusion. *Journal of the American Medical Association* **249**: 244–5.

Kreier J. P., ed. (1980) *Malaria*, 3 vols. New York and London: Academic Press.

Kreer, J. P., Ristic M., Baker J. R. (1989) *Malaria and Babesiosis.* 3rd International Congress on Malaria and Babesiosis, Annecy, France, September 1987. *Royal Society of Tropical Medicine and Hygiene* **83** (Supplement), 1–107.

Krotoski W. A., Bray R. S., Garnham P. C. C. *et al.* (1982) Observations on early and late post-sporozoite tissue stages in primate malaria II. The hypnozoite of *P. cynomolgi. American Journal of Tropical Medicine and Hygiene* **31**: 211–25.

Krotoski W. A., Garnham P. C. C., Bray R. S. *et al.* (1982) Observations on early and late post-sporozoite tissue stages in human malaria, I Discovery of a new latent form of *P. cynomolgi. American Journal of Tropical Medicine and Hygiene* **31**: 24–35.

Kwiatkowski D., Cannon J. G., Manogue K. R., Cerami A., Dinarello C. A., Greenwood B. M. (1989) Tumour necrosis factor production in falciparum malaria and its association with schizont rupture. *Clinical & Experimental Immunology* **77**: 361–6.

Kwiatkowski D., Hill A. V. S., Sambou I., Twumasi P., Castracane J., Manogue K. R., Cerami A., Brewster D. R., Greenwood B. M. (1990) TNF concentration in fatal cerebral, non-fatal cerebral and uncomplicated *Plasmodium falciparum* malaria. *Lancet* **336**: 1201–4.

Kwiatkowski D., Molyneux M. E., Stephens S., Curtis N., Klein N., Pontaire P., Smit M., Allan R., Brewster D. R., Gray G. E., Greenwood B. M. (1993) Anti-TNF therapy inhibits fever in cerebral malaria. *Quarterly Journal of Medicine* **86**: 91–8.

Laird M. (1988) *The Natural History of Larval Mosquito Habitats.* London: Academic Press.

Laird M., Miles J. W. (1985) *Integrated Mosquito Control Methodologies*, Vols 1 and 2. London: Academic Press.

Lanar D. E., McLaughlin G. L., Wirth D. F., Barker R. J., Zolg W., Chulay J. D. (1989) Comparison of thick films, *in vitro* culture and DNA hybridization probes for detecting *Plasmodium falciparum* malaria. *American Journal of Tropical Medicine and Hygiene* **40**: 3–6.

Langreth S. G., Jensen J. B., Rise, R. T., Trager W. (1978) Fine structure of human malaria *in vitro. Journal of Protozoology* **25**: 443–51.

Lawson J. B. (1967) Malaria in pregnancy. In *Obstetrics and Gynaecology in the Tropics* (Lawson J. B., Steward D. B., eds) pp. 59–72. London: Edward Arnold.

Lee D. J., Hicks M. M., Griffiths M., Debenham M. L., Bryan J. H., Russell R. C., Geary M., Marks E. N. (1987) *The Culicidae of the Australian Region*, Vol. 5, *Nomenclature, Synonyms, Literature, Distribution, Biology and Relation to Disease. Genus Anopheles. Subgenera Anopheles, Cellia.* Monograph Series, Entomology Monograph No. 2. Canberra: Commonwealth Department of Health, School of Public Health and Tropical Medicine, Australian Government Publishing Service.

Lee D. J., Woodhill A. R. (1944) *The Anopheline Mosquitoes of the Australian Region.* Zoological Publication No. 2, Sydney University.

Lee S. H., Looareesuwan S., Wattanagoon Y., Ho M., Wuthiekanun V., Vilaiwanna N., Weatherall D. J., White N. J. (1989) Antibody dependent red cell removal during *P. falciparum* malaria: the clearance of red cells sensitized with IgG anti-D. *British Journal of Haematology* **73**: 396–402.

Lindsay S. W., Gibson M. E. (1988) Bednets revisited – old idea, new angle. *Parasitology Today* **4**: 270–2.

Lines J. D. (1978) Do agricultural insecticides select for insecticide resistance in mosquitoes? A look at the evidence. *Parasitology Today* **4**: 517–20.

Linthicum K. J. (1988) A revision of the *argyritarsis* section of the subgenus *Nyssorhynchus* of *Anopheles* (Diptera: Culicidae). *Mosquito Systematics* **20**: 98–271.

Lobel H., Campbell C. C. (1983) Trends in imported malaria in USA. *Morbidity and Mortality Weekly Report, Surveillance Summary* **32**: 15–18.

Looareesuwan S., Warrell D. A., White N. J. *et al.* (1983) Retinal haemorrhages, a common sign of prognostic significance in cerebral malaria. *American Journal of Tropical Medicine and Hygiene* **32**: 911–15.

Looareesuwan S., Ho M., Wattanagoon Y., White N. J., Warrell D. A., Bunnag D., Harinasuta T., Wyler D. J. (1987) Dynamic alteration in splenic function during acute falciparum malaria. *New England Journal of Medicine* **317**: 675–9.

Looareesuwan S., Merry A. H., Phillips R. E., Pleehacinda R., Wattanagoon Y., Ho M., Charoenlarp P., Warrell D. A., Weatherall D. J. (1987) Reduced erythrocyte survival following clearance of malarial parasitaemia in Thai patients. *British Journal of Haematology* **67**: 473–8.

Looareesuwan S., Phillips R. E., Karbwang J., White N. J., Flegg P. J., Warrell D. A. (1900) *Plasmodium falciparum* hyperparasitaemia: use of exchange transfusion in seven patients and a review of the literature. *Quarterly Journal of Medicine* **75**: 471–81.

Looareesuwan S., Phillips R. E., White N. J., Kietinun S., Karbwang J., Rackow C., Turner R. C., Warrell D. A. (1985) Quinine and severe falciparum malaria in late pregnancy. *Lancet* **ii**: 4–8.

Looareesuwan S., Viravan C., Vanijanonta S., Wilairatana P., Suntharoisamai P., Charoenlarp P., Arnold K., Kyle D., Canfield C., Weboter K. (1992). Randomised trial of artesunate and mefloquine alone and in sequence for acute uncomplicated falciparum malaria. *Lancet* **339**: 821–4.

Looareesuwan S., Warrell D. A., White N. J., Suntharasamai P., Chanthavanich P., Sundaravej K., Juel-Jensen B. E., Bunnag D., Harinasuta T. (1983) Do patients with cerebral malaria have cerebral oedema? A computed tomography study. *Lancet* **i**: 434–7.

Luzzato L. (1979) Genetics of red cells and susceptibility to malaria. *Blood* **54**: 961–7.

Lysenko A. Y., Semashko I. N. (1968) Geography of malaria. In *Medical Geography* (Lebedev A. W., ed.). Moscow: Academy of Sciences USSR.

MacCormack C. P., Lwihula G. (1983) Failure to participate in a malaria chemosuppression programme: North Mara, Tanzania. *Journal of Tropical Medicine and Hygiene* **86**: 99–108.

MacCormack C. P. *et al.* (1989) Use of insecticide impregnated bed nets in Gambian primary health care: economic aspects. *Bulletin of the World Health Organization* **67**: 209–14.

Macdonald G. (1957) *The Epidemiology and Control of Malaria.* London, New York, Toronto: Oxford University Press.

Macdonald G. (1973) *Dynamics of Tropical Disease* (Bruce-Chwatt L. J., Glanville V., eds). London: Oxford University Press.

Mackey L. J., McGregor I. A., Paounova N., Lambert P. H. (1982) Diagnosis of *P. falciparum* infection in man: Detection of parasite antigens by ELISA. *Bulletin of the World Health Organization* **60**: 69–75.

MacPherson G. G., Warrell M. J., White N. J., Looareesuwan S., Warrell D. A. (1985) Human cerebral malaria: a quantitative ultrastructural analysis of parasitized erythrocyte sequestration. *American Journal of Pathology* **119**: 385–401.

Maegraith B. G. (1948) *Pathological Processes in Malaria and Blackwater Fever.* Oxford: Blackwell Scientific Publications.

Mahler H. (1983) Primary health care: Health for all and the role of doctors. *Tropical Doctor* **13**: 146–8.

Malaria Commission, Committee of Medical Sciences, Chinese Peoples Republic (1983) Epidemiological status of malaria in the Peoples Republic of China in 1981. *Journal of Parasitology and Parasitic Diseases* **1**: 2–21.

Mann R. D., Phillips-Howard P. A. (1989) Malaria in Britain. *Journal of the Royal Society of Medicine* **82** (Supplement No. 17): 1–70.

Manson P. (1898) *Tropical Diseases. A Manual of the Diseases of Warm Climates.* London: Cassell.

Manson-Bahr C. (1987) *Manson's Tropical Diseases*, 19th edition (Bell D. R., ed.). London: Baillière Tindall.

Marchi A., Munstermann L. E. (1987) The mosquitoes of Sardinia: species records 35 years after the malaria eradication campaign. *Medical and Veterinary Entomology* **1**: 89–96.

Marchiafava E., Bignami A. (1894) *On Summer, Autumn Malarial Fevers.* Translated from the 1st Italian edition by J. H. Thompson. London: The New Sydenham Society.

McGregor I. A. (1972) Immunology of malarial infection and its possible consequences. *British Medical Bulletin* **28**: 12–17.

McGregor I. A. (1983) Current concepts concerning man's resistance to infection with malaria. *Bulletin de la Société de Pathologie Exotique* **76**: 433–45.

McGregor I. A., Billewicz W. Z., Thomson A. M. (1961) Growth and mortality in children in an African village. *British Medical Journal* **2**: 1661–6.

McGregor I. A., Rahman A. R., Thomson A. M. *et al.* (1970) The health of young children in a West African (Gambian) village. *Transactions of the Royal Society of Tropical Medicine and Hygiene* **64**: 48–77.

McGregor I. A., Wilson M. E., Billewicz W. Z. (1983) Malaria infection of the placenta in the Gambia, West Africa; its incidence and relationship to stillbirth birthweight and placental weight. *Transactions of the Royal Society of Tropical Medicine and Hygiene* **77**: 232–44.

Médecine Tropicale (1982) Le paludisme. *Proceedings of a Symposium on Malaria* **42**: 363–462.

Merry A. H., Looareesuwan S., Phillips R. E., Chanthavanich P., Supanaranond W., Warrell D. A., Weatherall D. J. (1986) Evidence against immune haemolysis in falciparum malaria in Thailand. *British Journal of Haematology* **64**: 187–94.

Miller J. E., Lindsay S. N., Armstrong J. R. (1991) Experimental hut trials of bed nets impregnated with synthetic pyrethroid or organophosphate insecticide for mosquito control in the Gambia. *Medical and Veterinary Entomology* **5**: 465–76.

Miller K. D., Greenberg A. E., Campbell C. C. (1989) Treatment of severe malaria in the United States with continuous infusions of quinidine gluconate and exchange transfusion. *New England Journal of Medicine* **321**: 65–70.

Miller K. D., Lobel H. O., Satriale R. F., Kuritsky J. N., Stern R., Campbell C. C. (1986) Severe cutaneous reactions among American travellers using pyrimethamine–sulfadoxine (Fansidar) for malarial prophylaxis. *American Journal of Tropical Medicine and Hygiene* **35**: 451–8.

Miller L. H. (1991) Postscript. In *Waiting for the Vaccine* (Targett G. A. T., ed.) pp. 220–4. Chichester: John Wiley.

Miller L. H., Chien S., Usami S. (1972) Decreased deformability of *Plasmodium coatneyi* infected red cells and its possible relation to cerebral malaria. *American Journal of Tropical Medicine and Hygiene* **21**: 133–7.

Miller L. H., Fremount H. N., Luse S. A. (1971) Deep vascular schizogony of *Plasmodium knowlesi* in *Macaca mulatta.* Distribution in organs and ultrastructure of parasitized red cells. *American Journal of Tropical Medicine and Hygiene* **20**: 816–24.

Miller L. H., Usami S., Chien S. (1971) Alteration in the rheologic properties of *Plasmodium knowlesi*-infected red cells. A possible mechanism for capillary obstruction. *Journal of Clinical Investigation* **50**: 1451–5.

Milligan P. J. M., Phillips A., Molyneux D. H., Subbarao S. K., White G. B. (1986) Differentiation of *Anopheles culicifacies* Giles (Diptera: Culicidae) sibling species by analysis of cuticular components. *Bulletin of Entomological Research* **76**: 529–37.

Mills A. (1991) Economics of malaria control. In *Malaria – Waiting for the Vaccine* (Targett G. A. T., ed.) pp. 140–68. Chichester: John Wiley.

Molineaux L., Gramiccia G. (1980) *The Garki Project.* Research on epidemiology and control of malaria in the Sudan Savannah of West Africa. Geneva: World Health Organization.

Molyneux M. E., Looareesuwan S., Menzies I. S., Grainger S. L., Phillips R. E., Wattanagoon Y., Thompson R. P. H., Warrell D. A. (1989) Reduced hepatic blood flow and intestinal malabsorption in severe falciparum malaria. *American Journal of Tropical Medicine and Hygiene* **40**: 470–6.

Molyneux M. E., Taylor T. E., Wirima J. J., Borgstein A. (1989) Clinical features and prognostic indicators in paediatric cerebral malaria: a study of 131 comatose Malawian children. *Quarterly Journal of Medicine* **71**: 441–59.

Morray J. P., Tyler D. C., Jones T. K., Stuntz J. T., Lemire R. J. (1984) Coma scale for use in brain-injured children. *Critical Care Medicine* **12**: 1018–20.

Mosha F. W., Petrarca V. (1983) Ecological studies on *Anopheles gambiae* complex sibling species on the Kenya Coast. *Transactions of the Royal Society of Tropical Medicine and Hygiene* **77**: 344–8.

Most H. (1940) Malignant malaria among drug addicts. Epidemiological, clinical and laboratory studies. *Transactions of the Royal Society of Tropical Medicine and Hygiene* **34**: 139–72.

Mpofu S. H., Kanyimo K. H., Masendu H. (1991) Potential use of bendiocarb (FICAM VC) for malaria control in an area of Zimbabwe. *Journal of the American Mosquito Control Association* **7**: 536–42.

Murphy G. S., Basri H., Purnomo E. M. *et al.* (1993) Vivax malaria resistant to treatment and prophylaxis with chloroquine. *Lancet* **341**: 96–100.

Mutabingura T. K. (1993) *Studies on Malaria Chemosuppression During Pregnancy in Tanzania.* Amsterdam: M.D. Thesis.

Najera J., Liese B., Hammer J. S. (1991) Malaria. In *Disease Control Priorities in Developing Countries* (Jameson

D. T., Mosley W. H., eds). New York: Oxford University Press for the World Bank.

Nash G., O'Brien E., Gordon-Smith E. C., Dormandy J. A. (1989) Abnormalities in the mechanical properties of red blood cells caused by *Plasmodium falciparum*. *Blood* **74**: 855–61.

Newton C. R. J. C., Kirkham F. J., Winstanley P. A., Pasvol G., Peshu N., Warrell D. A., Marsh K. (1991) Intracranial pressure in African children with cerebral malaria. *Lancet* **337**: 573–6.

Newton C. R. J. C., Pasvol G., Winstanley P. A., Warrell D. A. (1990) Cerebral malaria: what is unarousable coma. *Lancet* **i**: 472.

Nguyen-Dinh P., Chemangey-Masaba S., Harrison Spencer C., Campbell C. C., Chin W., Collins W. E. (1981) *Comparative Studies on the Cryopreservation of Malaria Parasites*. WHO/Mal document 81.941. Geneva: World Health Organization.

Nguyen-Dinh P., Spencer H. C., Masaba S. C., Churchill F. C. (1982) Susceptibility of *P. falciparum* to pyrimethamine and sulfadoxine–pyrimethamine in Kisumu, Kenya. *Lancet* **1**: 823–5.

Ockenhouse C. F., Tegoshi T., Maeno Y., Benjamin C., Ho M., Khin-Ei-Kan, Ye-Thuray, Kyan Win, Aikawa M., Lobb R. R. (1992) Human vascular endothelial cell adhesion receptors for *Plasmodium falciparum*-infected erythrocytes: roles for endothelial leukocyte adhesion molecule 1 and vascular cell adhesion molecule 1. *Journal of Experimental Medicine* **176**: 1183–9.

Ogunmekan D. A. (1983) Control of malaria with special reference to socio economic factors. *Tropical Doctor* **13**: 186.

Olatunde A., Obih P. O. (1981) Use and misuse of 4-aminoquinoline antimalarials in tropical Africa and re-examination of itch reaction to these drugs. *Tropical Doctor* **11**: 97–101.

Onori E. (1986) Malaria. *Clinics in Tropical Medicine and Communicable Diseases* **1**: 463–512.

Onori E., Grab B. (1980) Indicators for the forecasting of malaria epidemics. *Bulletin of the World Health Organization* **58**: 91–8.

Onori E., Grab B., Ambroise-Thomas P., Thelu J. (1982) Incipient resistance of *P. falciparum* to chloroquine among a semi-immune population of Tanzania. *Bulletin of the World Health Organization* **60**: 899–906.

Onori E., Muir D. (1985) Malaria vector species complexes and intra specific variations: Relevance for malaria control and orientation for future research. Mimeographed document. Special Programme for Research and Training in Tropical Diseases. TDR/FIELDMAL/BANGKOK/WP/85.4, Geneva: World Health Organization.

Pampana E. Y. (1969) *A Textbook of Malaria Eradication*, 2nd edition. London, New York, Toronto: Oxford University Press.

Pan-American Health Organization (1990) Status of malaria programmes in the Americas. XLII Regional Committee Meeting, Washington DC.

Pant C. P., Houba V., Engers H. D. (1987) Bloodmeal identification in vectors. *Parasitology Today* **3**: 324–6.

Pasvol G., Newton C. R. J. C., Winstanley P. A., Watkins W. M., Peshu N. M., Were J. B. O., Marsh K., Warrell D. A. (1992) Quinine treatment of severe falciparum malaria in African children; a randomized comparison of three regimens. *American Journal of Tropical Medicine and Hygiene* **45**: 702–13.

Pasvol G., Wilson R. J. M. (1982) Malaria and the red cells. *British Medical Bulletin* **38**: 133–40.

Patarroyo M. E. *et al.* (1988) A synthetic vaccine protects humans against challenge with asexual blood stage of *P. falciparum* malaria. *Nature* (London) **332**: 158–61.

Pattanayak S., Roy R. G., Samnotra K. G., Bendley M. S. (1981) Urban malaria scheme of the national Malaria Eradication Programme of India. *Indian Journal of Malariology* **18**: 21–7.

Payet M., Coulaud J. P. (1976) *Les Maladies d'Importation*. Paris: Masson.

Payne D. (1982) Practical aspects of the *in vivo* testing for sensitivity of human plasmodia to antimalarials. WHO/Mal documents 82.988. Geneva: World Health Organization.

Payne D. (1988) Use and limitations of light microscopy for diagnosing malaria at the primary health care level. *Bulletin of the World Health Organization* **66**: 621–6.

Pène O., André L. J., Rougemont A., Bourgeade A., Barabé P. (1981) *Santé et Médecine en Afrique Tropicale*. Paris: Doin.

Perrin L. H., Dayal R. (1982) Immunity to asexual erythrocytic stages of *P. falciparum*: Role of defined antigens in the humoral response. *Immunological Review* **61**: 245–69.

Perrin L. H., Ramirez E., Lambert P. H., Miescher P. A. (1982) Inhibition of *P. falciparum* growth in human erythrocytes by monoclonal antibodies. *Nature* (London) **289**: 301–3.

Perring F. H., Mellanby K. (1978) *Ecological Effects of Pesticides*. London: Academic Press.

Persing D. H., Landry M. L. (1989) *In vitro* amplification techniques for the detection of nucleic acids: new tools for the diagnostic laboratory. *Yale Journal of Biology and Medicine* **62**: 159–71.

Peters W. (1987) *Chemotherapy and Drug Resistance in Malaria*, 2nd edition, Vols 1 and 2. London: Academic Press.

Peters W., Richards W. H. G., eds (1984) *Antimalarial Drugs*, 2 vols. Berlin, Heidelberg, New York, Tokyo: Springer-Verlag.

Peto T. E. A., Gilks C. F. (1986) Strategies for the prevention of malaria in travellers: comparison of drug regimens by means of risk–benefit analysis. *Lancet* **i**: 1256–61.

Phillips R. E., Looareesuwan S., Warrell D. A., Lee S. H., Karbwang J., Warrell M. J., White N. J., Swasdichai C., Weatherall D. J. (1986) The importance of anaemia in cerebral and uncomplicated falciparum malaria: role of complications, dyserythropoiesis and iron sequestration. *Quarterly Journal of Medicine* **227**: 305–23.

Phillips R. E., Warrell D. A., Looareesuwan S., Turner R. C., Bloom S. R., Quantrill D., Moore A. R. (1986) Effectiveness of SMS201–995, a synthetic, long-acting somatostatin analogue in treatment of quinine-induced hyperinsulinaemia. *Lancet* **i**: 713–16.

Phillips R. E., Warrell D. A., White N. J., Looareesuwan S., Karbwang J. (1985) Intravenous quinidine for the treatment of severe falciparum malaria. Clinical and pharmacokinetic studies. *New England Journal of Medicine* **312**: 1273–8.

Phillips R. S. (1983) *Malaria*. London: Edward Arnold.

Picq J. J. (1982) Epidemiologie du paludisme-première endemie mondiale. *Médecine Tropicale* **42**: 365–81.

Playfair J. H. L. (1982) *Immunology at a Glance*. Oxford: Blackwell Scientific Publications.

Playfair J. H. L. (1982) Immunity to Malaria. *British Medical Bulletin* **38**: 153–9.

Pull J. H., Grab B. (1974) A simple epidemiological model for evaluating the malaria inoculation rate and the risk of infection in infants. *Bulletin of the World Health Organization* **51**: 507–16.

Qari S. H., Shi Y-P., Goldman I. F., Udhayakumar V., Alpers M. P., Collins W. E., Lal A. A. (1993) Identification of *Plasmodium vivax*-like human malaria parasite. *Lancet* **341**: 780–3.

Ramalingaswami V., Satyarvati G. V., eds (1979) Hundred years of malaria research. *Indian Journal of Medical Research* (Supplement) **70**: 1–127.

Ramsdale C. D., de Zulueta J. (1983) Anophelism in the Algerian Sahara and some implications of the construction of the trans-Saharan highway. *Journal of Tropical Medicine and Hygiene* **86**: 51–8.

Ramsey J. M., Baudoin R. L., Bawden M. P., Espinal C. A. (1983) Specific identification of *Plasmodium* sporozoites using an indirect fluorescent antibody method. *Transactions of the Royal Society of Tropical Medicine and Hygiene* **77**: 378–83.

Ramsey J. M., Bown D. N., Aron J. L., Baudoin R. L., Mendez J. F. (1986) Field trial in Chiapas, Mexico, of a rapid detection method for malaria in anopheline vectors with low infection rates. *American Journal of Tropical Medicine and Hygiene* **35**: 234–8.

Ranque J. (1976) Le paludisme post-transfusionnel en France. *Revue Française de Transfusion et Immunohématologie* **19**: 315–24.

Rao T. R. (1981) Problems in malaria research. *Indian Journal of Malariology* **18**: 4–11.

Rao T. R. (1983) *The Anophelines of India*, revised edition. Delhi: Malaria Research Centre.

Ray A. P. (1979) Some aspects of *P. falciparum* containment programme. *Indian Journal of Medical Research* **70**: 1–13.

Ray A. P. (1981) Some aspects of the socio-economic impact of malaria and its control. *Indian Journal of Malariology* **18**: 12–20.

Ray A. P., Sharma G. K., eds (1984) The socio-economic aspects in the context of malaria and its control. In *Indo-UK Workshop on Malaria*. Delhi: Malaria Research Centre.

Reacher M., Freeman J., Campbell C. C., Robertson E. B., Bennett A. D. (1981) Drug therapy for *P. falciparum* malaria resistant to Fansidar in Eastern Thailand. *Lancet* **ii**: 1066–8.

Reid J. A. (1968) *Anopheline Mosquitoes of Malaya and Borneo*. Studies from the Institute for Medical Research, No. 21. Kuala Lumpur: Government of Malaysia.

Reilly P. L., Simpson D. A., Sprod R., Thomas L. (1988) Assessing the conscious level in infants and young children: a paediatric version of the Glasgow coma scale. *Child's Nervous System* **4**: 30–3.

Richards W. H. G. (1979) Some promising leads in experimental antimalarial drugs. *Advances in Pharmacology and Therapeutics* **10**: 71–8.

Richards W. H. G., Maples B. K. (1979) Studies on *P. falciparum* in continuous cultivation I. The effects of chloroquine and pyrimethamine on parasite growth and viability. *Annals of Tropical Medicine and Parasitology* **73**: 99–108.

Rieckmann K. H. (1982) Visual *in vitro* test for determining the drug sensitivity of *P. falciparum*. *Lancet* **1**: 1333–4.

Rieckmann K. H., Campbell G. H., Sax L. J., Mrema J. E. (1978) Drug sensitivity of *P. falciparum*: An *in vitro* technique. *Lancet* **1**: 22–3.

Riganti M., Pongponratn E., Tegoshi T., Looareesuwan S., Punpoowong B., Aikawa M. (1990) Human cerebral malaria in Thailand: a clinicopathological correlation. *Immunology Letters* **25**: 199–206.

Robert V., Ouari B., Ouedraogo V., Carnevale P. (1988) Etudes ecologiques des Culicidae adultes et larvaires dans une riziére en vallée du Kou, Burkina Faso. *Acta Tropica* **45**: 351–9.

Robert V., Petrarca V., Carnevale P., Ovazza L., Coluzzi M. (1989) Analyse cytogénetique du complexe *Anopheles gambiae* dans la région de Bobo-Dioulasso (Burkina Faso). *Annales de Parasitologie Humaine et Comparée* **64**: 290–311.

Robert V., Verhave J. P., Ponnudurai T., Louwe L., Scholtens P., Carnevale P. (1988) Study of the distribution of circumsporozoite antigen in *Anopheles gambiae* infected with *Plasmodium falciparum* using the enzyme-linked immunosorbent assay. *Transactions of the Royal Society of Tropical Medicine and Hygiene* **82**: 389–91.

Roberts D., Beck L., Rodriguez M. *et al.* (1992) *Options and Priorities in the Use of Remote Sensing for Human Health Applications; The NASA Experience.* Abstracts, 13th International Congress of Tropical Medicine and Malaria, Vol. 1.

Roberts D. J., Craig A. G., Berendt A. R., Pincher R., Nash G., Marsh K., Newbold C. I. (1992) Rapid switching to multiple antigenic and adhesive phenotypes in malaria. *Nature* **357**: 689–92.

Roberts D. W., Daoust R. A., Wraight S. P. (1983) *Bibliography of Pathogens of Medically Important Arthropods: 1981.* WHO/VBC/83.1. Geneva: World Health Organization.

Roberts D. W., Strand M. A. (1977) Pathogens of medically important arthropods. *Bulletin of the World Health Organization* **55** (Supplement): 1–419.

Rodhain F., Perez C. (1985) *Précis d'Entomologie Médicale et Vétérinaire. Notions d'Épidémiologie des Malades à Vecteurs.* Paris: Maloine S. A. Editeur.

Rodriguez da Silva L., Locke M., Dayal R., Perrin L. H. (1983) *P. falciparum* polypeptides released during *in vitro* cultivation. *Bulletin of the World Health Organization* **61**: 105–12.

Roitt I. (1980) *Essential Immunology*, 4th edition. Oxford: Blackwell Scientific Publications.

Rojas W., Northrop J., Gallo O., Monyoya A. E., Restrepo M., Nimnich G., Arango M., Echavarria M. (1987) Reduction in malaria prevalence after introduction of *Romanomermis culicivorax* (Mermithidae: Nematoda) in larval habitats in Colombia. *Bulletin of the World Health Organization* **65**: 331–7.

Roncoroni A. J., Martino D. A. (1979) Therapeutic use of exchange transfusion in malaria. *American Journal of Tropical Medicine and Hygiene* **28**: 490–544.

Rosenfield P., Widstrand C. G., Ruderman A. P. (1981) Social and Economic Research in the UNDP/World Bank/WHO special programme for Research and Training in Tropical Diseases. *Social Science and Medicine* **15A**: 529–38.

Roux J., Baudon D., Carnevale P., Guigemde T. R., Picq J. J. (1983) La chimioprophylaxie collective du paludisme, ses limites, ses difficultés. *Médecine Tropicale* **43**: 347–52.

Rozendaal J. A. (1989) Impregnated mosquito nets and curtains for self-protection and vector control. *Tropical Diseases Bulletin* **86**: R1–R41.

Russell P. F. (1952) *Malaria: Basic Principles Briefly Stated.* Oxford: Blackwell Scientific Publications.

Russell P. F. (1955) *Man's Mastery of Malaria.* New York, Toronto: Oxford University Press.

Russell P. F., Rozeboom L. E., Stone A. (1943) *Keys to the Anopheline Mosquitoes of the World.* Philadelphia: American Entomological Society.

Russell P. F., West, L. S., Manwell R. D., Macdonald G. (1963) *Practical Malariology*, 2nd edition. London, New York, Toronto: Oxford University Press.

Sandosham A. A., Thomas V. (1983) *Malariology, with Special Reference to Malaya*, 3rd edition. Singapore: University Press.

Saul A. (1992) Towards a malaria vaccine: riding the roller coaster between unrealistic optimism and lethal pessimism. *Southeast Asian Journal of Tropical Medicine and Public Health* **23**: 656–71.

Schmidt L. H. (1978) *Plasmodium falciparum* and *Plasmodium vivax* infections in the owl monkey (*Aotus trivirgatus*) I. The courses of untreated infections. *American Journal of Tropical Medicine and Hygiene* **27**: 671–702.

Schmidt L. H. (1978) *Plasmodium falciparum* and *Plasmodium vivax* infections in the owl monkey (*Aotus trivirgatus*) II. Responses to chloroquine, quinine, and pyrimethamine. *American Journal of Tropical Medicine and Hygiene* **27**: 703–17.

Schmidt L. H. (1978) *Plasmodium falciparum* and *Plasmodium vivax* infections in the owl monkey (*Aotus trivirgatus*) III. Methods employed in the search for new blood schizonticidal drugs. *American Journal of Tropical Medicine and Hygiene* **27**: 718–37.

Schmidt L. H. (1983) Relationships between chemical structures of 8-amino-quinolines and their capacities for radical cure of infections with *P. cynomolgi* in rhesus monkeys. *Antimicrobial Agents and Chemotherapy* **24**: 615–52.

Schmidt L. H., Crosby R., Rasco J., Vaughan D. (1978) The antimalarial activities of various 4-quinolinemethanols with special attention to WR-142,490 (mefloquine). *Antimicrobial Agents and Chemotherapy* **13**: 1011–30.

Sénevet G., Andarelli G. (1955) *Les Anophèles de l'Afrique du Nord et du Bassin Mediterranéen.* Paris: Maloine.

Sergiev P. G., ed. (1968) *Multivolume Manual on the Microbiology, Clinical Aspects and Epidemiology of Infectious Diseases*, Vol. 9. *Malaria* (in Russian). Moscow: Medicina.

Service M. W. (1976) *Mosquito Ecology; Field Sampling Methods.* London: Applied Science Publishers.

Service M. W. (1978) Some problems in the control of malaria. In *Ecological Effects of Pesticides* (Perring F. H., Mellanby K., eds) pp. 151–64. London: Academic Press.

Service M. W. (1980) *A Guide to Medical Entomology.* London: Macmillan.

Service M. W. (1981) Ecological considerations in the biocontrol strategies against mosquitoes. In *Biocontrol of Medical and Veterinary Pests* (Laird M., ed.) pp. 173–95. New York: Praeger Publishers.

Service M. W. (1983) Biological control of mosquitoes – has it a future? *Mosquito News* **43**: 113–20.

Service M. W. (1986) *Lecture Notes on Medical Entomology.* Oxford: Blackwell Scientific Publications.

Service M. W., ed. (1989) *Demography and Vector-Borne Diseases.* Boca Raton: CRC Press.

Service M. W. (1993) Mosquitos (Culicidae). In *Medical Insects and Arachnids* (Lane R. P., Crosskey R. W., eds) (in press). London: The Natural History Museum.

Service M. W. (1993) *Mosquito Ecology. Field Sampling Methods*, 2nd edition. London: Elsevier.

Service M. W., Voller A., Bidwell D. (1986) The use of the ELISA technique for the identification of blood meals of mosquitoes and other haematophagous insects. *Bulletin of Entomological Research* **76**: 321–30.

Sharma V. P. (1984) *Proceedings of the Indo-UK Workshop on Malaria*, November 1983. Delhi: Malaria Research Centre.

Sharma V. P. (1991) Environmental management in malaria control in India. In *Malaria Waiting for the Vaccine* (Targett G. A. T., ed.) pp. 49–66. Chichester: John Wiley.

Sharma V. P., Kondrashin A. V. (1991) *Proceedings of an Informal Consultative Meeting*. New Delhi: WHO/MRC.

Shepard D. S. (1991) Economic impact of malaria in Africa. *Tropical Medicine and Parasitology* **42** (Supplement 1): 197–224.

Shortt H. E. (1983) Relapse in primate malaria: Its implications for the disease of man. *Transactions of the Royal Society of Tropical Medicine and Hygiene* **77**: 734–6.

Shute P. G., Maryon M. (1960) *Laboratory Technique for the Study of Malaria*. London: J. A. Churchill.

Sinden R. E., Canning G. V., Bray R. S., Smalley M. E. (1978) Gametocyte and gamete development in *P. falciparum*. *Proceedings of the Royal Society* **B 201**: 375–99.

Singh J., Tham A. S. (1988) Case history on malaria vector control through the application of environmental management in Malaysia. Mimeographed document. WHO/VBC/88. Geneva: World Health Organization.

Sitprija V. (1988) Nephropathy in falciparum malaria. *Kidney International* **34**: 867–77.

Slater A. F., Cerami A. (1992) Inhibition by chloroquine of a novel haem polymerase enzyme activity in malaria trophozoites. *Nature* **355**: 167–9. (Also Comment *Nature* **355**: 108–9, 1992.)

Smith H., Nelson J. A., Gatimberg C. G., Crandall I., Sherman I. W. (1992) *Plasmodium falciparum*: cytoadherence of malaria-infected erythrocytes to human brain capillary and umbilical vein endothelial cells – a comparative study of adhesive ligands. *Experimental Parasitology* **75**, 269–80.

Sotiroff-Junker J. (1978) *A Bibliography on the Behavioural, Social and Economic Aspects of Malaria and its Control*. Geneva: WHO Offset Publications No. 42.

Sornmani S., Fungladda W. (1991) *Social and Economic Aspects of Malaria Control*. Bangkok: Museum and Reference Centre (MRC-Tropmed).

de Souza J. M. (1983) A phase I clinical trial of mefloquine in Brazilian male subjects. *Bulletin of the World Health Organization* **61**: 809–14.

de Souza J. M. (1983) A phase II clinical trial of mefloquine in Brazilian male subjects. *Bulletin of the World Health Organization* **61**: 815–20.

Spencer H. C., Chemengay-Masaba S., Chulay J. D., Nguyen-Dinh P. (1983) Field evaluation in Kenya of a 48-hour test for *P. falciparum* sensitivity to chloroquine. *American Journal of Tropical Medicine and Hygiene* **32**: 916–21.

Spencer H. C., Karobki D. M. (1983) *In vivo* and *in vitro* chloroquine resistance in *P. falciparum* from Kenya infants. *American Journal of Tropical Medicine and Hygiene* **32**: 922–5.

Spencer H. C., Kaseje D. C., Koech D. K. (1983) The Kenya Saradidi Community Malaria Project I. Response of *Plasmodium falciparum* isolates to chloroquine in 1981 and 1982. *Transactions of the Royal Society of Tropical Medicine and Hygiene* **77**: 689–92.

Spira D. T., Greenblatt C. L., eds (1978) *Malaria – Immunology and Immunopathology*. Basel: Karger.

Spitz S. (1946) The pathology of acute falciparum malaria. *Military Surgery* **99**: 555–72.

Stoker N. G. (1990) The polymerase chain reaction and infectious diseases: hopes and realities. *Transactions of the Royal Society of Tropical Medicine and Hygiene* **84**: 755–8.

Strickland G. T. (1986) *Clinics in Tropical Medicine and Communicable Diseases*, Vol. 1, Number 1, *Malaria*. London: W. B. Saunders.

Subbarao S. K., Vasantha K., Sharma V. P. (1988) Cytotaxonomy of certain malaria vectors. In *Biosystematics of Haematophagous Insects* (Service M. W., ed.) pp. 25–37. The Systematics Association Special Volume No. 37. Oxford: Oxford University Press.

Sucharit P., Suntharasamai P., Chintana T., Harinasuta T. (1979) *In vivo* and *in vitro* studies of quinine sensitivity of *P. falciparum* in Thailand. *Southeast Asian Journal of Tropical Medicine and Public Health* **10**: 137–41.

Sucharit S., Supavej S. (1987) *Practical Entomology. Malaria and Filariasis*. Bangkok: Mahidol University.

Swaroop S. (1966) (Revised by Gilroy A. B., Uemura K.). *Statistical Methods in Malaria Eradication*, Monograph Series No. 51. Geneva: World Health Organization.

Taylor A. R., Muller R. (1980) *Vaccines against Parasites*. Oxford: Blackwell Scientific Publications.

Taylor D. (1982) *Medicines, Health and the Poor World*. London: Office of Health Economics.

Taylor T. E., Wills B. A., Kazembe P., Chisale M., Wirima J. J., Ratsma E. Y. E. C., Molyneux M. E. (1993) Rapid coma resolution with artemether in Malawian children with cerebral malaria. *Lancet* **341**: 661–2.

Teasdale G., Jennett B. (1974) Assessment of coma and impaired consciousness. A practical scale. *Lancet* **ii**: 81–4.

Tennessee Valley Authority (1974) *Malaria Control in Impounded Waters*. Washington: US Government Printing Office.

Theru J., Ambroise-Thomas P., Contat M., Kupka P. (1982) Antigènes excretés-secretés par *Plasmodium falciparum* en cultures *in vitro*. *Bulletin of the World Health Organization* **60**: 761–6.

Thompson P. E., Werbel R. M. (1972) *Antimalarial Agents*. New York and London: Academic Press.

Toro G., Roman G. (1978) Cerebral malaria. *Journal of the American Medical Association* **35**: 271–6.

Trager W. (1979) Cultivation of erythrocytic stages of malaria. In *The* in vitro *Cultivation of the Pathogens of Tropical Diseases*, Tropical Diseases Research Series. Schwabe, Basel: UNDP/World Bank/WHO.

Trager W. (1980) Cultivation of malaria parasites *in vitro*: Its application to chemotherapy, immunology and the study of parasite–host interactions. In *The Host–Invader Interplay* (Van den Bossche H., ed.) pp. 537–48. Amsterdam: Elsevier.

Trager W. (1982) Cultivation of malaria parasites. *British Medical Bulletin* **38**: 129–32.

Trager W., Jensen J. B. (1976) Human malaria parasites in continuous culture. *Science* **193**: 673–5.

Trager W., Tershakovic M., Lyanduert L. *et al.* (1981) Clones of the malaria parasite *Plasmodium falciparum* obtained by microscopic selection: Their characterization with regard to knobs, chloroquine sensitivity and formation of gametocytes. *Proceedings of the National Academy of Sciences* **78**: 6527–30.

Trenholme G. M. *et al.* (1975) Mefloquine. *Science* **190**: 792–4.

UNDP/World Bank/WHO (1978) *Role of the Spleen in the Immunology of Parasitic Diseases*. Proceedings of a Meeting, Geneva.

UNDP/World Bank/WHO (1978) *The Membrane Pathobiology of Tropical Diseases*. Proceedings of a Meeting, Geneva.

UNDP/World Bank/WHO (1979) *The* in vitro *Cultivation of the Pathogens of Tropical Diseases*. Proceedings of a Workshop, Geneva.

UNDP/World Bank/WHO (1979) *Role of Spleen in the Immunology of Parasitic Diseases*, Tropical Diseases Research Series No. 1. Basel: Schwabe.

UNDP/World Bank/WHO (1980) *Modern Genetic Concepts and Techniques in the Study of Parasites*, Proceedings of a Symposium, Geneva.

UNDP/World Bank/WHO (1981) Immunodiagnostic Techniques in Malaria, Special Programme for Research and Training in Tropical Diseases, Geneva.

UNDP/World Bank/WHO (1982) *Drug-resistant Malaria*. Report of a meeting (Wernsdorfer W. H., ed.). Geneva.

UNDP/World Bank/WHO (1982) *Sixth Programme Report*, Special Programme (1981–82) for Research and Training in Tropical Diseases, Geneva.

UNDP/World Bank/WHO (1983) Development of mefloquine as an antimalarial drug. *Bulletin of the World Health Organization* **61**: 169–78.

UNDP/World Bank/WHO (1983) *Modern Design of Antimalarial Drugs* (Wernsdorfer W. H., Trigg P. I., eds). Proceedings of a Meeting, Geneva.

UNDP/World Bank/WHO (1983) *Report of the Steering Committees of the Scientific Working Groups on Malaria (1980–83)*, TDR/Mal/Sc-SWG (80–3) (Cyclostyled). Geneva.

UNDP/World Bank/WHO (1989) *Ninth Programme Report*, Tropical Diseases Progress in International Research, 1987–88. Geneva.

US Public Health Service (1947) *Malaria Control in Impounded Waters* (Bishop E. G., ed.). Washington DC: US Government Printing Office.

Valero M. V., Amador L. R., Galindo C., *et al.* (1993) Vaccination with SPF66, a chemically synthesized vaccine, against *Plasmodium falciparum* malaria in Colombia. *Lancet* **341**: 705–10.

Van den Bossche H., ed. (1976) *Biochemistry of Parasites and Host–Parasite Relationships*. Amsterdam: North Holland.

Vercruysse J., Jancloes M., Van de Velden L. (1983) Epidemiology of seasonal falciparum malaria in an urban area of Senegal. *Bulletin of the World Health Organization* **61**: 821–31.

Voller A. (1976) Applications of immunofluorescence to seroepidemiology of malaria. *Annals of the New York Academy of Sciences* **254**: 326–30.

Voller A., Bartlett A., Bidwell S. E. (1976) Enzyme immunoassays for parasitic diseases. *Transactions of the Royal Society of Tropical Medicine and Hygiene* **70**: 98–106.

Voller A., Draper C. C. (1982) Immunodiagnosis and seroepidemiology of malaria. *British Medical Bulletin* **38**: 173–7.

Voller A., Meuwissen H. E., Verhave J. P. (1980) Methods for measuring the immunological response to plasmodia. In *Malaria* Vol. 3 (Kreier J. P., ed.) pp. 67–110. New York and London: Academic Press.

Walliker D. (1982) Genetic variation in malaria parasites. *British Medical Bulletin* **38**: 123–8.

Ward R. A. (1984) Second supplement to 'A catalog of the mosquitoes of the world: (Diptera: Culicidae)'. *Mosquito Systematics* **19**: 227–70.

Warhurst D. C. (1986) Antimalarial drugs: mode of action and resistance. *Journal of Antimicrobial Chemotherapy* **18**: 51–9.

Warhurst D. C. (1987) Antimalarial drugs. An update. *Drugs* **33**: 50–65.

Warrell D. A. (1987) Pathophysiology of severe falciparum malaria in man. *Parasitology* **94**: S53–S76.

Warrell D. A. (1989) Cerebral malaria. *Quarterly Journal of Medicine* **71**: 369–71.

Warrell D. A., Looareesuwan S., Phillips R. E., White N. J., Warrell M. J., Chapel H. M., Areekul S., Tharavanij S. (1986) Function of the blood–cerebrospinal fluid barrier in human cerebral malaria: rejection of the permeability hypothesis. *American Journal of Tropical Medicine and Hygiene* **35**: 882–9.

Warrell D. A., Looareesuwan S., Warrell M. J., Kasemsarn P., Intaraprasert R., Bunnag D., Harinasuta T. (1982) Dexamethasone proves deleterious in cerebral malaria. *New England Journal of Medicine* **306**: 313–19.

Warrell D. A., Molyneux M. E., Beales P. F., eds (1990) Severe and complicated malaria, 2nd edition World Health Organization Malaria Action Programme. *Transactions of the Royal Society of Tropical Medicine and Hygiene* **84** (Supplement 2): 65.

Warrell D. A., Phillips R. E., Garrard C. S. (1991) Intensive care unit management of severe malaria. *Clinical Intensive Care* **2**: 86–96.

Warrell D. A., White N. J., Veall N., Looareesuwan S., Chanthavanich P., Phillips R. E., Karbwang J., Krishna S., Pongpaew P. (1988) Cerebral anaerobic glycolysis and reduced cerebral oxygen transport in human cerebral malaria. *Lancet* **ii**: 534–8.

Waters A. P., McCutchan T. F. (1990) Ribosomal DNA: nature's own polymerase-amplified target for diagnosis. *Parasitology Today* **6**: 56–9.

Wattanagoon Y., Phillips R. E., Warrell D. A., Silamut K., Looareesuwan S., Nagachinta B., Black D. J. (1986) Intramuscular quinine loading dose for falciparum malaria: pharmacokinetics and toxicity. *British Medical Journal* **293**: 11–13.

Weatherall D. J., Abdalla S. (1982) The anaemia of *Plasmodium falciparum* malaria. *British Medical Bulletin* **38**: 147–51.

Weidanz W. P. (1982) Malaria and alterations in immune reactivity. *British Medical Bulletin* **38**: 167–72.

Wellems T. E. *et al.* (1991) Genetic mapping of the chloroquine-resistance locus on *P. falciparum* chromosome 7. *Proceedings of the National Academy of Sciences* **88**: 3382–6.

Wernsdorfer W. H. (1980) Field evaluation of drug resistance in malaria; *In vitro* micro-test. *Acta Tropica (Basel)* **37**: 222–7.

Wernsdorfer W. H. (1980) The importance of malaria in the world. In *Malaria*, Vol I (Kreier J. P., ed.) pp. 1–93. New York and London: Academic Press.

Wernsdorfer W. H. (1981) Prospects for development of malaria vaccines. *Bulletin of the World Health Organization* **59**: 335–41.

Wernsdorfer W. H., Kouznetsov R. L. (1980) Drug resistant malaria – occurrence control and surveillance. *Bulletin of the World Health Organization* **58**: 341–52.

Wernsdorfer W. H., McGregor I., eds (1988) *Malaria: Principles and Practice of Malariology*, Vols 1 and 2. Edinburgh: Churchill Livingstone.

Wernsdorfer G., Wernsdorfer W. H. (1988) Social and economic aspects of malaria and its control. In *Principles and Practice of Malariology* (Wernsdorfer W. H., McGregor Sir I., eds) pp. 1421–72. Edinburgh: Churchill Livingstone.

Wéry M., Coosemans M. (1980) La résistance medicamenteuse dans le paludisme. *Annales de la Société Belge de Médecine Tropicale* **60**: 137–62.

White G. B. (1974) *Anopheles gambiae* complex and disease transmission in Africa. *Transactions of the Royal Society of Tropical Medicine and Hygiene* **68**: 278–98.

White G. B. (1978) Systematic reappraisal of the *Anopheles maculipennis* complex. *Mosquito Systematics* **7**: 14–44.

White G. B. (1982) Malaria vector ecology and genetics. *British Medical Bulletin* **38**: 207–12.

White N. J. (1992) Antimalarial pharmacokinetics and treatment regimens. *British Journal of Clinical Pharmacology* **34**: 1–10.

White N. J., Ho M. (1992) The pathophysiology of malaria. *Advances in Parasitology* **31**: 83–173.

White N. J., Looareesuwan S., Warrell D. A., Chongsuphajisiddhi T., Bunnag D., Harinasuta T. (1981) Quinidine in falciparum malaria. *Lancet* **ii**: 1069–71.

White N. J., Miller K. D., Churchill F. C., Berry C., Williams S. B., Brown J., Greenwood B. M. (1988) Chloroquine treatment of severe malaria in children: pharmacokinetics, toxicity and revised dosage recommendations. *New England Journal of Medicine* **319**: 1493–500.

White N. J., Miller K. D., Marsh K., Berry C. D., Turner R. C., Williamson D. H., Brown J. (1987) Hypoglycaemia in African children with severe malaria. *Lancet* **i**: 708–11.

White N. J., Waller D., Crawley J., Nosten F., Chapman D., Brewster D., Greenwood B. M. (1992) Comparison of artemether and chloroquine for severe malaria in Gambian children. *Lancet* **339**: 317–21.

White N. J., Warrell D. A. (1983) Clinical management of chloroquine-resistant *P. falciparum* malaria in Southeast Asia. *Tropical Doctor* **13**: 153–8.

White N. J., Warrell D. A. (1988) The management of severe malaria. In *Textbook of Malaria* (Wernsdorfer W. H., McGregor I. A., eds) Chapter 32, pp. 865–84. Edinburgh: Churchill Livingstone.

White N. J., Warrell D. A., Bunnag D. *et al.* (1981) Quinidine in falciparum malaria. *Lancet* **2**: 1069–71.

White N. J., Warrell D. A., Chanthavanich P., Looareesuwan S., Warrell M. J., Krishna S., Williamson D. H., Turner R. C. (1983) Severe hypoglycemia and hyperinsulinemia in falciparum malaria. *New England Journal of Medicine* **309**: 61–6.

White N. J., Warrell D. A., Looareesuwan S., Chanthavanich P., Phillips R. E., Pongpaew P. (1985)

Pathophysiological and prognostic significance of cerebrospinal fluid-lactate in cerebral malaria. *Lancet* **i**: 776–8.

Wilcox A. (1960) *Manual for the Microscopical Diagnosis of Malaria in Man*, 2nd edition. Washington DC: US Department of Health, Education and Welfare, Public Health Services.

Willmoth S. (1987) Malaria and urbanisation in Central Africa: the example of Brazzaville (People's Republic of Congo). *Transactions of the Royal Society of Tropical Medicine and Hygiene* **81** (Supplement 2): 42.

Winstanley P. A. (1992) Treatment and prevention of falciparum malaria in Africa. *Journal of the Royal College of Physicians* **26**: 445–9.

World Health Organization (1961) *Malaria: Eighth Report of the Expert Committee*. Technical Reports Series No. 243. Geneva.

World Health Organization (1962) *Malaria: Ninth Report of the Expert Committee*. Technical Reports Series No. 243. Geneva.

World Health Organization (1963) *Terminology of Malaria and of Malaria Eradication*. Monograph Series No. 13. Geneva.

World Health Organization (1965) *Integration of Mass Campaigns against Specific Diseases into General Health Services*. Technical Reports Series No. 294. Geneva.

World Health Organization (1966) *Haemoglobinopathies and Allied Disorders*. Technical Reports Series No. 338. Geneva.

World Health Organization (1967) *Malaria: Thirteenth Report of the Expert Committee*. Technical Reports Series No. 357. Geneva.

World Health Organization (1967) *Prevention of the Reintroduction of Malaria*. Technical Reports Series No. 374. Geneva.

World Health Organization (1967) *The Education of Engineers in Environmental Health*. Technical Reports Series No. 376. Geneva.

World Health Organization (1969) *Parasitology of Malaria*. Technical Reports Series No. 433. Geneva.

World Health Organization (1969) *Re-examination of the Global Strategy of Malaria Eradication*, Annex 13. Official Records No. 176, pp. 106–26. Geneva.

World Health Organization (1971) *Malaria: Fifteenth Report of the Expert Committee*. Technical Reports Series No. 467. Geneva.

World Health Organization (1972) *Human Development and Public Health*. Technical Reports Series No. 485. Geneva.

World Health Organization (1972) *Vector Control in International Health*. Geneva.

World Health Organization (1973) *Cell-mediated Immunity and Resistance to Infection*. Technical Reports Series No. 519. Geneva.

World Health Organization (1973) *Interrelationship Between Health Programmes and Socioeconomic Development*. Public Health Papers No. 49. Geneva.

World Health Organization (1973) *Manual on Larval Control Operations in Malaria Programmes*, WHO Offset Publications No. 1. Geneva: Offset Publications.

World Health Organization (1974) *Malaria Control in Countries where Time-limited Eradication is Impracticable at Present*. Technical Reports Series No. 537. Geneva.

World Health Organization (1974) *Manual on Personal and Community Protection against Malaria in Development Areas and New Settlements*. WHO Offset Publications No. 10. Geneva: Offset publications.

World Health Organization (1974) Serological testing in malaria (Memorandum). *Bulletin of the World Health Organization* **50**: 527–35.

World Health Organization (1975) *Manual on Practical Entomology in Malaria: Part I – Vector Bionics and Organization of Antimalaria Activities; Part II – Methods and Techniques*. WHO Offset Publications No. 13. Geneva: Offset publications.

World Health Organization (1978) Malaria control – a reoriented strategy. *WHO Chronicle* **32**: 226–32.

World Health Organization (1978) *The Membrane Pathobiology of Tropical Diseases*. Tropical Diseases Research Series No. 2. Schwabe, Basel: UNDP/World Bank/WHO Special Programme for Research and Training in Tropical Diseases.

World Health Organization (1979) *Seventeenth Report of the Expert Committee on Malaria*. Technical Reports Series No. 640. Geneva.

World Health Organization (1981) *Characterisation of Strains of Malaria Parasites, their Cryoconservation and Isolation*. Memorandum of a Scientific Group. *Bulletin of the World Health Organization* **59**: 537–48.

World Health Organization (1982) *Malaria Control and National Health Goals*. Report of Seventh Asian Malaria Conference. Technical Report Series No. 680. Geneva.

World Health Organization (1984) *Malaria Control as Part of Primary Health Care*. Technical Report Series No. 712. p. 73. Geneva.

World Health Organization (1984) Applied field research in malaria in Africa. *Bulletin of the World Health Organization* **62** (Supplement): 1–128.

World Health Organization (1984) *Chemical Methods for the Control of Arthropod Vectors and Pests of Public Health Importance*. Geneva.

World Health Organization (1985) *Specification for Pesticides Used in Public Health*, 6th edition. Geneva.

World Health Organization (1985) *Specifications for Pesticides Used in Public Health. Insecticides – Molluscicides – Repellents – Methods*, 6th edition. Geneva.

World Health Organization (1986) *Eighteenth Report of the Expert Committee on Malaria*. Technical Report Series No. 735. Geneva.

World Health Organization (1986) *Resistance of Vectors of Disease to Pesticides*. Technical Report Series No. 737. Geneva.

World Health Organization (1986) *Resistance of Vectors and Reservoirs of Diseases to Insecticides*. Technical Reports Series No. 737. Geneva.

World Health Organization (1986) The use of DNA probes for malaria diagnosis: Memorandum from a WHO Meeting. *Bulletin of the World Health Organization* **64**: 641–52.

World Health Organization (1987) *Vector Control in Primary Health Care*. Technical Report Series No. 755. Geneva.

World Health Organization (1987) *The Use of Impregnated Bednets and Other Materials for Vector-borne Disease Control*. Mimeographed document. WHO/VBC/89.981. Geneva.

World Health Organization (1988) Malaria diagnosis: Memorandum from a WHO Meeting. *Bulletin of the World Health Organization* **66**: 575–94.

World Health Organization (1988) *Bench Aids for the Diagnosis of Malaria*. Geneva.

World Health Organization (1989) *The Use of Impregnated Bed Nets and Other Materials for Vector-borne Disease Control*. WHO/VBC/89.981. Geneva.

World Health Organization (1989) *Specifications for Equipment for Vector Control*. Geneva.

World Health Organization (1989) *Geographical Distribution of Arthropod-borne Diseases and their Principal Vectors*. WHO/VBC/89.967. Geneva.

World Health Organization (1990) *Practical Chemotherapy of Malaria*. WHO Technical Report Series No. 805. Geneva.

World Health Organization (1990) *Equipment for Vector Control*, 3rd edition. Geneva.

World Health Organization (1990). *Pesticide Application Equipment for Vector Control. Twelfth Report of the WHO Expert Committee on Vector Biology and Control*. Technical Report Series No. 791. Geneva.

World Health Organization (1991) *Expert Committee on Insecticide Resistance*. WHO Technical Report Series No. 813. Geneva.

World Health Organization (1991) *Basic Malaria Microscopy*. Part I. *Learner's Guide*. Part II. *Tutor's Guide*. Geneva.

World Health Organization (1991) Risk of transmission of AIDS and other blood related diseases during malaria activities. *Bulletin of the World Health Organization* **69**: 242–3.

World Health Organization (1991) *Practical Chemotherapy of Malaria*. WHO Technical Report Series No. 805. Geneva.

World Health Organization (1991) *Synopsis of the World Malaria Situation*. Weekly Epidemiological Record No. 22.

World Health Organization (1992) *Entomological Field Techniques for Malaria Control*. Part I. *Learner's Guide*. Geneva.

World Health Organization (1992) *Entomological Field Techniques for Malaria Control*. Part II. *Tutor's Guide*. Geneva.

World Health Organization (1992) *International Travel and Health: Vaccination Requirements and Health Advice*. Geneva.

World Health Organization (1992) *WHO Expert Committee on Malaria. Nineteenth Report*. WHO/CTD/92.1. Geneva.

World Health Organization (1992) *The WHO Recommended Classification of Pesticides by Hazard and Guidelines to Classification 1992–1993*. WHO/PCS/92.14. Geneva.

World Health Organization (1992) *World Declaration on the Control of Malaria*, Ministerial Conference on Malaria, Amsterdam, 26–27 October 1992.

World Health Organization (1992) *Vector Resistance to Pesticides. Fifteenth Report of the WHO Expert Committee on Vector Biology and Control*. WHO Technical Report Series No. 818. Geneva.

World Health Organization (1992) *Vector Resistance to Pesticides*. WHO Technical Report Series No. 815. Geneva.

Wyler D. J. (1983) Malaria: Resurgence, resistance and research. *New England Journal of Medicine* **308**: 875–8; 934–40.

Yang Tsun Hsing (1983) A review of literature on *A. balabacensis balabacensis*. WHO/Mal/83.999; WHO/VBC/83.873 (Cyclostyled). Geneva.

Yap H. H. (1985) Biological control of mosquitoes, especially malaria vectors, *Anopheles* species. *Southeast Asian Journal of Tropical Medicine and Public Health* **16**: 163–72.

Yekutiel P. (1980) *Eradication of Infectious Diseases – A Critical Study*. Basel: S. Karger.

Zahar A. R. (1984) *Vector Bionomics in the Epidemiology and Control of Malaria*, Part I, *The WHO African Region and the Southern WHO Eastern Mediterranean Region*, Sections I and II. Mimeographed document. VBC/84.6 and MAP/84.3. Geneva: World Health Organization.

Zahar A. R. (1985) *Vector Bionomics in the Epidemiology and Control of Malaria*, Part I, *The WHO African Region and the Southern WHO Eastern Mediterranean Region*, Section III. Mimeographed document. VBC/85.1 and MAP/85.1; VBC/85.2 and MAP/85.2; VBC/85.3 and MAP/85.3. Geneva: World Health Organization.

Zahar A. R. (1988) *Vector Bionomics in the Epidemiology and Control of Malaria*, Part II, *The WHO European Region and the WHO Eastern Mediterranean Region*, Volume I. VBC/88.5 and MAP/88.2. Geneva: World Health Organization.

Zahar A. R. (1990) *Vector Bionomics in the Epidemiology and Control of Malaria. Part II. The WHO European Region and the WHO Eastern Mediterranean Region*, Volume II. Applied Field Studies. Section I: An Overview of the Recent Malaria Situation and Current Problems. Section II: Vector Distribution.

Zahar A. R. (1990) *Vector Bionomics in the Epidemiology and Control of Malaria. Part II. The WHO European Region and the WHO Eastern Mediterranean Region*, Volume II. Applied Field Studies. Section III. Vector Bionomics, Malaria Epidemiology and Control by Geographical Areas. (A) The Mediterranean Basin. VBC/90.2 and MAP/90.2. Geneva: World Health Organization.

Zahar A. R. (1990) *Vector Bionomics in the Epidemiology and Control of Malaria. Part II. The WHO European Region and the WHO Eastern Mediterranean Region*. Volume II. Applied Field Studies. Section III. Vector Bionomics, Malaria Epidemiology and Control by Geographical Areas. (B) Asia West of India. VBC/90.3 and Mal 90.3. Geneva: World Health Organization.

Zainiev S. A., Muminov M. S. (1983) Effectiveness of Gambusia on rice-fields in the Uzbek S.S.R. *Meditsinskaya Parasitologia* (Moscow) **61**: 76–9.

Zhou Z. J. (1981) Malaria in China. *Bulletin of the World Health Organization* **59**: 931–5.

Zulueta de J. (1973) Malaria eradication in Europe; The achievements and difficulties ahead. *Journal of Tropical Medicine and Hygiene* **76**: 279–82.

Zulueta de J., Ramsdale C. W., Coluzzi M. (1975) Receptivity to malaria in Europe. *Bulletin of the World Health Organization* **52**: 109–11.

Appendix I

International non-proprietary names of antimalarial drugs and some synonyms or proprietary names*

Quinine (sulfate, bisulfate, dihydrochloride, hydrochloride)
Adaquin; Adquin; Bichinine; Biquin; Biquinate; Chinine; Coquelusédal quinine; Dentojel; Grisotets; Kinin; Kinine; Myoquin; Quinamm; Quinate; Quinbisul; Quindan; Quine; Quinimax; Quinoctal; Quinoforme (formate); Quinsan; Quiphile

Acridines

Mepacrine (dihydrochloride)
Acrichin; Acriquine; Atabrin; Atabrine; Erion; Metoquina; Quinacrine (and other names)

Mepacrine (methanesulfonate)
Atebrine musonate; Quinacrine soluble (For injection)

4-Aminoquinolines

Chloroquine
Aralen; Avloclor; Bemaphate; Chinamine; Chlorquim; Cidanchin; Delagil; Gontochin; Imagon; Iroquine; Klorokin; Luprochin; Malarex; Matalets; Nivaquine; Nivaquine B; Resochin; Resochine; Resoquine; Sanoquin; Tanakan; Tresochin; Trochin

Hydroxychloroquine
Ercoquin; Plaquenil; Quensyl

Amodiaquine (dihydrochloride)
Basoquin; Cam-aqi; Camoquin; Camoquinal; Flavoquine; Fluroquine; Miaquine

Amopyroquine (dihydrochloride)
Propoquin (For injection)

8-Aminoquinolines

Primaquine (diphosphate)
Neo-Quipenyl

Quinocide (dihydrochloride)
Chinocid

Quinolinemethanols

Mefloquine, Lariam; Mephaquine
Mefloquine with pyrimethamine sulfadoxine, Fansimef

Phenanthrenemethanol

Halofantrine, Halfan

Dihydrofolate reductase inhibitors (antifolic compounds)

Proguanil (hydrochloride)
Balusil; Bigumal; Chlorguanide; Chloriguane; Diguanyl; Drinupal; Guanatol; Lepadina; Paludrine; Paludrinol; Palusil; Plasin; Proguanide; Tirian

Chlorproguanil (hydrochloride)
Lapudrine

Cycloguanil embonate (For injection)
Camolar; Cycloguanil pamoate

Pyrimethamine (base)
Chloridin; Darapram; Daraprim; Erbaprelina; Malocide; Pirimecidan; Tindurin (and other names)

***This list is based on *Chemotherapy of Malaria and Resistance to Antimalarials*, World Health Organization, Technical Reports Series No. 529, Geneva, 1973, and on *Chemotherapy of Malaria*, 2nd edition, World Health Organization, 1981.**

Trimethoprim
Ipral; Motrim; Polytrim; Syraprim; Tiempe; Trimogal; Trimopan (and many other names)

Sulfones

Dapsone (DDS)
Avlosulfone; Avlosulfon; Croysulfone; Damitone; Daphone; DAPS; Dermosone; Diphenason; Diaphenylsulfone; Diatox; Diphone; Disulone; Dubronax; Eporal; Novophone; Servidapson; Sulfadione; Sulfona Oral; Udolac

Acedapsone (For injection)
Camilan; Hansolar; Rodilone; Sulfadiamine

Sulfonamides

Sulfadiazine
Adiazine; Codiazine; Cremodiazine; Debenal; Diazine; Diazyl; Eskadiazine; Eustral; Keladiazine; Pirimal; Pyrimal; Sterazine; Sulfazine

Sulfadimethoxine
Levisul; Madribon; Madriquid; Sulfadimethoxypyrimidine

Sulfamethoxypyridazine
Davosin; Deposulfal; Depovernil; Kynex; Lederkyn; Midicel; Midikel; Myasul; Spofadiazine; Sulfadurazin; Sulfalex; Sultirène; Unosulf

Sulfadoxine
Fanasil; Fanasulf; Fanzil; Sulformethoxine; Sulforthodimethoxine; Sulforthomidine

Sulfalene
Kelfizina; Kelfizine; Sulfamethoxypyrazine; Sulfametopyrazine

Combinations of sulfones or sulfonamides with antifolic compounds (such as pyrimethamine)
Maloprim; Fansidar; Metakelfin; Kelfimet

Tetracycline, Lincomycin and Derivatives

Tetracyline (and its salts)
Achromycin; Cyclomycin; Polycycline; Tetracyn (and many other names)

Doxycycline (and its salts)
Biociclina; Doxacin; Nordox; Vibramycin; Vibramycin-D (and many other names)

Minocycline (and its salts)
Minocin

Lincomycin
Lincocin

Clindamycin
Cleocin

Artemisinin

Artemether, Injectio Artemetheri, Paluther

Appendix II

Characteristics of some major *Anopheles* vectors of human malaria*

Mainly after Service (1986).

1. Malaria vectors of Africa south of the Sahara

Anopheles gambiae *complex*

Consists of six very similar species, separated by banding of their polytene chromosomes. They differ in certain aspects of their biology and behaviour.

Anopheles gambiae (formerly called species A of the *gambiae* complex) is widespread in nearly all African countries south of the Sahara and is the world's most efficient malaria vector. Larvae occur mainly in temporary habitats such as pools, puddles, hoof prints, borrow pits, but also rice fields. The adult bites humans both indoors and outdoors; in some areas it also feeds on domestic animals. It rests predominantly indoors after feeding but may rest outdoors.

Anopheles arabiensis (formerly species B of the *gambiae* complex) is also widespread in most African countries, but often prefers drier savannah areas. Larval habitats the same as those of *A. gambiae*. Adults bite humans and animals, indoors and outdoors, and afterwards rest indoors or outdoors. This species usually has a greater tendency than *A. gambiae* to bite animals and rest outdoors. It is an important malaria vector, but not as efficient as *A. gambiae*.

Anopheles quadriannulatus (formerly species C of the *gambiae* complex) occurs in Ethiopia, Tanzania, Zimbabwe, Mozambique and southern Africa. It is not a malaria vector as it feeds mainly on cattle.

Anopheles bwambae (formerly species D of the *gambiae* complex) is known only from mineral springs in the Semliki forest of Uganda. It is a rare species and is not considered an important malaria vector, although it can transmit malaria within a very restricted area.

Anopheles melas, a salt-water breeding species of the *gambiae* complex, occurs along the coast of West Africa to Angola. It is very common in lagoons and mangrove swamps and does not breed in fresh water. Adults behave very similarly to *A. gambiae*. It is a malaria vector in many coastal areas.

Anopheles merus, the East African equivalent to *A. melas*, breeds in salt-water lagoons and swamps along the coast of East Africa. Occasionally it is found in inland habitats such as in Tanzania, South Africa and Zimbabwe. The biting behaviour of adults is similar to that of *A. gambiae*, but it is often more exophilic. It is a vector in certain coastal areas.

Anopheles funestus

Anopheles funestus is widespread in Africa south of the Sahara. It is the most important vector after *A. gambiae* and *A. arabiensis*. Larvae occur in more or less permanent waters, especially with vegetation, such as swamps, marshes, edges of streams, rivers, ditches. It prefers shaded habitats. The adult bites humans predominantly, but also domestic animals. It feeds both indoors and outdoors, and after feeding rests mainly indoors.

Other Anopheles

Anopheles nili, *Anopheles moucheti*, *Anopheles hargreavesi*, *Anopheles hancocki* and *Anopheles pharoensis* may also be malaria vectors of minor importance in certain localities.

***This tabulation of main larval habitats and feeding/resting behaviour of adults of some of the more important malaria vectors, cannot indicate all the countries in which these occur. Moreover, their importance as vectors and their behaviour may differ in some areas of their distribution. As stressed by Service (1986) such notes are merely a guide. For greater detail of the behaviour and importance of *Anopheles* as malaria vectors in different countries other reference works and books should be consulted.**

2. Malaria vectors of Europe, North Africa and the Middle East

Anopheles claviger

It is found in England through Europe to North Africa, Syria, Iran, Iraq and Asia Minor, to Afghanistan, but it is a vector only in countries of the Middle East. It likes ponds, marshes, wells, cisterns, rock pools, and either sunlight or shade. The adult bites humans and domestic animals indoors and outdoors, and after feeding rests indoors or outdoors.

Anopheles labranchiae

It is found in Italy, Sicily, Corsica, Sardinia to Morocco, Algeria and Tunisia, but is now a vector only in North Africa. It prefers brackish waters in coastal marshes, fresh waters of rice fields, marshes and edges of grassy streams and ditches, and prefers sunlight. The adult bites humans and also domestic animals indoors and outdoors, and rests mainly in houses or animal shelters after feeding.

Anopheles maculipennis *complex (including* atroparvus *and* messeae*)*

It is found in Europe, mainly in the coastal areas of the Netherlands, northern Germany, France, Portugal and farther to central Europe and north of the Caspian sea, extending eastwards to the Commonwealth of Independent States (formerly the USSR) and Mongolia. Larvae are found in fresh or brackish marshes, lagoons and rice fields. The adult bites humans and domestic animals both inside and outside. During the winter females enter partial hibernation, sheltering in houses and animal sheds, periodically emerging to bite people and livestock. There has been no malaria transmission since eradication in endemic areas, but potential capacity is present.

Anopheles pharoensis

It is found in Egypt, Sudan, Saudi Arabia, Yemen and most of Africa south of the Sahara. It is a vector of importance in Egypt. It prefers marshes, swamps, rice fields and ponds especially those with abundant grassy or floating vegetation. The adult bites humans and animals indoors and outdoors, and rests outdoors after feeding.

Anopheles sacharovi

It is found in Italy, Greece, Eastern Europe, Turkey, Syria, Jordan, Lebanon, Iran, Iraq and to Central Russia; it is a malaria vector in Middle East countries. Larvae occur in fresh or brackish waters of coastal or inland marshes, pools and ponds, especially those with vegetation. They prefer sunlit habitats. The adult bites humans and animals indoors and outdoors, and usually rests in houses or animal shelters after feeding.

Anopheles sergentii

It is found in Algeria, Tunisia, Egypt, Syria, Palestine, Saudi Arabia, Turkey, Afghanistan and Pakistan to north-west India. Larvae occur in rice fields, borrow pits, ditches, seepages, slow-flowing streams, and sunlit or partially shaded habitats. The adult bites humans and animals indoors or outdoors, and rests in houses and caves after feeding.

Anopheles stephensi

It is found in Egypt, Iraq, Iran, Saudi Arabia, Oman, Bahrain, Afghanistan, Pakistan, Sri Lanka, India, Union of Myanmar, Thailand and China. It is an important vector over much of its range, especially in and around towns. It breeds in man-made habitats associated with towns, such as cisterns, wells, gutters, water-storage jars and containers, drains, fresh water or brackish waters, and even polluted waters, and in rural situations in grassy pools and alongside rivers. Adults bite humans indoors and outdoors and rest mainly indoors after feeding.

Anopheles superpictus

It is found in the Mediterranean area, Iran, Iraq, Saudi Arabia, Palestine, Jordan, Turkey, Afghanistan and Pakistan. It prefers flowing waters such as torrents of shallow water over rocky streams, pools in rivers, muddy hill streams and where vegetation may be present. It prefers sunlight. The adult bites humans and animals indoors and outdoors, and after feeding rests mainly in houses and animal shelters, but also in caves.

3. Malaria vectors of the Indian subcontinent and parts of South-east Asia

Anopheles culicifacies

It is found in Oman, Iran, Iraq, Bahrain, Afghanistan, Pakistan through India, Sri Lanka, Bangladesh, Union of Myanmar, Thailand, Indonesia and southern China. It is probably the most important vector in much of Pakistan, India, Bangladesh and Sri Lanka. Larvae occur in a great variety of clean and polluted habitats, irrigation ditches, rice fields, swamp pools, wells, borrow pits, edges of streams, even occasionally brackish waters, and in sunlit or partially shaded habitats. The adult prefers domestic animals but commonly bites humans indoors or outdoors, and rests mainly indoors after feeding.

Anopheles dirus See section 4.

Anopheles fluviatilis
It is found in Oman, Bahrain, Iran, Iraq, eastern Saudi Arabia, Pakistan, Afghanistan, India, Sri Lanka, Bangladesh, Union of Myanmar, Thailand, Indonesia and Indochina. It is an important vector in Pakistan, India and Bangladesh. Larvae can occur in most flowing waters, such as hill streams, pools in river beds and irrigation ditches. They prefer sunlight. The adult bites humans and domestic animals indoors and outdoors, and rests both indoors and outdoors after feeding.

Anopheles minimus *(includes* flavirostris*)*
It is found in India, Sri Lanka, Union of Myanmar, Malaysia, Thailand, Indochina, Taiwan, Sumatra, Java and the Philippines to southern China. Larvae occur in flowing waters, such as foothill streams, springs, irrigation ditches, seepages, also rice fields and borrow pits. They prefer shaded areas of sunlit habitats. Adults feed mainly on humans, but also domestic animals, mainly feeding and resting indoors. In the Philippines subspecies *flavirostris* bites indoors but rests outdoors after feeding. Some authorities regard *flavirostris* as a distinct species, not a subspecies of *A. minimus*.

Anopheles stephensi See Section 2.

Anopheles sundaicus
It is found in India, Union of Myanmar, Malaysia, Thailand, Indonesia, Java, Sumatra, Borneo, China and Indochina. Larvae occur in salt or brackish waters, lagoons, marshes, pools, seepages, especially with putrifying algae and aquatic weeds. It is mainly a coastal species, but is also found in fresh water inland pools in Java and Sumatra. Larvae prefer sunlight. The adult bites humans and domestic animals indoors and outdoors, and rests mainly indoors after feeding.

Anopheles superpictus See Section 2.

Anopheles varuna
It is found in India, Sri Lanka, Nepal, Union of Myanmar and possibly Thailand. This species is similar to *A. minimus* and has often been confused with it. It may be a malaria vector in central and northern India. Larvae occur in stagnant ditches, pools, slow-running streams and wells in sunlit or shaded conditions. Adults bite humans and animals indoors and outdoors, and commonly rest indoors after feeding.

4. Malaria vectors of South-east Asia

Anopheles aconitus
It is found in India, Sri Lanka, Malaysia, Indochina, Indonesia, Sumatra, Borneo and southern China. Larvae occur in rice fields, swamps, irrigation ditches, pools and streams with vegetation and prefer sunlit habitats. Adults feed indoors or outdoors on humans but also commonly on animals; adults rest indoors or outdoors after feeding.

Anopheles leucosphyrus *group*
There has been confusion concerning the identity of three very similar species within this group, namely, *A. leucosphyrus*, *A. balabacensis* and *A. dirus*. *Anopheles leucosphyrus* occurs in Indonesia, Sumatra, Malaysia and Sarawak. Larvae commonly occur in clear seepage pools in forests. Adults bite humans inside or outside houses, but afterwards rest outdoors. It is a vector in Sumatra and Sarawak and possibly elsewhere. *Anopheles balabacensis* occurs in Sabah, Java, Borneo, Balabac island and Palawan island in the Philippines. It is also a forest species. Larvae colonize muddy and shaded forest pools, animal hoof prints and vehicle ruts. Adults bite humans and cattle and feed and rest outdoors. *Anopheles dirus*, a species very similar both morphologically and biologically to *A. balabacensis*, is found in western India, Bangladesh, Thailand, southern China, Hainan island, Vietnam, Kampuchea, Laos, Union of Myanmar, northern Malaysia, Sumatra and Java. It is an important malaria vector in most of these areas. Like *A. balabacensis* it is a forest species and adults rest out of doors.

Anopheles campestris
There has been considerable confusion over the identity of this species, it has sometimes been misidentified as *A. donaldi* but more frequently as *A. barbirostris*. Many references in the literature refer to *A. barbirostris* as an important vector of both malaria and filariasis, but *A. barbirostris* is predominantly zoophilic, although it bites humans in Timor and the Celebes where it can be a malaria vector. Most references giving *A. barbirostris* as a vector refer in fact to *A. campestris*, a species found along the coasts and deltas of Malaysia and Thailand, and possibly in other main-

land areas of South-east Asia, or to *A. donaldi*, found in Malaysia and Borneo. Larvae are usually found in swamps or ponds having some vegetation. Partial shade is preferred. Larvae often accumulate in shaded corners of rice fields, and also ditches, earthern wells and sometimes in brackish waters. Adults bite humans and animals indoors and outdoors, with substantial numbers resting indoors after feeding.

Anopheles culicifacies See Section 3.

Anopheles hyrcanus
This mosquito has been reported from Europe, the northern Mediterranean, North Africa, across central and northern Asia to Japan, but what was formerly considered a single species is now known to consist of a species group. Many records incriminating *A. hyrcanus* in the transmission of malaria refer to closely related species such as *A. anthropophagus*, *A. sinensis* and *A. nigerrimus*, and in these brief notes these species are given as malaria vectors, although *A. hyrcanus* sensu stricto may be a vector in some areas.

Anopheles anthropophagus *and* Anopheles sinensis
Anopheles sinensis is often considered an important vector in China, but this is in part based on misidentification, although it is an important vector in the plains of China and is the main or only vector north of 34°N. It breeds extensively in rice fields. Adults are mainly zoophilic but also bite humans. They rest mainly outdoors. The most important vector in the group is probably *A. anthropophagus*. This species occurs in Thailand, Malaysia, Borneo, Philippines, Korea and southern China to Japan. It is an important vector in the central plains and eastern China. Larvae occur in cool, clean waters, including rice fields; some forms can occur in brackish water. *Anopheles anthropophagus* is mainly anthropophilic and endophilic, but will also bite cattle, and adults sometimes rest outdoors.

Anopheles letifer
It is found in Thailand, Indonesia, Malaysia, Philippines, Sumatra, Java and Borneo. This species is very similar to *A. umbrosus*, which has a similar distribution and has in the past been confused with it. *Anopheles umbrosus*, however, is not as formerly supposed an important malaria vector because many sporozoites found in the salivary glands are of animal malarias. *Anopheles letifer* bites humans more often than *A. umbrosus*, but also commonly feeds on animals; it seems to be a malaria vector in certain areas. Larvae are often found in stagnant waters, especially on coastal plains, such as pools, swamps and ponds. They prefer shade. Adults bite animals and humans mainly outdoors, and rest outdoors after feeding.

Anopheles maculatus
It is found in India, Malaysia, Indonesia, Indochina, Borneo, Philippines, Sumatra, Java and southern China. It occurs in or near hilly areas, in seepage waters, pools formed in streams, edges of ponds, ditches, rice fields, and prefers sunlight. Adults bite domestic animals and also humans indoors and outdoors, and rest mainly outdoors after feeding. *Anopheles maculatus* in fact comprises a species complex of at least four and possibly seven species.

Anopheles minimus See Section 3.

Anopheles nigerrimus
Formerly regarded as a subspecies of *A. hyrcanus* it is found in India, Sri Lanka, Union of Myanmar, Thailand, Malaysia, Indochina, Borneo and China. Larvae like deep ponds, rice fields, irrigation ditches and swamps with much vegetation, and prefer sunlight. Adults bite humans and animals mainly outdoors, and rest mainly outdoors after feeding.

Anopheles pattoni
It is found in China, north of about the 30th parallel. Larvae occur in pools in or near streams, rock pools, especially habitats with algae, and prefer sunlight. Adults bite humans indoors and outdoors.

Anopheles subpictus
It is found in Iran, Pakistan, India, Sri Lanka, Union of Myanmar, Malaysia, Thailand, Indochina, China, Papua New Guinea, Java and Sulawesi. It may be an important malaria vector in Sulawesi, Java and Indochina. Larvae occur in muddy pools near houses, gutters, borrow pits and also in brackish waters. Adults bite animals mainly, but also humans indoors and outdoors, and rest indoors and outdoors after feeding.

Anopheles sundaicus See Section 3.

5. Malaria vectors of Mexico and Central America

Anopheles albimanus
It is found in Texas and Florida in the USA, through Central America to Colombia, Ecuador, Venezuela

and the Antilles. Larvae occur in fresh or brackish waters such as pools, puddles, marshes, ponds, lagoons, especially those containing floating or grassy vegetation, and prefer sunlight. Adults feed on humans and domestic animals, indoors and outdoors; after feeding they rest mainly outdoors. It is a very important malaria vector in Mexico and Central America.

Anopheles albitarsis
It is found in Central America to South America and Trinidad. Larvae nearly always occur in sunlit ponds, large pools and marshes with filamentous algae. Adults bite almost indiscriminately humans and domestic animals, outdoors and also indoors, and usually rest outdoors after feeding.

Anopheles aquasalis
It is found in the Lesser Antilles, Trinidad, Tobago and other nearby islands, Central America to northern parts of Brazil. Larvae occur in tidal salt-water marshes, lagoons, salt-water regions of rivers and estuaries, rarely in fresh water. They occur in sunlit or shaded habitats. Adults bite humans and domestic animals, indoors and outdoors, and rest mainly outdoors.

Anopheles aztecus
It is found in Mexico at an altitude of 1500–2200 m. Larvae occur in pools, ponds, lakes, especially with vegetation, canals and even polluted waters. Adults bite humans indoors and outdoors, and rest mainly outdoors after feeding.

Anopheles darlingi
It is found in Mexico through Central America to Argentina and Chile. Larvae occur in fresh-water marshes, lagoons, rice fields, swamps, lakes and ponds, pools, edges of streams, especially with vegetation, and prefer shaded habitats. Adults feed mainly on humans indoors, and remain indoors after feeding.

Anopheles pseudopunctipennis See Section 6.

Anopheles punctimacula
It is found in Mexico through Central America to Peru, Brazil, Argentina and Trinidad. Larvae occur in small pools, swamps, grassy pools at edges of streams, and prefer shade. Adults bite humans and domestic animals, indoors and outdoors, and rest indoors or outdoors after feeding.

6. Malaria vectors of South America

Anopheles albimanus See Section 5.

Anopheles albitarsis See Section 5.

Anopheles aquasalis See Section 5.

Anopheles bellator
It is found in Trinidad, Venezuela, Surinam, Guyana and Brazil. Larvae occur only in water collected in leaf axils of bromeliads, which are epiphytes of trees; they prefer partially shaded habitats. Adults bite humans during the daytime in shaded forests, as well as at night, and may enter houses to feed and usually rest indoors after feeding. Although humans are the favoured host domestic animals are also attacked.

Anopheles cruzii
It is found in Costa Rica, Panama, Ecuador, Bolivia, Colombia, Peru, Brazil and Venezuela. Larvae occur in water collected in leaf axils of bromeliads, and partial shade is preferred. Adults bite humans indoors and outdoors, and after feeding rest indoors and outdoors. Its main importance is as a malaria vector in coastal areas of Brazil.

Anopheles darlingi See Section 5.

Anopheles nuneztovari
It is found in Guyana, Venezuela, Colombia, Brazil and Bolivia. Larvae occur in muddy waters of pools, vehicle tracks, hoof prints, small ponds, especially in and around towns, and prefer sunlight. Adults mainly feed on animals, but also bite humans outdoors; they rest outdoors after feeding. It is an important vector in Colombia and Venezuela.

Anopheles pseudopunctipennis
It is found in the Antilles, southern USA to Argentina. Larvae occur in pools, puddles, seepage waters, edges of streams, especially habitats with algae, and prefer sunlight. Adults feed almost indiscriminately on humans and domestic animals, indoors or outdoors, and rest outdoors after feeding.

Anopheles punctimacula See Section 5.

7. Malaria vectors of Australasia

Anopheles punctulatus *complex*

It is found in Moluccas, Papua New Guinea, Solomon Islands, New Hebrides to northern Australia. This is a species complex consisting of at least five species: *A. punctulatus*, species numbers 1, 2 and 3 of *A. farauti*, and *A. koliensis*. In general larval habitats are swamps, edges of flowing streams, springs, puddles, hoof prints and pools. *Anopheles farauti* s.l. also sometimes breeds in wells, water-storage containers and other man-made receptacles. Larvae may also occur in brackish waters. Adults bite humans indoors and outdoors and rest indoors or outdoors after feeding. Generally *A. punctulatus* is more anthropophilic and endophilic than *A. farauti* s.l. which is more zoophilic and exophilic. *Anopheles koliensis* seems to prefer to breed in marshy pools at edges of forest streams. Adults usually both bite humans and rest outdoors after feeding. *Anopheles punctulatus*, *A. koliensis* and at least species No. 1 of *A. farauti* are malaria vectors.

Appendix III

Some common insecticides used in mosquito control

Common name	Other names	Chemical type	Usage
Abate	Temephos	OP	Larvae
Allethrin	—	PY	Mosquito coils
Baytex	Fenthion	OP	Larvae, adults–residual–aerosol
Bendiocarb	Ficam	C	Adults–residual–aerosol
Bioresmethrin	NRDC 107	PY	Adults–aerosol
BHC	HCH, Benzene hexachloride	OC	Adults–residual
Chlorphoxim	Baythion C Bayer AG	OP	Larvae, adults–residual
Chlorpyrifos	Dursban	OP	Larvae, adults–aerosols
Cypermethrin	Barricade, Ambush Cymbush Ripcord	PY	Adults–residual
Bacillus thuringiensis israelensis	*B.t.i.* *B. thuringiensis* H-14, Bactimos, Bactal Teknar	MIC	Larvae
DDT	Numerous	OC	Adults–residual
Deltamethrin	Decamethrin, NDRC 161	PY	Larvae, adults–residual–aerosol–mosquito nets
Dichlorvos	DDVP, Vapona, Nuvan	OP	Adults–fumigant
Diflubenzuron	Dimilin	IGR	Larvae
Fenitrothion	Sumithion Bayer 41831 Folithion	OP	Larvae Adults–residual–aerosol
Fenthion	Baytex, Entex	OP	Larvae, adults–residual–aerosol
Fuel oil	—	—	Larvae
Gamma-HCH	Lindane	OC	Adults–residual
HCH	BHC	OC	Adults–residual
Jodofenphos	Iodofenphos Nuvanol	OP	Larvae, adults–aerosol

Common name	Other names	Chemical type*	Usage
Lamda-cyhalothin	Icon	PY	Adults–residual–aerosol
Lindane	γ-HCH	OC	Adults–residual
Malathion	Numerous	OP	Larvae, adults–residual–aerosol
Methroprene	Altosid	IGR	Larvae
Monomolecular oils, and surfactants	Arosurf	—	Larvae
Naled	Bromchlorphos Dibrom	OP	Adults–aerosol
Paris green	—	CA	Larvae
Permethrin	Ambush Coopex Pounce	PY	Larvae, adults–residual–aerosol–mosquito nets
Phoxim	Baythion Bayer 77488	OP	Larvae
Pirimiphos–methyl	Actellic Cooperfos	OP	Larvae, adults–residual–aerosol
Propoxur	Arprocarb Baygon	C	Adults–residual–aerosol
Pyrethrum	—	P	Adults–aerosol
Resmethrin	Crossfire Synthrin	PY	Adults–aerosol
Temephos	Abate	OP	Larvae

C, carbamate; CA, copper acetoarsenite; IGR, insect growth regulator; MIC, microbial; OC, organochlorine; OP, organophosphate; P, pyrethrum; PY, pyrethroids; BCH and HCH, hexachlorocyclohexane; DDT, dichloro–diphenyl–trichloroethane

Appendix IV

Information on malaria risk by country or geographical area*

Health administrations are required by the World Health Assembly resolution of 1969 to provide the World Health Organization twice yearly with information on the malaria situation in their countries. From these data, WHO prepares *Information on Malaria Risk for International Travellers* to give an indication of parts of the world where malaria may be contracted. The list of countries given in this Appendix has been prepared from the booklet *Vaccination Certificate Requirements for International Travel and Health Advice to Travellers* of 1992 and the *WHO Weekly Epidemiological Record*, No. 23, 1991, 167–70; they refer only to countries where any degree of malaria risk is present. It should be understood that such risk is not uniform within the country concerned, and depends on varying local conditions such as weather, altitude, prevalence of the infection, density of *Anopheles* vectors etc. Moreover, the degree of any individual's personal protection from mosquito bites plays an important role.

In many malarious areas, centres of main towns are often free of transmission, although the risk is greater at the periphery. There is usually more risk at altitudes below 1500 m, although malaria may occur at altitudes up to 3000 m. The degree of risk of infection varies generally with the season of the year; warm and rainy periods increase the number of mosquitos and thus the chance of infection. The present information, based on the recent data collected by the WHO, is as accurate as possible in the circumstances, but subject to unforeseen changes. The indication of chloroquine resistance of malaria parasites refers only to *P. falciparum*. Since the degree of resistance may undergo rapid changes no attempt was made to provide this quantitative information in this list.

***Malaria risk is with *P. falciparum* unless otherwise stated.**

For detailed reports on areas where resistance to chloroquine has been reported see *WHO Weekly Epidemiological Record* 1991, No. 23, 167–70.

There are only a few countries from which resistance of *Plasmodium falciparum* to drugs has not been reported. Chloroquine resistance has now been *extensively* reported from Africa; most recently in West Africa, while in East and Central Africa the level has increased. However, in many of the countries in Africa, resistance is predominantly of the RI and RII type. Therefore, chloroquine can still be an effective drug which can reduce morbidity and mortality from malaria in large areas of the world providing one bears in mind that in children *anaemia* can occur with RII resistance and a second line drug (sulfadoxine–pyrimethamine) must be given as soon as anaemia is clinically detected. Resistance to sulfadoxine–pyrimethamine has developed in South-east Asia, South America and focally in Africa. In South-east Asia sensitivity to quinine is diminishing in certain areas, e.g. Thailand, Vietnam, and mefloquine resistance is on the increase.

North Africa and the Near East ranging from Morocco in the extreme West to Pakistan in the extreme East is an epidemic-prone zone. Two efficient vectors – *Anopheles arabiensis* and *Anopheles culicifacies* – are widely distributed.

In the Western Pacific and East Asia 115 million people live in areas where there is risk of exposure to *P. falciparum* and *P. vivax* infections. A further 360 million in China are exposed to *P. vivax*.

Afghanistan
Malaria risk exists from May through November below 2000 m. Resistance to chloroquine has been reported.

Algeria
Malaria risk is extremely small. Only three cases (all *P. vivax*) were reported in 1989.

Angola
Malaria risk exists throughout the year in most of the country. Resistance to chloroquine has been reported.

Argentina
Malaria risk exists from October through May below 1200 m in rural areas of Iruya, Orán, San Martin, Santa Victoria Dep. (Salta Province) and Ledesma Dep. (Jujuy Province). Predominantly *P. vivax*.

Bangladesh
Malaria risk exists throughout the year in the whole country, excluding Dhaka City. Resistance to chloroquine has been reported.

Belize
Malaria risk exists throughout the year excluding Belize District and urban areas. Predominantly *P. vivax*.

Benin
Malaria risk exists throughout the year in the whole country. Resistance to chloroquine has been reported.

Bhutan
Malaria risk exists throughout the year in the southern belt of five districts: Chirang, Gaylegphug, Samchi, Samdrupjongkhar, Shemgang. Resistance to chloroquine has been reported.

Bolivia
Malaria risk (predominantly *P. vivax*) exists throughout the year below 2500 m, excluding urban areas and excluding Oruro Department, the provinces of Ingavi, Los Andes, Omasuyos, and Pacajes (La Paz Department), and Southern and Central Potosi Department. Resistance to chloroquine has been reported.

Botswana
Malaria risk exists from November through May in the northern part of the country (north of 21°S). Resistance to chloroquine has been reported.

Brazil
Malaria risk exists throughout the year below 900 m in: Acre and Rondônia States, Territories of Amapá and Roraima, and in part of rural areas of Amazonas, Mato Grosso, and Pará States. Resistance to chloroquine has been reported.

Burkina Faso
Malaria risk exists throughout the year in the whole country. Resistance to chloroquine reported.

Burundi
Malaria risk exists throughout the year in the whole country. Resistance to chloroquine has been reported.

Cambodia
Malaria risk exists throughout the year in the whole country. Resistance to chloroquine reported.

Cameroon
Malaria risk exists throughout the year in the whole country. Resistance to chloroquine reported.

Cape Verde
Malaria risk exists throughout the year only in some rural parts of Concelho de Santa Cruz (São Tiago Island).

Central African Republic
Malaria risk exists throughout the year in the whole country.

Chad
Malaria risk exists through the year in the whole country. Resistance to chloroquine has been reported.

China
Malaria risk exists throughout the country below 1500 m except in Heilong Jiang, Jilin, Nei Monggol, Gansu, Beijing, Shanxi, Ningxia, Qinghai, Xinjiang (except along the valley of the Yili river), and Xizang (except along the valley of the Zangbo river in the extreme south-east). North of 35°N latitude transmission occurs from July to November, between 33°N and 25°N, from May to December and south of 25°N latitude, throughout the year. Falciparum malaria is confined to Hainan, Yunnan, Guizhou, Guangxi and Anhui. Resistance to chloroquine has been reported.

Colombia
Malaria risk exists throughout the year in rural areas below 800 m of Uraba (Antioquia Department), Bajo Cauca-Nechi (Cauca and Antioquia Department), Magdalen Medio, Caqueta (Caqueta Intendencia), Sarare (Arauca Intendencia), Catatumbo (Norte de Santander Department), Pacifico Central and Sur, Putumayo (Putumayo Intendencia), Ariari (Meta Department), Alto Vaupes (Vaupes Comisaria) and Amazonas. Resistance to chloroquine has been reported.

Comoros
Malaria risk exists throughout the year in the whole country. Resistance to chloroquine has been reported.

Congo
Malaria risk exists throughout the year in the whole country. Resistance to chloroquine has been reported.

Costa Rica
Malaria risk (predominantly *P. vivax*) exists throughout the year in rural areas below 500 m of: Alajuela, Guanacaste, Limon, and Puntarenas Province.

Djibouti
Malaria risk exists throughout the year in the whole country. Resistance to chloroquine has been reported.

Dominican Republic
Malaria risk exists throughout the year in rural aras of Pedernales Municipio (Pedernales Provincial); Elias Piña, El Llano, Banica Mun. (Elias Piña Province): Dajabon, Partido Mun. (Dajabon Province); Pepillo Salcedo Mun. (Monte Cristi Province).

Ecuador
Malaria risk exists throughout the year below 1500 m in Esmeraldas, Guayas, Manabi and El Oro Provinces: and in rural areas of Loja, Morona Santiago, Napo, Pastaza, Portoviejo, Puyo and Zamora (Chinchipe Province). Resistance to chloroquine has been reported.

Egypt
Malaria risk exists from June through October in rural areas of the Nile Delta, El Faiyûm area, the oases and part of Upper Egypt.

El Salvador
Malaria risk (predominantly *P. vivax*) exists throughout the year in the whole country, but is greater below 600 m in the rainy season.

Equatorial Guinea
Malaria risk exists throughout the year in the whole country. Resistance to chloroquine has been reported.

Ethiopia
Malaria risk exists throughout the year in the whole country below 2000 m. Resistance to chloroquine has been reported.

French Guyana
Malaria risk exists throughout the year in the whole area. Resistance to chloroquine has been reported.

Gabon
Malaria risk exists throughout the year in the whole country. Resistance to chloroquine has been reported.

Gambia
Malaria risk exists throughout the year in the whole country. Resistance to chloroquine has been reported.

Ghana
Malaria risk exists throughout the year in the whole country. Resistance to chloroquine has been reported.

Guatemala
Malaria risk (predominantly *P. vivax*) exists throughout the year below 1500 m in Department of (*a*) (excluding urban areas) Baja Verapaz, Chiquimula, Escuintla, Jalapa, El Peten, El Progreso, El Quiche, Santa Rosa, Suchitpequez, Zacapa; (*b*) Alta Verapaz, Huehuetenango, Izabal, Jutiapa, Retalhuleu; and in the Municipios of Coatepeque (Quetzaltenango Department), and Ocos (San Marcos Department).

Guinea
Malaria risk exists throughout the year in the whole country. Resistance to chloroquine has been reported.

Guinea-Bissau
Malaria risk exists throughout the year in the whole country. Resistance to chloroquine has been reported.

Guyana
Malaria risk exists throughout the year in the North West Region and in the Rupununi Region. Resistance to chloroquine reported.

Haiti
Malaria risk exists throughout the year below 300 m in suburban and rural areas.

Honduras
Malaria risk (predominantly *P. vivax*) exists throughout the year (from May through December in Departments of Atlántida, Cholutecca, Colón, El Paraiso, Gracias a Dios, Olancho, Valle, and Yoro) especially in rural areas.

India
Malaria risk exists throughout the year in the whole country excluding parts of the States of Himachal Pradesh, Jammu and Kashmir, and Sikkim. Resistance to chloroquine reported mainly in eastern states.

Indonesia
Malaria risk exists throughout the year in the whole country excluding Jakarta municipality and big cities. Resistance to chloroquine has been reported.

Iran (Islamic Republic of)
Malaria risk exists from March through November in the provinces of Sistan-Baluchestan and Hormozgan, the southern parts of the provinces of governorates of Fars, Kohgiluych-Boyar, Lorestan, and Chahar Mahal-Bakhtiari, and the north of Khuzestan. Resistance to chloroquine has been reported.

Iraq
Malaria risk exists from May through November in the Northern Region below 1500 m: Duhok, Erbil, Kirkuk, Ninawa, Sulaimaniya Province. Resistance to chloroquine has been reported.

Ivory Coast
Malaria risk exists throughout the year in the whole country. Resistance to chloroquine has been reported.

Kenya
Malaria risk exists throughout the year in the whole country. There is normally little risk in the city of Nairobi and in the highlands (above 2500 ml) of Central, Rift Valley, Eastern, Nyanza and Western Provinces. Resistance to chloroquine has been reported.

Lao People's Democratic Republic
Malaria risk exists throughout the year in the whole country, excluding Vientiane. Resistance to chloroquine has been reported.

Liberia
Malaria risk exists throughout the year in the whole country. Resistance to chloroquine has been reported.

Madagascar
Malaria risk exists throughout the year in all coastal areas. There is normally little risk in the outskirts of Antananarivo and in the towns of Antsirable, Manjakandriana, Andramasina, and almost no risk in the town of Antananarivo. Resistance to chloroquine has been reported.

Malawi
Malaria risk exists throughout the year in the whole country. Resistance to chloroquine has been reported.

Malaysia
Malaria risk exists only in limited foci in the deep hinterland. Urban and coastal areas are free from malaria except in Sabah, where there is risk throughout the year. Resistance to chloroquine has been reported.

Mali
Malaria risk exists throughout the year in the whole country. Resistance to chloroquine has been reported.

Mauritania
Malaria risk (predominantly *P. vivax*) exists throughout the year in the whole country, except in the following areas: Dakhlet-Nouadhibou, Inchiri, Adrar, Tiris-Zemour.

Mauritius
Malaria risk in the vivax form exists throughout the year in several rural areas in the north, except Rodrigues Island.

Mayotte
Malaria risk throughout the year.

Mexico
Malaria risk (*P. vivax*) exists in some areas that are not often visited by travellers: throughout the year in Chiapas, Guerrero, Michoacán, Nayarit, Oaxaca and parts of Campeche, Quintana Roo, Tabasco and Veracruz States; from June through to October in Morelos, Puebla (part) States and Alamos Mun. (Sonora State); from May through to October in Sinalo and parts of Chihuahua, Durango, Jalisco States; from May through to December in part of Yucatan State.

Morocco
Limited malaria risk (*P. vivax*) cannot be excluded from May to October in certain rural areas of the Garb (Provinces of Kenitra and Sidi Kacem) and in the area of Tiouzgui (Assa sector of Guelmim Province).

Mozambique
Malaria risk exists throughout the year in the whole country. Resistance to chloroquine has been reported.

Myanmar
Malaria risk exists (*a*) from April through December in rural areas (part) of Tenasserim Division; (*b*) from May through December in Irrawaddy Division (part) and rural areas (part) of Mandalay Division; (*c*) from June through December in rural areas (part) of Pegu and Rangoon Division and in rural areas of Arakan, Chin, Kachin, Karen, Kayah, Mon and Shan States; (*d*) from June through October in rural areas (part) of Magwe Division and in Sagaing Division (part). Resistance to chloroquine has been reported.

Namibia
Malaria risk exists in Ovamboland and the Caprivi Strip from November through to May. Resistance to chloroquine has been reported.

Nepal
Malaria risk exists throughout the year in rural areas of the Terai districts (including forested hills and forest areas) of Dhanukha, Mahotari, Sarlahi, Rautahat, Bara, Parsa, Rupendehi, Kapilvastu, and especially along the Indian border. Resistance to chloroquine has been reported.

Nicaragua
Malaria risk (predominantly *P. vivax*) exists from May through to December in rural areas as well as in the outskirts of Chinandega, León, Granada, Managua, Nandaime, and Tipitapa towns.

Niger
Malaria risk exists throughout the year in the whole country. Resistance to chloroquine has been reported.

Nigeria
Malaria risk exists throughout the year in the whole country. Resistance to chloroquine has been reported.

Oman
Malaria risk exists throughout the year in the whole country. Resistance to chloroquine has been reported.

Pakistan
Malaria risk exists throughout the year in the whole country below 2000 m. Resistance to chloroquine has been reported in some states.

Panama
Malaria risk (predominantly *P. vivax*) exists throughout the year in rural areas in: Darién, Bocas del Toro, and Colón (excluding Ciudad Colón) Provinces; Santa Fé (Veraguas Province), Chepo, Chiman (Panama Province) District and Comarca de San Blas. Resistance to chloroquine has been reported.

Papua New Guinea
Malaria risk exists throughout the year in the whole country below 1800 m. Resistance to chloroquine has been reported.

Paraguay
Malaria risk exists (predominantly *P. vivax*) from October through to May in some rural parts of Alto Paraná, Amambay and Canendiyú Departments.

Peru
Malaria risk exists (predominantly *P. vivax*) throughout the year in rural areas below 1500 m of:

Department of Amazonas. Cajamarca (excluding Hualgayoc Province), La Libertad (excluding Otuzco, Santiago de Chuco Province), Lambayeque, Loreto, Piura (excluding Talara Province), San Martin, and Tumbes: Province of Santa (Ancash Department); and parts of: Province of La Convención (Cuzco Department), Tayacaja (Huancavelica Department), and Satipo (Junin Department). Resistance to chloroquine has been reported.

Philippines
Malaria risk exists throughout the year in areas below 600 m, except in the provinces of Bohol, Catanduanes (Cebu, Leyte and Misamis Occidental). No risk is considered to exist in urban and flat areas. Resistance to chloroquine has been reported.

Rwanda
Malaria risk exists throughout the year in the whole country. Resistance to chloroquine has been reported.

São Tome and Principe
Malaria risk exists throughout the year. Resistance to chloroquine has been reported.

Saudi Arabia
Malaria risk exists throughout the year in areas other than Alhasa, Arar, Jauf, Quraiya (Gurayyat), Riyad, Tabuk, Taif, and the urban areas of Jeddah, Mecca, Medina and Qatif. Resistance to chloroquine has been reported.

Senegal
Malaria risk exists throughout the year in the whole country. There is less risk from January through June in the Cap-Vert region. Resistance to chloroquine has been reported.

Sierra Leone
Malaria risk exists throughout the year in the whole country. Resistance to chloroquine has been reported.

Solomon Islands
Malaria risk exists throughout the year except in some eastern and southern outlying islets. Resistance to chloroquine has been reported.

Somalia
Malaria risk exists throughout the year in the whole country. Resistance to chloroquine has been reported.

South Africa
Malaria risk exists throughout the year in the north, east and western low altitude areas of Transvaal and in Natal coastal areas north of 28°S (Richards Bay). Resistance to chloroquine has been reported.

Sri Lanka
Malaria risk exists throughout the year in the Districts of Amparai, Anuradhapura, Badulla (part), Batticaloa, Hambantota, Jaffna, Kandy, Kegalle, Kurunegala, Mannar, Matale, Matara, Moneragala, Polonnaruwa, Puttalam, Ratnapura, Trincomalee, and Vavuniya. Resistance to chloroquine has been reported.

Sudan
Malaria risk exists throughout the year in the whole country. Resistance to chloroquine has been reported.

Surinam
Malaria risk exists throughout the year in the whole country excluding Paramaribo District and the coastal areas north of 5°N. Resistance to chloroquine has been reported.

Swaziland
Malaria risk exists from December through March in the northern border areas: Bordergate, Lomahasha, Mhlume, Tshaneni. Resistance to chloroquine has been reported.

Syrian Arab Republic
Malaria risk exists (exclusively *P. vivax*) from May through to October in the whole country, excluding urban areas and the districts of Damascus, Deir-es-Zor, Homs, Sweida, and Tartus.

Tanzania
Malaria risk throughout the year in the whole country below 1800 m. Resistance to chloroquine has been reported.

Thailand
Malaria exists throughout the year in rural, especially forested and hilly, areas of the whole country. Resistance to chloroquine is widespread.

Togo
Malaria risk exists throughout the year in the whole country. Resistance to chloroquine has been reported.

Turkey
Potential malaria risk (exclusively *P. vivax*) exists from March to the end of November in the Çukurova Amikova areas and from mid-May to mid-October in south-east Anatolia.

Uganda
Malaria risk exists throughout the year in the whole country including the main towns of Fort Portal, Jinja, Kampala, Mbale and parts of Kigezi. Resistance to chloroquine has been reported.

United Arab Emirates
Malaria is not considered to be a risk in the Emirate of Abu Dhabi and the cities of Dubai, Sharjah, Ajman, and Umm at Quaiwain. There is malaria risk in the foothill areas and valleys in the mountainous regions of the northern Emirates.

Vanuatu (New Hebrides)
Malaria risk exists throughout the year in the whole country excluding Futuna Island. Resistance to chloroquine has been reported.

Venezuela
Malaria risk exists throughout the year in rural areas in part of: Apure, Bolivar, Barinas, Mérida, Táchira, and Zulia States. Resistance to chloroquine has been reported.

Vietnam
Malaria risk exists in the whole country excluding urban centres and the deltas. Resistance to chloroquine is widespread.

Yemen
Malaria risk exists throughout the year in the whole country excluding the First Governorate (Aden and airport perimeter). Resistance to chloroquine has been reported.

Zaire
Malaria risk exists throughout the year in the whole country. Resistance to chloroquine has been reported.

Zambia
Malaria risk exists from November through to May in the whole country. Resistance to chloroquine has been reported.

Zimbabwe
Malaria risk exists from November through to May in the whole country below 1200 m. Resistance to chloroquine has been reported.

See Figure 11.7 and Plate 28 for details.

Appendix V

Formulation of suspensions, emulsions, concentrates and sprays for malaria control

Reproduced from WHO, 1970, Technical Report Series no. 443 *Insecticide Resistance and Vector Control.*

Requirements for spray formulations

Dosage (weight per unit area)	Litres* of spray required per 100 m^2 (1000 ft^2) using following concentrations of technical insecticide:				
	0.25%	0.5%	1.0%	2.5%	5.0%
2 g/m^2 (200 mg/ft^2)	—	—	20	8	4
1 g/m^2 (100 mg/ft^2)	—	20	10	4	2
0.5 g/m^2 (50 mg/ft^2)	20	10	5	2	1
0.2 g/m^2 (20 mg/ft^2)	8	4	2	0.8	0.4

*1 litre is approximately equal to 0.25 USgal or 0.2 UKgal.

Amount of water-dispersible power (w.d.p.) required for preparation of spray suspensions

Percentage of toxicant in w.d.p.	kg (lb) of w.d.p. required for about 380 litres (100 USgal; 83 UKgal) of finished spray suspension with concentrations of:				
	5%	2.5%	1%	0.5%	0.25%
90	21.0 (46.3)	10.5 (23.1)	4.2 (9.3)	2.1 (4.6)	1.0 (2.3)
75	25.2 (55.6)	12.6 (27.8)	5.0 (11.1)	2.5 (5.6)	1.3 (2.8)
50	37.8 (83.3)	18.9 (41.7)	7.6 (16.7)	3.8 (8.3)	1.9 (4.2)
25	75.6 (166.7)	37.8 (83.3)	15.1 (33.3)	7.6 (16.7)	3.8 (8.3)

Preparation of emulsion from concentrates of different strengths

Percentage of toxicant in emulsion concentrate	Parts of water to be added to 1 part of emulsion concentrate when concentration of final form is:				
	5%	2.5%	1%	0.5%	0.25%
80	15	31	79	159	319
60	11	23	50	119	239
50	9	19	49	99	199
25	4	9	24	49	99
10	1	3	9	19	39

Preparation of emulsion concentrates from technical material

Concentration desired (%)	Weight of technical material required to make the following volumes of concentrate:*		
	100 litres	100 USgal	100 UKgal
35	35 kg	292 lb	350 lb
25	25 kg	208 lb	250 lb
15	15 kg	125 lb	150 lb
12.5	12.5 kg	104 lb	125 lb
6.25	6.25 kg	52 lb	62.5 lb

*To every 100 parts of concentrate 2 parts of emulsifier should be added.

Index